Cardiovascular Prevention and Rehabilitation

Joep Perk, Peter Mathes, Helmut Gohlke, Catherine Monpère,
Irene Hellemans, Hannah McGee, Philippe Sellier,
and Hugo Saner, *Editors*

Cardiovascular Prevention and Rehabilitation

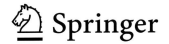 Springer

Joep Perk, FESC
Public Health Department
Kalmar County
Oskarshamn
Sweden

Helmut Gohlke, FACC, FESC
Klinische Kardiologie II
Herz-Zentrum Bad Krozingen
Germany

Irene Hellemans, MD, (Speciality
    Cardiology), PhD
Institute of Health Sciences
Department of Earth Sciences
Vrije University
and
Department of Cardiology
Vrije University Medical Center
Amsterdam
The Netherlands

Philippe Sellier, MD
Hôpital Broussais-HEGP
Assistance Publique-Hôpitaux de Paris
Paris
France

Peter Mathes, MD, FACC, FESC
Department of Cardiology
Technical University of Munich
Munich Rehabilitation Center
München
Germany

Catherine Monpère, MD
Cardiac Rehabilitation Center
Bois Gilbert
Ballan Miré
France

Hannah McGee, BA(Mod), PhD, RegPsycholFPsSI
Department of Psychology
Royal College of Surgeons in Ireland
Dublin
Ireland

Hugo Saner, MD
Swiss Cardiovascular Center Bern
Cardiovascular Prevention and Rehabilitation
    University
Hospital Inselspital
Switzerland

British Library Cataloguing in Publication Data
Cardiovascular prevention and rehabilitation
    1. Cardiovascular system – Diseases – Patients – Rehabilitation   2. Cardiovascular system – diseases –
    Prevention
    I. Perk, Joep
    616.1′2
ISBN-13: 9781846289934

Library of Congress Control Number: 2006926876

ISBN-13: 978-1-84628-993-4   e-ISBN-13: 978-1-84628-502-8   Printed on acid-free paper

9 8 7 6 5 4 3 2 1

Springer Science+Business Media
springer.com

Preface

Over the past decades the medical care of the patient with cardiovascular disease (CVD) has shown an impressive development, with marked positive consequences for mortality, morbidity, and the quality of life of coronary patients. This improvement has profoundly changed the arena in which cardiac rehabilitation (CR) has been acting over the past 40 years. The younger patient from the 1970s with uncomplicated myocardial infarction without ventricular dysfunction was joined in the early 1990s by patients with advanced heart failure, and the transition continues: modern cardiac rehabilitation is increasingly faced with a generation of patients who have been diagnosed and adequately treated early with minimal residual cardiovascular damage. The focus of CR is changing from physical rehabilitation to lifestyle counseling. But this development is paradoxical indeed: with more cardiac patients surviving the acute event, the numbers of elderly patients have grown and the total need for comprehensive CR has not been reduced. The elderly were rarely enrolled in the early years of exercise-based training programs. Therefore, this large population presents a new challenge, especially as CR has proved to be particularly beneficial for patients with congestive heart failure.

Other factors play a role in the changing arena for CVD prevention and rehabilitation: the worldwide pandemic of obesity is expected to again raise the numbers of young cardiac patients and the disease is now extending into other parts of the globe. Thus CVD will remain the main cause of premature death in the first half of this century. Preventive public health measures are required. The relative weight of different risk factors appears to be altering, with disturbances in the psychosocial sphere becoming more important. With new diagnostic methods atherosclerosis can be detected well before an acute event, which creates a greater demand for preventive cardiology, as has been appreciated in the 2003 European Guidelines on Cardiovascular Prevention. Prevention and rehabilitation are gradually becoming a united and intertwined multidisciplinary service.

Furthermore, the theoretical basis for prevention and rehabilitation has been strengthened over past years and the medical, social and economic benefits have now been well established, contributing to their incorporation in standard cardiac care in many countries.

In the context of this scenario, the aim of the textbook is to give guidance in prevention, lifestyle counseling and rehabilitation for cardiologists, other physicians, and many different categories of health professionals in CR teams. For this purpose we have gathered over 60 experts from all parts of the globe, many of them members of the recently founded network, the European Association for Cardiovascular Prevention and Rehabilitation, a registered branch of the European Society of Cardiology.

Commencing with an introduction on the rationale for prevention and rehabilitation and its application worldwide, the book continues with two sections on the cornerstone of CR: exercise testing and training. Thereafter the other key elements of a multidisciplinary service are described: nutrition, smoking cessation, behavioral and social support and the caring aspects of CR. Special attention has been given to adapted programs for newer groups with specific demands, such as the elderly, patients with implantable devices, and patients after cardiac transplantation. In the final section, a concise overview of CVD pharmacology is given and the organizational aspects of CR, including quality assurance and economic evaluation, are addressed. We do hope that the textbook will be of value to CR teams around the world and thereby contribute to a high quality, comprehensive service for the cardiovascular patient of the 21st century.

Joep Perk
Peter Mathes
Helmut Gohlke
Catherine Monpère
Irene Hellemans
Hannah McGee
Philippe Sellier
Hugo Saner

Contents

Contributors

Stamatis Adamopoulos, MD, PhD
Onassis Cardiac Surgery Centre
and
Attikon University Hospital
Athens, Greece

Silvia Aepli
Swiss Heart Foundation
Switzerland

Agneta Andersson, MD
Department of Cardiology
Karolinska University Hospital Solna
Stockholm, Sweden

Dan Atar, MD, FESC, FACC FAHA
Department of Cardiology
Aker University Hospital
Oslo, Norway

A. Avram, MD
Cardiac Rehabilitation Clinic
University of Medicine and Pharmacy
   "Victor Babes" Timisoara
Timisoara, Romania

Guy de Backer, MD, PhD
Department of Public Health
Ghent University
Ghent, Belgium

Florence Beauvais
Service de Cardiologie
Hôpital Beaujon
Clichy, France

S. Beloka, MSc
Cardiovascular Rehabilitation Unit
Department of Rehabilitation Sciences
K.U. Leuven
Leuven, Belgium

Paul Bennett, PhD
Health and Social Care Research Center
University of Cardiff
Cardiff, UK

Birna Bjarnason-Wehrens
Institute for Cardiology and Sports Medicine
German Sport University Cologne
Cologne, Germany

Hans H. Bjørnstad, MD PHD
Department of Heart Disease
Haukeland University Hospital
Bergen, Norway

Tor H. Bjørnstad, MD
Institute of Circulation and Imaging
St. Olav University Hospital
Trondheim, Norway

K. Brockmeier
Pediatric Cardiology
University Hospital
University of Cologne
Cologne, Germany

Stephen J. Bunker
St.Vincent's Hospital Melbourne
and
National Heart Foundation of Australia
Australia

Gunilla Burell
Behavioral Medicine and
    Health Promotion
Department of Public Health
    and Caring Sciences
Uppsala University
Sweden

Alison Cahill
Cardiac Rehabilitation
Beaumont Hospital
Dublin, Ireland

Douglas Carroll, PhD
School of Sport and Exercise Psychology
University of Birmingham
Edgbaston
Birmingham, UK

Alain Cohen-Solal
Service de Cardiologie
Hôpital Beaujon
Clichy, France

Carsten B. Cordes, MD
Cardiac Rehabilitation Centre
Gollwitzer-Meier-Klinik
Bad Oeynhausen, Germany

Ugo Corrà, MD
Divisione di Cardiologia,
Fondazione "Salvatore Maugeri"
(NO), Italy

Wayne E. Derman, MBchB, PhD, FACSM
MRC/UCT Research Unit
    for Exercise Science and
    Sports Medicine
University of Cape Town
Sport Science Institute of South Africa
Cape Town, South Africa

Sigrid Dordel
Institute for School Sports and
    School Development
German Sport University Cologne
Cologne, Germany

L. Dorian Dugmore, PhD
Wellness International
Hazel Grove
Stockport
Nr Manchester,
Cheshire, UK

Katerina Fountoulaki, MD
Onassis Cardiac Surgery Center
and
Attikon University Hospital
Athens, Greece

Dan Gaita, MD, PhD
Cardiac Rehabilitation Clinic
University of Medicine and Pharmacy "Victor
    Babes" Timisoara
Timisoara, Romania

Pantaleo Giannuzzi, MD
Salvatore Maugeri Foundation
Institute for Clinical Care and Research (IRCCS)
Scientific Institute of Veruno
(NO), Veruno, Italy

Stephen Gielen, MD
Department of Internal Medicine/Cardiology
University of Leipzig
Leipzig
Saxony, Germany

Helmut Gohlke, FACC, FESC
Klinische Kardiologie II
Herz-Zentrum Bad Krozingen
Germany

Christa Gohlke-Bärwolf
Herz-Zentrum Bad Krozingen
Germany

Rainer Hambrecht, MD
Department of Internal Medicine/Cardiology
University of Leipzig
Leipzig
Saxony, Germany

Bo Hedbäck, MD, PhD
Department of Cardiology
University Hospital
Linköping, Sweden

**Irene Hellemans, MD, (Speciality
    Cardiology), PhD**
Institute of Health Sciences
Department of Earth Sciences
Vrije University
and
Department of Cardiology
Vrije University Medical Center
Amsterdam, The Netherlands

David Hevey, BA, MA, PhD
Department of Psychology
Trinity College Dublin
Dublin, Ireland

Asle Hirth, MD
Department of Heart Disease
Haukeland University Hospital
Bergen, Norway

John H. Horgan
Cardiac Rehabilitation Programme
Beaumont Hospital
Dublin, Ireland

Tiny Jaarsma, PhD, RN
Department of Cardiology
University Hospital Groningen
Groningen, Netherlands

**Michael V. Jelinek, MBBS, MD, FRACP,
FACC, FCSANZ**
Department of Cardiology
St.Vincent's Hospital Melbourne
and
National Heart Foundation of Australia
Australia

Kate Jolly, MBChB, MSc
Department of Public Health and Epidemiology
University of Birmingham
Edgbaston, Birmingham, UK

Therese Junker
Swiss Heart Foundation
Switzerland

Terence Kavanagh, MD, FRCPC
Faculty of Medicine, Graduate Program in
Exercise Science
University of Toronto
Ontario, Canada

Ulrich Keil, FESC
Institute of Epidemiology
Institute of Social Medicine
University of Munster
Munster, Germany

Deirdre A. Lane, BSc, PhD
University Department of Medicine
Sandwell and West Birmingham Hospitals
NHS Trust
Birmingham, UK

Robert J. Lewin
Department of Health Sciences
University of York
York, UK

Susanne Løgstrup
European Heart Network
Brussels, Belgium

Michel de Lorgeril, MD
School of Medicine
University of Grenoble
Domaine de la Merci
La Tronche, France

M. Martens, MSc
Cardiovascular Rehabilitation Unit
Department of Rehabilitation Sciences
K.U. Leuven
Leuven, Belgium

Peter Mathes, MD, FACC, FESC
Department of Cardiology
Technical University of Munich
Munich Rehabilitation Center
München, Germany

**Hannah McGee, BA(Mod.), PhD,
RegPsycholFPsSI**
Department of Psychology
Royal College of Surgeons in Ireland
Dublin, Ireland

Miguel F. Mendes, MD
Instituto Do Coraçao
Hospital Santa Cruz
Carnaxide, Linda-a-Velha, Portugal

Catherine Monpère, MD
Cardiac Rehabilitation Center
Bois Gibert
Ballan Miré, France

Jonathan Myers, PhD
Department of Cardiology
VA Palo Alto Health Care System
Palo Alto, CA, USA

Saied Nadirpour, MD
Department of Medicine
Haugesund Hospital
Haugesund, Norway

Josef Niebauer, MD, PhD
Department of Internal Medicine/Cardiology
University of Leipzig
Leipzig
Saxony, Germany

N.B. Oldridge, PhD
College of Health Sciences
University of Wisconsin-Milwaukee
Milwaukee, WI, USA

Yngvar Ommundsen, PhD
Department of Coaching and Psychology
Norwegian School of Sports Sciences
Oslo, Norway

Nicolas Paquot, MD, PhD
Head Associate Division of Diabetes
Nutrition and Metabolic Disorders
Department of Medicine
University of Liège
Academic Hospital Sart Tilman
Liège, Belgium

John T. Parissis, MD
Onassis Cardiac Surgery Center
and
Attikon University Hospital
Athens, Greece

Jill F. Pattenden, BA, PGCE, MSc
Department of Health Sciences
University of York
Heslington
York, UK

Ulla-Riitta Penttilä
Finnish Heart Association
Helsinki, Finland

Joep Perk, MD, FESC
Public Health Department
Kalmar County
Oskarshamn, Sweden

Annika Rosengren
Department of Medicine
Sahlgrenska University Hospital/Ostra
Goteborg, Sweden

Patricia Salen, BSc
School of Medicine
University of Grenoble
Domaine de la Merci
La Tronche, France

Hugo Saner, MD
Swiss Cardiovascular Center Bern
Cardiovascular Prevention and Rehabilitation
     University
Hospital Inselspital
Switzerland

André J. Scheen
Division of Diabetes
Nutrition and Metabolic Disorders
Department of Medicine
CHU Sart Tilman
Liège, Belgium

Karin Schenck-Gustafsson, MD, PhD, FESC
Department of Cardiology
Karolinska University Hospital Solna
Stockholm, Sweden

Jean-Paul Schmid, MD
Department of Cardiovascular Prevention
     and Rehabilitation
Swiss Cardiovascular Centre
Bern, Switzerland

Philippe Sellier, MD
Hôspital Broussais-HEGP
Assistance Publique-Hôpitaux de Paris
Paris, France

P.J. Senden
Department of Cardiology
Ziekenhuis Eemland (Hospital)
Amersfoort, The Netherlands

Sigmund Silber, MD, FACC, FESC
Department of Cardiology
Cardiology Practice and Hospital
Munich, Germany

Narayanswami Sreeram
Pediatric Electrophysiology
University Hospital
University of Cologne
Cologne, Germany

Elaine E. Steinke, BSN, MN, PhD
School of Nursing
Wichita State University
Wichita, KS, USA

A. Stevens, MSc
Cardiovascular Rehabilitation Unit
Department of Rehabilitation Sciences
K.U. Leuven
Leuven, Belgium

Anna Strömberg, RN, PhD, NFESC
Department of Cardiology
Linköping University Hospital
Linköping, Sweden

Jean Yves Tabet
Service de Cardiologie
Hôpital Beaujon
Clichy, France

Rod S. Taylor, MSc, PhD
Department of Public Health and Epidemiology
University of Birmingham
Edgbaston, Birmingham, UK

David R. Thompson, BSc, MA, PhD, MBA, RN, FRCN, FESC
The Nethersole School of Nursing
The Chinese University of Hong Kong
Shatin, New Territories
Hong Kong SAR
People's Republic of China

Serena Tonstad, MD, PhD
Department of Preventive Cardiology
Ullevål University Hospital
Oslo, Norway

Trudi P.G. Tromp-Beelen
Jellinek Medical Center
Amsterdam, The Netherlands

Britt Undheim MD
Department of Heart Disease
Haukeland University Hospital
Bergen, Norway

L. Vanhees, PhD, FESC
Cardiovascular Rehabilitation Unit
Department of Rehabilitation Sciences
K.U. Leuven
Leuven, Belgium

Bruno Vergès
Endocrinology-Diabetology Department
University Hospital Dijon
France

Bénédicte Vergès-Patois
Cardiac Rehabilitation Unit
University Hospital Dijon
France

Nanette K. Wenger, MD
Department of Cardiology
Emory University School of Medicine
Grady Memorial Hospital
Emory Heart and Vascular Center
Atlanta, GA, USA

David A. Wood
Cardiovascular Medicine
National Heart and Lung Institute
Imperial College
London, UK

Cheuk-Man Yu, MD, FRACP, FRCP, FHKAM
Division of Cardiology
Department of Medicine and Therapeutics
The Chinese University of Hong Kong
Shatin, New Territories
Hong Kong SAR
People's Republic of China

Section I
Introduction

The concept of exercise as a fundamental part of a healthy lifestyle has its origin in ancient Greece. Lost for many hundred years, it re-emerged in the British Isles, rapidly spreading into Western societies. As a therapeutic modality, the preventive aspect was discovered early. As a treatment concept for heart patients, it was a controversial issue for many years, now even being accepted in heart failure, a condition regarded as a strict contraindication only a few years ago.

Cardiac rehabilitation programs improve outcome, recent meta-analyses have revealed. A reduction in cardiac events, increase in functional status, and an improvement of the quality of life are the sustained beneficial effects. Initially reserved for the patient with an uncomplicated myocardial infarction, these programs are now extended to all cardiac patients with a condition that endangers their functional capacity.

Although the interventions vary considerably in the different parts of the world, rehabilitation programs improve the process of care, coronary risk factor profiles, functional status, and the quality of life. Particularly in aging societies, but also beginning in the developing world, such programs are a means of preserving an independent lifestyle for the elderly, thus preventing an overuse of nursing services, which the majority of countries are unable to provide.

Risk factor profiles give us a good guideline for the management of the coronary patient. In the field of prevention, they are helpful in targeting the high-risk individual. Since the majority of patients fall into the average category of risk, it will be mandatory to identify those at risk in this large group more clearly. Newer diagnostic concepts such as the coronary calcium score or the intima–media thickness of the carotid artery as determined by ultrasound are promising steps in this direction.

Main Messages

Chapter 1: From Exercise Training to Comprehensive Cardiac Rehabilitation

Following the initial description of the gradual healing of a myocardial infarction, utmost care was taken to avoid any exercise for the patient. Much to the surprise of the medical profession, it turned out that a sizeable portion of the patients who had survived this treatment reached their previous functional level. Gradually, a more active approach was adopted, including a formal exercise prescription as a therapeutic aspect. Later, educational counseling and psychosocial support were added. The current is best defined by the WHO definition: "The rehabilitation of cardiac patients is the sum of activities required to influence favourably the underlying cause of the disease, as well as the best possible physical, mental and social conditions, so that they may by their own efforts, preserve or resume when lost, as normal a place as possible in the society."

Chapter 2: The Evidence Base for Cardiac Rehabilitation

Cardiac rehabilitation programs improve outcomes for patients with coronary disease.

Meta-analyses confirm that rehabilitation programs not only reduce the risk of recurrent myocardial infarction and death, but also improve risk factor profiles, use of therapies, functional status, and quality of life. Benefits did not differ among the types of programs, those that incorporated education and counseling about coronary risk factors with or without a supervised exercise program, and those that consisted of a structured exercise program only. Rehabilitation and secondary prevention programs improve processes of care, coronary risk factor profiles, functional status, and quality of life.

Chapter 3: Indications for Cardiac Rehabilitation

Cardiovascular diseases constitute the leading cause of morbidity and premature mortality in Western societies, while they are increasing in numbers in developing countries. Whereas rehabilitation and secondary prevention were once seen as valuable only to patients with an uncomplicated myocardial infarction, they are now regarded as a treatment option for all patients with heart disease. Improvement in functional status, reduction in morbidity, improvement of the quality of life, and maintenance of an independent lifestyle are valuable aims in the treatment of any form of heart disease.

Chapter 4: Prevention Guidelines: Management of the Coronary Patient

The effective prevention of myocardial infarction and death from coronary disease requires accurate identification of persons at risk. Risk factor stratification has recently been redefined to allow a more precise identification for the different areas in Europe.

Chapters 5 to 10: Practice Worldwide

Different programs and approaches have been developed in the different areas of the world,

all aiming at a similar outcome, utilizing a variety of methods. The Anglo-Saxon countries have largely preferred a primarily ambulatory approach, favoring long-term exercise-based rehabilitation programs, to which educational, psychological, and social components are being added in a stepwise fashion. Countries with a long-standing spa tradition such as Germany, Austria, and some eastern and southern European countries including Italy have adopted an inpatient residential center approach, with a rather short duration, consisting of an intense, gradually increasing exercise program, where educational, psychological, and social components are begun during the very first days of the program. Formidable differences in availability, distance, funding, and acceptance have led to an increasing diversity of rehabilitation services worldwide.

Chapter 5: Cardiac Rehabilitation: Europe
Chapter 6: Cardiac Rehabilitation: United States
Chapter 7: Cardiac Rehabilitation: Canada
Chapter 8: Cardiac Rehabilitation: Australia
Chapter 9: Cardiac Rehabilitation: South Africa
Chapter 10: Cardiac Rehabilitation: China

Chapter 11: New Concepts for Early Diagnosis of Coronary Artery Disease

In the effort to identify the person at risk of myocardial infarction and death, an ideal and valuable additional tool should be a proven independent risk factor, providing additional information without inherent risk and with wide availability. A sizeable number of studies have shown that a high calcium score is a predictor of cardiac events, independent of the traditional risk factors, thus providing additional information. The two approaches – conventional risk estimation and calcium scoring – should enable the physician to better delineate the individual risk in the "intermediate-risk category," which is of such an importance because of the sheer number of people in this category.

1
From Exercise Training to Comprehensive Cardiac Rehabilitation

Peter Mathes

The WHO definition of cardiac rehabilitation from 1968[1] refers to a "process by which a person is restored to an optimal physical, medical, psychological, social, emotional, sexual, vocational and economic status." Over the ensuing years this statement of intent has remained remarkably similar. The World Health Organization's current definition addresses the cardiovascular status of the patient before, during, and after the event:

The rehabilitation of cardiac patients is the sum of activities required to influence favourably the underlying cause of the disease, as well as the best possible physical, mental and social conditions, so that they may by their own efforts, preserve or resume when lost, as normal a place as possible in the society. Rehabilitation cannot be regarded as an isolated form of therapy but must be integrated within the entire treatment.[2]

Current cardiac rehabilitation programs strive to involve the patient's family in the whole process, thereby deploying health promotion intervention in a wider section of the community.

Objectives of cardiac rehabilitation include:

- a significant improvement in the patient's functional capacity
- psychological adaptations to the chronic disease process
- a foundation for long-term behavior and lifestyle changes to favorably influence the long-term prognosis
- maintenance of an independent lifestyle for as long as possible.

This was not always the case. Initially, the emphasis was put on physical training as the mainstay of cardiac rehabilitation, primarily with the intent of improving symptoms and physical capacity.

Physical conditioning in reference to heart disease is actually far from new. Fully 200 years ago Heberden observed the beneficial effects in a patient he advised to saw wood for 30 minutes daily over a 6-month period. Although that was long before the first mention of acute myocardial infarction in the medical literature, no doubt some of Heberden's patients had sustained an infarct as the condition is understood today.

The first person to introduce exercise systematically into the therapy of cardiovascular disease was M. Oertel in 1875.[3] He successfully treated a patient with overweight and shortness of breath with an increasing number of steps in a hilly terrain, the "Terrain-Kur," which became popular in the ensuing years. Later he used an arm ergometer for this purpose. As early as 1875, Stokes recommended physical activity for the treatment of angina pectoris. This counsel was all but forgotten following Herrick's original clinical description of acute myocardial infarction in 1912: the worry that physical exertion heightens the risk of ventricular aneurysm or rupture, or aggravates myocardial ischemia, kept patients virtually immobilized in bed for 6 or 8 weeks. On discharge, anything as strenuous as stair-climbing was forbidden for at least a year. A few patients returned to work many months after hospital discharge; for most, all chance of a normal life was past.

Credit is due to Samuel Levine for questioning the wisdom of enforced bedrest and inactivity for a prolonged period following the onset of infarction; his "armchair" method, recommended largely on an empiric basis to avoid thromboembolic or respiratory complications, has since been well supported and extended on both a clinical and research basis. When Leonard Goldwater and colleagues assessed their experience at the first cardiac work classification clinic in the US in the 1940s, it came as a surprise to many that fully 50–70% of patients could return to work, although not necessarily to the same job as before.

The first inpatient progressive physical activity program for patients with acute myocardial infarction was described by Newman et al. in 1952.[4] Physical activity began during the second week of hospitalization and gradually increased until discharge at 6 weeks. During the 1950s, a concept of utilization of residual functional capacity and an occupational classification by energy expenditure was popular.[5] Later in the decade, detailed physical activity programs for inpatients were formalized. This was promoted by Wilhelm Raab and P.D. White in the US, Beckmann and Knipping in Germany, and Gottheiner in Israel.[6] Beckmann started the first systematic inpatient training program for the prevention of cardiovascular disease.

In the 1960s, with the proliferation of coronary care units involving continuous electrocardiographic (ECG) monitoring, progressively earlier mobilization after acute myocardial infarction was practiced. It was realized that the belief that there would be measurable physical invalidism after a coronary event was largely unfounded. Many patients with healed myocardial infarctions were found to have exercise capacities that were equal to those of presumably healthy, sedentary middle-aged men. Rehabilitation was dominated by exercise training and included some vocational readjustment. It was recognized that such measures resulted in an earlier return to normal activities as a result of improvements in both physical and psychological capabilities.[7] Early mobilization helped reduce the fear of disability, although a restrictive attitude still hampered patient progress.[8]

During the 1970s, the multidimensional aspects of cardiac rehabilitation were acknowledged, and the team approach became popular.[9] Established methods were developed, which resulted in a proliferation of hospital-based inpatient and outpatient programs.[8] Guidelines for cardiac exercise programs were established by the American College of Sports Medicine[10] and the American Heart Association.[11] During the 1970s, public awareness of the individual's potential role in his or her own health destiny grew. Rehabilitation and secondary prevention gained widespread support as an integral component of comprehensive coronary care.

Developments in Rehabilitation Care

Enormous changes in the rehabilitative approach to the care of patients with cardiovascular disease have occurred since the WHO Expert Committee on the Rehabilitation of Patients with Cardiovascular Disease was organized by WHO in 1963. At that time, rehabilitation was concerned predominantly with individuals recovering from acute, essentially uncomplicated, myocardial infarction; the rehabilitative interventions recommended for such patients were considered to encompass "the sum of activities required to ensure them the best possible physical, mental and social conditions so that they may, by their own efforts, resume and maintain as normal a place as possible in the community." Now, however, rehabilitation is considered to be an essential part of the care that should be available to all cardiac patients. Its goals are to improve functional capacity, alleviate or lessen activity-related symptoms, reduce unwarranted invalidism, and enable the cardiac patient to return to a useful and personally satisfying role in society.

Cardiovascular disease is the number one medical problem in the Western world. It is becoming an increasing problem in developing countries; rheumatic heart disease, hypertension, and cardiomyopathy are already prevalent, and coronary heart disease is assuming growing significance. Despite differences in patterns of cardiac disease between and within developing countries, current concepts of cardiac rehabilitative care can be applied even in societies with minimal medical personnel and equipment resources. Guidelines are essential for their application. Rehabilitative care should be incorporated into the existing healthcare system, and should conform to cultural traditions and social norms. Guidance is also needed on maintenance of cardiovascular health, particularly for societies undergoing social transition, with consequent changes in culture, foods, lifestyle, and economics.

Demographic factors have had a radical influence on the range of cardiac patients considered eligible for exercise therapy during rehabilitation. Among patients with coronary heart disease, it is not only those who have recovered from uncomplicated myocardial infarctions, but also patients with complications of the acute episode, those with angina pectoris of varying severity, and those who have undergone coronary artery bypass surgery and coronary angioplasty who are now considered candidates for rehabilitative care. The spectrum of coronary disease is extensive. At one end are the patients treated by acute myocardial reperfusion with coronary thrombolysis and/or early coronary angioplasty or coronary bypass surgery, who exhibit a lesser severity of disease, minimal residual symptoms, little functional impairment, and a characteristically excellent prognosis. At the other end are patients who, having survived several acute infarctions and surgical procedures, often have severe end-stage coronary heart disease characterized by varying combinations of myocardial ischemia, ventricular dysfunction, and ventricular arrhythmias. For all these patients, one of the most significant advances has been the emergence of a variety of test procedures designed to identify both the risk of early recurrent coronary events and the long-term prognosis. These assessments are typically exercise-based, and are designed to distinguish patients who can perform reasonable levels of activity without adverse consequences (low-risk patients) from those with a very limited exercise capacity in whom there is early onset of myocardial ischemia, ventricular dysfunction, or serious arrhythmias. An intermediate-risk group can also be identified. This delineation can serve as a basis for recommending not only medical and surgical therapies but also exercise (including the need for and intensity and duration of professional supervision of exercise). It can also serve as a guide to the resumption of work and other pre-illness activities.[12–14]

At the extremes of the coronary risk profile, computation of morbidity and mortality is unlikely to be a sensitive measure of the outcome of rehabilitative or other interventions. For very low-risk coronary patients, the morbidity and mortality are so low, at least in the short term, that any intervention is unlikely to affect the outcome. On the other hand, the outlook in end-stage coronary disease is so uniformly poor that other measures are required to ascertain the benefits of any intervention. Prominent among these are likely to be quality of life measures, which are related to an individual patient's perception of improvements in physical, social, and emotional status, and the value he or she places on such improvements.[15,16]

Other categories of patients now considered candidates for rehabilitation include those who have undergone cardiac valvular surgery, those (both adults and children) who have undergone surgical correction or amelioration of congenital heart disease, those with cardiomyopathy and ventricular dysfunction of other etiology, those with implanted cardiac pacemakers and cardioverter-defibrillators, and individuals who are recovering form cardiac or cardiopulmonary transplantation.[12,17]

These categories include large numbers of elderly cardiac patients. In both developed and developing countries, the numbers of "frail elderly" – the oldest members of society – are increasing more rapidly than any other population group. For many elderly patients with cardiovascular disease, return to remunerative work is often not an appropriate outcome measure of rehabilitation: rather, the attainment and maintenance of an independent lifestyle is an outcome that is valued both personally and, given the high cost of institutional care, by society. Thus, small improvements in capacity for physical work may exert a major and favorable impact on the quality of life of elderly cardiac patients.[14,18]

Current Concepts

In addition to the more favorable functional status and prognosis in a variety of cardiovascular illnesses, which reflect improved medical and surgical therapies, changes in a number of aspects of rehabilitative care per se have substantially influenced its application.

First, there is evidence that patients classified by stratification procedures as being at low risk can safely exercise without medical supervision and safely and promptly return to pre-illness activities, including remunerative work. Further, it is now accepted that exercise training of lower intensity can produce improvements in functional capacity comparable to those produced by higher-intensity exercise. The lower-intensity exercise is characterized by greater safety, which is particularly important if exercise sessions are unsupervised; it causes less discomfort and is more enjoyable, and thus makes adherence to the recommended exercise regime more likely. Among patients who can safely perform modest levels of dynamic exercise, the relative safety and substantial value of low-intensity isometric or resistive (strength training) exercise have also been identified.[26] That patients receiving all types of antianginal drugs can benefit from exercise training has been extensively documented. Cardiac enlargement and compensated heart failure are no longer considered contraindications to physical activity, and rehabilitation has improved functional status. Another important observation is the lack of correlation between the extent of ventricular dysfunction and physical work capacity.[19–21]

Greater attention is now being devoted to the educational and counseling components of rehabilitative care, with new techniques being applied in these areas as well. Prominent among these is the behavioral approach to reducing coronary risk; this comprises not only transmission of information, but also practical training in the skills needed for adoption of a healthy lifestyle, and provision of opportunity to practice and reinforce these skills. To achieve successful lifestyle changes, patients must actively participate in the management of their disease. Evidence that favorable modification of coronary risk factors can not only limit progression of the disease but even induce regression of the underlying atherosclerosis has encouraged efforts of this area. This is particularly true for individuals with accelerated atherosclerosis, manifest as myocardial infarction or a requirement for myocardial revascularization procedures. The importance of the family – and often the workplace – in encouraging and reinforcing efforts to reduce coronary risk is increasingly acknowledged. It is thus essential that healthcare professionals at all levels are trained to be effective teachers to their patients.[15,22]

Perception of health status is recognized as having an influence on clinical outcomes; for example, the perceived ability to exercise correlates better with resumption of work than do objective measurements of exercise capacity during formal testing. There is also substantial correlation between perception of health status and return to usual family and community activities, and recreational and occupational pursuits. Importantly, this perception can be favorably altered by education and counseling.[23,24]

Psychological problems, predominantly anxiety and depression, are recognized as greater obstacles to the resumption of pre-illness activities by coronary patients than physical incapacity. Return to work is increasingly viewed as an outcome measure that is economically, physically, and socially relevant to a wide variety of coronary patients, but one that may relate poorly to restoration of functional capacity. Total restoration of functional status, occupational as well as physical, remains a challenge to be met.

Practice Worldwide

Different programs and approaches have been developed in different areas of the world, all aiming at a similar outcome, utilizing a variety of different ways.

The Anglo-Saxon countries have largely preferred a primarily ambulatory approach, favoring long-term exercise-based rehabilitation programs, to which educational, psychological, and social components are being added in a stepwise fashion (R. Mulcahy[16]).

Countries with a long-standing spa tradition such as Germany, Austria, some eastern European countries and some of the southern European countries including Italy have adopted an inpatient, residential rehabilitation center approach, with a rather short duration (up to 4 weeks), consisting of intense, gradually increasing exercise programs, where educational, psychological and social components are begun during the very first days of the program.

In Germany, the initial, primarily exercise oriented-rehabilitation programs were begun by Oertel,[3] followed by Peter Beckmann.[6] Patients were put together in groups of similar physical fitness, and the goal to be achieved was to make a proper mountain climbing tour at the end of this rehabilitation period. Koenig and Halhuber added psychological counseling and social support as essential components.[16] In the days of a booming economy with the ever-present need for a large workforce, such rehabilitation centers proliferated within Germany and neighboring countries. Now that the economy is lagging, the number of centers is declining, being replaced in a less comprehensive way by ambulatory programs.[16,25]

Rehabilitative interventions are increasingly undertaken in children and young adults with a variety of cardiovascular disorders. The growing quantity of information about appropriate interventions in these age groups warrants wider dissemination. Medical and surgical treatments have significantly improved life expectancy in children with cardiovascular disease; subsequent comprehensive rehabilitation will thus have long-term economic and social benefits.[25] Surgical treatment is available for over 95% of congenital cardiac lesions, yet post-operative results after successful surgery show that these children fail to achieve the same functional capacity as their healthy peers. Children with cardiac disease require significantly different physical activities from adults, and the educational and counseling requirements for both the children and their families are also different. Comprehensive cardiac rehabilitation for children is cost-effective and prudent, benefiting individual patients and the society in which they live. Moreover, a large percentage of cardiac patients in developing countries are children and adolescents. Specific attention should therefore be directed to disseminating rehabilitative guidelines and promulgating the implementation of appropriate programs for this section of the population.

References

1. Rehabilitation of patients with cardiovascular disease. Report of WHO Expert Committee. Geneva: WHO, 1964. WHO Technical Report Series No 270.
2. Rehabilitation after cardiovascular disease with special emphasis on developing countries. Geneva: WHO, 1993. WHO Technical Report Series No 831.
3. Oertel M. Allgemeine Therapie der Kreislaufstörungen. In: Ziemssen J. Handbuch der allgemeinen Therapie. Leipzig: Vogel; 1891.
4. Newman LB, Andrews MF, Koblish MO, et al. Physical medicine and rehabilitation in acute myocardial infarction. Arch Intern Med 1952;89:552–561.
5. Chapman CB, Fraser RS. Studies of the effect of exercise on cardiovascular function. III. Cardiovascular response to exercise in patients with healed myocardial infarction. Circulation 1954;9:347–351.
6. Hellerstein HF, Ford AB. Rehabilitation of the cardiac patient. JAMA 1957;164:225–231.
7. Naughton J, Balke B, Poarch A. Modified work capacities studies in individuals with and without coronary artery disease. J Sports Med Phys Fitness 1964;4:208–212.
8. Hellerstein HK. Cardiac rehabilitation: a retrospective view. In: Pollock ML, ed. Heart Disease and Rehabilitation. Boston: Houghton Mifflin Professional; 1987:509–520.
9. Hayes JR. Evaluating the efficacy of cardiac rehabilitation. Psychiatr Ann 1978;8(Oct):100–110.
10. American College of Sports Medicine. Guidelines for Graded Exercise Testing and Exercise Prescription. Philadelphia: Lea & Febiger; 1975:1–48.
11. American Heart Association. The Exercise Standards Book. Dallas: American Heart Association; 1979.
12. Foxworth GD. Rehabilitation for hospitalized adults after open-heart procedures: the team approach. Heart Lung 1978;7:834–839.
13. Gau GT. Cardiac rehabilitation. I. A cardiologist's view: Psychiatr Ann 1978;8(Oct):31–43.
14. Squires RW, Lavie CJ, Brandt TR, et al. Cardiac rehabilitation in patients with severe ischemic left ventricular dysfunction. Circulation 1979;60:1519–1536.
15. Wenger NK. Patient and family education and counseling: a requisite component of cardiac rehabilitation. In: Mathes P, Halhuber MJ, eds. Controversies in Cardiac Rehabilitation. New York: Springer-Verlag; 1982:108–114.
16. Mathes P, Halhuber MJ. Controversies in Cardiac Rehabilitation. New York: Springer-Verlag; 1982.
17. Rod JL, Squires RW, Pollock ML, et al. Symptom-limited graded exercise testing soon after myocardial revascularization surgery. J Cardiac Rehabil 1982;2:199–205.

18. Sullivan MJ, Higginbotham MB, Cobb FR. Exercise training in patients with severe left ventricular dysfunction: hemodynamic and metabolic effects. Circulation 1988;78:506–515.
19. Théroux P, Waters DD, Halphen C, et al. Prognostic value of exercise testing soon after myocardial infarction. N Engl J Med 1979;301:341–334.
20. Smith JW, Dennis CA, Gassmann A, et al. Exercise testing three weeks after myocardial infarction. Chest 1979;75:12–16.
21. Starling MR, Crawford MH, Kennedy GT, et al. Exercise testing early after myocardial infarction: predictive value for subsequent unstable angina and death. Am J Cardiol 1980;46:909–914.
22. Cassem NH, Hackett TP. Psychological rehabilitation of myocardial infarction patients in the acute phase. Heart Lung 1973;2:382–388.
23. Hackett TP, Cassem NH. The psychologic reactions of patients in the pre- and post-hospital phases of myocardial infarction. Postgrad Med 1975;57:43–46.
24. Friedman M, Thoresen CE, Gill JJ, et al. Alteration of type A behavior and its effect on cardiac recurrences in post myocardial infarction patients: summary results on the recurrrent coronary prevention project. Am Heart J 1986;112:653–665.
25. Oldridge NB, Guyatt GH, Fischer ME, et al. Cardiac rehabilitation after myocardial infarction: combined experience of randomized clinical trials. JAMA 1988;260:945–950.
26. Hollmann W, Rost R, Dufaux B, Liesen H. Prävention und Rehabilitation von Herz-Kreislaufkrankheiten durch körperliches Training. Stuttgart: Hippokrates; 1983.

2
The Evidence Base for Cardiac Rehabilitation

Rod S. Taylor and Kate Jolly

Introduction

- How effective is cardiac rehabilitation?
- Are particular interventions in cardiac rehabilitation more effective than others?
- Does cardiac rehabilitation offer benefits over and above other secondary prevention measures, such as drug therapy?
- Are there groups of patients in which cardiac rehabilitation is more (or less) effective?
- Is home-based cardiac rehabilitation as effective a method of delivering cardiac rehabilitation as supervised center- or hospital-based programs?
- Does cardiac rehabilitation provide good value for money?

These are the principal questions raised by healthcare administrators, hospital managers, and regional and national healthcare policy makers involved in the commissioning of cardiac rehabilitation (CR) services. This chapter examines the evidence for CR in order to address each of these questions. The question of value for money (or "cost-effectiveness") will be dealt with in Chapter 60, Economic Evaluation of Cardiac Rehabilitation.

Before we examine the evidence for CR, we need to determine what constitutes "good" evidence and, specifically, consider the concept of the "hierarchy of evidence."

The Evidence Hierarchy – the Randomized Controlled Trial and the Systematic Review

It is well accepted that the gold standard study design for establishing the effect of a therapy (or collection of therapies as in the case of cardiac rehabilitation) is the randomized controlled trial (RCT).[1] For example, let's say we want to know the effectiveness of a 12-week outpatient cardiac rehabilitation program for patients with New York Heart Association (NYHA) class II and III heart failure (HF). According to this design, patients would be randomly assigned (usually by means of a computer-generated random number sequence) to receive usual medical care (e.g. drug therapy, advice etc.) or outpatient CR plus usual medical care. Patients would undergo an assessment battery (e.g. exercise test, questionnaires of psychological well-being, number of hospitalizations for HF in last 3 months) prior to randomization and, then again, at various follow-up points thereafter. The strength of the RCT (assuming that the study size is large enough) is that the process of randomization ensures that the characteristics of the two groups (e.g. age, sex, severity of disease) are identical. Thus it can be assumed that any difference in the outcome at follow-up is due to CR rather than selection bias, that is, a difference in the patient characteristics of the two groups. Such is this bias, that it is well documented that non-randomized studies tend to overestimate the effect of therapies by some 20% to 30% compared to RCTs.[2]

Nevertheless, one RCT is rarely enough evidence on its own. A single study may well not be large enough to have the statistical power to detect the effect of the treatment being tested, particularly if that effect is fairly small – as most modern day therapies are. A single study may not be representative of the range of real world practice. For example, returning to the example RCT, it may be that your practice includes patients with NYHA class IV heart failure. It may be that your CR practice only includes exercise training while the RCT is based on exercise training plus stress management training and education. By looking for all RCTs that have investigated the question of the impact of CR on patients with HF, it is more likely that this overall body of evidence will reflect the range of real world practice than will one RCT alone.

The systematic review is a methodology that comprehensively gathers studies (RCTs or other design) together in as unbiased a manner as possible to address a particular healthcare question.[3] Many systematic reviews include a "meta-analysis," that is, a statistical technique that allows the results of several studies to be combined into a single numerical estimate. Meta-analyses provide greater statistical power than a single RCT alone. One of the best sources of good quality systematic reviews and meta-analyses over the last decade has become the Cochrane Library.[4] The Cochrane Library is the output of the Cochrane Collaboration, an international movement with the bold mission of "Preparing, maintaining and disseminating systematic reviews of the effects of (whole of) health care."

At the time of writing this chapter, three Cochrane systematic reviews were published that directly examine the effectiveness of CR.[5–10] The remainder of this chapter discusses the findings of these three systematic reviews in the context of the questions posed above.

How Effective Is CR?

Although the question "how effective is my therapy?" appears a simple one, for CR a careful framing of the question is required in order to provide a meaningful answer. In contrast to taking a drug, CR is a "complex intervention" – one "made up of various interconnecting parts."[11] CR is complex in a number ways. First, it is a multi-faceted intervention that can consist of exercise training, psychological therapy (e.g. stress management), education, and other interventions (e.g. occupational counseling) and is usually delivered by a multidisciplinary team. It can be delivered in a variety of different settings (hospital, community center, or patient's own home) and at different points in the disease continuum (phase I to IV programs). Finally, CR is often targeted at/to a population of patients that include a variety of cardiac diagnoses, usually post acute myocardial infarction, post coronary artery bypass grafting (CABG) or percutaneous transluminal coronary angioplasty (PTCA) and, increasingly, heart failure.

Each of three Cochrane systematic reviews has been scoped to address specific aspects of the question of the effectiveness of cardiac rehabilitation.

1. Effectiveness of Exercise-Based Cardiac Rehabilitation for Coronary Heart Disease (CHD) – Taylor et al.[6]

This Cochrane review examines the question of the effectiveness of exercise-based CR (exercise training alone or exercise training combined with other therapies, such as education or psychological interventions) compared to usual care in patients with CHD (post myocardial infarction, angina pectoris, or following CABG and PTCA).

The latest version of this review was published in 2004 by Taylor and colleagues and updates the original Cochrane review on this subject performed in 2000 by Jolliffe et al. and previous systematic reviews in 1988 by Oldridge et al. and 1989 by O'Connor et al. The 2004 review identified a total of 48 RCTs in 8940 CHD patients. A total of 19 RCTs assessed exercise training only, 30 RCTs combined exercise with other interventions

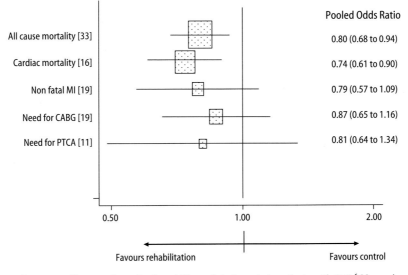

FIGURE 2-1. Summary of impact of exercise-based CR on clinical events in patients with CHD.[6] [ ], number of trials.

("comprehensive CR") and one RCT assessed both exercise only and comprehensive CR. The review reported three groups of outcomes – clinical endpoints (mortality and morbidity), risk factor levels, and health-related quality of life. The meta-analysis of clinical endpoints is shown in Figure 2-1. Compared to usual care, exercise-based CR significantly reduced total mortality by 20% and cardiac mortality by 26%, although there was no significant reduction in nonfatal MI events or the need for recurrent CABG or PTCA. Exercise-based

cardiac rehabilitation was associated with improvements in a number of primary risk factors including lipid profile and smoking behavior (Table 2-1). A total of nine RCTs assessed patient health-related quality of life (HRQoL) using a validated outcome measure. Given the range of HRQoL instruments used, the authors were not able to pool results across studies. However, all RCTs reported an improvement in HRQoL (total or domain score) with exercise-based CR. Nevertheless, and perhaps

TABLE 2-1. Summary of impact of exercise-based[6] and psychology-based CR[7] on primary risk factors

Outcome	Exercise-based CR	Psychology-based CR
	Mean difference+	
Total cholesterol (mmol/L)	−0.34 (−0.56 to −0.11)*	−0.27 (−0.55 to 0)*
HDL cholesterol (mmol/L)	0.03 (−0.06 to 0.11)	0.05 (−0.10 to 0.08)
LDL cholesterol (mmol/L)	−0.32 (−0.55 to −0.10)*	−0.16 (−0.69 to 0.37)
Triglycerides (mmol/L)	−0.28 (−0.49 to −0.06)*	Not reported
Systolic blood pressure (mmHg)	−0.5 (−6.5 to 5.5)	0.05 (0.01 to 0.08)*
Diastolic blood pressure (mmHg)	−0.6 (4.5 to 2.8)	−1.9 (−4.8 to −1.1)*
	Relative risk++	
Smoking	0.77 (0.62 to 0.94)*	0.81 (0.53 to 1.25)

*Statistically significant at $P \leq 0.05$.
+Mean difference <0: indicates reduced in the CR group than usual care.
++Relative risk <1.00 indicates lower probability of outcome in the CR group than usual care group.

surprisingly, only one RCT reported an improvement that exceeded that observed in the usual care controls.

2. Effectiveness of Psychology-Based CR – Rees et al.[7]

In the 2004 Cochrane review, Rees et al. examined the question of the effectiveness of psychology-based CR compared to usual care in patients with CHD.

This Cochrane review updates two previous systematic reviews by Linden et al. in 1996 and Dusseldorp et al. in 1999 that assessed this question. These latter two reviews have been criticized as being both non-systematic and including non-randomized evidence.[7]

Rees et al. identified a total of 36 RCTs across 12,841 CHD patients. The authors reported clinical endpoints, risk factor levels, psychological well-being and HRQoL. Meta-analysis showed a 28% reduction in the number of nonfatal MI events with psychological CR but no significant change in either all cause or cardiac mortality (Figure 2-2). Significant improvements in lipid profile and diastolic blood pressure

were observed with psychological CR (Table 2-1). The authors reported improvement in anxiety (−0.07 standard deviation units, 95% CI: −0.15 to: 0.01) and depression (SMD: −0.032, 95% CI: −0.56 to −0.08) with CR. Two out of five RCTs reported improvements in HRQoL with CR.

3. Effectiveness of Exercise-Based CR for Heart Failure – Rees et al.,[8] Smart et al.,[9] and ExTraMATCH[10]

Three meta-analyses have recently been published that examine the effectiveness of exercise-based CR (aerobic training alone or combined aerobic and resistance training) compared to usual care in patients with heart failure – the Cochrane review by Rees et al. in 2003, a systematic review and meta-analysis by Smart and colleagues, and a meta-analysis performed by a collaboration of the trial authors (the ExTraMATCH group, 2004).

Because of their different timings (Rees et al. searched up to March 2001 while Smart et al. searched up to May 2003) and use of

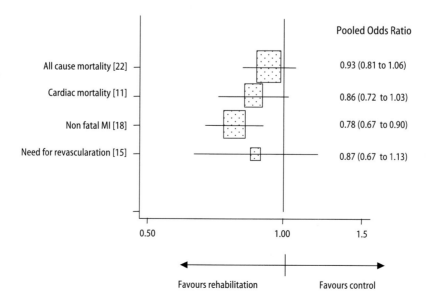

FIGURE 2-2. Summary of psychology-based CR on clinical events in patients with CHD.[7]

TABLE 2-2. Summary of scope of meta-analyses of exercise-based CR for heart failure

	ExTraMATCH (2004)[10]	Smart et al. (2004)[9]	Rees et al. (2003; Cochrane)[8]
Diagnosis	Ejection fraction <50%	Ejection fraction <40%	Clinical diagnosis
RCTs (n)	12	39	29
Aerobic alone	7	Not reported	23
Aerobic + resistance	2		6
Patients (n)	801	1394	1126
Outcomes	Mortality Hospitalization	Exercise tolerance Mortality Hospitalization	Exercise tolerance Mortality Morbidity Hospitalization Quality of life

systematic review methods (ExTraMATCH did not explicitly search for all published RCTs but used all those RCTs known to the authors) the comprehensiveness of these three studies varied (Table 2-2) as did, to some extent, their conclusions.

The main point of departure in the results of the three meta-analyses was total mortality. Compared to usual care, no significant difference in total mortality with CR was reported by either Rees et al. (pooled odds ratio 1.13, 95% CI: 0.58 to 2.22) or Smart et al. (pooled odds ratio 0.85, 95% CI: 0.51 to 1.41). However, ExTraMATCH reported a statistically significant 35% reduction in total mortality with exercise training (pooled hazard ratio 0.65, 95% CI: 0.46 to 0.92). Why the difference in result? ExTraMATCH was a meta-analysis where the authors had access to individual patient outcome data from each RCT. This more positive result of ExTraMATCH was due to the inclusion of the recent 3-year follow-up of the Belardinelli et al. trial, a large and positive trial not included at the time of the Cochrane review by Rees et al. in 2003. The greater number of events in the trials included in the ExTraMATCH review suggested that the authors might have had access to unpublished outcome results collected over a longer follow-up period. In view of the potentially non-systematic selection of evidence by the ExTraMATCH authors, the positive conclusion of exercise-based CR on total mortality should be interpreted cautiously.

Exercise-based CR appeared to have benefit for both exercise tolerance and HRQoL. Rees et al. reported a significant increase in maximum oxygen consumption of 2.1 mL/kg/min (95% CI: 2.8 to 1.4). Seven out of the nine RCTs reported a significant improvement HRQoL following CR. In five of these trials the improvement exceeded that of the usual care group.

Are Particular Interventions Within Cardiac Rehabilitation More Effective Than Others?

Few RCTs have that been designed to directly assess the ("subgroup") question of whether there are differences in the relative effectiveness of the different components of CR, for example exercise-training versus psychological interventions; dose "x" of exercise training versus dose "y"; or comprehensive rehabilitation versus exercise training only.

However, some (albeit indirect) evidence on this question is available from the Cochrane reviews. Meta-analyses potentially provide an opportunity to compare the results of one group of trials to another, so-called "meta-regression," and thereby allow these subgroup questions to be examined. Such subgroup analyses were reported by the meta-analyses of Taylor et al. (2004) and ExTraMATCH.

Taylor et al. found no significance in the impact of CR on total mortality when comparing trials of exercise-only CR to comprehensive CR or when comparing trials of different exercise doses (based on overall duration, session frequency, and session duration) of exercise (Figure 2-3). Similarly, the ExTraMATCH group reported no difference in total mortality with CR comparing trials of less than 28 weeks exercise training to trials of 28 weeks or more (Figure 2-4).

Therefore it appears that there is little evidence that one form or method of CR intervention is better than another. Nevertheless, given the indirect nature of these comparisons there is a need for caution in this conclusion[12]

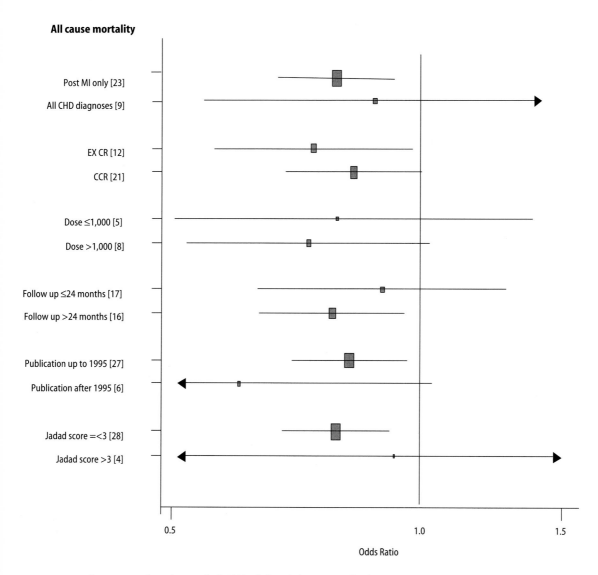

All cause mortality

Dose: amount of exercise prescribed: 1,000 units is equivalent to 3 months of 3 sessions/week for 30 mins/session

FIGURE 2-3. Exercise-based CR for CHD: subgroup analyses I.[7]

	Training		Control			Hazard ratio (95% CI)	χ^2	P value	
	No of events /	No at risk	No of events /	No at risk	Death			Effect	Interaction
Sex									
Male	79/349		95/354			0.60 (0.41 to 0.87)	7.30	0.01	
Female	9/46		10/52			1.17 (0.41 to 3.34)	0.09	0.77	0.27
Age									
>60 years	52/202		65/205			0.64 (0.41 to 0.99)	3.97	0.05	
<60 years	36/193		40/201			0.65 (0.36 to 1.18)	2.02	0.16	0.74
Functional class									
NYHA I–II	45/206		43/206			0.69 (0.40 to 1.20)	1.75	0.19	
NYHA III–IV	43/189		62/200			0.63 (0.40 to 0.99)	4.03	0.05	0.84
Cause									
Ischaemic	54/256		75/253			0.54 (0.35 to 0.83)	7.78	0.01	
Non-ischaemic	34/139		30/153			0.93 (0.52 to 1.68)	0.06	0.81	0.10
Left ventricular ejection traction									
>27%	38/193		36/187			0.83 (0.45 to 1.50)	0.40	0.53	
<27%	50/202		69/219			0.59 (0.38 to 0.92)	5.54	0.02	0.30
Peak oxygen consumption									
>15 ml/kg/min	36/177		32/173			0.74 (0.39 to 1.40)	0.86	0.35	
<15 ml/kg/min	52/218		73/233			0.63 (0.42 to 0.96)	4.59	0.03	0.43
Duration of training									
>28 weeks	41/216		60/219			0.64 (0.41 to 0.99)	4.08	0.04	
<28 weeks	47/179		45/187			0.66 (0.37 to 1.19)	1.88	0.17	0.53
Total	**88/395**		**105/406**			**0.65 (0.46 to 0.92)**	**5.92**	**0.015**	

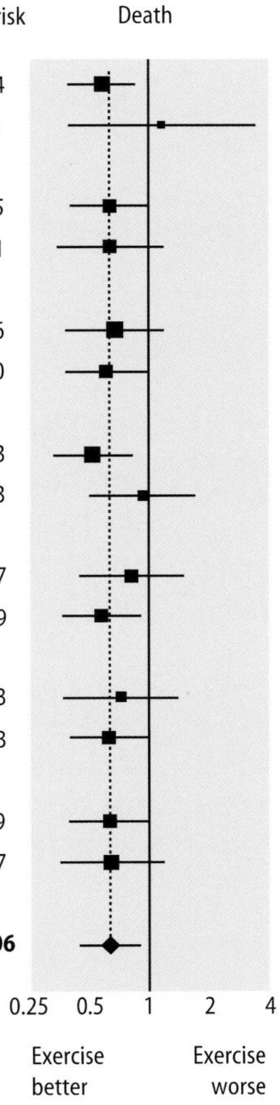

0.25 0.5 1 2 4

Exercise better — Exercise worse

FIGURE 2-4. Exercise-based CR for HF – subgroup analyses.[10] (Reproduced with permission of the *BMJ*.)

and further direct evidence on this issue is needed.

Does Cardiac Rehabilitation Offer Benefits over and above Other Secondary Prevention Measures, Such as Drug Therapy?

In the last 10 to 15 years, there has been a large increase in the use of drug therapies in secondary preventive management in patients with CHD, notably lipid-lowering agents, such as statins, and beta-blockers. Meta-analyses show that the im-provement in survival with exercise-based CR appears to be similar to that of many accepted cardiac drug therapies (Table 2-3). However, the early systematic reviews of CR have been criticized because the usual care arm included RCTs that are not reflective of current practice. Indeed, it has been argued that the benefits of exercise and psychology-based interventions used in CR would be substantially reduced in the context of current therapy. In response, many rehabilitation specialists argue it is artificial to attempt to partition secondary prevention (including drug therapy) and CR. Nevertheless, what evidence do we have to support the benefits of CR over and above current cardiac drug therapy? To answer this question,

TABLE 2-3. Comparison of the mortality benefits of CR* versus cardiac therapies

	No. of trials (no. of patients)	Relative reduction in all cause mortality	Reduction in all cause mortality per 1000 per year
Beta-blockers[17]	31 trials (24,974)	23% (15–31%)	12 (6–17)
ACE inhibitors[18]	22 trials (102,476)	17% (2–11%)	4 (1–6)
Statins[19]	3 trials (17,617)	23% (15–30%)	4 (2–6)
Antiplatelets[20]	11 trials (18,773)	24% (16–32%)	7 (1–3)
Cardiac rehabilitation*	44 trials (8700)	16% (4–27%)	9 (15 to 116)

*Exercise-based CR.
Source: From Taylor et al.[6]

Taylor et al. (2004) compared the magnitude of all cause mortality reduction with exercise-based CR in more recent trials (1995 and later) to that found in older trials (before 1995) (Figure 2-3). It was assumed that the more recent trials would include standard care and current secondary preventative drugs. As Taylor et al. found no significant difference between the two time periods (Figure 2-4), they concluded that the benefits of exercise-based CR "are not limited to particular CHD patient subgroups or particular models of exercise intervention."[6]

Are There Groups of Patients in Which Cardiac Rehabilitation Is More (or Less) Effective?

CR is increasingly being extended beyond the traditional patient groups of CHD and post PTCA and CABG and, more recently, heart failure. Patients with valvular disease, with an implanted intracardiac defibrillator or biventricular pacemaker, and unstable angina, including acute coronary syndrome, can now receive CR in some

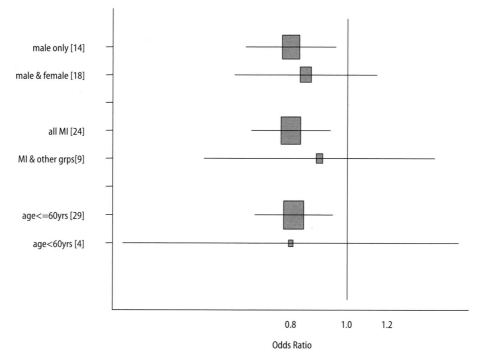

FIGURE 2-5. Exercise-based CR for CHD – subgroup analyses II.[7]

centers. It is beyond the scope of this section to discuss the evidence for the role of CR in these later patient groups. However, there remains the question of whether there are patients within the more traditional groups of CHD, post PCI and HF, in which CR is more (or less effective). Targeting of therapies to particular patient subgroups is often used to optimize the cost-effectiveness of a therapeutic regime.

The meta-analyses by Taylor et al. and ExTra-MATCH used meta-regression to examine the effect of a number of patient characteristics (e.g. age, sex, diagnoses, NYHA classification) on the impact of exercise-based CR for CHD and HF, respectively. Both groups reported no significant difference in the benefit of CR across these patient subgroups (Figures 2-4 and 2-5). Thus there appears to be little evidence, at this time, to limit the use of CR in any particular CHD or HF subgroups.

Is Home-Based Cardiac Rehabilitation as Effective a Method of Delivering Cardiac Rehabilitation as Supervised Center- or Hospital-Based Programs?

Home-based CR provision has become more commonplace in number of countries. For example, a number of healthcare providers in the UK have purchased the *Heart Manual*, a self-help resource designed for the home-based CR of CHD patients following a myocardial infarction. There are a number of reasons for the development of home-based programs: increasing pressure on hospital-based services; the difficulty in patient transportation; patients' dislike of group-based CR sessions, and the belief that home-based rehabilitation may facilitate a faster return to normal life and may better sustain an increase in activity.[13]

The question therefore arises as to whether home-based and hospital- (or center-) based programs are equally effective.

This question was not addressed by the three Cochrane reviews. Indeed, most, if not all, of the RCT evidence in these reviews came from the traditional hospital setting. However, Jolly and colleagues in 2005 have undertaken a systematic review of home-based CR.

In this review, they identified 18 RCTs that compare home-based CR to usual care and 6 RCTs that compare home-based to center-based CR. The authors reported significant improvements in systolic blood pressure (4 mmHg, 95% CI: 6.5, 1.5) and a reduced relative risk (RR) of being a smoker at follow-up (RR: 0.71, 95% CI: 0.51, 1.00) in home program participants. Nonsignificant improvements in exercise capacity, total cholesterol, and psychological well-being were all in favor of the home-based CR compared to usual care. There was insufficient evidence to comment on the impact on clinical events. When directly compared to center-based CR, the effects of home-based CR on exercise tolerance and risk factors appeared to be similar. However, only 750 patients have been included in these later trials to date. Recent RCTs of home-versus-hospital-based cardiac rehabilitation confirm that outcomes and overall costs of the two approaches are similar.[14,15]

Conclusions

1. Three Cochrane systematic reviews/meta-analyses have assessed the effectiveness of cardiac rehabilitation.[5-8]

2. These reviews provide level I evidence[16] that, when compared to usual care alone: (a) exercise-based cardiac rehabilitation reduces mortality and improves the risk factor profile of CHD patients; (b) psychology-based cardiac rehabilitation improves psychological well-being and risk factor profile of CHD patients; and (c) exercise-based cardiac rehabilitation improves exercise tolerance and HRQoL of heart failure patients. The impact of CR on total mortality at the time of writing remains uncertain. Further evidence is needed on the effects of cardiac rehabilitation on health-related quality of life in CHD patients and total mortality of heart failure patients.

3. There is currently little evidence to support the belief that particular cardiac rehabilitation interventions are more effective than others or that cardiac rehabilitation should be limited to any particular CHD or HF patient subgroups. However, given the increasing resource and financial limitations of providing cardiac rehabil-

itation to all patients, there is a need for additional effectiveness and cost-effectiveness evidence on this issue.

4. Cardiac rehabilitation appears to have similar effects whether provided in a hospital- (or center-) based facility or at home. Therefore, where possible, patients should be offered hospital- or home-based CR. However, more evidence is needed, particularly as to the cost-effectiveness of CR provision in different settings.

References

1. Sackett DR, Haynes B, Tugwell P, Guyatt GH. Clinical Epidemiology: A Basic Science for Clinical Medicine, 2nd edn. London: Lippincott Williams & Wilkins; 1991.
2. MacLehose RR, Reeves BC, Harvey IM, Sheldon TA, Russell IT, Black AM. A systematic review of comparisons of effect sizes derived from randomised and non-randomised studies. Health Technol Assess 2000;4(34):1–154.
3. Oxman AD, Cook DJ, Guyatt GH. Users' guides to the medical literature. VI. How to use an overview. Evidence-Based Medicine Working Group. JAMA. 1994;272:1367–1371.
4. The Cochrane Library 2005, Issue 2 http://www3. interscience.wiley.com/cgi-bin/mrwhome/ 106568753/HOME [last accessed 1 May 2005].
5. Jolliffe JA, Rees K, Taylor RS, Thompson D, Oldridge N, Ebrahim S. Exercise-based rehabilitation for coronary heart disease. The Cochrane Database of Systematic Reviews 2001, Issue 1. Art. No.: CD001800. DOI: 10.1002/14651858.CD001800.
6. Taylor RS, Brown A, Ebrahim S, et al. Exercise based rehabilitation for patients with coronary heart disease: Systematic review and meta-analysis of randomized controlled trials. Am J Med 2004; 116:682–692.
7. Rees K, Bennett P, West R, Davey SG, Ebrahim S. Psychological interventions for coronary heart disease. Cochrane Database Syst Rev 2004;(2): CD002902. Review.
8. Rees K, Taylor RS, Singh S, Coats AJS, Ebrahim S. Exercise based rehabilitation for heart failure. (Cochrane Review). In: The Cochrane Library, Issue 3. Chichester, UK: John Wiley; 2004.
9. Smart N, Marwick TH. Exercise training for patients with heart failure: a systematic review of factors that improve mortality and morbidity. Am J Med 2004 15;116:693–706.
10. Piepoli MF, Davos C, Francis DP, Coats AJ. ExTraMATCH Collaborative. Exercise training meta-analysis of trials in patients with chronic heart failure (ExTraMATCH). BMJ 2004;328:189.
11. Campbell M, fitzpatrick R, Haines A, et al. Framework for design and evaluation of complex interventions to improve health. BMJ 2000;321: 694–696.
12. Song F, Altman DG, Glenny A-M, Deeks JJ. Validity of indirect comparison of competing interventions: Empirical evidence from published meta-analysis. BMJ 2003;326:472.
13. King AC, Haskell WL, Young DR, Oka RK, Stefanick ML. Lipids/glucose intolerance/sudden death: long-term effects of varying intensities and formats of physical activity on participation rates, fitness, and lipoproteins in men and women aged 50 to 65 years. Circulation 1995;91:2596–2604.
14. Jolly K, Taylor RS, Lip GY, Stevens A. Home-based cardiac rehabilitation compared with centre-based rehabilitation and usual care: A systematic review and meta-analysis. Int J Cardiol. 2005 Nov 26 (e-publication).
15. Jolly K, Lip GY, Taylor RS, et al. Recruitment of ethnic minority patients to a cardiac rehabilitation trial: The Birmingham Rehabilitation Uptake Maximisation (BRUM) study [ISRCTN72884263]. BMC Medical Research Methodology 2005;5:18.
16. Harbour R, Miller J. A new system for grading recommendations in evidence based guidelines. BMJ 2001;323:334–336.
17. Freemantle N, Cleland J, Young P, Mason J, Harrison J. Beta blockade after myocardial infarction: systematic review and meta regression analysis. BMJ 1999;318:1730–1737.
18. Domanski MJ, Exner DV, Borkowf CB, Geller NL, Rosenberg Y, Pfeffer MA. Effect of angiotensin converting enzyme inhibition on sudden cardiac death in patients following acute myocardial infarction. A meta-analysis of randomized clinical trials. J Am Coll Cardiol. 1999;33:598–604.
19. LaRosa JC, He J, Vupputuri S. Effect of statins on risk of coronary disease: a meta-analysis of randomized controlled trials. JAMA 1999;282:2340–2346.
20. Collins R, Baigent C, Sandercock P, Peto R. Antiplatelet therapy for thromboprophylaxis: the need for careful consideration of the evidence from randomised trials. Antiplatelet Trialists' Collaboration. BMJ;309(6963):1215–1217.

3
Indications for Cardiac Rehabilitation

Peter Mathes

Cardiovascular diseases constitute the leading cause of morbidity and premature mortality in industrialized parts of the world, and now pose a growing public health problem in developing countries. Where rehabilitation and secondary prevention were once seen as valuable only to patients recovering from uncomplicated acute myocardial infarction, they are now regarded as essential to all cardiac patients. Rehabilitation in appropriate exercise programs, education, and counseling are emerging as the most effective means of restoring patients' quality of life and independence and promoting their social integration.[1,2]

Entry Assessment for Rehabilitation

Assessment of a patient for entry into a cardiac rehabilitation program requires:

- a diagnosis of the cardiac condition, prescription of appropriate medical or surgical treatment, and an opinion on further prognosis and risks
- identification of the appropriate type of cardiac rehabilitation
- evaluation of the patient's condition as a basis for future surveillance and further evaluation.[3–5]

Diagnostic Groups Suitable for Rehabilitation

The categories of patients with coronary heart disease and its complications who may need rehabilitation services include the following:

- those who have been admitted to a hospital for unstable angina
- those with chronic ischemic heart disease who are starting an exercise program
- those who have undergone coronary bypass surgery and percutaneous transluminal coronary angioplasty.

The largest group will be patients who have sustained acute myocardial infarction, and this should be taken into consideration in planning personnel training and facilities for exercise programs.[6–8]

Risk assessment of patients entering exercise programs is essential, as is the identification of any factors that would contraindicate exercise. Individually prescribed exercises should take account of the degree and type of surveillance necessary for safety and for assessment of results. It is also important to assess patients' educational needs and to develop plans for secondary prevention. Any special needs (e.g. psychological or vocational) must also be considered.[9–10]

In many countries, rheumatic heart disease is a problem of childhood, adolescence, and young adulthood. The disease progresses rapidly and few of those affected survive into middle age without proper medical and surgical treatment. In both rheumatic heart disease and coronary heart disease, many of the common residual defects and hemodynamic derangements leave post-surgical patients with varying degrees of disability. This is further confounded by problems of chronic anticoagulation in patients with mechanical prosthetic valves.[11–14]

Patients who need rehabilitation generally belong to one of the following categories:

- those who have become inoperable or whose lesions are too complex for the available surgery
- postoperative patients in whom results and prognosis are good
- postoperative patients with significant residual defects
- those who need chronic anticoagulation and prophylaxis for rheumatic fever.

While patients with rheumatic heart disease and congenital heart disease may have to be cared for in the same rehabilitation facility as those with other cardiac problems, they may be very different in age from other cardiac patients and will need special care and assessment.[15,16]

Valvular Heart Disease

Mitral Valve Disease

Mitral valve disease is the most common problem among patients with rheumatic heart disease. In dominant mitral stenosis, closed valvular mitral commissurotomy reduces the symptoms, improves function, and provides cost-effective rehabilitation.

Patients in classes III and IV with mitral valve disease are candidates for surgery and subsequent exercise training programs. Such patients usually have a long history of disability and severely limited activity.

Exercise after Heart Valve Replacement

When exercise is prescribed after heart valve replacements, four major factors must be considered:

- the type of valve prosthesis used or reconstructive procedure undertaken, as it affects valve gradient
- the anticoagulant treatment
- the extent of myocardial dysfunction
- prior physical deconditioning.

Aortic Valve Replacement

After aortic valve replacement for aortic stenosis, exercise testing is a useful guide to prescribing appropriate exercise. Long-term prognosis for valve replacement for aortic stenosis differs from that for aortic regurgitation: the more favorable prognosis in aortic stenosis relates to preserved ventricular function. The recommendation for exercise after aortic valve replacement for aortic regurgitation depends on residual left ventricular dysfunction and on residual aortic regurgitation. In all patients with a valve prosthesis, anticoagulation will substantially increase the risk of complications from exercise- or activity-related trauma.[2,17,18]

Mitral Valve Replacement or Repair

After surgery for the repair or replacement of the mitral valve, the following hemodynamic abnormalities remain:

- An average gradient of 6–10 mmHg (0.833–1.33 kPa) persists across the valve at rest. This gradient is substantially increased by exercise-induced tachycardia.
- Atrial fibrillation is frequently present and superimposes its adverse effects on cardiac output, giving rise to rapid heart rate and loss of atrial contribution to ventricular filling.

The extent of postoperative ventricular dysfunction determines whether or not exercise recommendations should be as for left ventricular dysfunction (see Section III). Early mobilization and progressive ambulation reduce the likelihood of postoperative venous thromboembolism.

There are few systematic studies dealing with physical rehabilitation of patients who have had valvular surgery. Postoperative physical activity involves low-intensity muscular conditioning that does not impose an undue load on the heart. This includes walking, calisthenics (with due care taken of the sternal incision), and supervised treadmill or bicycle exercise. A symptom-limited exercise test is useful in assessing ability to return to work and for recommending levels of occupational and recreational activities.

Soon after surgery patients should receive advice and counseling about anticoagulation treatment (and keeping records of this), other medical therapy, the type of valve prosthesis, prophylaxis against infectious endocarditis, and response to recurrence of symptoms.[2,5,17,18]

Return to work and appropriate social reintegration depend on many variables, including the patient's motivation, cardiac status, prognosis and risk, competent vocational counseling, and – very importantly – the opinion and influence of the training physician. The longer a patient has been out of work, the less likely it is that he or she will resume a remunerative occupation.[5]

Septal Defects

Atrial Septal Defect

Atrial arrhythmias and, rarely, sick sinus syndrome may occur in patients with atrial septal defect. Evaluation before sports activities should therefore include an ambulatory ECG recording and an exercise test in an attempt to elicit dysrhythmias and to document a normal heart rate response to exercise.

Ventricular Septal Defect

A small residual ventricular septal defect without hemodynamic consequences is not a reason to limit activity. Since ventricular dysrhythmias can occur, especially after operative ventriculotomy to close the defect, patients should be evaluated in the same way as those with atrial septal defect before being allowed to take part in sports.[16,19,20]

Cardiomyopathy

The most common cardiomyopathies are the dilated and hypertrophic varieties, while the restrictive variety, though rarer in many countries, is common in Africa and South America. All ages and both sexes are affected. The disease may be very mild and chronic, or severe enough to result in death in a short period of time. There is increasing evidence that some form of exercise is of benefit to patients with dilated cardiomyopathy. Careful exercise training may result in sufficient peripheral cardiovascular and musculoskeletal adaptation for there to be significant improvement in effort tolerance; it can thus transform a totally dependent person into one capable of independent self-care and even of training for a sedentary job.[21-25]

It has become apparent that exercise capacity may not correlate with left ventricular function in the individual patient. The special needs of patients with cardiomyopathies include strict medical management of congestive failure and arrhythmias. Some patients with dilated cardiomyopathy will need long-term anticoagulation.

Requirements for trained personnel, facilities and equipment, patient evaluation, exercise programs, and surveillance are no different from those discussed previously for medically complex cardiac patients.[26-29]

Hypertrophic Cardiomyopathy

Only low-intensity exercise should be undertaken by patients with hypertrophic cardiomyopathy because of the increased risk of sudden death if they have:

- significant outflow gradient (identified by echocardiography or catheterization)
- severe left ventricular hypertrophy
- history of syncope
- history of sudden death in relatives
- exercise-induced complex ventricular arrhythmias.[9]

Exercise Training in Patients with Implanted Pacemakers

Many patients who are pacemaker-dependent at rest show a reappearance of atrioventricular conduction when they exercise, although many others remain pacemaker-dependent. In patients with pacemakers that are atrioventricular-synchronized and/or rate-responsive, exercise testing can be used both to set the pacing rate of the pacemakers and to prescribe exercise training based on heart rate.[30,31]

Rehabilitation of Patients with Serious Arrhythmias

Rehabilitation of patients with serious arrhythmias poses complex problems. Beta-blocking agents seem to reduce the incidence of sudden death after myocardial infarction among patients for whom their use is suitable; in many patients, the negative inotropic effect of these drugs reduces exercise capacity. An evaluation of the effect of anti-arrhythmic drugs by an exercise test and/or ambulatory ECG monitoring should be conducted before the patient enters a rehabilitation program.[30]

Atrial fibrillation is the most common supraventricular arrhythmia, and makes a heart rate parameter during exercise unreliable. In patients with atrial fibrillation, the Borg scale of rate of perceived exertion (see Section III) may be a valuable guide to exercise training.[32]

Implanted cardioverter defibrillators are increasingly used for management of life-threatening arrhythmias. Although the number of patients with these devices who will undergo exercise training is limited, the following points should be emphasized:

– Exercise testing can identify the patients with exercise-induced arrhythmias who should not undergo exercise training.
– Exercise testing can be a guide to heart rate settings, ensuring that a device responds to life-threatening arrhythmias but is not triggered by heart rates achieved during exercise.
– Other patients who share the same exercise sessions should be reassured that no harm will result from touching patients with cardioverter defibrillators during discharge of the devices.

Rehabilitation of Elderly Patients

As populations age in both developed and developing countries, more elderly patients with cardiac disease will be enrolled in rehabilitation programs. Coronary heart disease is the most common problem. Elderly coronary patients are medically complex because of the frequent complications of coronary disease and concomitant problems of diabetes, cerebral and peripheral vascular disease, hypertension, and chronic obstructive pulmonary disease.

The exercise capacity of elderly cardiac patients reflects the nature of their disease, other concomitant diseases, and, frequently, the deconditioning resulting from a sedentary lifestyle, all superimposed on the physiological effects of aging. Exercise training may help reduce the consequent limitations of activity and provide the sense of well-being and self-esteem necessary to prolong active and independent life.

Important considerations for exercise training in elderly cardiac patients include the following:

– High impact activities should be avoided.
– Prolonged warm-up and cool-down periods are necessary.
– Training should begin at low intensity and progress gradually.
– Repeated short periods of activity may be as beneficial as a single, more prolonged session.
– Exercise intensity should be reduced in hot and humid environments because of patients' impaired thermoregulation.
– Exercise-related orthostatic hypotension resulting from delayed baroreceptor responsiveness should be assessed.
– Specific muscle-strengthening activities can aid in self-care.[33–35]

Patients with Severe Cardiac Failure

Heart failure is not a disease entity but a manifestation of many causes of heart disease, including dilated cardiomyopathy, hypertensive cardiac failure, valvular heart disease, endomyocardial fibrosis, and ischemic ventricular dysfunction.

Comprehensive Rehabilitation Programs for Patients with Compensated Heart Failure and Severely Impaired Left Ventricular Function

Patients with chronic stable heart failure are disabled by breathlessness and fatigue. There is no constant correlation between these symptoms, which limit exercise tolerance, and the degree of left ventricular dysfunction. The decreased muscular function may be due either to hypoperfusion during exercise or to prolonged deconditioning. Respiratory discomfort is caused both by hyperventilation, which provokes premature fatigue of the respiratory muscles, and to some extent by an increase in pulmonary vascular pressures, which gives rise to a feeling of suffocation.[11,24–27]

Thus, to improve exercise tolerance, maximal blood flow should be increased, muscle vasodilation improved, and deconditioning avoided. The drugs normally used to compensate heart failure result in improved exercise tolerance. Studies of the effects of exercise training in patients with heart failure are limited, but results have been encouraging. A training-induced decrease in lactate accumulation, a consequent delay in onset of anaerobic threshold, and an increase in exercise endurance favorably affect the submaximal exercise level involved in patients' day-to-day activities.

Rehabilitation after Large Myocardial Infarction

After large myocardial infarction, even patients in NYHA functional class III or IV may achieve some relative benefit from an exercise program. Clinical studies have shown that, although patients with left ventricular dysfunction, especially those with ischemic heart disease, are at potentially high risk of exercise-related arrhythmias, the actual risk is relatively small when compared with the high incidence of non-exercise-related sudden death. Patients with large infarction should be considered with caution for long-term exercise therapy. Serial clinical evaluation of heart size and left ventricular function should be carried out; in case of worsening, physical training should be reduced or stopped.[35-38]

Rehabilitation in Cardiac Transplantation

Pre-Transplantation Patients

Patients awaiting transplantation are often deconditioned and exhibit severe cardiac impairment, breathlessness on exertion, and cardiac cachexia; they are also at increased risk of sudden cardiac death. The goal of exercise is to prevent further deconditioning and, in some patients, to improve skeletal muscle status. Standard exercise testing or cardiopulmonary exercise testing is valuable in formulating recommendations for physical activity.[39]

Education and counseling can introduce the concept of reducing coronary risk factors after transplantation, improve patients' motivation and encourage family support.

Post-Transplantation Patients

After transplantation, patients receive immunosuppressive medication. They are at high risk of infection, and exhibit a predisposition to atherosclerosis, susceptibility to transplant rejection, diastolic dysfunction of the transplanted heart, chronic effects of medication-related hypertension on cardiac function and exercise, wasting of skeletal muscle, weakness resulting from corticosteroid therapy, and a blunted heart rate response and lower cardiac output with exercise because of cardiac denervation.

Once these patients are stabilized postoperatively, exercise training carries intermediate or low risk. They generally remain in a supervised rehabilitation program at the transplant center, as a component of intensive early postoperative treatment and rehabilitation.

Subsequent rehabilitation services will vary according to where the patient receives primary long-term care. Rehabilitative exercise training may take place in a community-based facility or be undertaken without supervision at home.[1,36,39,40]

References

1. Haskell WL. Populations with special needs for exercise rehabilitation. Cardiac transplantation patients. In: Wenger NK, Hellerstein HK, eds. Rehabilitation of the Coronary Patient, 3rd edn. New York: Churchill Livingstone; 1992.
2. Wenger NK, et al. Ad Hoc Task Force on Cardiac Rehabilitation. Cardiac rehabilitation services following PTCA and valvular surgery: guidelines for use. Cardiology 1990;19:4–5.
3. Goble AJ, et al. Effect of early programmes of high and low intensity exercise on physical performance after transmural infarction. Br Heart J 1991;65(3): 126–131.
4. Hämäläinen H, et al. Long-term reduction in sudden deaths after a multifactorial intervention programme in patients with myocardial infarction. 10-years results of a controlled investigation. Eur Heart J 1989;10(10):55–62.

5. Position Report on Cardiac Rehabilitation. Recommendations of the American College of Cardiology. J Am Coll Cardiol 1986;7:451–453.

6. Blumenthal JA, et al. Comparison of high- and low-intensity exercise training early after acute myocardial infarction. Am J Cardiol 1988:61(1):26–30.

7. O'Connor GT, et al. An overview of randomized trials of rehabilitation with exercise after myocardial infarction. Lancet 1979;ii(8152):1091–1094.

8. Hedback B, Perk J. five years' results of a comprehensive rehabilitation programme after myocardial infarction. Eur Heart J 1978;8:234–242.

9. American Association of Cardiovascular and Pulmonary Rehabilitation. Guidelines for Cardiac Rehabilitation. Champaign, IL: Human Kinetics Publishers; 1991.

10. Wasserman K. Measures of functional capacity in patients with heart failure. Circulation, 1990, 81(1, Suppl):II1–4.

11. Goldberg SJ, Weiss R, Adams FH. A comparison of the maximal endurance of normal children and patients with congenital disease. J Pediatr 1966; 69(19):46–55.

12. James FW, et al. Responses of normal children and young adults with cardiovascular disease. Circulation 1980;61(5):902–912.

13. Longmuir PE, et al. Postoperative exercise rehabilitation benefits children with congenital heart disease. Clin Invest Med 1985;8(3):232–238.

14. National Heart, Lung and Blood Institute. Report of the Task Force on Blood Pressure Control in Children. Pediatrics 1977;59(5, 2, Suppl):I–II, 797–820.

15. Kellermann JJ. Rehabilitation of coronary patients. Prog Cardiovasc Dis 1975;17(14):303–328.

16. Beekman RH. Exercise recommendations for adolescents after surgery for congenital heart disease. Pediatrician 1986;13(4):210–219.

17. Kellermann JJ, et al. Functional evaluation of cardiac work capacity by spiroergometry in patients with rheumatic heart disease. Arch Phys Med Rehabil 1969;50:189–193.

18. Newell J, et al. Physical training after heart valve replacement. Br Heart J 1980;44(6):638–649.

19. Goldberg B, et al. Effect of physical training on exercise performance of children following surgical repair of congenital heart disease. Pediatrics 1981; 68(5):691–699.

20. James FW, et al. Response to exercise in patients after total surgical corrections of tetralogy of Fallot. Circulation 1976;54(4):671–679.

21. Coats AJS, et al. Effects of physical training in chronic heart failure. Lancet 1990;81(1, Suppl II):115–113.

22. Franciosa JA, Park M, Levine TB. Lack of correlation between exercise capacity and indexes of resting left ventricular performance in heart failure. Am J Cardiol 1981;47(1):33–39.

23. Lichtfield RL, et al. Normal exercise capacity in patients with severe left ventricular dysfunction. Compensatory mechanisms. Circulation 1982; 66(1):129–134.

24. Wilson JR, et al. Exercise intolerance in patients with chronic heart failure: role of impaired nutritive flow to skeletal muscle. Circulation 1984;69(6):1079–1087.

25. Sullivan MJ, et al. Relation between central and peripheral hemodynamics during exercise in patients with chronic heart failure: muscle blood flow is reduced with maintenance of arterial perfusion pressure. Circulation 1989;80(4):769–781.

26. Conn EH, Williams RS, Wallace AG. Exercise responses before and after physical conditioning in patients with severely depressed left ventricular function. Am J Cardiol 1982;49(2):296–300.

27. Cody EV, et al. Early exercise testing, physical training and mortality in patients with severe left ventricular dysfunction. J Am Coll Cardiol 1983;1(2):718.

28. Ehsani AA. Adaptations to training in patients with exercise-induced left ventricular dysfunction. Adv Cardiol 1986;34:148–155.

29. Mathes P. Physical training in patients with left ventricular dysfunction: choice and dosage of physical exercise in patients with pump dysfunction. Eur Heart J 1988;9(Suppl F):67–69.

30. Pashkow FJ. Populations with special needs for exercise rehabilitation. Patients with implanted pacemakers or implanted cardioverter defibrillators. In: Wenger N, Hellerstein HK, eds. Rehabilitation of the Coronary Patient, 3rd edn. New York: Churchill Livingstone; 1992.

31. Superko HR. Effects of cardiac rehabilitation in permanently paced patients with third-degree heart block. J Card Rehabil 1983;3:561–568.

32. Borg G, Linderholm E. Exercise performance and perceived exertion in patients with coronary insufficiency, arterial hypertension and vasoregulatory asthenics. Acta Med Scand 1970;187(17):17–26.

33. Kellermann JJ, et al. Arm exercise training in the rehabilitation of patients with impaired ventricular function and heart failure. Cardiology 1990;77(2):130–138.

34. Oldridge NB, et al. Cardiac rehabilitation after myocardial infarction: combined experience and randomized clinical trials. JAMA 1988;260(7): 9445–9950.

35. Wenger NK. Rehabilitation of the coronary patient. Arch Intern Med 1989, 149(7):1504–1506.

36. Wenger NK, et al. Cardiac rehabilitation services after cardiac transplantation. In: Guidelines for Cardiac Rehabilitation. Champaign, IL: Human Kinetic Publishers; 1991.

37. Jugdutt BI, Michorowski BL, Kappagoda CT. Exercise training after anterior Q-wave myocardial infarction: importance of regional left ventricular function and topography. J Am Coll Cardiol 1988;12:362–372.

38. Sullivan MJ, Higginbotham MB, Cobb FR. Exercise training in patients with chronic heart failure delays ventilatory anaerobic threshold and improves submaximal exercise performance. Circulation 1989;79(2):324–329.

39. Kavanagh T, et al. Cardiorespiratory responses to exercise training after orthotopic cardiac transplantation. Circulation 1988;77(1):162–171.

40. Savin WM, et al. Cardiorespiratory responses of cardiac transplant patients to graded, symptom-limited exercise. Circulation 1980;62(1):55–60.

4
Prevention Guidelines: Management of the Coronary Patient

Guy de Backer

Guidelines on prevention of coronary heart disease (CHD) in clinical practice have been issued by Joint Task Forces of European and other Societies[1-3] and the latest update was released in 2003 by the Third Joint Task Force.[3]

The objectives of these guidelines are the prevention of disability and early death from cardiovascular disease (CVD) through lifestyle changes, management of risk factors and when needed the prophylactic use of certain drugs.

The guidelines represent a state of the art regarding what is known on effective and safe preventive strategies applicable in clinical practice.

Resources available for preventive cardiology are generally limited; therefore one should use them as efficiently as possible and this requires priority setting. Patients with established CVD are the top priority; they should receive all the attention one can give for the prevention of recurrent events.

Next in priority are asymptomatic subjects at high risk for developing CVD in the coming years. To identify them an estimate of total coronary or cardiovascular risk should be used. The first and Second Joint Task Forces in Europe have recommended the use of the risk estimation model based on results from the Framingham study[4]; in the guidelines from the Third Joint Task Force a new model based on the results from the SCORE project[5] is recommended.

One of the reasons why the risk estimation model was changed is that the SCORE model predicts cardiovascular events, not merely coronary events, and the latest update of the guidelines is now focused on CVD, and not just CHD.

The reason for moving from prevention of CHD to prevention of CVD is that the etiology of myocardial infarction, ischemic stroke, and peripheral arterial disease (PAD) is similar and, indeed, recent intervention trials have shown that several forms of therapy prevent not only coronary events and revascularizations but also ischemic stroke and PAD. Hence, decisions about whether to initiate specific preventive action should be guided by an estimation of the risk of suffering any such vascular event not just a coronary event.

However, in the management of coronary patients there is no need for total CV risk estimation. The fact that they have already suffered a CV event places them in the highest risk category and therefore secondary prevention should contain all aspects of effective and safe strategies.

The goals that one should try to achieve are summarized in Table 4-1: they relate to lifestyle, to risk factor management, and to the prophylactic use of certain drugs.

The greatest challenge and failure in rehabilitation and secondary prevention relate to lifestyle changes. Therefore the guidelines pay great attention to behavioral change models and to the consideration of psychosocial factors as possible barriers for lifestyle changes.

Strategies to make behavioral counseling more effective have been developed and tested and have been described in detail.[3] In Table 4-2 10

TABLE 4-1. Goals for CVD prevention in patients with established cardiovascular disease

Lifestyle:	No smoking
	Make healthy food choices
	Be physically active
Risk factors:	
Blood pressure	<140/90 mmHg in most
	<130/80 mmHg in some
Total cholesterol	<4.5 mmol/L (175 mg/dL)
LDL cholesterol	<2.5 mmol/L (100 mg/dL)

Good glycemic control in all persons with diabetes
Prophylactic drug therapy in particular groups

strategies identified in the Report of the US Preventive Services Task Force[6] are given. The physician/caregiver–patient interaction is a powerful tool to enhance patients' ability to cope with stress and illness and their adherence to recommended lifestyle change.

Multimodal behavioral interventions integrate educational efforts with practical training sessions, combining learning with practical implementation and skills training. All this fits very well within the framework of a comprehensive multidisciplinary rehabilitation program for patients with CHD.

Regarding smoking of tobacco, results from EUROASPIRE[7,8] have shown that 1 in 4 to 1 in 5 of our patients continue to smoke after an acute event. They should be encouraged by health professionals to permanently stop smoking all forms of tobacco. The momentum for smoking cessation is particularly strong at the time of an acute event, an invasive treatment, or vascular surgery. However, relapse occurs frequently. Therefore this problem should be identified at all possible occasions.

If necessary, the patient's capacity to change should be identified in order to adapt the necessary action accordingly. The value of the simple advice of a doctor or other health professional should not be underestimated. But, if needed, there are nowadays different techniques that can help in assisting patients during the difficult period of withdrawal. And there is a need for follow-up visits; relapses are frequent and should be dealt with as soon as possible.

On making healthy food choices the guidelines remain very general because it was realized that adaptations are necessary according to local culture. But obesity seems to have become a global problem and therefore energy balances through diet and physical activity strategies are needed everywhere.

Other general recommendations are not new but should be re-emphasized:

– Foods should be varied.
– The consumption of certain foods should be encouraged: fruits and vegetables, whole grain cereals and bread, low fat dairy products, fish and lean meat.
– Oily fish and omega-3 fatty acids have particular protective properties, especially in patients with established CHD.
– Total fat should account for no more than 30% of energy intake and the intake of saturated fats should not exceed a third of total fat intake; the intake of cholesterol should be less than 300 mg/day.
– In an isocaloric diet, saturated fat can be replaced partly by complex carbohydrates, and partly by monounsaturated and polyunsaturated fats from vegetables and marine animals.

Patients with arterial hypertension, with severe dyslipidemias, and/or with diabetes should receive specialist dietary advice.

All patients with CVD should be encouraged and supported to increase their physical activity safely to the level associated with the lowest risk of suffering new events. For patients with established disease advice must be based on a comprehensive clinical judgment including the results of an exercise test. Detailed recommendations for

TABLE 4-2. How to achieve intensive lifestyle change in patients with coronary heart disease?

Strategies to make behavioral counseling more effective include:
• Develop a therapeutic alliance with the patient
• Counsel all patients
• Gain commitments from the patient to achieve lifestyle change
• Ensure the patient understands the relationship between lifestyle and disease
• Help the patient overcome barriers to lifestyle change
• Involve the patient in identifying the risk factor(s) to change
• Design a lifestyle modification plan
• Use strategies to reinforce the patient's own capacity to change
• Monitor progress of lifestyle change through follow-up contacts
• Involve other healthcare staff wherever possible

CVD patients have been given by other expert committees[9,10] or are available elsewhere in this book.

Regarding the management of the classical risk factors, the guidelines for patients with established CVD can be summarized as follows: regarding blood pressure the goal is in general to maintain the blood pressure below 140/90 mmHg; however, in patients with type 2 diabetes, we should aim at lower levels below 130/80 mmHg. But patients with CVD and a systolic blood pressure of 130–140 mmHg and/or a diastolic pressure 85–89 mmHg may also qualify for further blood pressure reduction depending on the overall risk profile, the presence of target organ damage, and the effects of non-pharmacological interventions.

In terms of blood lipid levels, goals are set for total and low-density lipoprotein (LDL) cholesterol; for patients with CVD these goals are <175 mg/dL or <4.5 mmol/L for total cholesterol and <100 mg/dL or <2.5 mmol/L for LDL cholesterol. The first clinical trials which documented the clinical benefits of lipid-lowering therapy with statins were restricted to patients <70 years old and total cholesterol levels >5 mmol/L (190 mg%). Now published trials indicate that such treatment can also be effective in the elderly and in patients with lower cholesterol levels.

In patients with established CVD, polypharmacy can become a major problem and good clinical management is required to resolve it. In some patients goals cannot be reached even on maximal therapy but they will still benefit from treatment to the extent to which cholesterol has been lowered.

Recommended treatment targets for patients with type 1 diabetes and type 2 diabetes have been defined by the International Diabetes Federation Europe.[11,12] Treatment targets should, however, always be individualized particularly, in patients with other competing diseases such as CVD, with severe late diabetic complications, and in the elderly patients. As mentioned above, the treatment goals for blood pressure and for lipids are generally more ambitious in patients with diabetes.

Secondary prevention includes besides lifestyle changes, risk factor management also the use of prophylactic drugs other than those needed to control blood pressure, lipids, and diabetes.

In the guidelines four different categories are considered:

- Aspirin or other platelet-modifying drugs in virtually all patients with CVD. The most recent meta-analysis of antiplatelet trials provides convincing evidence of a significant reduction in all cause mortality, vascular mortality, nonfatal reinfarction and nonfatal stroke in patients with unstable angina, acute myocardial infarction, stroke, transient ischemic attacks, or other clinical evidence of vascular disease.[13] The available evidence supports daily doses of aspirin in the range of 75–150 mg for the long-term prevention of vascular events. Although there is no clinical trial evidence of treatment beyond a few years, it would be both prudent and safe to continue aspirin therapy for life.
- Beta-blockers in patients following a myocardial infarction or with left ventricular (LV) dysfunction due to CHD are associated with a reduction in total mortality and cardiovascular death as well as non fatal reinfarction. Beta-blockers should be considered in all patients with CHD, providing there are no contraindications, for the following reasons: to relieve symptoms of myocardial ischemia, to lower blood pressure to <140/90 mmHg, as prophylaxis following myocardial infarction, and in the treatment of heart failure;
- ACE inhibitors in patients with symptoms or signs of LV dysfunction due to CHD and/or arterial hypertension. More recently ACE inhibition has been shown to reduce the risk of cardiovascular morbidity and mortality in patients with stable CHD without apparent heart failure.[14]
- Anticoagulants in those patients with CVD who are at increased risk of thromboembolic events.

References

1. Pyörälä K, De Backer G, Graham I, Poole-Wilson P, Wood D. Prevention of coronary heart disease in clinical practice: recommendations of the Task Force of the European Society of Cardiology, European Atherosclerosis Society and European Society of Hypertension. Atherosclerosis 1994;110(2):121–161.

2. Wood D, De Backer G, Faergeman O, Graham I, Mancia G, Pyörälä K. Prevention of coronary heart disease in clinical practice. Recommendations of the Second Joint Task Force of European and other Societies on coronary prevention. Eur Heart J 1998;19(10):1434–1503.

3. Third Joint Task Force of European and other Societies. European guidelines on cardiovascular disease prevention in clinical practice. Eur J Cardiovasc Prev Rehabil 2003;10(Suppl 1):S1–S78.

4. Anderson KM, Wilson PW, Odell PM, Kannel WB. An updated coronary risk profile. A statement for health professionals. Circulation 1991;83(1):356–362.

5. Conroy R, Pyörälä K, fitzgerald A, et al. Prediction of ten-year risk of fatal cardiovascular disease in Europe: the SCORE project. Eur Heart J 2003;24: 987–1003.

6. US Preventive Services Task Force. Guide to clinical services. Baltimore: Williams & Wilkins; 1996.

7. EUROASPIRE. A European Society of Cardiology survey of secondary prevention of coronary heart disease: principal results. EUROASPIRE Study Group. European Action on Secondary Prevention through Intervention to Reduce Events. Eur Heart J 1997;18(10):1569–1582.

8. Lifestyle and risk factor management and use of drug therapies in coronary patients from 15 countries; principal results from EUROASPIRE II Euro Heart Survey Programme. Eur Heart J 2001;22(7): 554–572.

9. Long-term comprehensive care of cardiac patients. Recommendations by the Working Group on Rehabilitation of the European Society of Cardiology. Eur Heart J 1992;13(Suppl C):1–45.

10. American Association of Cardiovascular and Pulmonary Rehabilitation. Guidelines for cardiac rehabilitation and secondary prevention programs. Champaign, IL: Human Kinetics; 1995.

11. A desktop guide to Type 1 (insulin-dependent) diabetes mellitus. European Diabetes Policy Group 1998. Diabet Med 1999;16(3):253–266.

12. A desktop guide to Type 2 diabetes mellitus. European Diabetes Policy Group 1999. Diabet Med 1999;16(9):716–730.

13. Collaborative meta-analysis of randomised trials of antiplatelet therapy for prevention of death, myocardial infarction, and stroke in high risk patients. BMJ 2002;324(7329):71–86.

14. Smith P, Arnesen H, Holme I. The effect of warfarin on mortality and reinfarction after myocardial infarction. N Engl J Med 1990;323(3):147–152.

5
Cardiac Rehabilitation: Europe

L. Vanhees, M. Martens, S. Beloka, A. Stevens, A. Avram, and Dan Gaita

Introduction

Cardiac rehabilitation (CR) has been defined as the sum of interventions required to ensure the best possible physical, psychological, and social conditions so that patients with subacute or chronic disease may, by their own efforts, preserve or resume as normal a place as possible in the life of the community.[1–5]

This definition implies a clear need for a multidisciplinary approach over a long time period. Cardiac rehabilitation was therefore divided by the World Health Organization into three phases: (I) the acute phase, (II) the reconditioning phase, and (III) the maintenance phase.[4,6]

Nowadays, acute rehabilitation starts in the hospital from the first days after an acute heart attack. Phase II CR exists in a multidisciplinary program requiring a range of knowledge and skills to bring together medical treatment, education, exercise training, and counseling for all people with coronary heart disease (CHD).[7]

Comparison of phase II and III programs in Europe, more specifically in 15 member states of the European Union, was first performed in the Carinex Survey (1999).[6] Phase II is the reconditioning phase that starts after the acute coronary event and has a multidisciplinary base including exercise training, risk factor modification, educational programs, and psychosocial counseling. Phase III is the maintenance phase conducted in sports clubs and cardiac groups focused on adapting physical activity and the modification of risk factors, such as smoking, sedentary lifestyle, hypertension, and hyperlipidemia.

Following the enlargement of the European Union, new member states have given us a new motive for further European research on the occurrence of cardiac disease, the existing rehabilitative services, and the advancements that have been occurring in recent years. Central and eastern European countries are characterized by heterogeneity due to their national conditions, resources, priorities, economic level, and political trends. Since health follows a social gradient, many inequalities are also noticed in the medical system.[8]

At European level, there is the same problem as in the entire world – the increasing burden of cardiovascular disease. Recent studies show that central and eastern Europe has higher cardiovascular disease mortality compared with the rest of Europe. The cardiovascular mortality rate varies from 5 per 1000 inhabitants in Poland to 9 per 1000 inhabitants in Bulgaria and Ukraine; this is two to three times more than in the West, where the advanced treatments for coronary heart disease have increased the survival rates by 50%.[9]

Multidisciplinary Rehabilitation

Cardiac rehabilitation is an important aspect of cardiac care strategies. From the Carinex Survey it is obvious that cardiac rehabilitation programs vary between countries in western Europe, but most programs are well organized. In this survey,[6] information on staff involvement, duration and content of programming, costs and other organizational activities were reported. Wide variations between countries were reported, but variation within each country was as great as or even greater than that reported between countries. Most programs contain exercise testing and training, psychosocial interventions, diet and smoking counseling, family and spouse involvement, and some other components. All these programs have the same aims: functional adaptation, an increase in exercise capacity, and improvement of quality of life and psychosocial status. The most striking difference in the phase II programs studied in the Carinex Survey was probably the type of organization: institution-based versus outpatient versus home-based programs. The Carinex Survey demonstrated that there is a moderate range of duration for phase II from 4 weeks to 13 weeks (Table 5-1).[6] The duration of phase II in countries where an inpatient rehabilitation model was used was limited to 4 weeks. When outpatient rehabilitation was performed the duration of phase II programs ranged from 7 to 26 weeks.

A short duration of the reconditioning phase requires a well-organized follow-up in phase III. Most countries try to maintain phase III "as long as possible." The continuity of the program depends on individual motivation to continue the program and the social security system that reimburse patients. Physical training during phase III, so far, is limited but it leads to reinforcement of previous condition and lifestyle.[10]

Regarding cardiac rehabilitation programs in eastern Europe, few international data are recorded, although all these countries had more than 20 years' experience in this field and all recognized the crucial role of comprehensive management of cardiac patients. In eastern Europe most often an in-hospital rehabilitation program is used. It comprises cardiological management and psychosocial interventions during a residential stay in a specific rehabilitation clinic. It is based on the individual's requirements aiming at the improvement of exercise capacity and quality of life, and medical, educational, and psychological interventions. It may enhance compliance, resulting in a better long-term implementation of secondary prevention. Nevertheless, there are few specific clinics for phase II and III cardiac rehabilitation.[11,12]

Frequently, home-based programs follow on from hospital rehabilitation or are used in the period between hospital discharge and ambulatory cardiac rehabilitation, or sometimes even after an outpatient programme.[13,14] These home-based programs aim to maintain the patient's motivation for lifestyle change at a time when there is limited contact with healthcare professionals. Home-based rehabilitation programs usually include education, exercise schedules, written booklets, and psychosocial interventions. A disadvantage of home-based rehabilitation is that the main part of the program consists of exercise with taped counseling of education and psychosocial interventions and telephone contact or visits every 2 months.[15] Specialized sports clubs or specifically designed heart groups may be better at facilitating the long-term secondary preventive lifestyle.[10]

Special Groups

Participation in CR is less evident in women, the elderly, and socially deprived and ethnic minorities.[15] People who do not participate in a program often have greater degrees of functional impairment and are the ones most in need of and most likely to benefit from rehabilitation. The problem of low patient adherence in these groups includes lack of information from professionals, reduced motivation, and increased anxiety feelings. Further socio-demographic reasons such as education level, deprivation,

TABLE 5-1. Duration of phase II cardiac rehabilitation across Europe (weeks)

Ireland	8.8 ± 2.17
United Kingdom	9.15 ± 3.32
The Netherlands	7.0 ± 2.07
Belgium	12.71 ± 7.50
Germany	3.87 ± 0.30
Italy	6.97 ± 5.51
France	3.00 ± 0.0
Spain	10.33 ± 3.20
Portugal	13.0 ± 6.86
Greece	8.00 ± 0.00
Austria	3.70 ± 0.67
Finland	7.51 ± 11.85
Sweden	10.0 ± 0.0
Total	8.44 ± 5.31

and the family environment should be considered.[16]

The cardio-rehabilitation service should be available for all CHD patients according to their needs and the level of impairment. A cardiac rehabilitation system should be available on a common European cross-border basis for every country instead of by selection procedures such as medical needs, rehabilitation center, and the duration and implementation of the rehabilitation program.[17]

In some European countries, CR is still in the early stages of development with low rates of patient participation, limited encouragement and introductions from medical doctors, and social health systems that do not support such innovations. It is clear that a lot of changes must be undertaken to advance the socio-political base so that all cardiac patients receive the appropriate information and rehabilitation treatment.[18]

Organization

In 1964, cardiac rehabilitation was for the first time described and discussed in a WHO report.[4] In October 1967, the first meeting of the WHO Regional Office for Europe on Cardiac Rehabilitation was held at Noordwyk aan Zee in the Netherlands. The leading organization in Europe concerning cardiology, the European Society of Cardiology, started to restructure itself into working groups. The Working Group on Epidemiology and Prevention was founded in 1976 and their first scientific meeting was held in Dublin in 1977. In 1980, the Working Group on Exercise Physiology was founded by Jean Marie Detry from Belgium and Bruno Caru from Italy, followed by the Working Group on Cardiac Rehabilitation in 1984, founded by Peter Mathes from Germany and Risteard Mulcahy from Ireland. In 1994, the latter two working groups amalgamated into the Working Group on Cardiac Rehabilitation and Exercise Physiology.

In the meantime, in the period 1987–1992, experts with different professional backgrounds in cardiac rehabilitation from various European countries discussed in several meetings the long-term approach and the multidisciplinary aspects of cardiac rehabilitation. These meetings have revealed great variation in the development and structure of cardiac rehabilitation activities within the member states of the European Union (EU). In 1992, the European Association of Cardiovascular Rehabilitation (EACVR) was established, with the aims to represent and to promote the multidisciplinary organization and the long-term approach in CR throughout Europe. In 1999, the EACVR joined the Working Group on Cardiac Rehabilitation and Exercise Physiology.

The European Association for Cardiovascular Prevention and Rehabilitation was launched in 2004 and was formed through the merger of the ESC Working Groups no. 1 (cardiac rehabilitation and exercise physiology) and no. 13 (epidemiology and prevention). Its mission statement is "to promote excellence in research, practice, education and policy in cardiovascular prevention and rehabilitation in Europe."

Conclusion

After the end of the acute phase, all patients should be able to follow a multidisciplinary CR program. Thereafter, everyone should be advised to maintain an active lifestyle and adherence to secondary preventive measures. This lifelong secondary preventive lifestyle must be promoted by all healthcare providers and can be facilitated by specialized sports clubs or by specifically designed heart groups.

Professionals who are responsible for rehabilitation programs need to develop a European action plan for the inclusion of all cardiac patients who are eligible to participate and benefit. Future challenges to cardiac rehabilitation include developing patient-focused services across the boundaries of primary, secondary and social care, and increasing patient and public involvement in services.[19] The application of socio-political interventions concerning all parts of society – global, European, national, regional, local, familial, and individual – will amplify the benefit of modern medical interventions.[20]

References

1. Wenger NK, Gilbert CA. Rehabilitation of the Myocardial Infarction Patient. In: Hurst JW, ed. The Heart. New York: McGraw Hill; 1978: 1303–1310.

2. Morris JN, Kagan A, Pattison DC, Gardner MJ. Incidence and prediction of ischaemic heart-disease in London busmen. Lancet 1966;2:553–559.

3. Berlin JA, Colditz GA. A meta-analysis of physical activity in the prevention of coronary heart disease. Am J Epidemiol 1990;132(4):612–628.

4. Rehabilitation of patients with cardiovascular disease: Report of a WHO expert committee. WHO Technical Report Series 1964:240.

5. Task force of the working group on cardiac rehabilitation of the European Society of Cardiology. Long-term comprehensive care of cardiac patients. Eur Heart J 1991;13:1–45.

6. Vanhees L, McGee H, Dugmore D, Vuori I, Pentilla UR, on behalf of the Carinex group. The Carinex Survey: Current Guidelines and Practices in Cardiac Rehabilitation within Europe. Leuven: Acco; 1999.

7. Giannuzzi P, Saner H, Björnstad H, et al. Secondary prevention through cardiac rehabilitation: position paper of the Working Group on Cardiac Rehabilitation and Exercise Physiology of the European Society of Cardiology. Eur Heart J 2003;24(13):1273–1278.

8. Marmot M, Bobak M. International comparators and poverty and health in Europe. BMJ 2000;321:1124–1128.

9. Quittan M, Resch KL, Lukacs P, et al. The concept of myocardial infarct rehabilitation in phase III. Wien Med Wochenschr 1994;144(4):74–77.

10. Vanhees L, McGee H, Dugmore D, Schepers D, Van Daele P. A representative study of cardiac rehabilitation activities in European Union member states. The Carinex Survey. J Cardiopulm Rehabil 2002;22(4):264–272.

11. Gaita D, Branea I, Dragulescu S, et al. Benefit of exercise training in patients with valve protheses and chronic heart failure. XXI Congress of The European Society of Cardiology. Monduzzi Editore 1999:665–669.

12. Baessler A, Hengstenberg C, Holmer S, et al. Long-term effects of in-hospital cardiac rehabilitation on the cardiac risk profile. A case-control study in pairs of siblings with myocardial infarction. Eur Heart J 2001;22:1111–1118.

13. Arthur H, Smith K, Kodis J, McKelvie R. A controlled trial of hospital versus home-based exercise in cardiac patients. Med Sci Sports Exerc 2002; 34(10):1544–1550.

14. Beswick AD, Rees K, West RR, et al. Improving uptake and adherence in cardiac rehabilitation: literature review. J Adv Nurs 2005;49(5):538–555.

15. Jolly K, Lip G, Sandercock J, et al. Home-based versus hospital-based cardiac rehabilitation after myocardial infarction or revascularisation: design and rationale of the Birmingham Rehabilitation Uptake Maximisation Study (BRUM): a randomised controlled trial. BMC Cardiovasc Disord 2003;3:10.

16. Rees K, Victory J, Beswick A, et al. Cardiac rehabilitation in the UK: Uptake among under-represented groups. Heart 2005;91:375–376.

17. Farin E, Follert P, Gerdes N, Jackel W, Thalaus J. Quality assessment in rehabilitation centres: the indicator system 'Quality Profile'. Disabil Rehabil 2004;26(18):1096–1104.

18. Block P, Weber P, Kearny P. On behalf of the Cardiology Section of the UEMS. Manpower in cardiology II in western and central Europe (1999–2000). Eur Heart J 2003;24:299–310.

19. Child A. Cardiac rehabilitation: goals, interventions and action plans. Br J Nurs 2004;13(12):734–738.

20. Shelley E. Promoting heart health – a European consensus. Eur J Cardiovasc Prev Rehabil 2004; 11(2):85–86.

6
Cardiac Rehabilitation: United States

Nanette K. Wenger

The Clinical Practice Guideline *Cardiac Rehabilitation*, prepared for and promulgated by the US Department of Health and Human Services,[1] characterizes cardiac rehabilitation as the provision of comprehensive long-term services involving medical evaluation; prescribed exercise; cardiac risk factor modification; and education, counseling, and behavioral interventions. The goal of this multifactorial process is to limit the adverse physiologic and psychologic effects of cardiac illness, to reduce the risk of sudden death or reinfarction, to control cardiac symptoms, to stabilize or reverse progression of the atherosclerotic process, and to enhance the patient's psychosocial and vocational status. The guideline defines that provision of cardiac rehabilitation services is directed by a physician, but can be implemented by a variety of healthcare professionals.

Although many patients with coronary heart disease are appropriate candidates for cardiac rehabilitation services, only 11–20% of eligible patients in the US currently participate in supervised, structured cardiac rehabilitation programs. Major barriers to cardiac rehabilitation include the low patient referral rate; poor patient motivation; inadequate insurance reimbursement; and geographic limitations as to the accessibility of structured program sites. Typical insurance reimbursement covers 36 exercise sessions (three times weekly for 12 weeks) and the associated education and counseling.

Although traditionally most candidates for cardiac rehabilitation were patients following myocardial infarction or coronary artery bypass graft surgery, contemporary use also includes patients after percutaneous coronary interventions; heart transplantation recipients; patients with stable angina or stable chronic heart failure; those with peripheral arterial disease with claudication; and patients following other cardiac surgical procedures such as those for valvular heart disease.

Components of Cardiac Rehabilitation

The components of cardiac rehabilitation analyzed in the guideline include exercise training; education, counseling, and behavioral interventions; and organizational issues, including consideration of alternative approaches to the delivery of cardiac rehabilitative care (to be discussed subsequently). Highlighted by the guideline is the effectiveness of multifactorial cardiac rehabilitation services, integrated in a comprehensive approach.

The physiologic parameters targeted by cardiac rehabilitation interventions include an improvement in exercise tolerance and in exercise habits; optimization of coronary risk factors, including improvement in lipid and lipoprotein profiles, body weight, blood glucose levels and blood pressure levels, and cessation of smoking. There should be attention to the emotional responses to living with heart disease, specifically reduction of stress and anxiety and lessening of depression. An essential goal, particularly for elderly patients, is functional independence. Return to appropriate and satisfactory occupation is thought to benefit both patients and society.

Benefits of Cardiac Rehabilitation

The most substantial evidence-based benefits of cardiac rehabilitation include an improvement in exercise tolerance, improvement in symptoms, improvement in blood lipid levels, reduction in cigarette smoking, improvement in psychosocial well-being and reduction of stress, and reduction in mortality. These are addressed in turn.

Appropriately prescribed and conducted exercise training is an integral component of cardiac rehabilitation, particularly for patients with decreased exercise tolerance. Specific activity recommendations are available for women, for older adults, for patients with chronic heart failure and after cardiac transplantation, for stroke survivors, and for patients with claudication as a reflection of peripheral arterial disease. Strength training can improve skeletal muscle strength and endurance. Smoking cessation can be achieved by specific strategies. Lipid management requires intensive nutrition education, counseling, and behavioral interventions to improve dietary fat and cholesterol intake. Optimal lipid control typically entails pharmacologic management, in addition to diet and exercise training. Diet and exercise are recommended for weight management. A multifactorial education, counseling, behavioral, and pharmacologic approach is the recommended strategy for the management of hypertension. Increased attention is currently directed to management of diabetes and the precise control of other coronary risk factors in diabetic patients. Specific national guidelines address the goals and recommended strategies for lipid management, blood pressure control, management of diabetes, and of obesity and smoking cessation.[2-6]

Common psychosocial problems in patients referred for cardiac rehabilitation include depression, anger, anxiety disorders, and social isolation. Education, counseling, and/or psychosocial interventions, either alone or as a component of multifactorial cardiac rehabilitation, can improve psychosocial well-being and quality of life; these are recommended to complement the psychosocial benefits of exercise training. To date, psychosocial interventions have not been documented to alter the prognosis of coronary patients.

Rehabilitation of Elderly Patients

Specific attention has been directed to the rehabilitation of elderly coronary patients; they have exercise trainability comparable to younger patients, with elderly women and men showing comparable improvement. Unfortunately, referral to and participation in exercise rehabilitation is less frequent at elderly age, especially among elderly women, suggesting that elderly patients of both genders should be strongly encouraged to participate in exercise-based cardiac rehabilitation.

2005 AHA Scientific Statement

A 2005 Scientific Statement of the American Heart Association,[7] in collaboration with the American Association of Cardiovascular and Pulmonary Rehabilitation, updates prior scientific statements from these professional organizations and reviews the recommended components for effective cardiac rehabilitation/secondary prevention programs, including alternative ways to deliver these services.

It reinforces that the safety of medically-supervised cardiac rehabilitation exercise training is well established, with contemporary risk stratification procedures guiding the intensity of required surveillance. The benefits of both exercise training and regular daily physical activities are defined as improvement in peak oxygen uptake by 11–36%, with the greatest improvement occurring in the most deconditioned individuals. Improved fitness increases the activity threshold before the onset of myocardial ischemia in patients with advanced coronary heart disease. Resistance training can improve muscular strength.

Clinical Trial Data

Meta-analyses of randomized trials of exercise training in patients with coronary heart disease, alone or as a component of a multidisciplinary cardiac rehabilitation program, have been updated in a recent review. The current study[8] involved women as one-fifth of the cohort and included an increased number of patients older than 65 years and those following myocardial revascularization procedures. Exercise-based cardiac rehabilitation was associated with lower total and cardiac mortality rates compared with usual medical care, with favorable trends for nonfatal myocardial infarction and the need for myocardial revascularization procedures. Potentially cardioprotective mechanisms presented included improvement in endothelial function, decrease in the biomarkers of inflammation, favorable effects on multiple coronary risk factors including all components of the metabolic syndrome, potential anti-ischemic effects, ischemic preconditioning, and favorable hemostatic effects.

In addition to the exercise benefits for patients with coronary heart disease, a recent meta-analysis of patients with stable heart failure documented an improvement in functional capacity, reduction in cardiorespiratory symptoms and a trend toward increased survival to result from exercise training.[9]

Alternative Modes of Delivery of Cardiac Rehabilitation Services

Alternative approaches to the delivery of cardiac rehabilitation services, other than traditional supervised group interventions, were considered effective and safe for stable cardiac patients.[1] Transtelephonic and other means of monitoring and surveillance were advocated to extend cardiac rehabilitation services beyond the setting of supervised, structured, and group-based rehabilitation. The American Heart Association 2005 Scientific Statement[7] further offered models that included home-based programs for which a nurse serves as a case manager to supervise and monitor patient care and progress; and community-based group program guidance by nurses or non-physician healthcare providers. Electronic media programs are also considered an alternative method for home-based comprehensive risk modification education and instruction, as well as for guidance of a structured exercise regimen. An unmet need is the long-term assessment of the effectiveness of these approaches and determination of the optimal mode of delivery of these services. The attractiveness of these alternative approaches is the potential to provide cardiac rehabilitation to low- and moderate-risk patients, who comprise the majority of contemporary US patients with stable coronary heart disease, most of whom currently do not participate in structured, supervised cardiac rehabilitation.

References

1. Wenger NK, Froelicher ES, Smith LK, et al. Cardiac Rehabilitation. Clinical Practice Guideline No. 17. Rockville, MD: US Department of Health and Human Services, Public Health Service, Agency for Health Care Policy and Research, and the National Heart, Lung, and Blood Institute, AHCPR Publication No. 96-0672, October 1995.
2. National Cholesterol Education Program (NCEP) Expert Panel on Detection, Evaluation, and Treatment of High Blood Cholesterol in Adults (Adult Treatment Panel III). Third Report of the National Cholesterol Education Program (NCEP) Expert Panel on Detection, Evaluation, and Treatment of High Blood Cholesterol in Adults (Adult Treatment Panel III) final report. Circulation 2002;106:3143–3421.
3. Chobanian AV, Bakris GL, Black HR, et al. National Heart, Lung, and Blood Institute Joint National Committee on Prevention, Detection, Evaluation, and Treatment of High Blood Pressure; National High Blood Pressure Education Program Coordinating Committee. The Seventh Report of the Joint National Committee on Prevention, Detection, Evaluation, and Treatment of High Blood Pressure: the JNC7 Report. JAMA 2003;289:2560–2572. [Published erratum in: JAMA 2003;290:197.]
4. NHLBI Obesity Education Initial Expert Panel. Clinical Guidelines on the Identification, Evaluation, and Treatment of Overweight and Obesity in Adults: The Evidence Report. Rockville, MD: National Heart, Lung and Blood Institute in cooperation with the National Institutes of Diabetes and Digestive and Kidney Diseases; September 1998. NIH Publication 98-4083.
5. American Diabetes Association. Clinical practice recommendations 2004. Diabetes Care 2004;27:S1–S145.
6. Murray EW. Smoking cessation clinical practice guidelines update and Agency for Healthcare Research and Quality tobacco resources. Tob Control 2000;9(Suppl 1):I72–I73.
7. Leon AS, Franklin BA, Costa F, et al. Cardiac rehabilitation and secondary prevention of coronary heart disease. An American Heart Association Scientific Statement from the Council on Clinical Cardiology (Subcommittee on Exercise, Cardiac Rehabilitation, and Prevention) and the Council on Nutrition, Physical Activity, and Metabolism (Subcommittee on Physical Activity), in collaboration with the American Association of Cardiovascular and Pulmonary Rehabilitation. Circulation 2005;111:369–376.
8. Taylor RS, Brown A, Ebrahim S, et al. Exercise-based rehabilitation for patients with coronary heart disease: systematic review and meta-analysis of randomized trials. Am J Med 2004;116:682–697.
9. Smart N, Marwick TH. Exercise training for patients with heart failure: a systematic review of factors that improve mortality and morbidity. Am J Med 2004;116:693–706.

7
Cardiac Rehabilitation: Canada

Terence Kavanagh

Cardiac rehabilitation had its beginnings in Canada in the late 1960s; since then it has gained in strength and stature until today there are 130 comprehensive multidisciplinary programs across the country. The province of Ontario, with 11 million inhabitants, most of whom live within 200 km of the United States border, is the most populated and has the largest number of full-service and partial-service programs. Of the remainder, the majority are in western Canada (the provinces of British Columbia, Alberta, and Manitoba), with fewer in Quebec and the Maritime Provinces.

Unfortunately, as is the case in most countries, only about 20–30% of potential candidates for cardiac rehabilitation services in Canada actually receive them. Apart from the customary prejudices against referral, e.g. female sex, age over 70 years, co-morbid conditions, there is also the skepticism (or lack of awareness) of some physicians as to the efficacy of cardiac rehabilitation. Obviously for those living in rural or remote northern communities, difficult access to rehabilitation services is a major obstacle, although the introduction of a telehealth system, involving 34 different networks across Canada, may help in this regard.

The need for a national body to document and validate all programs as well as establish best-practice guidelines was realized in 1990 with the formation of the Canadian Association of Cardiac Rehabilitation (CACR). The Guidelines document, drawn up in accordance with the European Appraisal of Guidelines Research and Evaluation (AGREE) formula, was first published in 1998, with the second edition in 2004.[1] This has become the CACR reference for those working in the field, and thus much of what follows is based on its content.

The very close working relationships between Canadian and American health professionals result in similar approaches to cardiac rehabilitation, and there is inevitably considerable overlap in program fundamentals. Nevertheless, there are dissimilarities, driven largely by philosophical differences in healthcare funding.

The Canada Health Act legislates that the provinces provide access to universal healthcare. Consequently, most large hospital or rehabilitation center-based programs are supported by an allocation from the various provincial Ministry of Health institutional budgets. Additional monies may be obtained through fund-raising events or, in the case of maintenance programs, direct patient payments; these supplemental sources of income are essential in those provinces where cardiac rehabilitation is a low medical priority.

Program Structure

This varies slightly across the country depending upon a particular province's population distribution and availability of appropriate health professional staff. However, despite regional differences there are broad principles which apply to all programs. Shorter hospital stays have tended to curtail the relevance and effectiveness of in-hospital programs for the vast majority of patients recovering from an uncomplicated myocardial infarction or coronary artery bypass graft surgery.

In the short time available, often only 5 or 6 days, the emphasis has to be on mobilization as well as identification of risk factors and the steps to eliminate them. The latter is achieved largely by the use of audiovisual aids and handouts. Patients are given advice on the principles of exercise training, encouraged to gradually increase their level of physical activity after discharge, and provided with information on cardiac rehabilitation services in the community.

Currently, outpatient programs predominate. The major sources of referrals are family physicians, cardiologists, and cardiac surgeons; a minority of programs allow self-referral. Typically, attendance is two to three times weekly for an average of 6 months, with a range of 2 months to 1 year. The Toronto program, the largest in Canada with 1400 to 1600 new referrals annually, is "hybrid" in structure. Over a 6-month period patients attend the center once weekly for education, counseling, behavioral modification, a supervised exercise training session, and then work out a further four times weekly away from the center. Thereafter, attendance is monthly for between 3 and 6 months. This approach has been shown to be at least as effective and no more costly than the typical 12-week, three attendances weekly, regimen.[2]

The case management approach is an alternative outpatient model. A cardiovascular trained nurse interfaces with the patient, specialist physician, and rehabilitation team, and assumes responsibility for the patient's care. This method has been shown to be very effective in some American jurisdictions, but does not lend itself to the Canadian healthcare system of funding, and therefore is rarely seen.

Historically, cardiac rehabilitation had its origins in the care of myocardial infarction survivors, and these individuals still constitute a significant proportion of all referrals. However, as the treatment of cardiovascular disease has advanced, the spectrum of patients referred to cardiac rehabilitation has broadened to include patients who have undergone revascularization procedures and cardiac transplantation. Chronic heart failure patients, previously advised to avoid all forms of physical exertion, are now found to benefit from an aerobic, and in some cases, a resistance training program. As the population ages, the number of patients receiving pacemakers is rising, and this is also a group suitable for exercise-based rehabilitation. The use of implantable cardioverter defibrillators to prevent sudden death is increasing, and with it the referral of such patients to cardiac rehabilitation. Most programs are still gaining experience in this area,[3] but it is becoming apparent that the training benefits include an improvement in self-confidence, increased functional capacity, and an enhanced quality of life.

Program Staffing

Comprehensive full-service programs which are located in hospitals have ready access to professional, technical, and administrative staff. Community free-standing clinics or rehabilitation centers, however, typically appoint a full-time or part-time medical director, nurse coordinator/manager, health professionals trained in the exercise sciences, exercise testing technicians, and a part-time dietician, psychologist, and social worker (or make provision for access to these latter three). Each of these individuals, in addition to a high level of competence in their profession, is required to possess a core of knowledge common to all and specific to the discipline of cardiac rehabilitation. This is usually gained in the practical setting, and is similar to the core functions and program personnel recommendations published by the American Association of Cardiovascular and Pulmonary Rehabilitation (AACVPR), the American Heart Association (AHA), and the American College of Sports Medicine (ACSM).

Program Content

Inasmuch as the essence of comprehensive cardiac rehabilitation is to determine the patient's level of cardiovascular risk, and then intervene to reduce that risk, it is essential to set treatment goals which are accepted nationally and are scientifically sound. Accordingly, the targets set out in the Canadian Guidelines were arrived at in close collaboration with the Canadian Associations for diabetes, hypertension, dyslipidemia, exercise physiology, and tobacco control. This ensured that the guidelines' targets are consistent with recommendations published by each of the major cardiovascular health and risk factor interest groups. As for the lifestyle interventions and behavior modification techniques, it is now apparent that these are essentially the same for each of the major risk factors. The various approaches recommended include the transtheoretical model of behavior change, motivational interviewing, and a variety of counseling styles, e.g. preacher, director, educator/instructor, counselor/consultant.

Current Canadian practice calls for all entrants to a cardiac rehabilitation program to undergo a risk stratification procedure. The guidelines propose that, after a full clinical assessment, the degree of disease progression is calculated using the Framingham Risk Score (FRS),[4] which takes into account age, gender, lipid profile, systolic blood pressure, smoking history, as well as presence or absence of diabetes. The Duke Treadmill Score[5] is then obtained from a graded exercise test, and this is then combined with the FSHSRS to estimate whether the patient is at high, intermediate, or low risk for a recurrent event. This approach allows for the matching of the degree of cardiovascular disease to the level of intervention, and thus a cost-effective application of rehabilitation resources. It also provides the patient with information conducive to program adherence and successful lifestyle modification.

An alternative to the FRS is the European Systematic Coronary Risk Evaluation Score (SCORE) equation.[6] The 2004 Canadian Guidelines discuss the relative merits of both and, on balance, find SCORE to have more merit. Advantages include the use of only fatal cardiovascular disease endpoints, separate prediction models in high- and low-risk populations, the ability to show changes in outcomes based on changes in risk factor values, and the fact that the model can be calibrated to specific populations if outcomes data and major risk factor data are available for the population of interest. However, its disadvantages are that it is unfamiliar to North American healthcare professionals, is not currently calibrated for Canadian populations, and has not been validated in people with documented cardiovascular disease. The FRS system is simple, and has recently been adjusted for age, gender, and the presence of cardiovascular disease; for these

reasons it is included in the current recommendations. However, it is important to point out that the Canadian Cardiovascular Society is currently sponsoring an evaluation of SCORE in Canada, and this therefore remains an attractive option for future guidelines.

Cardiopulmonary exercise testing is practiced in only a handful of programs, although measured peak oxygen intake has been shown to be a powerful predictor of survival in over 12,000 men with coronary heart disease referred for rehabilitation and followed for a median of 8 (4–29) years.[7]

Depression has been shown to be a risk factor for cardiovascular disease, and the presence of persistent depression following a myocardial infarction may be a marker for a recurrence. The mechanism may be physiological and/or the adverse influence depression has on behavior modification and program adherence. Anxiety, chronic psychological stress, social isolation, and a high hostile/anger personality profile have all been associated in various degrees with adverse cardiovascular outcomes. In light of this it is recommended that patients undergo a psychosocial screening. This need not be time-consuming, and can be incorporated into the initial assessment. As part of a pilot project conducted in the province of Ontario in 2002,[8] the use of various questionnaires such as the Beck Depression Scale, the Hospital Anxiety and Depression Scale, and the Medical Outcomes Study (MOS) Short Form 36 was found to be expeditious and effective.

Progressive aerobic type training is the cornerstone of the cardiac rehabilitation process. With regard to the mode intensity, frequency, and duration aspects of the training prescription, Canadian practice adheres closely to the recommendations of the ACSM, the AACVPR, and the AHA. Similarly with resistance training, although original work in this area carried out by researchers from McMaster University has engendered even greater enthusiasm for this approach.[9]

Program Safety

The initial risk stratification helps to identify patients at risk for sudden cardiac death, and thereby allows for a proactive approach. Consideration can be given to pharmacological interventions, revascularization procedures, or implantation of a cardioverter defibrillator. While not recommended for routine use, telemetry can provide valuable information when exercising high-risk patients. Furthermore, these individuals should be seen in classes where the ratio of staff to patient is no greater than 1 to 5. In the final analysis, however, ensuring that patients adhere strictly to their exercise prescription, are familiar with the Borg rating of perceived exertion, can take an accurate pulse, and can recognize the significance of adverse signs and symptoms such as an erratic pulse, excessive breathlessness, lightheadedness, "blackouts," etc. is probably the greatest insurance against adverse events.

Conclusions

Exercise-based comprehensive cardiac rehabilitation has made steady progress in Canada over the past 50 years, and its place in the continuum of cardiovascular care is now largely accepted. However, programs are unevenly distributed across the country and in some areas are disproportionate to population requirements. Provincial health networks need to consider their cardiac rehabilitation needs and develop a delivery infrastructure based on health service funding. Greater attention has to be given to the elderly, especially women, and different ethnic groups. Currently, program length has been chosen empirically and more research is required to determine optimal duration, cost-effectiveness, and outcomes.[2] When one realizes that, despite the efforts of public health authorities, 8 out of 10 adult Canadians suffer from one risk factor, and 1 in 10 has three or more, the need for cardiac rehabilitation and secondary prevention programs can only increase.

References

1. Stone JA, ed. Canadian Association of Cardiac Rehabilitation Guidelines for Cardiac Rehabilitation and Cardiovascular Disease Prevention. Winnipeg: Canadian Association of Cardiac Rehabilitation; 2004.
2. Hamm LF, Kavanagh T, Campbell RB, et al. Timeline for peak improvements during 52 weeks of outpatient cardiac rehabilitation. J Cardiopulm Rehabil 2004;24:374–382.
3. Kamke W, Dovifat C, Schranz M, et al. Cardiac rehabilitation in patients with implantable defibrillators: Feasibility and complications. Z Kardiol 2003;92(10): 869–875.
4. Califf RM, Armstrong PW, Carver JR, et al. Task force 5. Stratification of patients into high, medium, and low risk subgroups for purposes of risk factor management. J Am Coll Cardiol 1996;27(5):1007–1019.
5. Mark DB, Shaw L, Harrell FE Jr, et al. Prognostic value of a treadmill exercise score in outpatients with suspected coronary artery disease. N Engl J Med 1991;325(12);849–853.
6. Conroy RM, Pyorala K, Fitzgerald AP, et al. Estimation of ten-year risk of fatal cardiovascular disease in Europe: The SCORE project. Eur Heart J 2003;24(11):987–1003.
7. Kavanagh T, Mertens DJ, Hamm LF, et al. Prediction of long-term prognosis in 12,169 men referred for cardiac rehabilitation. Circulation 2002;106:666–671.
8. Suskin, N, MacDonald S, Swabey T, et al. Cardiac rehabilitation and secondary prevention services in Ontario: Recommendations from a consensus panel. Can J Cardiol 2003;19(7):833–838.
9. McCartney N. Role of resistance training in heart disease. Med Sci Sports Exerc 1998;30(Suppl):S396–S402.

8
Cardiac Rehabilitation: Australia

Michael V. Jelinek and Stephen J. Bunker

Evolution of Cardiac Rehabilitation in Australia

The concept of cardiac rehabilitation (CR) was introduced into Australia by the National Heart Foundation (NHF) in 1961 when it began establishing CR clinics in each of the major cities. Medical Directors of the four pioneer CR clinics were Dr Alan Goble, Melbourne, Dr Tony Seldon, Sydney, Dr Graeme Neilson, Brisbane, and Dr Robert Cutforth, Hobart. By 1964 over 1000 patients were attending these clinics.

The success of these clinics, together with the establishment of coronary care units, led to a greater interest in the principles of CR among cardiologists, physicians, and general practitioners. Gradually the clinics were phased out in favor of structured exercise and education programs that were being established in hospital outpatient departments. Multidisciplinary hospital- and community-based programs of group light–moderate exercise, combined with education and discussion, have become the predominant model throughout most of Australia.[1] These programs incorporated the essential components of CR without reducing efficacy, thereby providing greater access for patients and improving cost-effectiveness.[2]

Factors Influencing Development of Cardiac Rehabilitation in Australia

Research

From 1980 to 1985 a landmark study, undertaken at the Austin Hospital, Melbourne, compared the high-intensity exercise component of CR to a light–moderate exercise program. It was demonstrated that a light–moderate exercise program achieved the same benefits gained from high-intensity exercise.[3,4] This had important implications for CR in Australia. The advantage of a light–moderate exercise program is that it can be conducted in community settings, as well as hospitals, because it needs no special equipment or medical supervision and is therefore much cheaper to run. It is also much more acceptable to older patients and females. As a result, high-intensity exercise programs typically recommended overseas are uncommon in Australia.

The important role that psychosocial factors play in the recovery and prognosis of patients with heart disease was recognized early in the development of CR in Australia.[5] The early NHF clinics included a social worker and psychiatrist as part of the rehabilitation team.

As evidence has emerged for the benefits of risk factor reduction and adherence to certain medications (secondary prevention), CR programs in Australia have increasingly incorporated the principles of identification and management of risk factors through lifestyle change and compliance with medical therapies.

Role of the National Heart Foundation (NHF)

In addition to establishing the NHF CR clinics during the early 1960s, the NHF maintained a National Cardiac Rehabilitation Committee responsible for providing expert advice to the Foundation, as well as developing policies, guidelines, and professional education resources. During the late 1980s and early 1990s, the growth and development of a decentralized network of hospital- and community-based programs throughout Australia was facilitated by NHF staff who had been employed to work with multi-disciplinary health professionals and assist with the planning and establishment of programs. The NHF also encouraged and supported the establishment of state-based Cardiac Rehabilitation Associations, as well as the Australian Cardiac Rehabilitation Association, which provide forums and support for health professionals with an interest in, or working in, the field.

Funding Model

With the exception of the privately funded health sector, there has been no formal funding base for CR in Australia. Health professionals contribute their time to the program as part of their wider role and responsibilities within the hospital or primary care setting. Only in the case of larger centers are coordinators employed and then usually only on a part-time basis. This model has contributed to both the low cost of CR in Australia and its sustainability.

Current Status and Future Directions

Through its CR policy and guidelines[6] the NHF promotes the routine referral of all patients with cardiovascular disease to an appropriate CR program. Patients are encouraged to attend as soon as possible after discharge. Currently, there are almost 300 structured post-discharge CR programs throughout Australia, mainly in urban areas. Programs vary in length from a minimum of one session a week for 6 weeks through to more comprehensive programs.

Despite the abundant evidence supporting the benefits of CR, only a minority of patients attend a structured CR service in Australia.[7-9] CR is more likely to be performed by patients after coronary artery bypass surgery than after percutaneous coronary intervention. Reasons for poor attendance at CR include lack of available CR services[10] as well patient under-referral and underutilization.[8,11]

To address issues such as the lack of CR services in rural and remote areas, the NHF has called for the development of alternative models of CR to reach a greater number of patients, particularly disadvantaged populations. For example, Aboriginal and Torres Strait Islander people are known to die from cardiovascular disease at twice the rate of other population groups but they are under-represented in CR and there is a strong need to develop flexible methods of CR delivery.[6]

The delivery of home-based programs, which have been shown to be as safe and cost-effective as hospital-based CR programs, has been growing overseas, particularly in the UK. However, no such model is currently being evaluated in Australia.

The Coaching Patients on Achieving Cardiovascular Health (COACH) Program is a training program for patients with coronary heart disease. Health professionals use the telephone to train patients to vigorously pursue the target levels for their particular coronary risk factors while working with their usual doctor(s). Coaching emphasizes both lifestyle measures and drug treatment. The COACH Program has been shown to be effective in achieving secondary prevention goals and targets[12,13] and reducing hospital readmissions.[14]

Conclusion

CR in Australia is predominantly based on group light–moderate exercise and education programs. As is true elsewhere, only a minority of patients with coronary heart disease attend CR. New models are being developed, particularly the COACH Program, which potentially can reach all patients in Australia by the telephone.

References

1. Hare DL, fitzgerald H, Darcy F, Race E, Goble AJ. Cardiac rehabilitation based on group light exercise and discussion. An Australian hospital model. J Cardiopulm Rehabil 1995;15(3):186–192.
2. Hare DL, Bunker SJ. Cardiac rehabilitation and secondary prevention. Med J Aust 1999;171:433–439.
3. Goble AJ, Hare DL, Macdonald PS, Oliver RG, Reid MA, Worcester MC. Effect of early programmes of high and low intensity exercise on physical perfor-

mance after transmural acute myocardial infarction. Br Heart J 1991;65:126–131.

4. Worcester MC, Hare DL, Oliver RG, Reid MA, Goble AJ. Early programmes of high and low intensity exercise and quality of life after acute myocardial infarction. BMJ 1993;307:1244–1247.

5. Wynn A. Unwarranted emotional distress in men with ischaemic heart disease. Med J Aust 1967;2: 847.

6. National Heart Foundation of Australia. Recommended Framework for Cardiac Rehabilitation. 2004. (Available at: www.heartfoundation.com.au/downloads/CR_04_Rec_final.pdf_)

7. Bunker S, McBurney H, Cox H, Jelinek M. Identifying participation rates at outpatient cardiac rehabilitation programs in Victoria, Australia. J Cardiopulm Rehabil 1999;19(6):334–338.

8. Scott IA, Lindsay KA, Harden HE. Utilisation of outpatient cardiac rehabilitation in Queensland. Med J Aust 2003;179:341–345.

9. Sundararajan V, Bunker SJ, Begg S, Marshall R, McBurney H. Attendance rates and outcomes of cardiac rehabilitation in Victoria, 1998. Med J Aust 2004;180:268–271.

10. Dollard J, Smith JR, Thompson D, Stewart S. Broadening the reach of cardiac rehabilitation to rural and remote Australia. Eur J Cardiovasc Nurs 2004;3:27–42.

11. Bunker SJ, Goble AJ. Cardiac rehabilitation: under-referral and underutilisation. Med J Aust 2003;179: 332–333.

12. Vale MJ, Jelinek MV, Best JD, Santamaria JD. Coaching patients with coronary heart disease to achieve the target cholesterol: a method to bridge the gap between evidence-based medicine and the 'real world'. Randomized controlled trial. J Clin Epidemiol 2002;55:245–252.

13. Vale MJ, Jelinek MV, Best JD, et al. Coaching Patients on Achieving Cardiovascular Health (COACH); a multicenter randomized trial in patients with coronary heart disease. Arch Intern Med 2003;163: 2775–2783).

14. Vale MJ, Sundararajan V, Jelinek MV, Best JD. Four-year follow-up of the multicenter RCT of Coaching Patients on Achieving Cardiovascular Health (The COACH Study) shows that The COACH Program keeps patients out of hospital. Oral presentation at the 77th Scientific Sessions of the American Heart Association, November 7–10, 2004, New Orleans, Louisiana, USA. Circulation 2004;110: Suppl: III-801.

9
Cardiac Rehabilitation: South Africa

Wayne E. Derman

Introduction

The population of South Africa totals approximately 46 million people and is ethnically and economically diverse. The diversity is reflected in the patterns of urbanization with nearly 50% of the black population residing primarily in rural or peri-urban areas compared to fewer than 20% of white South Africans or those of mixed ancestral or Asian origin (South African National Census 2001). However, urbanization of the black population has been increasing rapidly, particularly since 1994. Furthermore, this rapid urbanization combined with globalization has been accompanied by large shifts in the health patterns of South Africans, increasing the prevalence of non-communicable disease.[1] The South African National Burden of Disease study for the year 2000 estimated that 17% of all deaths were due to cardiovascular diseases.[2] Of these deaths, ischemic heart disease and stroke each accounted for 35% of cardiovascular deaths, hypertensive heart disease 15%, inflammatory heart disease 6%, and other causes including rheumatic heart disease accounted for 9%. It is of interest to note that in South Africa HIV/AIDS is the leading cause of death and accounts for 30% of all deaths.

Prevalence of Risk Factors for Heart Disease

Along with the increased burden of non-communicable diseases, there has been an associated increase in the prevalence of a number of known risk factors associated with heart disease including smoking, sedentary lifestyle, and increased intake of dietary fat.[3-5] Furthermore, South Africans have a high prevalence of overweight and obesity, with over 50% of women and more than 20% of men considered overweight by World Health Organization (WHO) standards (body mass index (kg/m^2) >25). Indeed, the World Health Survey 2003, published by the WHO, suggests that the prevalence of physical inactivity in South African adults is greater than 60% for both males and females. In fact, nearly 60% of all South African adults have at least one major reversible factor. Thus, the need for both secondary and indeed primary intervention initiatives including cardiac rehabilitation is large.

Historical Perspective

Cardiac rehabilitation was officially started in Johannesburg by Dr John Sim in 1970. This program began with a handful of patients who used a parking lot in the premises of the Johannesburg Civic Centre to conduct their exercises. This initiative was shortly followed by the University of Cape Town program, initiated under the guidance of Professor Tim Noakes, who gained much local fame for encouraging cardiac patients to get fit and eventually run a full marathon.

In 1990 the South African Association of Cardiovascular and Pulmonary Rehabilitation was initiated. This association was recently incorporated into the South African Sports Medicine Association (www.sasma.co.za).

Contemporary Cardiac Rehabilitation Programs in South Africa

South Africa is divided into nine provinces. Formal cardiac rehabilitation programs exist in most of these provinces associated with academic universities or private hospitals. Although there have been initiatives to arrange rehabilitation services at governmental hospitals, these services have been fragmented and severely limited due to staff and financial shortages. Some provincial government hospitals' physiotherapy units provide some phase I rehabilitation following cardiac surgery.

Most outpatient cardiac rehabilitation programs are conducted from private gymnasia, gymnasia or biokinetic practices associated with private hospitals or private practices under the auspices of Universities or Sports Science/Sports Medicine departments. These programs vary in size and have an attendance of typically between 10 and 100 patients per day. Services can vary from provision of exercise rehabilitation only to exercise rehabilitation, patient education, dietary and psychological intervention.

The programs which provide medical monitoring and comprehensive services as listed above tend to be costly and quite exclusive whilst the university-based programs tend to be less expensive and have a wider patient base.

However, despite an increasing worldwide trend for cardiac rehabilitation to be considered an important part of patient care, it is estimated that only 15–20% of eligible private cardiac patients are referred to rehabilitation services. This figure is even less in the public sector.

Although cardiac rehabilitation services are underutilized in South Africa, the increasing demand for these services has come to the attention of the health insurance industry and medical insurance schemes. In general most schemes recognize patient claims for reimbursement for cardiac rehabilitation. However, a few still refuse to assist their members in paying for cardiac rehabilitation.

One medical insurance scheme leads the way in South Africa by encouraging members with an incentive-based system based on rewards for attending cardiac rehabilitation or indeed undertaking a primary intervention program to lower and manage their risk factors. It is interesting to note that this company has in a short period become the largest medical insurance company in South Africa.

This company has also promoted the teaching and science of cardiac rehabilitation by initiating "best practice teaching symposia" around the country and has a committee which assesses and rates the practices in the established network. This has assisted the standards of cardiac rehabilitation throughout South Africa. For example, it is not possible to practice cardiac rehabilitation as part of this network if one does not have the necessary skilled staff, required emergency drugs, and an automated external defibrillator or similar device.

Shift of Emphasis in Cardiac Rehabilitation Programs in South Africa

Although the practice of cardiac rehabilitation in South Africa is conducted according to international guidelines and is considered successful,[6,7] an observation from our Cardiac Rehabilitation Program is that patients attending the program for rehabilitation of a cardiac condition often also present with additional co-morbidities and musculoskeletal injuries. Thus we recently undertook a descriptive study to determine the profile of patients attending the Cardiac Rehabilitation Program at the Sports Science Institute of South Africa.[8]

This descriptive retrospective analysis evaluated the medical records of 313 patients who entered the program during the period of January 1996 to August 2000. Of the total population, 80% had documented coronary artery disease (CAD). The remaining 20% attended the program for rehabilitation of another chronic lifestyle disease. Of the group of patients presenting with CAD, only 31% presented with CAD as the sole disorder, 14% presented with CAD and another chronic lifestyle disease, 26% with CAD and a chronic musculoskeletal injury, and a last group of 14% required rehabilitation for CAD plus another co-morbidity and a musculoskeletal injury. Furthermore, 11% presented with two or more risk factors, attending the program for primary prevention of CAD only, whilst 6% attended the program for primary prevention and the rehabilitation of another chronic disease.

Musculoskeletal rehabilitation was required in 57% of the total population. Of the total 286 musculoskeletal injuries noted, back injuries were the most common musculoskeletal condition (49%), with grade I motion segment abnormality the most common back injury (63% of back injuries). Other common injuries included knee injuries (18%), shoulder injuries (13%), and hip injuries (7%).

These findings suggest that the focus of cardiac rehabilitation programs should be shifted to "chronic disease" rehabilitation. Furthermore, as previous musculoskeletal injury is so common, staff who possess musculoskeletal rehabilitation skills should be employed in such programs. Indeed, we suggest that lumbar "prehabilitation" be taught to all patients enrolled in the program. These factors may necessitate an evaluation of the current status of cardiac rehabilitation programs in general, including provisions for musculoskeletal rehabilitation, variety in exercise forms, adequate supervision, the necessary testing and exercise equipment, and adequate reimbursement by medical aid schemes.

Challenges in South Africa

The economic diversity in South Africa makes the provision of cardiac rehabilitation services very challenging, particularly at the state or provincial hospitals where budget and staff shortages have made exercise rehabilitation programs seem a less important priority.

Initiating programs into the poorer community is also a significant challenge. One successful model used by the Community Health Intervention Programmes (CHIPs) Division of the Sports Science Institute of South Africa has been to initiate low-cost, community-led rehabilitation and primary prevention projects in the Western Cape and Gauteng regions in South Africa. Members of the community are encouraged to contact this division of the Institute and, once a core group of thirty community members, a safe venue (e.g. a church or school hall) and three to four community leaders volunteer, the Institute provides leadership and training as well as supervision for the initial 8 weeks of the program. A small amount of essential equipment (balls, rubber resistance bands, and blood pressure monitoring equipment) are donated to the group by a sponsor. The four community leaders are then trained by our staff regarding low-intensity exercise training, safety issues during exercise, and patient monitoring. The initial 8 weeks of training is followed by a co-implementation period of 6 weeks, where community leaders and Institute staff together lead the program. Once the training is complete and our team are convinced the group is running smoothly and safely, the project is then handed over to the community at a celebratory function. The Institute provides ongoing back-up help for problem solving and guidance for the community leaders. This has proved to be a successful model and to date over 30 such programs have been created within the community.

References

1. Bradshaw D, Groenewald P, Laubscher R, et al. Initial Burden of Disease Estimates for South Africa, 2000. Cape Town: South African Medical Research Council; 2003 (http://www.mrc.ac.za/bod/bod.htm).
2. Bradshaw D. What do we know about the burden of cardiovascular disease in South Africa. Cardiovasc J S Afr 2005;16(3):140–141.
3. Bourne LT, Langenhoven ML, Steyn K, Jooste PL, Laubscher JA, van der Vyver E. Nutrient intake in the urban African population of the Cape Peninsula, South Africa. The Brisk study. Cent Afr J Med 1993;39(12):238–247.
4. Yach D, Townshend G. Smoking and Health in South Africa: the need for Action. Cape Town: South African Medical Research Council; 1988.
5. Reddy SP, Panday S, Swart D, et al. The South African Youth Risk Behaviour Survey 2002. Cape Town: South African Medical Research Council; 2003.

6. Joughin HM, Digenio AG, Daly L, Kqare E. Physiological benefits of a prolonged moderate-intensity endurance training programme in patients with coronary artery disease. S Afr Med J 1999; 89(5):545–550.

7. Digenio AG, Cantor A, Noakes TD, et al. Is severe left ventricular dysfunction a contraindication to participation in an exercise rehabilitation programme? S Afr Med J 1996;86(9):1106–1109.

8. Dreyer L, Schwellnus M, Noakes TD, Derman EW. Physiological and medical considerations of patients attending cardiac rehab programmes: implications for staffing and equipment. Med Sci Sports Exerc 2001;33(5, Suppl);S320.

10
Cardiac Rehabilitation: China

David R. Thompson and Cheuk-Man Yu

Introduction

The concept of cardiac rehabilitation is comparatively new in mainland China and has received scant attention until recently. Indeed, in most parts of the country it is underdeveloped. This is not surprising when one considers the enormity of the country (9 million km^2) and its population (1.3 billion), and the fact that heart disease has only recently, although rapidly, become a major cause of death and disability. This is partly a reflection of the rapid increases in urbanization, population mobility and aging, environment deterioration and economic growth and, as a consequence, growing income disparities and rising unemployment. The population of China with coronary heart disease is now estimated to be at least 20 million and there are major challenges, such as hypertension and tobacco smoking. For instance, at least 350 million people smoke, of which 50 million are teenagers. Thus, there is a growing recognition that cardiac rehabilitation services should be established and developed.

Evolution of Cardiac Rehabilitation in China

It is difficult to pinpoint a specific epoch in the evolution of cardiac rehabilitation in China because of its size and diversity. China is divided into 23 provinces, five autonomous regions, and four municipalities, and has 320,000 hospitals and clinics, 1.4 million doctors and 1.3 million nurses.

Formal cardiac rehabilitation programs (many at a crude stage of development) exist in many of these provinces associated with university or private hospitals. Public hospitals are comparatively poorly served and services are relatively fragmented and limited. Reasons why cardiac rehabilitation programs in China are underdeveloped include limited medical resources, priority being given to acute cardiac rather than rehabilitation services, and lack of training in cardiac rehabilitation as part of general cardiology training as a result of which physicians' understanding of and enthusiasm for promoting cardiac rehabilitation is low.

The patient demand for cardiac rehabilitation is low due to the medical system in China, which is reliant on patients paying for services. There is no established scheme of medical reimbursement for the majority of people and medical insurance is in its infancy.

However, in some parts of China, notably Hong Kong, rehabilitation services are comparatively well developed and are seen as an important aspect of health service provision. For instance, in Hong Kong, six of the 44 public hospitals and one of the 12 private hospitals run cardiac rehabilitation programs. Most have been running for around 10 years (though some as long as 17 years), and are located in the hospital or community clinic. Most hospital-based programs accept only referrals from cardiologists, though one group has open access, and all community-based programs accept self-referrals.

There are some very good models of cardiac rehabilitation in Hong Kong. For example, one well-established comprehensive hospital-based program that provides a clinical and research perspective is run by two cardiologists, a rehabilitation physician, four cardiac rehabilitation nurses, two physiotherapists, two occupational therapists, a clinical psychologist, a dietician, and a research assistant.[1-3] This program consists of four phases: (1) inpatient ambulation program for 7–14 days; (2) a twice weekly outpatient education and exercise program lasting for 8 weeks; (3) a community-based home exercise program; and (4) long-term maintenance for another 12 months. However, such programs are the exception rather than the rule.

Program Structure, Staffing, and Content

The program structure varies widely across each province, depending upon a particular province's population distribution and availability of appropriate health professionals. In the vast majority of cases, cardiac rehabilitation is in the form of verbal information supplemented by leaflets and booklets emphasizing early mobilization and the identification and control of risk factors. The focus is invariably on patients with myocardial infarction and coronary artery bypass surgery. The duration of most programs is usually two classes per week for 12 weeks. There is routine follow-up in a minority of programs (usually for 3–6 months) and the focus is usually solely on myocardial infarction patients. There is little systematic audit data and no outcome evaluation using standardized measures, nor is there any form of national benchmarking.

Most programs that do exist are coordinated by a nurse, though in some instances it is a cardiologist or social worker. In exceptional cases, such as Hong Kong, cardiac rehabilitation programs invariably involve a range of healthcare professionals, including nurse, physician (cardiologist and/or rehabilitation physician), physiotherapist, occupational therapist, dietician, clinical psychologist, and social worker. However, very few of these staff will have been trained to a high level of competence or be accredited in cardiac rehabilitation.

The program content comprises mainly education, diet, and exercise, though some include behavior and family therapy. Few programs in China use cardiovascular risk stratification or treatment goals determined by national guidelines. However, with the difference in epidemiology of risk factors between Chinese and Caucasian patients with coronary heart disease[4] and the limited applicability of some risk score scales in clinical practice (such as the Framingham score),[5] it is necessary to re-evaluate the impact of risk factor modification on the progression of the disease.

There is a paucity of community resources in China, though the Hong Kong Society for Rehabilitation Community Rehabilitation Network has been running cardiac rehabilitation programs for over 10 years. In Hong Kong there is also a "Care for your heart" self-support group and a HEART (health education and rehabilitation training) club.

There are genuine attempts to raise the profile and improve the provision of cardiac rehabilitation. For example, a well-established and growing forum for practitioners and researchers is the Asia Pacific Congress of Cardiac Rehabilitation who held their most recent meeting (8th) in Hong Kong in 2003.

Research

There is a dearth of studies on cardiac rehabilitation in China, although a few rigorous studies have been conducted, notably in Hong Kong.[1-3,6] These studies examined nearly 700 patients who were enrolled into the cardiac rehabilitation program in one of the cluster referral hospitals in Hong Kong, and observed the following unique findings. firstly, in a registry of 418 patients who had undergone cardiac rehabilitation, the two major determinants of clinical outcome (mortality or cardiovascular hospitalization) after acute myocardial infarction are the presence of diabetes mellitus and low exercise capacity (<4 metabolic equivalents by exercise treadmill test).[1] Secondly, in the clinical setting of Hong Kong, the implementation of cardiac rehabilitation is highly cost-effective since it actually saves money with gains in quality of life. In a randomized controlled study of 269 patients, the cost-utility analysis calculated a saving of US$640 per quality-adjusted life year

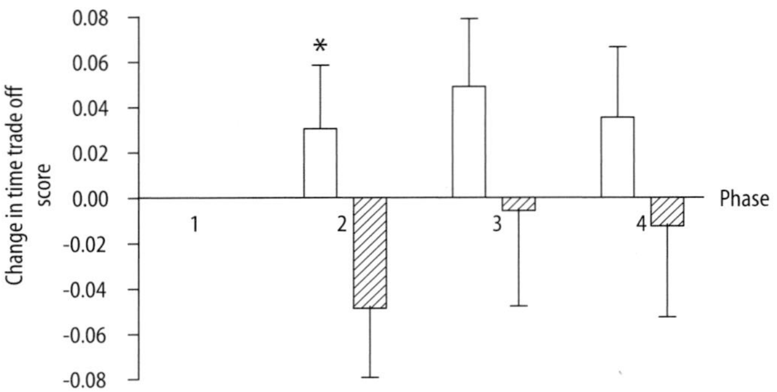

FIGURE 10-1. Changes in time trade-off scores after adjustment for baseline differences in patients who underwent cardiac rehabilitation (white bars) and controls (hatched bars). *$P < 0.005$ when compared between the two groups.

(QALY) gained (Figure 10-1).[2] This is possibly explained by a lower need for subsequent percutaneous coronary intervention.[2] Improvement in quality of life was clearly shown by more than one quality of life questionnaire.[2] Thirdly, Chinese subjects have a different body build and, therefore, the definition of obesity is more stringent (defined as a body mass index of $\geq 26 \, kg/m^2$) than the one adopted by the World Health Organization.[7] The cardiac rehabilitation conducted in patients ($N = 112$) with recent myocardial infarction or percutaneous coronary intervention was associated with early improvement in exercise capacity and quality of life, and better maintenance of a regular exercise habit when compared with the control group who only received education.[6] Lastly, the effect of cardiac rehabilitation on diastolic function has received little attention. Diastolic dysfunction refers to the abnormal process of left ventricular relaxation that is common after myocardial infarction.[8] A randomized controlled trial in Hong Kong Chinese patients found a preventive effect of exercise training on the progression of diastolic dysfunction.[3] Improvement in exercise capacity was observed which was persistent even at phase 4 of the rehabilitation program (Figure 10-2). Interestingly, the improvement in diastolic function predicted the gain in exercise capacity, implicating the pathophysiological basis of diastolic dysfunction on exercise intolerance in patients with heart diseases.[3]

Some other studies conducted in Hong Kong have attempted, with limited success, to assess quality of life in patients enrolled into a conventional cardiac rehabilitation program,[9] and others

have examined cardiac patients' and caregivers' experiences of a community rehabilitation network.[10]

Most of the literature on cardiac rehabilitation in China is, understandably, published in Chinese, which limits its accessibility and impact. That which can be identified and translated tends to be small-scale and have methodological limitations. These studies, typically, have focused on information on exercise and coronary risk factors and have had modest benefits. Whilst the body of research literature in China is growing in cardiac rehabilitation, the focus of efforts has been on early mobilization and exercise, with comparatively little attention being given to psychosocial, including quality of life, outcomes. Surprisingly

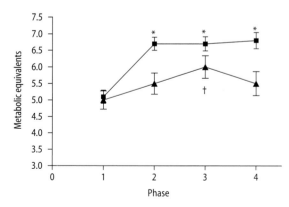

Figure 10-2. Plotting of exercise capacity as assessed by metabolic equivalents in 269 patients who were randomized to a cardiac rehabilitation program (■) and control group (▲). *$P < 0.001$ versus phase 1 for cardiac rehabilitation group. †$P < 0.001$ versus phase 1 for control group.

little attention has been given to more culturally suited rehabilitation interventions or adjuncts, such as tai chi, an avenue that appears to offer some promise for a Chinese population.[11,12]

In view of the massive population, much of it still rural, and scarce resources, there is a need for more creative, flexible and responsive cardiac rehabilitation service provision. For example, two trials are being undertaken at the moment in Xian and Beijing of a self-help, home-based, cardiac rehabilitation manual, and the results are awaited with interest.

Conclusion

Both the quantity and quality of cardiac rehabilitation programs in China are currently poor because of significant underinvestment. As a consequence, the vast majority of potential candidates who are likely to accrue benefits do not have the opportunity to access such services. There is growing interest in and support for establishing such programs, but these will need to be matched with sufficient commitment, funding, staff, and resources.

Many hospitals have been slow to institute provision and very few have developed specific guidelines. The spectrum of patients enrolled into cardiac rehabilitation needs to be broadened. Suggestions for improvement include a needs-led, menu-driven program with audit data to permit benchmarking. A minimum data set would be useful.

There is a need for a national body to coordinate, document, and validate cardiac rehabilitation programs as well as establish and benchmark best practice.

References

1. Yu CM, Lau CP, Cheung BM, et al. Clinical predictors of morbidity and mortality in patients with myocardial infarction or revascularization who underwent cardiac rehabilitation, and importance of diabetes mellitus and exercise capacity. Am J Cardiol 2000;85:344–349.

2. Yu CM, Lau CP, Chau J, et al. A short course of cardiac rehabilitation program is highly cost effective in improving long-term quality of life in patients with recent myocardial infarction or percutaneous coronary intervention. Arch Phys Med Rehabil 2004;85:915–922.

3. Yu CM, Li LSW, Lam MF, Siu DCW, Miu RKM, Lau CP. Effect of a cardiac rehabilitation program on left ventricular diastolic function and its relationship to exercise capacity in patients with coronary heart disease: experience from a randomized, controlled study. Am Heart J 2004;147:e24.

4. Gu D, Gupta A, Muntner P, et al. Prevalence of cardiovascular disease risk factor clustering among the adult population of China: results from the International Collaborative Study of Cardiovascular Disease in Asia (InterAsia). Circulation 2005; 112:658–665.

5. Liu J, Hong Y, D'Agostino RB Sr, et al. Predictive value for the Chinese population of the Framingham CHD risk assessment tool compared with the Chinese Multi-Provincial Cohort Study. JAMA 2004;291:2591–2599.

6. Yu CM, Li LS, Ho HH, Lau CP. Long-term changes in exercise capacity, quality of life, body anthropometry, and lipid profiles after a cardiac rehabilitation program in obese patients with coronary heart disease. Am J Cardiol 2003;91:321–325.

7. Ko GT, Tang J, Chan JC, et al. Lower BMI cut-off value to define obesity in Hong Kong Chinese: an analysis based on body fat assessment by bioelectrical impedance. Br J Nutr 2001;85:239–242.

8. Yu CM, Sanderson JE, Shum IO, et al. Diastolic dysfunction and natriuretic peptides in systolic heart failure. Higher ANP and BNP levels are associated with the restrictive filling pattern. Eur Heart J 1996;17:1694–1702.

9. Chan DS, Chau JP, Chang AM. Acute coronary syndromes: cardiac rehabilitation programmes and quality of life. J Adv Nurs 2005;49:591–599.

10. Holroyd E, Twinn S, Shiu A. Evaluating psychosocial nursing interventions for cardiac clients and their caregivers: a case study of the community rehabilitation network in Hong Kong. J Adv Nurs 2001; 35:393–401.

11. Taylor-Piliae RE. Tai Chi as an adjunct to cardiac rehabilitation exercise training. J Cardiopulmon Rehabil 2003;23:90–96.

12. Lan C, Chen SY, Lai JS, Wong MK. The effect of Tai Chi on cardiorespiratory function in patients with coronary artery bypass surgery. Med Sci Sports Exerc 1999;31:634–638.

11
New Concepts for Early Diagnosis of Coronary Artery Disease

Sigmund Silber and Peter Mathes

Background and Problem

Cardiovascular diseases are still the number one killer in developed countries. The term "death from cardiovascular disease," however, includes not only acute myocardial infarction, but also death from chronic ischemic heart disease, stroke, peripheral artery disease, and pulmonary embolism. A more detailed analysis shows that only approximately 18% of the cardiovascular deaths arise from *acute* myocardial infarction, while a continuously increasing percentage result from *chronic* ischemic heart disease. Although modern medicine significantly improved the short-term outcome of acute myocardial infarction, it shifted the problem from a decrease in mortality to an increase in morbidity. Therefore, the challenge of modern medicine is not only to further reduce the already declining cardiovascular mortality,[1,2] but also to reduce cardiovascular morbidity. The major goal is to thus prevent the first acute myocardial infarction to ensure not only a long life but also a life without cardiovascular events. This is even more important, since 31% to 72% of coronary occlusions developed from a previously "insignificant" coronary lesion by sudden and "unexpected" plaque rupture leading to a nonfatal or fatal coronary event.[3] To achieve this goal it is not only important to detect "atherosclerosis" per se, but also to identify the asymptomatic high-risk individual, then initiate intensive risk factor modification at this preclinical stage.[4,5]

Noninvasive Detection of the Presence of Atherosclerotic Disease

Asymptomatic atherosclerotic disease is defined as the presence of abnormal function or structure of the vessel wall due to atherosclerosis. In this early stage, patients cannot be warned by ischemic chest pain (angina pectoris). Also, functional tests, like exercise ECG, stress echocardiography, perfusion scintigraphy, or perfusion magnetic resonance imaging (MRI), will be negative, because there is not yet a critical lumen narrowing leading to inducible perfusion abnormalities or myocardial ischemia. Intravascular (intracoronary) ultrasound (IVUS) is an excellent tool to diagnose and follow up preclinical atherosclerosis.[6] It is, however, an invasive tool requiring arterial access (cardiac catheterization).

Pathology studies have documented that levels of traditional risk factors are associated with the extent and severity of atherosclerosis. However, at every level of risk factor exposure, there is substantial variation in the amount of atherosclerosis. This variation in disease is probably due to genetic susceptibility, combinations and interactions with other risk factors, including life habits, duration of exposure to the specific level of the risk factors and such factors as biological and laboratory variability. Therefore, no blood test exists that "proves" the presence of atherosclerotic disease. All the known traditional (e.g. hypercholesterolemia) and modern (e.g. elevated C-reactive protein) risk factors increase the likelihood of atherosclerosis, but they do not prove its existence in an individual person. Therefore functional and imaging techniques have to be used for diagnosing atherosclerosis at this early stage. A variety of noninvasive tests are available for determining the presence of asymptomatic atherosclerosis in various vascular beds.

Functional Tests for Early Detection of Atherosclerotic Disease

Endothelial Dysfunction and Forearm Blood Flow Testing

Endothelial cells play a central role in inhibiting the development of atherosclerosis and its thrombotic consequences. Endothelial dysfunction is secondary to the long-term impact of risk factors on endothelial cells. Conventional risk factors increase the oxidative stress in vascular tissue, giving oxidative stress a crucial role in endothelial dysfunction.[7] In patients undergoing either routine diagnostic catheterization for the evaluation of chest pain or percutaneous transluminal coronary angioplasty (PCI), a significantly increased vasoconstrictor response to acetylcholine predicted long-term atherosclerotic disease progression and cardiovascular event rates.[8] Noninvasive endothelial function testing is emerging as a biomarker of vascular disease.[9] The most frequently used endothelial-directed vasodilator stimulus is an increase in blood flow (brachial artery flow-mediated vasodilation, FMD). This is assessed by changes in brachial artery diameter (7–12 MHz linear array probe) after 5-minute blood pressure cuff arterial occlusion. Vasodilation is usually measured 1 minute after cuff release. To assess endothelium-independent vasodilation, the subject is given a single dose of nitroglycerin. Patients with risk factors for coronary heart disease (CHD) have impaired vasodilator responses.[10] Investigators are still seeking to improve the methods for ultrasonographic analysis of brachial artery vasomotion. More precise analysis techniques are now available in the form of automated continuous estimation of brachial artery responses. There is, however, significant biologic variability in measurement, greatly varying in response to factors such as size of the blood pressure cuff, baseline arterial diameter, a high-fat meal, and a women's menstrual cycle. The technique is skill- and labor-intensive and not yet easily used in routine clinical practice.[10]

Ankle–Brachial Index (ABI)

The measurement of the ankle–brachial blood pressure index (ABI) is an easy-to-perform, inexpensive, and reproducible noninvasive test to detect asymptomatic atherosclerotic disease. Technical requirements are a regular blood pressure cuff and a Doppler ultrasound device to measure the systolic blood pressures in left and right brachial arteries as well as both posterior tibial and dorsalis pedis arteries.[10] Usually, the highest systolic ankle pressure is used for calculation. Because of its high sensitivity and specificity (>90% respectively), an ABI <0.90 is considered a reliable sign of peripheral arterial disease (PAD). Its high specificity is partially explained by the fact that the ABI may paradoxically be elevated with age-dependent increased arterial stiffness, including arterial calcification. Therefore, an ABI >1.5 may be difficult to interpret.[11] ABI reflecting significant PAD adds additional validity to medical history, because 50% to 89% of patients with an ABI <0.9 do not have typical claudication.[12] The history of claudication alone "dramatically underestimates" the presence of large-vessel PAD.[13]

The presence of PAD is strongly related to a high incidence of coronary events and stroke. Therefore, ABI also correlates with further development of angina, myocardial infarction, congestive heart failure, coronary artery bypass graft surgery, stroke, or carotid surgery. However, ABI should not be considered as a continuous measure of generalized atherosclerosis.[11] In asymptomatic individuals over 55 years of age, an ABI < 0.9 may be found in 12% to 27%. Even in an elderly population (71–93 years), a low ABI further identifies a higher-risk CHD subgroup.[14] However, a normal ABI does not predict the absence of severe coronary artery disease (CAD).[15]

Imaging for Early Detection of Atherosclerotic Disease

Carotid Ultrasound

Sonography of superficial arteries is a relatively inexpensive means of noninvasively visualizing the lumen and walls of arteries which are involved in the ubiquitous process of atherosclerosis. Risk assessment using carotid ultrasound focuses on measurement of the intima–media thickness (IMT) and plaque characteristics.

Intima–Media Thickness (IMT)

Intima–media thickness is an integrated measurement of the involvement of both the intima and the media in the atherosclerotic process. Current ultrasound instrumentation with transducers ≥8 MHz is capable of identifying the borders between the vessel lumen and the intima as well as between the media and the adventitia. Although there is no uniformly accepted methodology, the common carotid IMT is determined as the average of 12 measurements (6 measurements each from the near and far wall of each of the three segments in both sides). As there is a graded increase of cardiovascular risk with increasing IMT, no cut-off value to distinguish between normal and abnormal has been defined. In young and healthy individuals with multiple traditional risk factors from the Bogalusa Heart Study, IMT increased significantly with the number of risk factors for both common carotid and carotid bulb segments, but not for the internal carotid segment.[16] Persons without known cardiovascular disease with higher IMT values (those in the highest quintile or ≥1 mm) are at increased risk for cardiac events and stroke.[17] When IMT is used to predict the incidence of subsequent stroke, the risk is graded but nonlinear, with hazards increasing more rapidly at lower IMTs than at higher IMTs.[18] Therefore, precision of measurements is of greatest importance in the submillimeter range, which poses high requirements on instruments and physicians. The risk of cardiac events in 4–7 years of follow-up in patients free of clinical coronary artery disease at baseline is also nonlinearly related to IMT.[19]

Plaque Characteristics

Plaque characteristics as assessed by carotid ultrasound were found to be predictive of subsequent cerebral ischemic[20] and coronary[21] events. Patients with echolucent stenotic plaques had a higher risk of cerebrovascular and coronary events than sub-

jects with other plaque types. On B-mode ultrasound assessments, lipids, thrombi, and hemorrhage will all appear as echolucent structures. As the Rotterdam Study showed, noninvasive measures of extracoronary atherosclerosis are predictors of myocardial infarction (MI).[22] The relatively crude measures directly assessing plaques in the carotid artery (and abdominal aorta) predicted MI equally well as the more precisely measured carotid IMT.[22]

Magnetic Resonance Imaging (MRI)

MRI offers direct visualization of the atherosclerotic plaque, allowing identification of plaque components such as the fibrous cap, lipid core, hemorrhage, and thrombosis. It has been evaluated as a means of in vivo imaging of the arterial wall by noninvasively depicting coronary plaques.[23,24] Using optimized three-dimensional (3D) imaging sequences to improve contrast between lumen and vessel wall, a spatial resolution of $0.66 \times 0.66 \times 2$ mm can be obtained. However, longer acquisition times are still a limitation. Regression of the lipid component of atherosclerotic plaques induced in animal models can now be demonstrated by serial in vivo MR examinations.[25] The current fast technical improvement has led to 3D black-blood vessel wall imaging which permits in vivo distinction between "normal" and diseased vessel walls.[26] MRI may identify the fibrous cap in the atherosclerotic aorta.[27] Carotid, aortic, and even coronary plaque assessment with MRI may lead to its use as a scanning tool for quantifying subclinical disease, predicting future cardiovascular events, and evaluating therapeutic interventions. For the present, MRI is a promising research tool, but its use is limited to only a small number of research laboratories. Further advances are needed to reduce the problems from cardiac and respiratory motion and the nonlinear course of the coronary arteries. Thus, MRI is not yet appropriate for use in identifying patients at high risk for CAD in clinical practice.

Ultrafast CT Imaging (EBCT, MSCT)

For cardiac CT imaging, ultrafast techniques are necessary: In Europe, predominantly very fast rotating mechanical CTs are used (MSCT with 16 or more slices simultaneously acquiring the data), while in the US, electron beam CT (EBCT, no mechanically moving parts) is the prevailing technology. Besides the considerably lower costs of MSCT, the spatial resolution of MSCT is superior to EBCT with the temporal resolution still a matter of debate using the "sector technology" for MSCT. In contrast to cardio-MR, cardio-CT easily depicts the presence of calcified plaques of more than 1 mg. In general, there is clinically good agreement between the calcium scores measured by EBCT and MSCT.[28-30] As regards radiation exposure, the effective dose for calcium scoring is 0.7 mSv for EBCT and 1.0 mSv for (prospectively triggered) MSCT.[31] For a practical comparison, the German government allows a radiation dose of 1.0 mSv during pregnancy for an unborn child.

The presence of coronary calcium is identical with "disease" – there is no "normal" calcium in the coronary vessel wall.[3,32] In an international multicenter study of 5345 individuals with no signs or history of CAD, calcified atherosclerotic plaques were present in 63% of men and in 41% of women.[33] The amount of calcified coronary plaques reflects the *total* coronary plaque burden, that is, the more calcified plaques are present, the higher is the amount of non-calcified plaques.[34] In an autopsy study of sudden-death coronary victims, all hearts of age >50 years showed some calcification.[35] A calcified plaque is not necessarily stable; stable and vulnerable plaques contain the same amount of calcium.[35,36]

The use of contrast media for the cardio-CT examination enables non-calcified plaques to be visualized and characterized. The density measurements of non-calcified plaques reflect echogenicity and plaque composition and may allow differentiation between soft and fibrous plaques.[37-39] Cardio-CT may one day be considered a "noninvasive IVUS." At the present time, the clinical role of non-calcified plaques, especially in persons without any calcified plaques, has not yet been determined. Nevertheless, the demonstration of coronary calcium for the first time offers the opportunity to *directly* and *noninvasively* visualize coronary atherosclerosis.

Modern Identification of the High-Risk Individual

In the RECALL Study "any form of atherosclerosis" was present in 53% of the individuals investigated (4814 persons, age 45–74 years), so atherosclerosis is a common finding in people over 45 years.[40,41] Although population-based, general recommendations for risk factor modification make sense, they have not been as successful as expected.[42] In recent years, there has been a shift of paradigm regarding the detection of early atherosclerotic disease. Whereas in the previous versions of the European and US guidelines the detection of "any atherosclerosis" was essential for decision making in further treatment,[43-45] the newer guidelines focus specifically on the assessment of the *individual* risk, particularly on detection of the "high-risk" individual.[4,5,46] The determination of a high "absolute" individual risk has been increasingly recognized as a critical determinant for making decisions about instituting pharmacological therapy for risk reduction in prevention of cardiovascular disease in the US[47] and in Europe.[48,49]

Today, there are two concepts for the definition of a "high-risk" individual, one based on morbidity *and* mortality, and the other on mortality only: For the combination of morbidity and mortality, traditionally the Framingham score[46] or, predominantly in Germany, the PROCAM score[50] are used. Both scores (based on approximately 5000 individuals each, from Framingham/US or industrial workers from Münster/Germany) have determined a "high risk" if the likelihood for a cardiovascular event is >20% per 10 years, that is, 2% per year. The question remains whether data from the US can be extrapolated to Europe.[51] The Framingham and PROCAM scores overestimated the absolute CHD risk of middle-aged men in Belfast and France.[52] These regional differences were considered when introducing the European SCORE system (based on more than 200,000 individuals), focusing only on the hard endpoint "cardiovascular death."[53] Thus, the "SCORE score" has defined "high risk" as a likelihood of >5% to die from cardiovascular disease within the next 10 years.

The Dilemma of Traditional Identification of High-Risk Patients

Two large cohort studies revealed that 80% to 90% of the patients with CHD had at least one of four traditional risk factors (cigarette smoking, hyperlipidemia, arterial hypertension, or diabetes).[54,55] In the clinical practice of prevention, however, we have the opposite problem: of course we treat arterial hypertension and diabetes anyway, but which asymptomatic patient without demonstrable myocardial ischemia with which risk factors is at high risk for developing a cardiovascular event? The identification of high-risk individuals based on a single laboratory parameter may be misleading: for example, only about 50% of patients having an MI demonstrated hypercholesterolemia.[56] Thus, predicting a heart attack based on hypercholesterolemia alone may be like flipping a coin. The diagnosis of a "metabolic syndrome" has not been shown to be of additional value in predicting events as compared to the Framingham score.[57] Adding abdominal obesity, triglycerides, and fasting glucose to these equations provides little or no increase in power of prediction.[57]

The usefulness of newer blood-laboratory parameters to identify high-risk patients is not yet established: There are newer promising data for plasma natriuretic peptide levels predicting cardiovascular events and death.[58] Elevated homocysteine has been shown to be an independent risk factor for MI in middle-aged women.[59] Among older adults, an elevated level of Lp(a) lipoprotein is an independent predictor of stroke, death from vascular disease, and death from any cause in men but not in women.[60] ApoB, apoB/apoA-I and apoA-I were also regarded as highly predictive in evaluation of cardiac risk.[61] The value of C-reactive protein (CRP) in identifying high-risk individuals is a matter of ongoing controversy, with reports describing CRP levels as a marker of atheromatous plaque vulnerability,[62,63] enhancing global risk assessment.[64] A recent study, however, questioned its predictive value and recommended a review of its use for predicting coronary events.[65] Measurement of CRP in elderly people has no additional value in coronary disease prediction when traditional cardiovascular risk factors are already present.[66] Thus, the clinical rel-evance of CRP measurements in the prediction of the risk of CHD remains unproven.[67] Although CRP, Lp(a), homocysteine, apoB, apoA-I, and fibrinogen may be associated with vascular disease risk, their optimal use in routine screening remains to be determined.[68] At the present time it is not clear how to integrate all these blood tests into an evidence-based risk score.

High-risk patients are traditionally identified using one of the three major risk scores, derived from the parameters listed in Table 11-1.

There is, however, one inherent problem in identifying individuals at high risk related to the prevalence. This is explained for the PROCAM score as follows: Figure 11-1 shows the actually observed 10-year coronary events based on the PROCAM score.[50] Taking the prevalence into consideration, the following calculations can be made: A score >61 was observed in 2% of the population with an event rate of 43.2%. Thus, out of 1000 persons, 20 persons (2%) would have a score >61, leading in 9 persons (43.2% of 20 persons) to an event. On the other hand, a score of 45–53 was observed in 15% of the population with an event rate of 14.8%. Thus, out of 1000 persons, 150 persons (15%) would have a score of 45–53, leading in 22 persons (14.8% of 150 persons) to an event. Thus, twice as many patients with a heart attack (62%) come from the "medium-risk" group as from the "high-risk" group (31%) (Figure 11-2). A similar problem has been shown for the Framingham score. Thus, the dilemma is that the guidelines primarily focus on the "high-risk" patients,

TABLE 11-1. Comparison of the parameters used for calculating the individual "absolute" risk according to the three major risk scores

Parameter	Framingham score	PROCAM score	SCORE score
Age	+	+	+
Gender	+	– (men only)	+
Systolic blood pressure	+	+	+
Smoking	+	+	+
Diabetes mellitus	–	+	–
Total cholesterol	+	–	+
HDL cholesterol	+	+	+
LDL cholesterol	–	+	–
Triglycerides	–	+	–
Positive family history	–	+	–

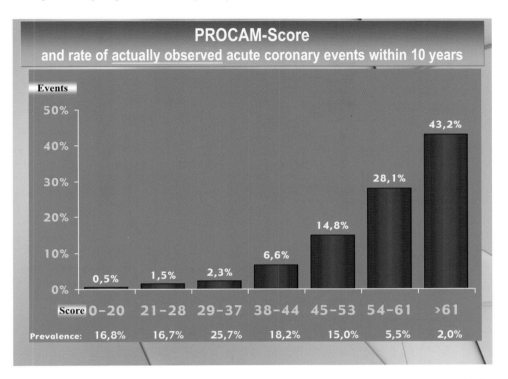

FIGURE 11-1. The PROCAM score, its prevalence, and the percentage of observed acute coronary events within each risk group.

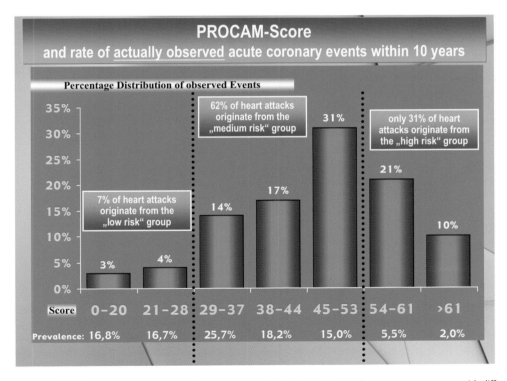

FIGURE 11-2. The PROCAM score, its prevalence, and the percentage distribution of observed acute coronary events with different risk groups.

but most events occur in the large intermediate-risk group. Therefore, an additional method is needed to identify the "true high-risk" individuals hidden in the medium-risk group.

Imaging Methods for the Detection of High-Risk Individuals

An ideal valuable additional tool should meet the following requirements:

- proven independent risk factor (= independent from the risk factors in Table 11.1)
- proven information additional to the traditional risk factors
- no inherent risk
- widely available.

Although MRI is a valuable research tool for assessing plaques in asymptomatic atherosclerotic disease (see above), there are no data proving that this imaging method delivers clinically important, independent, and additional information. Atherosclerosis of the carotid artery as detected by ultrasound (see above) is related to an increased hazard ratio. But neither for MRI nor for carotid ultrasound does data exist regarding how to additionally identify patients at high risk for cardiovascular events, that is, a risk of >2%/year.

Calcium Scoring for the Detection of High-Risk Patients

For the identification of high-risk individuals, the absolute calcium score has to be interpreted within the context of age and gender. Thus each interpretation of the calcium score (e.g. the Agatston score) should describe the percentile allocated to the score.[28,69,70] An overwhelming number of studies have shown that a calcium score, especially in the upper (usually >75%) percentile range, is a predictor of coronary/cardiovascular events, *independent* of the traditional risk factors.[70–81] There is in particular no correlation between the calcium score and LDL or HDL cholesterol,[82] nor any correlation with CRP,[83,84] even after adjusting for traditional risk factors.[85] In an unselected population of subjects older than 55 years, 30% of the men and 15% of the women without risk factors had extensive coronary calcification.[86] There is no or only a weak correla-

tion between calcium scoring and the Framingham risk estimate[87,88] as well as the PROCAM risk factor model.[89]

Three studies have shown that coronary calcium provides independent incremental information in addition to the Framingham score in the prediction of cardiovascular events.[71,76,90] Mortality data from 10,377 asymptomatic individuals with cardiac risk factors showed that when considering the receiver operating curve, the concordance index alone for cardiac risk factors increased from 0.72 to 0.78 ($P < 0.001$) when the calcium score was added to a multivariable model for prediction of death.[76] Another study including 1461 asymptomatic adults has shown that across all Framingham risk categories, calcium scoring was predictive of risk among patients with a Framingham score higher than 10%.[71] All three studies concluded that calcium scoring offers the most additional information among individuals in the Framingham intermediate-risk category. Therefore, the ESC guidelines recommended calcium scoring (with either EBCT or MSCT) as an independent method of incremental information for detecting a subset of high-risk patients.[4,5] Although calcium scoring does not identify an individual vulnerable plaque, it identifies the vulnerable individual.

According to the NCEP guidelines, diabetic patients are already a "CAD equivalent" and should therefore be treated like patients with established CAD.[46] An ABI <0.9 always represents an individual at high risk (see above). Chronic kidney disease is a risk factor for the development of cardiovascular disease. It has been recommended that chronic kidney disease be regarded as a high risk in the full prevention and treatment of CVD risk factors.[91] The role of carotid plaque imaging in ruling out high-risk coronary patients is not yet clear: In the RECALL Study, 52% of 1526 individuals (mean age 58 ± 8 years) with no carotid plaque did have coronary calcified plaques.[40]

The indications for calcium scoring in asymptomatic patients without evidence of myocardial ischemia are listed in Table 11-2.

If high-risk strategies are to have a major impact on CVD in the population, they need to be more widely used than previously envisaged.[49] Combining the two approaches – conventional

TABLE 11-2. Indications for calcium scoring in asymptomatic patients with no demonstrable myocardial ischemia. The highest additional information is obtained in individuals classified as "intermediate risk" according to conventional risk factor scoring

Conventional risk scoring (e.g. Framingham score, PROCAM score)	Calcium scoring
Low-risk patients	Not indicated (no screening method, radiation, not cost-effective)
Intermediate-risk patients:	Indicated (additional information, identification of individuals actually at high risk)
High-risk patients	Not indicated (not necessary, no additional information)
Diabetic patients, ABI < 0.9, chronic kidney disease (carotid plaques?)	Not indicated (not necessary, no additional information, because already at high risk)

risk estimation and calcification measurement – should enable clinicians to better assess the management of asymptomatic individuals.[92]

Once an individual patient has been detected as at "high-risk," an intensive risk factor modification including lifestyle changes and medical therapy should be initiated. An intensive nurse-based educational program, however, was not successful.[93] Obviously, more than patient education is necessary to reach these goals.[94] Fortunately, calcium scoring is helpful in patients' motivation.[95]

Conclusions

Although modern medicine significantly improved the short-term outcome of acute myocardial infarction, it shifted the problem from a decrease in mortality to an increase in morbidity. Therefore, the challenge of modern medicine is to reduce the cardiovascular morbidity, that is, to prevent the first event.

Asymptomatic atherosclerotic disease is defined as the presence of abnormal function or structure of the vessel wall without angina pectoris or demonstrable myocardial ischemia. Functional tests for early detection of asymptomatic atherosclerotic disease are forearm blood flow measurements (not yet clinically established) and the ankle–brachial index (ABI). An ABI <0.9

identifies patients with (even asymptomatic) peripheral artery disease. Carotid ultrasound detects increased intima–media thickness (IMT) and plaque characteristics. The relatively crude measures directly assessing plaques in the carotid artery (and abdominal aorta) predicted myocardial infarction equally well as the more precisely measured carotid IMT. Magnetic resonance imaging (MRI) has been evaluated as a means of in vivo imaging of the arterial wall by noninvasively visualizing coronary plaques, but MRI is not yet appropriate for use in additionally identifying patients at high risk for CAD in clinical practice.

In contrast, cardio-CT easily depicts the presence of calcified plaques. The presence of coronary calcium is identical with "disease" – there is no "normal" calcium in the coronary vessel wall. The amount of calcified coronary plaques reflects the *total* coronary plaque burden; that is, the more calcified plaques are present, the higher the amount of non-calcified plaques. The demonstration of coronary calcium offers for the first time the opportunity to directly visualize coronary atherosclerosis by noninvasive means.

In recent years, there has been a paradigm shift from the detection of "any atherosclerosis" to the assessment of the individual risk, particularly detecting the "high-risk" individual, defined as a risk of >2%/year. High-risk patients can be identified using the Framingham, PROCAM, or SCORE score. There is, however, one inherent problem in identifying individuals at high-risk related to the prevalence: twice as many patients with a heart attack (62%) arise from the "medium-risk" group as from the "high-risk" group. The dilemma is that the guidelines primarily focus on "high-risk" patients, but most events occur in the large intermediate-risk group. Therefore, an additional method is needed to identify the "true high-risk" individuals hidden in the medium-risk group:

An ideal and valuable additional tool should be a proven independent risk factor, provide additional information to the traditional risk factors with no inherent risk, and be widely available. An overwhelming number of studies have shown that a high (percentile) calcium score is a predictor of coronary/cardiovascular events, *independent* of the traditional risk factors. Three studies showed that coronary calcium provides independent incremental information in addition to the Framingham score in the prediction of cardiovascular events. Thus, in asymptomatic individuals with no demonstrable myocardial ischemia, the highest additional information from calcium scoring is obtained in individuals classified as "intermediate risk" according to conventional risk factor scoring. Combining the two approaches – conventional risk estimation and calcification measurement – should enable clinicians to better assess the management of asymptomatic individuals.

References

1. Cooper R, Cutler J, Desvigne-Nickens P, et al. Trends and disparities in coronary heart disease, stroke, and other cardiovascular diseases in the United States: findings of the national conference on cardiovascular disease prevention. Circulation 2000; 102:3137–3147.
2. Unal B, Critchley JA, Capewell S. Explaining the decline in coronary heart disease mortality in England and Wales between 1981 and 2000. Circulation 2004;109:1101–1107.
3. Silber S. Quantification of coronary artery calcifications in the risk stratification of cardiac events. Dtsch Med Wochenschr 2002;127:2575–2578.
4. De Backer G, Ambrosioni E, Borch-Johnsen K, et al. Executive Summary: European guidelines on cardiovascular disease prevention in clinical practice. Third Joint Task Force of European and Other Societies on Cardiovascular Disease Prevention in Clinical Practice (executive summary). Eur Heart J 2003;24:1601–1610.
5. De Backer G, Ambrosioni E, Borch-Johnsen K, et al. Full Version: European guidelines on cardiovascular disease prevention in clinical practice: third joint task force of European and other societies on cardiovascular disease prevention in clinical practice (full version). Eur J Cardiovasc Prev Rehabil 2003;10:S1–S10.
6. Nissen SE, Tsunoda T, Tuzcu EM, et al. Effect of recombinant ApoA-I Milano on coronary atherosclerosis in patients with acute coronary syndromes: a randomized controlled trial. JAMA 2003;290:2292–2300.
7. Heitzer T, Schlinzig T, Krohn K, Meinertz T, Münzel T. Endothelial dysfunction, oxidative stress, and risk of cardiovascular events in patients with coronary artery disease. Circulation 2001;104:2673–2678.
8. Schächinger V, Britten MB, Zeiher AM. Prognostic impact of coronary vasodilator dysfunction on adverse long-term outcome of coronary heart disease. Circulation 2000;101:1899–1906.
9. Verma S, Buchanan MR, Anderson TJ. Endothelial function testing as a biomarker of vascular disease. Circulation 2003;108:2054–2059.
10. Smith SC Jr, Greenland P, Grundy SM. AHA Conference Proceedings. Prevention conference V: Beyond secondary prevention: Identifying the high-risk patient for primary prevention: executive summary and full version. Circulation 2000;101: 111–116 (full version: e116–e122).
11. Oei HH, Vliegenthart R, Hak AE, et al. The association between coronary calcification assessed by electron beam computed tomography and measures of extracoronary atherosclerosis: the Rotterdam Coronary Calcification Study. J Am Coll Cardiol 2002;39:1745–1751.
12. Hirsch AT, Criqui MH, Treat-Jacobson D, et al. Peripheral arterial disease detection, awareness, and treatment in primary care. JAMA 2001;286: 1317–1324.
13. Criqui MH, Fronek A, Barrett-Connor E, Klauber MR, Gabriel S, Goodman D. The prevalence of peripheral arterial disease in a defined population. Circulation 1985;71:510–515.
14. Abbott RD, Petrovitch H, Rodriguez BL, et al. Ankle/brachial blood pressure in men > 70 years of age and the risk of coronary heart disease. Am J Cardiol 2000;86:280–284.
15. Otah KE, Madan A, Otah E, Badero O, Clark LT, Salifu MO. Usefulness of an abnormal ankle-brachial index to predict presence of coronary artery disease in African-Americans. Am J Cardiol 2004;93:481–483.
16. Urbina EM, Srinivasan SR, Tang R, Bond MG, Kieltyka L, Berenson GS. Impact of multiple coronary risk factors on the intima-media thickness of different segments of carotid artery in healthy young adults (The Bogalusa Heart Study). Am J Cardiol 2002;90:953–958.
17. O'Leary DH, Polak JF, Kronmal RA, Manolio TA, Burke GL, Wolfson SK, Jr. Carotid-artery intima and media thickness as a risk factor for myocardial infarction and stroke in older adults. Cardiovascular Health Study Collaborative Research Group. N Engl J Med 1999;340:14–22.
18. Chambless LE, Folsom AR, Clegg LX, et al. Carotid wall thickness is predictive of incident clinical stroke: the Atherosclerosis Risk in Communities (ARIC) study. Am J Epidemiol 2000;151:478–487.
19. Chambless LE, Heiss G, Folsom AR, et al. Association of coronary heart disease incidence with

carotid arterial wall thickness and major risk factors: the Atherosclerosis Risk in Communities (ARIC) Study, 1987–1993. Am J Epidemiol 1997;146: 483–494.

20. Mathiesen EB, Bonaa KH, Joakimsen O. Echolucent plaques are associated with high risk of ischemic cerebrovascular events in carotid stenosis: the Tromso study. Circulation 2001;103:2171–2175.

21. Honda O, Sugiyama S, Kugiyama K, et al. Echolucent carotid plaques predict future coronary events in patients with coronary artery disease. J Am Coll Cardiol 2004;43:1177–1184.

22. van der Meer IM, Bots ML, Hofman A, del Sol AI, van der Kuip DA, Witteman JC. Predictive value of noninvasive measures of atherosclerosis for incident myocardial infarction: the Rotterdam Study. Circulation 2004;109:1089–1094.

23. Botnar RM, Stuber M, Kissinger KV, Kim WY, Spuentrup E, Manning WJ. Noninvasive coronary vessel wall and plaque imaging with magnetic resonance imaging. Circulation 2000;102:2582–2587.

24. Fayad ZA, Fuster V, Fallon JT, et al. Noninvasive in vivo human coronary artery lumen and wall imaging using black-blood magnetic resonance imaging. Circulation 2000;102:506–510.

25. Helft G, Worthley SG, Fuster V, et al. Progression and regression of atherosclerotic lesions: monitoring with serial noninvasive magnetic resonance imaging. Circulation 2002;105:993–998.

26. Kim WY, Stuber M, Bornert P, Kissinger KV, Manning WJ, Botnar RM. Three-dimensional black-blood cardiac magnetic resonance coronary vessel wall imaging detects positive arterial remodeling in patients with nonsignificant coronary artery disease. Circulation 2002;106:296–299.

27. Kramer CM, Cerilli LA, Hagspiel K, DiMaria JM, Epstein FH, Kern JA. Magnetic resonance imaging identifies the fibrous cap in atherosclerotic abdominal aortic aneurysm. Circulation 2004;109:1016–1021.

28. Schmermund A, Erbel R, Silber S. Age and gender distribution of coronary artery calcium measured by four-slice computed tomography in 2,030 persons with no symptoms of coronary artery disease. The MUNICH registry. Am J Cardiol 2002;90:168–173.

29. Stanford W, Thompson BH, Burns TL, Heery SD, Burr MC. Coronary artery calcium quantification at multi-detector row helical CT versus electron-beam CT. Radiology 2004;230:397–402.

30. Becker CR, Jakobs TF, Aydemir S, et al. Helical and single-slice conventional CT versus electron beam CT for the quantification of coronary artery calcification. AJR Am J Roentgenol 2000;174:543–547.

31. Morin RL, Gerber TC, McCollough CH. Radiation dose in computed tomography of the heart. Circulation 2003;107:917–922.

32. Sangiorgi G, Rumberger JA, Severson A, et al. Arterial calcification and not lumen stenosis is highly correlated with atherosclerotic plaque burden in humans: a histologic study of 723 coronary artery segments using nondecalcifying methodology. J Am Coll Cardiol 1998;31:126–133.

33. Silber S, Shemesh J, Weg N, Yoon HC. Multicentre age and gender distribution of coronary artery calcification as measured by four-slice computed tomography in 5,345 people. Eur Heart J 2003; 24(Suppl):570.

34. Rumberger JA, Simons DB, Fitzpatrick LA, Sheedy PF, Schwartz RS. Coronary artery calcium area by electron-beam computed tomography and coronary atherosclerotic plaque area. A histopathologic correlative study. Circulation 1995;92:2157–2162.

35. Burke AP, Taylor A, Farb A, Malcom GT, Virmani R. Coronary calcification: insights from sudden coronary death victims. Z Kardiol 2000;89(Suppl 2):49–53.

36. Schmermund A, Erbel R. Unstable coronary plaque and its relation to coronary calcium. Circulation 2001;104:1682–1687.

37. Leber AW, Knez A, Becker A, et al. Accuracy of multidetector spiral computed tomography in identifying and differentiating the composition of coronary atherosclerotic plaques: a comparative study with intracoronary ultrasound. J Am Coll Cardiol 2004;43:1241–1247.

38. Achenbach S, Moselewski F, Ropers D, et al. Detection of calcified and noncalcified coronary atherosclerotic plaque by contrast-enhanced, submillimeter multidetector spiral computed tomography: a segment-based comparison with intravascular ultrasound. Circulation 2004;109:14–17.

39. Schroeder S, Kopp AF, Baumbach A, et al. Noninvasive detection and evaluation of atherosclerotic coronary plaques with multislice computed tomography. J Am Coll Cardiol 2001;37:1430–1435.

40. Erbel R, Schmermund A, Stang A, et al. The "Heinz Nixdorf RECALL Study": Improvement of prediction of risk for myocardial infarction based on known and newer risk factors as well on modern imaging and non-imaging methods. Z Kardiol 2004;93(Suppl. 3):III/244.

41. Schmermund A, Möhlenkamp S, Stang A, et al. Assessment of clinically silent atherosclerotic disease and established and novel risk factors for predicting myocardial infarction and cardiac death in healthy middle-aged subjects: rationale and design of the Heinz Nixdorf RECALL Study. Risk

Factors, Evaluation of Coronary Calcium and Lifestyle. Am Heart J 2002;144:212–218.

42. The EUROASPIRE I and II Group, Clinical reality of coronary prevention guidelines: a comparison of EUROASPIRE I and II in nine countries. EUROASPIRE I and II Group. European Action on Secondary Prevention by Intervention to Reduce Events. Lancet 2001;357:995–1001.

43. The NCEP Expert Panel, Summary of the second report of the National Cholesterol Education Program (NCEP) Expert Panel on Detection, Evaluation, and Treatment of High Blood Cholesterol in Adults (Adult Treatment Panel II). JAMA 1993;269:3015–3023.

44. The NCEP Expert Panel, National Cholesterol Education Program. Second Report of the Expert Panel on Detection, Evaluation, and Treatment of High Blood Cholesterol in Adults (Adult Treatment Panel II). Circulation 1994;89:1333–1445.

45. Wood D, De Backer G, Faergeman O, Graham I, Mancia G, Pyorala K. Prevention of coronary heart disease in clinical practice. Summary of recommendations of the Second Joint Task Force of European and other Societies on Coronary Prevention. Eur Heart J 1998;19:1434–1503.

46. The NCEP Expert Panel, Executive Summary of The Third Report of The National Cholesterol Education Program (NCEP) Expert Panel on Detection, Evaluation, and Treatment of High Blood Cholesterol in Adults (Adult Treatment Panel III). JAMA 2001;285:2486–2497.

47. Grundy SM, Bazzarre T, Cleeman J, et al. Prevention Conference V: Beyond secondary prevention: identifying the high-risk patient for primary prevention: medical office assessment: Writing Group I. Circulation 2000;101:e3–e11.

48. Hennekens CH, D'Agostino RB. Global risk assessment for cardiovascular disease and astute clinical judgement. Eur Heart J 2003;24:1899–1900.

49. Emberson J, Whincup P, Morris R, Walker M, Ebrahim S. Evaluating the impact of population and high-risk strategies for the primary prevention of cardiovascular disease. Eur Heart J 2004;25: 484–491.

50. Assmann G, Cullen P, Schulte H. Simple scoring scheme for calculating the risk of acute coronary events based on the 10-year follow-up of the prospective cardiovascular Munster (PROCAM) study. Circulation 2002;105:310–315.

51. Brindle P, Emberson J, Lampe F, et al. Predictive accuracy of the Framingham coronary risk score in British men: prospective cohort study. BMJ 2003; 327:1267.

52. Empana JP, Ducimetiere P, Arveiler D, et al. Are the Framingham and PROCAM coronary heart disease risk functions applicable to different European populations? The PRIME Study. Eur Heart J 2003;24:1903–1911.

53. Conroy RM, Pyorala K, Fitzgerald AP, et al. Estimation of ten-year risk of fatal cardiovascular disease in Europe: the SCORE project. Eur Heart J 2003;24:987–1003.

54. Greenland P, Knoll MD, Stamler J, et al. Major risk factors as antecedents of fatal and nonfatal coronary heart disease events. JAMA 2003;290:891–897.

55. Khot UN, Khot MB, Bajzer CT, et al. Prevalence of conventional risk factors in patients with coronary heart disease. JAMA 2003;290:898–904.

56. Böger GI, Hoopmann M, Busse R, Budinger M, Welte T, Böger RH, Drug therapy of coronary heart disease – are therapeutic guidelines being paid attention to? Z Kardiol 2003;92:466–475.

57. Grundy SM, Hansen B, Smith SC Jr, Cleeman JI, Kahn RA. Clinical management of metabolic syndrome: report of the American Heart Association/ National Heart, Lung, and Blood Institute/ American Diabetes Association conference on scientific issues related to management. Circulation 2004;109:551–556.

58. Wang TJ, Larson MG, Levy D, et al. Plasma natriuretic peptide levels and the risk of cardiovascular events and death. N Engl J Med 2004;350:655–663.

59. Zylberstein DE, Bengtsson C, Bjorkelund C, et al. 4-year follow-up of the population study of women in Gothenburg. Circulation 2004;109:601–606.

60. Ariyo AA, Thach C, Tracy R. Lp(a) lipoprotein, vascular disease, and mortality in the elderly. N Engl J Med 2003;349:2108–2115.

61. Walldius G, Jungner I, Holme I, Aastveit AH, Kolar W, Steiner E. High apolipoprotein B, low apolipoprotein A-I, and improvement in the prediction of fatal myocardial infarction (AMORIS study): a prospective study. Lancet 2001;358:2026–2033.

62. Arroyo-Espliguero R, Avanzas P, Cosin-Sales J, Aldama G, Pizzi C, Kaski JC. C-reactive protein elevation and disease activity in patients with coronary artery disease. Eur Heart J 2004;25:401–408.

63. Ridker PM, Cushman M, Stampfer MJ, Tracy RP, Hennekens CH. Inflammation, aspirin, and the risk of cardiovascular disease in apparently healthy men. N Engl J Med 1997;336:973–979.

64. Koenig W, Lowel H, Baumert J, Meisinger C. C-reactive protein modulates risk prediction based on the Framingham Score: implications for future risk assessment: results from a large cohort study in southern Germany. Circulation 2004;109:1349–1353.

65. Danesh J, Wheeler JG, Hirschfield GM, et al. C-reactive protein and other circulating markers of

inflammation in the prediction of coronary heart disease. N Engl J Med 2004;350:1387–1397.

66. van der Meer IM, de Maat MP, Kiliaan AJ, van der Kuip DA, Hofman A, Witteman JC. The value of C-reactive protein in cardiovascular risk prediction: the Rotterdam Study. Arch Intern Med 2003;163: 1323–1328.

67. Tall AR, C-reactive protein reassessed. N Engl J Med 2004;350:1450–1452.

68. Hackam DG, Anand SS. Emerging risk factors for atherosclerotic vascular disease: a critical review of the evidence. JAMA 2003;290:932–940.

69. Agatston AS, Janowitz WR, Hildner FJ, Zusmer NR, Viamonte M Jr, Detrano R. Quantification of coronary artery calcium using ultrafast computed tomography. J Am Coll Cardiol 1990;15:827–832.

70. Raggi P, Callister TQ, Cooil B, et al. Identification of patients at increased risk of first unheralded acute myocardial infarction by electron-beam computed tomography. Circulation 2000;101:850–855.

71. Greenland P, LaBree L, Azen SP, Doherty TM, Detrano RC. Coronary artery calcium score combined with Framingham score for risk prediction in asymptomatic individuals. JAMA 2004;291:210–215.

72. Arad Y, Spadaro LA, Goodman K, et al. Predictive value of electron beam computed tomography of the coronary arteries. 19-month follow-up of 1173 asymptomatic subjects. Circulation 1996;93:1951–1953.

73. Arad Y, Spadaro LA, Goodman K, Newstein D, Guerci AD. Prediction of coronary events with electron beam computed tomography. J Am Coll Cardiol 2000;36:1253–1260.

74. Kondos GT, Hoff JA, Sevrukov A, et al. Electron-beam tomography coronary artery calcium and cardiac events: a 37-month follow-up of 5635 initially asymptomatic low- to intermediate-risk adults. Circulation 2003;107:2571–2576.

75. Möhlenkamp S, Lehmann N, Schmermund A, et al. Prognostic value of extensive coronary calcium quantities in symptomatic males – a 5-year follow-up study. Eur Heart J 2003;24:845–854.

76. Shaw LJ, Raggi P, Schisterman E, Berman DS, Callister TQ. Prognostic value of cardiac risk factors and coronary artery calcium screening for all-cause mortality. Radiology 2003;228:826–833.

77. Vliegenthart R, Oudkerk M, Song B, van der Kuip DA, Hofman A, Witteman JC. Coronary calcification detected by electron-beam computed tomography and myocardial infarction. The Rotterdam Coronary Calcification Study. Eur Heart J 2002;23: 1596–1603.

78. Wayhs R, Zelinger A, Raggi P. High coronary artery calcium scores pose an extremely elevated risk for hard events. J Am Coll Cardiol 2002;39:225–230.

79. Wong ND, Hsu JC, Detrano RC, Diamond G, Eisenberg H, Gardin JM. Coronary artery calcium evaluation by electron beam computed tomography and its relation to new cardiovascular events. Am J Cardiol 2000;86:495–498.

80. Taylor AJ, Burke AP, O'Malley PG, et al. A comparison of the Framingham risk index, coronary artery calcification, and culprit plaque morphology in sudden cardiac death. Circulation 2000;101:1243–1248.

81. Taylor AJ, Feuerstein I, Wong H, Barko W, Brazaitis M, O'Malley PG. Do conventional risk factors predict subclinical coronary artery disease? Results from the Prospective Army Coronary Calcium Project. Am Heart J 2001;141:463–468.

82. Hecht HS, Superko HR, Electron beam tomography and National Cholesterol Education Program guidelines in asymptomatic women. J Am Coll Cardiol 2001;37:1506–1511.

83. Hunt ME, O'Malley PG, Vernalis MN, Feuerstein IM, Taylor AJ. C-reactive protein is not associated with the presence or extent of calcified subclinical atherosclerosis. Am Heart J 2001;141:206–210.

84. Reilly MP, Wolfe ML, Localio AR, Rader DJ. C-reactive protein and coronary artery calcification: The Study of Inherited Risk of Coronary Atherosclerosis (SIRCA). Arterioscler Thromb Vasc Biol 2003;23:1851–1856.

85. Schmermund A, Stang A, Moebus S, et al. Is there an association of high-sensitive C-reactive protein with coronary calcium? The Heinz Nixdorf RECALL Study. J Am Coll Cardiol 2004;43(Suppl A): 334A.

86. Oei HH, Vliegenthart R, Hofman A, Oudkerk M, Witteman JC. Risk factors for coronary calcification in older subjects. The Rotterdam Coronary Calcification Study. Eur Heart J 2004;25:48–55.

87. Schmermund A, Lehmann N, Möhlenkamp S, et al. Independent information provided by Framingham risk algorithm and coronary calcium scores in a large German population sample: Heinz Nixdorf RECALL Study. J Am Coll Cardiol 2004;43(Suppl. A):334A.

88. Desai MY, Nasir K, Braunstein JB, et al. Framingham risk estimate is weakly correlated with coronary artery calcification in asymptomatic population. J Am Coll Cardiol 2004;43(Suppl A):363A.

89. Achenbach S, Nomayo A, Couturier G, et al. Relation between coronary calcium and 10-year risk scores in primary prevention patients. Am J Cardiol 2003;92:1471–1475.

90. Arad Y, Newstein D, Roth M, Guerci AD. Rationale and design of the St. Francis Heart Study: a randomized clinical trial of atorvastatin plus antioxidants in asymptomatic persons with elevated coronary calcification. Control Clin Trials 2001;22:553–572.

91. Sarnak MJ, Levey AS, Schoolwerth AC, et al. Kidney disease as a risk factor for development of cardiovascular disease: a statement from the American Heart Association Councils on Kidney in Cardiovascular Disease, High Blood Pressure Research, Clinical Cardiology, and Epidemiology and Prevention. Circulation 2003;108:2154–2169.

92. Thompson GR, Partridge J, Coronary calcification score: the coronary-risk impact factor. Lancet 2004;363:557–559.

93. Lichtman JH, Amatruda J, Yaari S, et al. Clinical trial of an educational intervention to achieve recommended cholesterol levels in patients with coronary artery disease. Am Heart J 2004;147:522–528.

94. Kline-Rogers EM, Eagle KA. It takes more than patient education to reach low-density lipoprotein cholesterol goals. Am Heart J 2004;147:381–382.

95. Kalia NK, Miller LG, Budoff MJ. Higher coronary calcification scores improve adherence to cardiac risk factor-modifying behaviors. J Am Coll Cardiol 2004.43:363A (abstract).

Section II
Exercise Testing in Heart Disease

Main Messages

Chapter 12: The Molecular Base of Exercise

The pathogenesis of exercise intolerance in cardiovascular diseases is more complex than previously thought. In *coronary artery disease* (CAD) it was commonly believed that the degree of epicardial coronary stenoses correlated with the severity of myocardial ischemia. This is, however, not necessarily the case. With the increasing knowledge about endothelial dysfunction it has become evident that even mild stenoses may cause critical ischemia when combined with pathologic endothelial vasoconstriction in response to catecholamines or exposure to cold temperatures. Basically, regional myocardial hypoperfusion in CAD results from a combination of four basic pathogenetic components: vascular stenosis, coronary vasomotion, microrheology and hemostasis, and mobilization of endothelial progenitor cells (EPCs). Exercise training has the potential to affect all components. Although regression of vascular stenoses is rarely observed, exercise clearly retards the progression of atherosclerotic lesions. Endothelial function is dramatically improved by training interventions as a result of increased expression/activation of the key enzyme endothelial nitric oxide synthase (eNOS) and reduction of reactive oxygen species. Microrheology is improved and hemostasis reduced. Novel data from both animal experiments and clinical studies indicate that exercise enhances the release of EPCs from the bone marrow into the circulation. These cells contribute to the formation of new vessels in ischemic tissue areas and repair endothelial lesions in atherosclerotic vessels.

In *chronic heart failure* (CHF) the degree of left ventricular dysfunction is unrelated to the extent of exercise intolerance. Peripheral factors like the neurohormonal system, endothelial dysfunction, and an inflammatory peripheral myopathy play a much greater role in determining the exercise limitations associated with CHF. Exercise training programs favorably affect neurohormonal activation by reducing circulating catecholamines, angiotensin II, and aldosterone by up to one-third. Endothelial function is significantly improved, leading to reduced peripheral resistance and a hemodynamically relevant afterload reduction. Finally, the inflammatory/catabolic activation found in skeletal muscle biopsies of patients with CHF is reversed and muscle wasting halted by endurance training programs.

Thus, in both CAD and CHF exercise-based interventions have the potential to interfere with the underlying disease processes and to improve the patient's prognosis.

Chapter 13: Exercise and Fitness

The body of epidemiologic research demonstrating the health benefits of physical activity spans more than five decades. A sedentary lifestyle, lack of physical fitness, or both, are major precursors for cardiovascular disease (CVD). Even relatively modest increases in levels of fitness or physical activity patterns are associated with substantial health benefits. However, in countries that have reported evidence supporting the role of physical activity in health the majority of citizens do not get enough physical activity to achieve health benefits. Likewise, only a small percentage of patients who are eligible for cardiac rehabilitation are referred to a program.

The state of being sedentary and low levels of fitness are in and of themselves CVD risk factors. Therefore, mechanisms underlying the health benefits of regular exercise include counteracting the state of being sedentary, and the potential increases in fitness level that occur with activity. Other mechanisms are the favorable influence on CVD risk, including reductions in blood pressure and body weight, improved lipid profile, inflammatory markers and insulin sensitivity. Exercise training appears to have a profound effect on endothelial dysfunction and thus on the vasodilatory properties of the vasculature.

Western societies have become more sedentary in the last two decades, which has led to an increase in the prevalence of several chronic conditions. Efforts are required from government agencies, healthcare providers, and health organizations in order to offset this trend. This chapter provides an overview of the epidemiologic evidence associating physical activity and fitness level with better health outcomes, and the physiologic benefits of activity.

Chapter 14: Exercise Testing in Coronary Heart Disease

Exercise testing is probably the most often performed diagnostic test for persons with suspected coronary heart disease. It provides not only information about ST-segment depression, heart rate, and blood pressure during and after exercise but more importantly information also on the overall exercise performance in relation to the expected performance adjusted for age and gender, which is of greater prognostic importance than a limited look at the ST segments. Exercise testing provides additional prognostic information particularly in persons with an intermediate pretest probability of disease. This chapter provides a thorough overview of the different types of exercise testing from treadmill exercise to different imaging modalities, and is aimed at the interested new-

comer in this area as well as the expert, already familiar with the details of the most recent modifications. Introduction to exercise testing is an introduction to cardiology!

Chapter 15: Cardiopulmonary Exercise Testing in Chronic Heart Failure

Cardiopulmonary exercise testing (CPX) provides major insights regarding the degree of functional impairment, the overall circulatory response to exercise, the prognosis, and the effect of treatment in patients with heart failure. Although peak oxygen uptake (peak VO_2) is the most important variable used to evaluate exercise capacity and prognosis, CPX provides a lot of information besides peak VO_2. This chapter gives clues on how to utilize this information, which now has an important place in the evaluation of the patient with heart failure. It is a rather inexpensive and safe procedure with the potential to provide information that is of key importance for these patients and their physicians: how much oxygen can be delivered to the tissues and what are the potential best treatment modalities?

Chapter 16: Exercise Testing in Valvular Heart Disease

Although more often performed in patients with suspected or proven coronary artery disease, exercise testing is also of great value in patients with valvular heart disease. It has an important role in eliciting symptoms in asymptomatic patients, in evaluating atypical symptoms, and in assessing true exercise capacity. Exercise testing is not only of prognostic importance but is also useful for advising patients about their physical activities and exercise limits. It also gives clues about where and how to start medical therapy (heart rate or blood pressure control). After valve interventions or valve surgery an exercise test is advised prior to starting an exercise training program, to assess its safety but also to evaluate the medical management. Exercise testing should be used more often to optimize clinical management in patients with valvular heart disease.

12
The Molecular Base of Exercise

Rainer Hambrecht

The Causes of Exercise Intolerance in Cardiovascular Diseases

Exercise intolerance is a key feature of most cardiovascular diseases. Its value for describing the stage of the disease is so important that standardized classification systems of exercise limitation (i.e. the New York Heart Association Classification) were developed more than half a century ago. While the symptoms of reduced maximal exercise capacity may be similar, the underlying mechanisms causing exercise limitations are fundamentally different between major disease entities:

In stenotic *coronary artery disease* (CAD) the patient is limited by the mismatch between myocardial perfusion and oxygen demand during physical exertion. The onset of relative myocardial ischemia determines the exercise capacity and is typically characterized by the development of angina pectoris. However, coronary stenoses are not the only source of myocardial ischemia – frequently they only become hemodynamically relevant in the presence of endothelial dysfunction, where an additional vasoconstriction can critically diminish coronary blood flow in moderate stenoses. Alterations in coronary vascular endothelial function were first described in 1986 when Ludmer et al. observed a paradoxical vasoconstriction of atherosclerotic segments after infusing acetylcholine into the left coronary artery of patients with atypical chest pain.[1] It has been shown that a paradoxical response to acetylcholine is indicative of a greater vasoconstrictive effect of both endogenous and exogenous catecholamines (i.e. norepinephrine and phenylephrine). Sympathetic activation and consecutive release of catecholamines occurs during physical activity, exposure to cold, or mental stress. In all these contexts paradoxical epicardial coronary vasoconstriction has been described, which makes endothelial dysfunction a likely pathomechanism to explain stress- or exercise-induced angina pectoris in stable coronary artery disease.[2]

In *chronic heart failure* (CHF) exercise intolerance has traditionally been regarded as a consequence of either *forward failure* with inadequate rise in cardiac output during physical exertion or as secondary to *backward failure* with pulmonary congestion and dyspnea. However, this view was shattered in the 1980s when cardiologists found no correlation between the degree of left ventricular dysfunction (as measured by ejection fraction) and maximal exercise capacity.[3] If central hemodynamics were not the principal determining factor, alternative concepts needed to be generated. The first focus was on systemic alterations in CHF: In the *neurohormonal concept* CHF was viewed as a clinical process that was initiated by myocardial dysfunction but then affected virtually any organ system as a consequence of activation of the renin–angiotensin–aldosterone system (RAAS) and augmented circulating catecholamines.[4] This pathophysiological model of CHF is still valid today and has been extended by new findings of immune activation and inflammation in CHF in recent years.[5]

Building on this model, peripheral changes associated with neurohumoral and inflammatory activation have been systematically analyzed in the last decade. Characteristic changes of endothelial function, respiration, and skeletal muscle function – to name the factors most closely associated with exercise intolerance – have been found. Today we know that CHF causes a peripheral hypoperfusion due to impaired endothelium-dependent vasodilation,[6] reduces the strength of respiratory muscles,[7] and leads to profound morphologic,[8,9] metabolic,[10,11] and functional alterations in the skeletal muscles.[12] In the course of these scientific advances peripheral changes have become a new therapeutic target.

Over the last two decades the clinical application of physical exercise as a therapeutic strategy has developed from rehabilitation to exercise treatment of cardiovascular diseases. This shift in clinical application was accompanied by a more systematic research approach to the involved mechanisms and the objective clinical assessment of sport interventions using prospective randomized clinical trials. This ongoing process established physical exercise as an evidence-based and guideline-oriented treatment option.

In this chapter some important molecular mechanisms involved in the training response to exercise will be discussed. Training mechanisms will be presented for two clinically important disease entities, which together represent the largest proportion of patients enrolled in rehabilitation programs: stable coronary artery disease (CAD) and chronic heart failure (CHF).

Organ-Specific Adaptations to Exercise in Cardiovascular Diseases

Exercise Training in Coronary Artery Disease

Effects of Exercise on the Vascular Endothelium in Atherosclerotic Disease

Despite the clear prognostic benefits of exercise training in reducing cardiovascular events, the underlying mechanisms have long remained obscure. Basically, regional myocardial hypoperfusion in CAD results from a combination of four pathogenetic components: (A) vascular stenosis, (B) coronary vasomotion, (C) microrheology and hemostasis, and (D) mobilization of EPCs. All four components may be affected by exercise training in stable CAD.

(A) Vascular Stenosis

The initial hypothesis that training would lead to a regression of coronary artery stenosis was not substantiated in the majority of patients. Only those with vigorous training programs were able to actually reverse the process of atherosclerosis. However, training was effective in retarding disease progression.[13]

(B) Coronary Vasomotion

Coronary vasomotion is influenced by mechanical and agonist-mediated stimuli, both of which converge on endothelial nitric oxide synthesis/release as the final common pathway. Endothelial dysfunction occurs as a result of decreased bioactive nitric oxide concentrations at vascular smooth muscle cells.

Nitric oxide concentrations can be affected by alterations at different steps of the NO pathway:

1. Availability of the precursor molecule L-arginine.

2. Alterations in NO synthesis rate as determined by endothelial nitric oxide synthase (eNOS) conformational changes, expression, or genetic polymorphism.

3. Differences in NO breakdown velocity related to reactive oxidative species (ROS) once it is released (Figure 12-1).[14]

4. Finally, endothelial regeneration by circulating bone-marrow derived endothelial progenitor cells (EPCs) is increasingly recognized as an important contributing factor for the pathogenesis of endothelial dysfunction.

1. L-Arginine. The availability of L-arginine at the active site of eNOS depends on several factors: First, exogenous supply with L-arginine or endogenous synthesis. Second, intracellular accumulation of L-arginine, which depends on an active cytokine-regulated transmembraneous transport. Third, intracellular degradation of L-arginine. Fourth, nitric oxide synthesis from L-arginine may be blocked by its endogenous antagonist asymmetric dimethyl arginine (ADMA).[15] Today, there is little doubt that a relative L-arginine deficiency is involved in

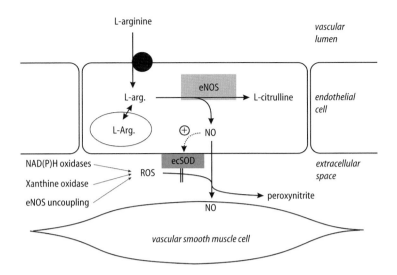

FIGURE 12-1. Endothelial dysfunction develops as a consequence of several changes: L-arginine uptake and intracellular substrate availability are reduced, eNOS expression is lowered, and extracellular inactivation of NO by reactive oxygen species (ROS) is increased. The major sources of ROS in the vascular wall are NAD(P)H oxidases, xanthine oxidase, and eNOS uncoupling. As a net effect, less NO reaches its target organ, the vascular smooth muscle cell.

reduced NO generation. A rare genetic disorder (lysinuric protein intolerance – LPI) serves as a proof-of-concept model: In a patient with LPI markedly reduced L-arginine serum levels and endothelial dysfunction were described. A 30 min intravenous L-arginine infusion led to a dramatic improvement of endothelial function.[16] Clinical intervention studies with oral L-arginine supplementation documented an improvement of endothelium-dependent vasodilation in several clinical situations like hypercholesterolemia, hypertension, diabetes, and chronic heart failure.[17–19] The effect of L-arginine supplementation on vascular function is dose-dependent as evidenced by diverging results of low-dose and high-dose studies in patients with stable CAD: While 9 g/day had no effect on vasomotion in patients with stable CAD,[20] studies with either high-dose intracoronary L-arginine administration or 21 g/day oral supplementation showed a significant improvement of endothelium-dependent vasodilation.[21]

In contrast to these encouraging results in pathologic situations, dietary L-arginine uptake was unrelated to the incidence of acute coronary events among 1981 men in the Kuopio Ischaemic Heart Disease Risk Factor Study.[22]

2. Endothelial Nitric Oxide Synthase. The activity of eNOS as the key enzyme for endothelial NO generation can be modulated on several different levels: gene polymorphisms, mRNA expression, conformational changes, phosphorylation, and cofactor availability.

Among patients with overt atherosclerosis a number of *gene polymorphisms* of the eNOS gene have been described in recent years. Recent clinical trials suggest that the T768C and the Glu298Asp polymorphism may be associated with an increased risk for premature development of CAD.[23,24] However, data are still controversial, with other studies failing to show an association between the Glu298Asp polymorphism and atherosclerotic heart disease.[25] Data from training studies with invasive measurement of endothelial function suggest that the improvement of vasomotion after exercise is attenuated or even abolished in eNOS promoter (T768C) polymorphisms.[26] These data may have important implications for exercise-based rehabilitation strategies.

In a proatherosclerotic setting with high levels of oxidized low-density lipoprotein (oxLDL), elevated serum cytokines like TNF-α, and hypoxia, eNOS *expression* is significantly reduced (reviewed in Harrison et al.[27]).

eNOS *phosphorylation* plays an important role in short-term regulation of enzyme activity in response to flow conditions. Increased shear stress leads to an increased phosphorylation at Ser[1177] with consecutive conformational changes leading to augmented NO generation.[28]

Finally, tetrahydrobiopterin (THB) is a necessary *cofactor* for NO production. However, in the absence of THB, eNOS uses molecular oxygen instead of L-arginine as a substrate, which leads to production of the toxic free radical superoxide O^{2-} turning the enzyme "from good to evil." This process is also referred to as eNOS uncoupling.

3. Nitric Oxide Breakdown.
The integrity of endothelial function depends on an intricate balance between endothelial NO production and extracellular NO degradation. To cause vasodilation NO must reach the vascular smooth muscle cells by diffusion. In this way NO can be prematurely degraded in the presence of reactive oxygen species (OH, H_2O_2) leading to the formation of toxic peroxynitrite (Figure 12-1), which in turn can induce endothelial cell damage and apoptosis by itself.

Several sources of ROS have been identified in endothelial dysfunction: (1) Adventitial NADPH oxidases, for example, produce quantities of superoxide high enough to affect endothelial function.[29] (2) Xanthine oxidase (XO) contributes to ROS generation especially in patients with CHF, where XO inhibition with oral or intra-arterial allopurinol led to significant improvements in endothelium-dependent vasodilation.[30]

The extracellular levels of ROS are also modulated by an antioxidative enzyme produced by the vascular smooth muscle cells: The extracellular superoxide dismutase (ecSOD) is induced by NO itself in a time- and dose-dependent fashion.[31] It may be that despite constant or even slightly increased SOD the prevalence of large amounts of ROS in atherosclerosis leads to a mismatch between oxidative stress and antioxidative enzyme capacity resulting in decreased NO half-life.

4. Endothelial Progenitor Cell.
The endothelium undergoes a constant process of cellular aging, apoptosis, and regeneration of endothelial cells. Contrary to previous concepts, regeneration of endothelial cells in areas of diseased/damaged endothelium occurs not only from neighboring endothelial cells by cell division but also from a pool of bone-marrow-derived circulating endothelial progenitor cells (EPCs). It has been documented that these cells are reduced in the presence of established cardiovascular risk factors.[32]

EPCs are also involved in collateral formation. In the past it was believed that sprouting of pre-existent vessels (i.e. angiogenesis) was the only way of forming new vessels in ischemic areas. In recent years it has become evident that EPCs are capable of forming entirely new vessels in a process termed *vasculogenesis*.

Exercise influences endothelial function on all four levels discussed above:

1. L-Arginine.
Shear stress increases L-arginine uptake by endothelial cells by modulating the velocity of the endothelial transmembraneous transport system for L-arginine.[33]

2. Endothelial Nitric Oxide Synthase.
Shear stress causes a dramatic increase in eNOS activity (up to 13 times basal levels) within only 60 minutes.[34] This increase seems to be mediated by both short-term enhancement of eNOS activity and activation of eNOS expression. Increases in eNOS expression were demonstrated in endothelial cell culture experiments after exposure to laminar shear stress[35] and in animal studies of exercise training.[36] However, both alleles of the eNOS gene seem to be necessary to increase eNOS expression in response to exercise training: In mice heterozygotic for a loss of the eNOS gene no increased eNOS protein expression could be observed in the aorta whereas wild-type eNOS$^{+/+}$ mice had a 2.5 ± 0.4-fold increase.[37]

Several different phosphorylation sites exist within the eNOS enzyme – some of them inhibitory (threonine-495, serine-116), others stimulatory (serine-617, serine-635, and serine-1177). Evidence from animal experiments confirmed that adenoviral transfection of a phosphomimetic serine-1179DeNOS (equivalent to the human serine-1177) to eNOS knockout mice completely restored endothelium-dependent vasodilation in response to acetylcholine whereas transfection with a non-phosphorylatable serine-1179AeNOS resulted in significant endothelial dysfunction.[38] These findings underline the physiologic relevance of serine-1177 phosphorylation for NO generation.

We are only beginning to understand how the complex phosphorylation status of the eNOS enzyme is affected by exercise training. Increases in eNOS phosphorylation at serine-1177 have recently been documented in patients with CAD after 4 weeks of ergometer training in left internal mammary artery rings.[28] Based on the data from this clinical study and other in vitro experiments shear-stress induced phosphorylation is mediated via phosphoinositide-3 (PI3) kinase and AKT (protein kinase B) in a calcium-independent manner and is maintained over a longer period of time (days) as compared to the short-term calcium-dependent changes in phosphorylation associated with exposure to bradykinin (for review refer to Fleming and Busse[39]).

3. Nitric Oxide Breakdown.

It has long been unclear why exercise training, which increases total oxygen uptake (VO_2) and in turn production of ROS, can yet improve endothelial function. As mentioned above, it has just recently been shown that endothelium-derived NO increases expression of ecSOD in vascular smooth muscle cells.[31] In the same publication the authors demonstrated that exercise training increased both eNOS and ecSOD in wild-type mice whereas ecSOD remained unchanged in mice lacking eNOS. This suggests that the effect of training on ecSOD is mediated via endothelium-derived NO.

ROS production is also affected by exercise: After 4 weeks of ergometer training the activity of NAD(P)H oxidase – a key ROS-generating enzyme in the vascular wall – and the expression of its components were significantly reduced (Figure 12-2).[40]

4. Endothelial Progenitor Cells.

A growing number of studies address the issue of how exercise – both acute and chronic – may affect circulating EPC levels. In the first such study, Adams documented a significant increase in circulating EPCs after a single maximal exercise test in patients with stenotic CAD and exercise-induced myocardial ischemia. Healthy subjects and non-ischemic CAD-patients showed no such increase.[41] The effects of chronic endurance exercise were investigated in a second study by Laufs et al. who described an NO dependence of EPC increases in a transgenic animal model: eNOS$^{-/-}$ mice showed lower EPC numbers at baseline and a significantly attenuated increase of EPC in response to physical activity.[42] Wild-type mice, on the other hand, showed a significant, nearly 3-fold increase in circulating EPCs after running training. In a prospective randomized training study in patients with peripheral arterial occlusive disease (PAOD) with and without prior revascularization, we were able to document that only ischemic training induced a significant increase in circulating EPCs while non-ischemic training in patients post successful percutaneous angioplasty had no effect.

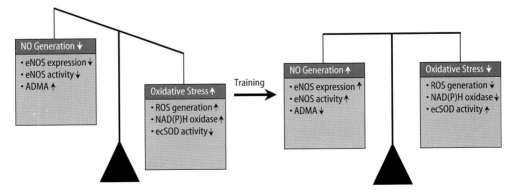

Figure 12-2. Imbalance between reduced NO generation and increased NO degradation as a result of higher oxidative stress in the vascular wall in atherosclerotic coronary artery disease. Exercise training and vascular shear stress augment endothelial NO production by increasing eNOS expression and activity; on the other hand, the local generation of ROS is reduced by exercise due to lower activity of ROS-producing enzymes like NAD(P)H oxidase and better antioxidative protection. As a result, endothelial function is improved.

(C) Microrheology and Hemostasis

Exercise training affects both functional and morphologic aspects of the microvascular bed: Resistance vessel sensitivity and maximal responsiveness to adenosine is improved and total vascular bed cross-sectional area increased by up to 37% after 16 weeks. While acute bouts of exercise may have thrombogenic side-effects, with platelet number and activity being increased, chronic exercise training has been shown to attenuate this potentiation of platelet function, to increase platelet cGMP content, and to suppress coagulability.

Exercise Training in Chronic Heart Failure

Exercise training in CHF is a nonspecific intervention which simultaneously affects several organ systems (Figure 12-3). As the focus of this

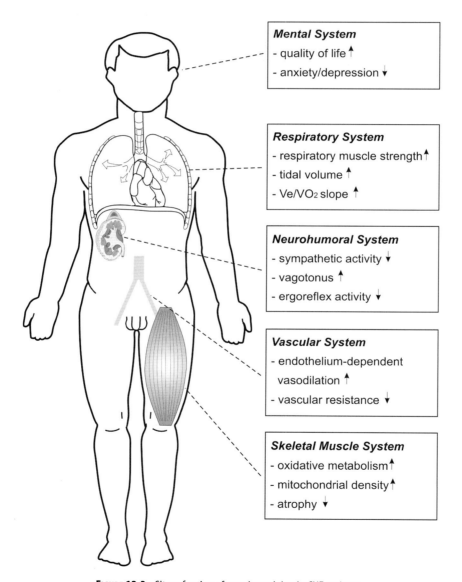

Figure 12-3. Sites of action of exercise training in CHF patients.

chapter is on molecular mechanisms rather than on functional changes, training effects on ventilation will be omitted.

Neurohormonal Adaptations

An aerobic training program in CHF patients regularly reduces the resting heart rate, which indicates a reduction in sympathoadrenergic drive. This has also been confirmed for serum catecholamine levels: Coats et al. showed a 16% reduction in radiolabeled norepinephrine secretion after 8 weeks of training. This reduction in adrenergic tone was accompanied by increase in heart rate variability.[43] In addition to the reduction in circulating catecholamines Braith et al. described a 25–30% reduction in angiotensin II, aldosterone, arginine vasopeptide, and atrial natriuretic peptide following 4 months of walking training in CHF patients.[44]

Vascular Adaptations

Exercise has a profound impact on peripheral endothelial dysfunction in CHF: It can improve basal nitric oxide production and enhance endothelium-dependent peripheral vasodilation.[45] There seems to be a close correlation between the increase in endothelium-dependent dilation and the change in peak VO_2 ($r = 0.64$, $P < 0.005$), suggesting that peripheral hypoperfusion might play a contributory role to exercise intolerance in CHF. Data from animal experiments suggest that exercise can upregulate endothelial nitric oxide synthase (eNOS)[36] and reduce NO breakdown by attenuating oxidative stress.[46]

Cardiac Adaptations

In a recently published randomized clinical trial[47] it was confirmed that exercise has no negative impact on cardiac function. On the contrary, after 6 months of a regular aerobic training program, a small but significant improvement of left ventricular ejection fraction was observed accompanied by a reduction in left ventricular end-diastolic diameter.[47]

Skeletal Muscle Adaptations

CHF causes profound alterations in skeletal muscle morphology, metabolism, and function,

which are not just a consequence of deconditioning but represent intrinsic changes induced by the systemic neurohumoral and inflammatory response in CHF.

Aerobic Energy Metabolism

All aspects of skeletal muscle characteristics can be positively influenced by training: On the ultrastructural level, the volume density of cytochrome-C positive mitochondria is increased,[48] permitting an enhanced oxidative phosphorylation. These changes are also reflected by a fiber type shift from anaerobic fast type II to aerobic slow type I fibers in skeletal muscle biopsies after 6 months of training.[48]

Anabolic–Catabolic Balance

As suggested by the association between low serum insulin-like growth factor I (IGF-I) levels and loss of lean muscle mass, patients with CHF suffer from a clinically relevant imbalance between anabolic and catabolic influences on the peripheral muscle.[49] In skeletal muscle biopsies of non-cachectic patients with CHF, the local IGF-I expression was substantially reduced despite normal growth hormone (GH) and IGF-I serum concentrations.[50] It has been previously shown that a state of GH resistance may develop in cardiac cachexia. Exercise training has the potential to increase local IGF-I expression and to reverse muscle catabolism.

Cytokines and Local Inflammation

Cytokine levels are elevated not only in the serum of patients with advanced CHF but also in skeletal muscle biopsies of patients with stable moderate heart failure where TNF-α, IFN-γ, and IL-1β are potent activators of iNOS expression.[51] The intracellular accumulation of NO is high enough to inhibit key enzymes of the oxidative phosphorylation.[52] In vitro experiments documented that NO can thus attenuate the contractile performance of the skeletal muscle, a finding which puts cytokine production and iNOS expression in perspective for the development of exercise intolerance in patients with severe heart failure. Regular exercise training can significantly reduce local cytokine expression and improve aerobic metabolism.[53]

Future Perspectives

Exercise training affects virtually every human organ system and we are just beginning to understand the complexity of the mechanisms involved. Two new frontiers are currently being investigated with great enthusiasm: (1) In ischemic heart disease the potential role of bone-marrow-derived EPCs in the focus of several studies involving either interventional administration or endogenous mobilization by exercise. (2) After aerobic endurance training has been successfully established in CHF, researchers are now assessing the potential benefits of adding resistance exercise to achieve greater increases in muscle mass.

Despite the advances of the last years our understanding of the complex molecular pathways activated by physical exercise is still in its infancy. A coordinated basic research approach is needed to shed more light on the physiological adaptations to exercise. Thus we will be able to recruit beneficial training effects for clinical applications on the basis of a better pathophysiological understanding as well as on empirical knowledge.

References

1. Ludmer PL, Selwyn AP, Shook TL, et al. Paradoxical vasoconstriction induced by acetylcholine in atherosclerotic coronary arteries. N Engl J Med 1986; 315(17):1046–1051.
2. Hasdai D, Gibbons RJ, Holmes DR, Higano ST, Lerman A. Coronary endothelial dysfunction in humans is associated with myocardial perfusion defects. Circulation 1997;96:3390–3395.
3. Franciosa JA, Park M, Levine TB. Lack of correlation between exercise capacity and indexes of resting left ventricular performance in heart failure. Am J Cardiol 1981;47:33–39.
4. Cohn JN. The management of chronic heart failure. N Engl J Med 1996;335(7):490–498.
5. Levine B, Kalman J, Mayer L, Fillit HM, Packer MP. Elevated circulating levels of tumor necrosis factor in severe chronic heart failure. N Engl J Med 1990; 323:236–241.
6. Kubo SH, Rector TC, Williams RE, Heifritz SM, Bank AJ. Endothelium dependent vasodilation is attenuated in patients with heart failure. Circulation 1991;84:1589–1596.
7. Mancini DM, Henson D, LaMacna J, Levine S. Respiratory muscle function and dyspnea in patients with chronic congestive heart failure. Circulation 1992;86(3):909–918.
8. Sullivan MJ, Green HJ, Cobb FR. Skeletal muscle biochemistry and histology in ambulatory patients with long-term heart failure. Circulation 1990;81: 518–527.
9. Simonini A, Long CS, Dudley GA, Yue P, McElhinny J, Massie BM. Heart failure in rats causes changes in skeletal muscle morphology and gene expression that are not explained by reduced activity. Circ Res 1996;79:128–136.
10. Mancini DM, Coyle E, Coggan A, et al. Contribution of intrinsic skeletal muscle changes to 31-P NMR Skeletal muscle metabolic abnormalities in patients with chronic heart failure. Circulation 1989;80: 1338–1346.
11. Okita K, Yonezawa K, Nishijima H, et al. Skeletal muscle metabolism limits exercise capacity in patients with chronic heart failure. Circulation 1998;98:1886–1891.
12. Opasich C, Ambrosino N, Felicetti G, et al. [Skeletal and respiratory muscle strength in chronic heart failure]. G Ital Cardiol 1993;23(8):759–766.
13. Niebauer J, Hambrecht R, Velich T, et al. Attenuated progression of coronary artery disease after 6 years of multifactorial risk intervention: Role of physical exercise. Circulation 1997;96:2534–2541.
14. Harrison DG. Cellular and molecular mechanisms of endothelial cell dysfunction. J Clin Invest 1997; 100(9):2153–2157.
15. Cooke JP. Asymmetrical dimethylarginine: the Uber marker? Circulation 2004;109(15):1813–1818.
16. Kamada Y, Nagaretani H, Tamura S, et al. Vascular endothelial dysfunction resulting from L-arginine deficiency in a patient with lysinuric protein intolerance. J Clin Invest 2001;108(5):717–724.
17. Creager MA, Gallagher SJ, Girerd XJ, Coleman SM, Dzau VJ, Cooke JP. L-arginine improves endothelium-dependent vasodilation in hypercholesterolemic humans. J Clin Invest 1992;90:1248–1253.
18. Drexler H, Zeiher AM, Meinzer K, Just H. Correction of endothelial dysfunction in coronary microcirculation of hypercholesterolaemic patients by L-arginine. Lancet 1991;338:1546–1550.
19. Hambrecht R, Hilbrich L, Erbs S, et al. Correction of endothelial dysfunction in chronic heart failure: additional effects of exercise training and oral L-arginine supplementation. J Am Coll Cardiol 2000; 35(3):706–713.
20. Blum A, Hathaway L, Mincemoyer R, et al. Oral L-arginine in patients with coronary artery disease on medical management. Circulation 2000;101:2160–2164.
21. Adams MR, McCredie R, Jessup W, Robinson J, Sullivan D, Celermajer DS. Oral L-arginine

improves endothelium-dependent dilatation and reduces monocyte adhesion to endothelial cells in young men with coronary artery disease. Atherosclerosis 1997;129(2):261–269.

22. Venho B, Voutilainen S, Valkonen VP, et al. Arginine intake, blood pressure, and the incidence of acute coronary events in men: the Kuopio Ischaemic Heart Disease Risk Factor Study. Am J Clin Nutr 2002;76(2):359–364.

23. Hingorani AD, Liang CF, Fatibene J, et al. A common variant of the endothelial nitric oxide synthase (Glu298→Asp) is a major risk factor for coronary artery disease in the UK. Circulation 1999;100: 1515–1520.

24. Nakayama M, Yoshimura M, Sakamoto T, et al. Synergistic interaction of T-786→C polymorphism in the endothelial nitric oxide synthase gene and smoking for an enhanced risk for coronary spasm. Pharmacogenetics 2003;13(11):683–688.

25. Rossi GP, Cesari M, Zanchetta M, et al. The T-786C endothelial nitric oxide synthase genotype is a novel risk factor for coronary artery disease in Caucasian patients of the GENICA study. J Am Coll Cardiol 2003;41(6):930–937.

26. Erbs S, Baither Y, Linke A, et al. Promoter but not exon 7 polymorphism of endothelial nitric oxide synthase affects training-induced correction of endothelial dysfunction. Arterioscler Thromb Vasc Biol 2003;23(10):1814–1819.

27. Harrison DG, Venema RC, Arnal JF, et al. The endothelial cell nitric oxide synthase: Is it really constitutively expressed? Agents Actions 1995;45: 107–117.

28. Hambrecht R, Adams V, Erbs S, et al. Regular physical activity improves endothelial function in patients with coronary artery disease by increasing phosphorylation of endothelial nitric oxide synthase. Circulation 2003;107(25):3152–3158.

29. Wang HD, Pagano PJ, Du Y, et al. Superoxide anion from the adventitia of the rat thoracic aorta inactivates nitric oxide. Circ Res 1998;82:810–818.

30. Doehner W, Schoene N, Rauchhaus M, et al. Effects of xanthine oxidase inhibition with allopurinol on endothelial function and peripheral blood flow in hyperuricemic patients with chronic heart failure: results from 2 placebo-controlled studies. Circulation 2002;105(22):2619–2624.

31. Fukai T, Siegfried MR, Ushio-Fukai M, Cheng Y, Kojda G, Harrison DG. Regulation of the vascular extracellular superoxide dismutase by nitric oxide and exercise training. J Clin Invest 2000;105(11): 1631–1639.

32. Hill JM, Zalos G, Halcox JP, et al. Circulating endothelial progenitor cells, vascular function, and cardiovascular risk. N Engl J Med 2003;348(7):593–600.

33. Posch K, Schmidt K, Graier WF. Selective stimulation of L-arginine uptake contributes to shear stress-induced formation of nitric oxide. Life Sci 1999;64(8):663–670.

34. Corson MA, James ML, Latta SE, Nerem RM, Berk BC, Harrison DG. Phosphorylation of endothelial nitric oxide synthase in response to fluid shear stress. Circ Res 1996;79(5):984–991.

35. Noris M, Morigi M, Donadelli R, et al. Nitric oxide synthesis by cultured endothelial cells is modulated by flow conditions. Circ Res 1995;76:536–543.

36. Sessa WC, Pritchard K, Seyedi N, Wang J, Hintze TH. Chronic exercise in dogs increases coronary vascular nitric oxide production and endothelial cell nitric oxide synthase gene expression. Circ Res 1994;74:349–353.

37. Kojda G, Burchfield JS, Cheng YC, Harrison DG. Exercise and eNOS expression: The effect of loss of one eNOS gene. Circulation 1999;100(18):I–337.

38. Scotland RS, Morales-Ruiz M, Chen Y, et al. Functional reconstitution of endothelial nitric oxide synthase reveals the importance of serine 1179 in endothelium-dependent vasomotion. Circ Res 2002;90(8):904–910.

39. Fleming I, Busse R. Molecular mechanisms involved in the regulation of the endothelial nitric oxide synthase. Am J Physiol Regul Integr Comp Physiol 2003;284(1):R1–12.

40. Adams V, Linke A, Kränkell N, et al. Impact of regular physical activity on the NAD(P)H oxidase and angiotensin receptor system in patients with coronary artery disease. Circulation 2005;111(5): 555–562.

41. Adams V, Lenk K, Linke A, et al. Increase of circulating endothelial progenitor cells in patients with coronary artery disease after exercise-induced ischemia. Arterioscler Thromb Vasc Biol 2004;24 (4):684–690.

42. Laufs U, Werner N, Link A, et al. Physical training increases endothelial progenitor cells, inhibits neointima formation, and enhances angiogenesis. Circulation 2004;109(2):220–226.

43. Coats AJS, Adamopoulos S, Radaelli A, et al. Controlled trial of physical training in chronic heart failure: Exercise performance, hemodynamics, ventilation, and autonomic function. Circulation 1992; 85:2119–2131.

44. Braith R, Welsch M, Feigenbaum M, Kluess HA, Pepine C. Neuroendocrine activation in heart failure is modified by endurance training. J Am Coll Cardiol 1999;34:1170–1175.

45. Hambrecht R, Fiehn E, Weigl C, et al. Regular physical exercise corrects endothelial dysfunction and

improves exercise capacity in patients with chronic heart failure. Circulation 1998;98:2709–2715.

46. Fukai T, Siegfried MR, Ushio-Fukai M, Cheng Y, Kojda G, Harrison DG. Regulation of the vascular extracellular superoxide dismutase by nitric oxide and exercise training. J Clin Invest 2000;105(11): 1631–1639.

47. Hambrecht R, Gielen S, Linke A, et al. Effects of exercise training on left ventricular function and peripheral resistance in patients with chronic heart failure. A randomised trial. JAMA 2000;283:3095–3101.

48. Hambrecht R, Fiehn E, Yu J, et al. Effects of endurance training on mitochondrial ultrastructure and fiber type distribution in skeletal muscle of patients with stable chronic heart failure. J Am Coll Cardiol 1997;29:1067–1073.

49. Niebauer J, Pflaum CD, Clark AL, et al. Deficient insulin-like growth factor I in chronic heart failure predicts altered body composition, anabolic deficiency, cytokine and neurohormonal activation. J Am Coll Cardiol 1998;32(2):393–397.

50. Hambrecht R, Schulze PC, Gielen S, et al. Reduction of insulin-like growth factor-I expression in the skeletal muscle of noncachectic patients with chronic heart failure. J Am Coll Cardiol 2002;39(7): 1175–1181.

51. Adams V, Nehrhoff B, Spate U, et al. Induction of iNOS expression in skeletal muscle by IL-1beta and NFkappaB activation: an in vitro and in vivo study. Cardiovasc Res 2002;54(1):95–104.

52. Gross SS, Wolin MS. Nitric oxide: pathophysiological mechanisms. Ann Rev Physiol 1995;57:737–769.

53. Gielen S, Adams V, Möbius-Winkler S, et al. Anti-inflammatory effects of exercise training in the skeletal muscle of patients with chronic heart failure. J Am Coll Cardiol 2003;42(5):861–868.

13
Exercise and Fitness

Jonathan Myers

Introduction

Since the late 1950s, numerous scientific reports have examined the relationships between physical activity, physical fitness, and cardiovascular health. Expert panels convened by organizations such as the Centers for Disease Control and Prevention (CDC), American College of Sports Medicine (ACSM), the European Working Group on Exercise Physiology and Rehabilitation, and the American Heart Association (AHA),[1–5] along with the US Surgeon General's Report on Physical Activity and Health,[6] have reinforced scientific evidence linking regular physical activity to various measures of cardiovascular health. The prevailing view in these reports is that more active or fit individuals tend to experience less coronary heart disease (CHD) than their sedentary counterparts, and when they do acquire CHD, it occurs at a later age and tends to be less severe. Cardiac rehabilitation, as both a science and an industry, has evolved in large part owing to the abundance of evidence indicating that regular exercise improves physical function, and reduces the risk of reinfarction and sudden death in patients with known CHD.[7–11] Despite this evidence, however, most adults in Western societies remain effectively sedentary,[3,6] and more than 80% of patients who sustain a myocardial infarction (MI) are not referred to a cardiac rehabilitation program. This is in part due to the fact that physical activity is not currently integrated into the Western healthcare paradigm, and the majority of physicians fail to prescribe exercise to their patients.[12]

Given the well-documented association between physical inactivity and adverse health outcomes worldwide, the prevalence of physical inactivity, and the growth in the prevalence of obesity in the US and Europe, the healthcare provider's role is more critical than ever in terms of encouraging societies to become more physically active, and to develop strategies that promote the adoption of physically active lifestyles in all their patients. This chapter provides an overview of the scientific evidence linking physical activity and health, and summarizes the physiologic changes that occur with a program of regular exercise.

Role of Exercise in Cardiovascular Health

Physiologic Fitness and Health

In the last two decades, a striking amount of data have been published demonstrating the importance of fitness level in predicting risk for adverse health outcomes.[2,3,13,14] A consistent observation in these studies is that after adjustment for age and other risk factors, exercise capacity has been shown to be a stronger marker of risk for cardiovascular morbidity or all-cause mortality than established risk factors such as hypertension, smoking, obesity, hyperlipidemia, diabetes, and obesity. In addition, exercise capacity has been shown to be a more powerful predictor of risk than other exercise test variables, including ST depression, symptoms, and hemodynamic

Table 13-1. Survival benefit per MET in recent epidemiologic studies using maximal exercise testing as a measure of fitness

Blair et al. JAMA 1995:
    Nearly 16% survival benefit per minute increase (roughly 1-MET) on the treadmill with serial testing
Dorn et al. Circulation 1999:
    NEHDP: 8–14% survival benefit per MET increase during cardiac rehabilitation over 19 years
Goraya et al. Ann Intern Med 2000:
    14% and 18% survival benefit per MET for younger and elderly subjects, respectively
Myers et al. N Engl J Med 2002:
    12% survival benefit per MET among patients referred for treadmill testing
Gulati et al. Circulation 2003:
    17% survival benefit per MET among healthy women
Mora et al. JAMA 2003:
    20% survival benefit per MET among women in the Lipid Research Clinics Trial
Balady et al. Circulation 2004:
    13% reduction in risk of events per MET among high risk men in Framingham Offspring Study
Myers et al. Am J Med 2004:
    20% survival benefit per MET, roughly equivalent to 1000 kcal/week adulthood activity

responses.[13,15–19] Moreover, the lower levels of fitness in these studies did not appear to be associated with subclinical disease. A number of recent studies have expressed exercise capacity in the context of survival benefit per MET (metabolic equivalent); these studies are presented in Table 13-1. These studies are noteworthy in that each increase in 1-MET (a small increment achievable by most individuals) is associated with large (10–25%) improvements in survival. The importance of exercise capacity in the risk paradigm has historically received inadequate attention because of the tendency for clinicians to focus on the ST segment.[20] Some of the major recent studies are reviewed in the following.

Blair and associates[14] assessed fitness by treadmill performance in >13,000 asymptomatic subjects and followed them for 110,482 person-years (averaging >8 years) for all-cause mortality. These results are presented in Table 13-2. Age-adjusted mortality rates were lowest (18.6 per 10,000 man-years) among the most fit and highest (64.0 per 10,000 man-years) among the least fit men, with the corresponding rates among women 8.5 and 39.5 per 10,000 woman-years, respectively. These findings closely parallel an earlier report among

Table 13-2. Rates and relative risks of death* among 10,244 men and 3120 women, by gradients of physical fitness

Quintiles of fitness†	Men			Women		
	No. of deaths	Deaths per 10,000 man-years	Relative risk of death‡	No. of deaths	Deaths per 10,000 woman-years	Relative risk of death‡
1 (low)	75	64.0	1.00	18	39.5	1.00
2	40	25.5	0.40	11	20.5	0.52
3	47	27.1	0.42	6	12.2	0.31
4	43	21.7	0.34	4	6.5	0.15
5 (high)	35	18.6	0.29	4	8.5	0.22

*Age-adjusted.
†Quintiles of fitness determined by maximal exercise testing.
‡*P* value for trend 0.05.
Source: From Blair et al.[14] © 1989 American Medical Association. All rights reserved. Reprinted with permission.

asymptomatic men from the Lipid Research Clinics (LRC) Mortality Follow-up,[18] in which each 2 SD decrement in exercise capacity was associated with a 2- to 5-fold higher CHD or all-cause death rate. More recent studies, including one from the LRC, have reinforced the fact that these findings also apply to women who are healthy at the time of evaluation.[18,19] Gulati et al.[19] suggested that the strength of exercise capacity in predicting risk of mortality was even greater among women than men, reporting a 17% reduction in risk for every 1-MET increase in fitness. In the LRC, nearly 3000 asymptomatic women underwent exercise testing and were followed for up to 20 years.[18] A 20% decrease in survival was observed for every 1-MET decrement in exercise capacity. This study also pointed out the relative weakness of ischemic ECG responses in predicting cardiovascular and all-cause mortality among women.

More recently, this issue has been addressed in clinical populations, e.g. patients referred for exercise testing for clinical reasons.[13,15–17] In a recent study performed among US Veterans, 6213 men underwent maximal exercise testing for clinical reasons and were followed for a mean of 6.2 years.[13] The subjects were classified into five categories by gradients of fitness. After adjustment for age, the researchers observed that the largest gains in terms of mortality were achieved between the lowest fitness group and the next lowest fitness group. Figure 13-1 illustrates the age-adjusted relative risks associated with the different categories of fitness. Among both normal subjects and those with cardiovascular disease, the least fit individuals had more than four times the risk of all-cause mortality compared to the most fit. Importantly, an individual's fitness level was a stronger predictor of mortality than established risk factors such as smoking, high blood pressure, high cholesterol, and diabetes. Over the last several years, other cohorts, such as those from the Cleveland Clinic[17] and the Mayo Clinic,[15,16] have documented the importance of exercise capacity as a predictor of

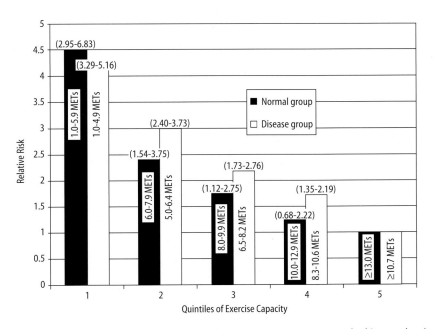

FIGURE 13-1. Age-adjusted relative risks of mortality by quintiles of exercise capacity among normal subjects and patients with cardiovascular disease. The subgroup with the highest exercise capacity (group 5) is the reference category. For each quintile, the range of values for exercise capacity represented appears within each bar; 95% confidence intervals for the relative risks appear above each bar. (From Myers et al.[13]) © 2002 Massachusetts Medical Society. All rights reserved. Reprinted with permission.

mortality among clinically referred populations. These clinically based studies confirm the observations of Blair et al.,[14] Framingham,[21] and the LRC trial[18,22] among asymptomatic populations, underscoring the fact that fitness level has a strong influence on the incidence of cardiovascular and all-cause morbidity and mortality.

Epidemiologic Evidence Supporting Physical Activity

In the United States alone, it has been estimated that roughly 250,000 deaths per year are attributed to lack of regular physical activity[3] (roughly one-quarter of all preventable deaths annually). However, others have suggested that these figures may be significantly underestimated.[23] Ongoing longitudinal studies have provided consistent evidence of varying strength documenting the protective effects of activity for a number of chronic diseases, including CHD, chronic heart failure (CHF), type 2 diabetes, hypertension, osteoporosis, and site-specific cancers.[2,3,6] In contrast, low levels of physical fitness or activity are consistently associated with higher cardiovascular and all-cause mortality rates.[2,3,13,14] Midlife increases in physical activity, fitness level, or both, through change in occupation or recreational activities, are associated with a decrease in mortality rates.[24,25] Considering the last few years alone (2000–2004), an impressive volume of data has been published throughout the European Union and the US confirming the association between physical activity and cardiovascular health; some notable examples of these cohorts are presented in Table 13-3.

The landmark epidemiologic work of Paffenbarger and associates among Harvard alumni[24,26] has been particularly persuasive in support of physical activity, and thus the development of the CDC, AHA, ACSM, and European Working Group guidelines. Table 13-4 illustrates the rates and relative risks of death over a 9-year period among 11,864 Harvard alumni by patterns of physical activity. Several findings in Table 13-4 are particularly noteworthy. The largest benefits in terms of mortality appear to accrue through engaging in moderate activity levels; *moderate* is generally defined as activity performed at an intensity of 3 to 6 METs, roughly equivalent to

TABLE 13-3. Recent cohorts (2000–2004) supporting the role of physical activity in predicting health outcomes

Framingham Heart Study (Boston)
Belgian Physical Fitness Study
Physicians Health Follow-up Study (Boston)
Nurses Health Study (Boston)
VA Health Care System (Palo Alto)
The Whitehall Study (London)
Seven Countries Study (US, Europe, multicenter)
National Center for Chronic Disease Prevention and Health Promotion (CDC, Atlanta)
The SENECA Study (Europe, multicenter)
Baltimore Longitudinal Study on Aging
Finnish Twin Study
Aerobics Center for Longitudinal Research (Dallas)
Honolulu Heart Study
Canada Health Survey
Harvard Alumni Health Study (Boston)
Copenhagen Male Study
Zutphen Elderly Study (Greece)
Osteoporotic Fractures Research Group (US, multicenter)
Caerphilly Wales Study
Puerto Rico Heart Health Program
Nordic Research Project on Aging (NORA)
Lipid Research Clinics Follow-up (Baltimore)

brisk walking for most adults. Note also that regular, moderate walking or sports participation is associated with 30% to 40% reductions in mortality (relative risk of death 0.60 to 0.70). Likewise, the physical activity index, expressed as kilocalories per week (the sum of walking, stair climbing, and sports participation), suggests that a 40% reduction in mortality occurs by engaging in modest levels of activity (1000 to 2000 kcal/week, equivalent to three to five 1-hour sessions of activity), whereas only minimal additional benefits are achieved by engaging in greater-intensity activity. These findings agree closely with earlier results among 16,936 Harvard alumni assessed in the early 1960s and followed for all-cause mortality for nearly 20 years.[26] Similar results have been reported from large studies that have followed cohorts for CHD morbidity and mortality in the range of 10 to 20 years among British civil servants, US railroad workers, San Francisco longshoremen, nurses, physicians, other healthcare workers, and other cohorts (for review, see Kohl[27] or Lee and Paffenbarger[28]). Clearly, the evidence linking a physically active lifestyle and cardiovascular health is substantial.

TABLE 13-4. Rates and relative risks of death* among Harvard alumni, by patterns of physical activity

Physical activity (weekly)		Man-years (%)	No. of deaths	Deaths per 10,000 man-years	Relative risk of death	P value of trend
Walking (km)	<5	26	228	86.2	1.00 ⎤	
	5–14	42	275	67.4	0.78 ⎬	<0.001
	15+	32	194	57.7	0.67 ⎦	
Stair-climbing (floors)	<20	37	341	80.0	1.00 ⎤	0.001
	20–54	48	293	62.9	0.79 ⎬	
	55+	15	80	59.6	0.75 ⎦	
All sportsplay	None	12	156	88.9	1.00 ⎤	
	Light only	10	152	97.4	1.10 ⎬	<0.001
	Light and moderate	36	208	59.7	0.67 ⎬	
	Moderate only‡	42	178	56.4	0.63 ⎦	
Moderate sportsplay (h)	<1	30	308	92.9	1.00 ⎤	
	1–2	41	126	58.2	0.63 ⎬	<0.001
	3+	29	64	43.6	0.47 ⎦	
Index (kcal)§	<500	12 ⎤	197	110.3 ⎤	1.00 ⎤	
	500–999	18 ⎥ 58	135	69.1 ⎥ 78.9	0.63 ⎥ 1.00	
	1000–1499	15 ⎥	111	68.9 ⎥	0.62 ⎥	
	1500–1999	13 ⎦	73	61.4 ⎦	0.56 ⎦	<0.001
	2000–2499	10 ⎤	51	52.4 ⎤	0.48 ⎤	
	2500–2999	8 ⎥ 42	44	64.6 ⎥ 55.4	0.59 ⎥ 0.70	
	3000–3400	6 ⎥	36	74.7 ⎥	0.68 ⎥	
	3500+	18 ⎦	82	48.1 ⎦	0.44 ⎦	

METs, metabolic equivalents.
*Age-adjusted.
†<4.5 METs intensity.
‡4.5+ METs intensity.
§Sum of walking, stair climbing, and all sportsplay.
Source: From Paffenbarger et al.[26] © 1994 Human Kinetics, Inc. All rights reserved. Reprinted with permission.

Specific Recommendations for Activity from Major Health Organizations

A variety of consensus reports from major health organizations worldwide have been published with specific recommendations for physical activity.[1-6] Consistent in these reports is the recommendation that all individuals participate in a minimum of 30 minutes of moderate activity on most, and preferably all, days of the week. Repeated intermittent or shorter bouts of activity (e.g. 10 minutes), including occupational, non-occupational, or tasks of daily living, have similar cardiovascular and health benefits if performed at a level of moderate intensity (e.g. brisk walking, cycling, swimming, home repair, and yard work) with an accumulated duration of at least 30 minutes per day. Individuals who already meet these standards receive additional benefits from increasing this amount to more vigorous activity.

The 30 minutes/day recommendation is generally consistent with an energy expenditure in the order of 1000 kcal/week. Energy expenditure of this magnitude has been associated with 20–30% reductions in all-cause and cardiovascular mortality.[2-6] The 30 minutes per day/1000 kcal/week recommendation is at the heart of a noteworthy theme that is consistent in each of the aforementioned consensus statements on physical activity and health. It is now appreciated that considerable health benefits are derived from *moderate* levels of activity. Many researchers have argued that it is generally not necessary to engage in vigorous, sustained activity to derive many of the health benefits of exercise. Prior to the release of these reports in the mid-1990s, guidelines generally promoted the concept that exercise was thought to be effective only if an improvement in some measure of cardiopulmonary fitness was observed, implying that only physically "trained" individuals benefited from physical activity. In recent years, the philosophy on exercise as a means to this end ("fitness" measured by exercise capacity) has changed significantly. Current guidelines reflect the concept that substantial health benefits can be achieved through modest amounts of regular exercise, regardless of whether exercise results in a measurable improvement in exercise capacity.

Physical Activity Pattern Versus Fitness Level in Defining Health Risk

Although physical activity status and physiologic fitness are clearly linked, the latter carries an important genetic component; that is, some people remain comparatively fit without engaging in a great deal of physical activity. The above-mentioned studies by Blair and colleagues,[14,25] those at the VA,[13] and elsewhere,[15-19] provide compelling evidence that one's fitness level has a profound influence on mortality. There has been some recent debate as to whether daily physical activity patterns largely determine one's fitness level and therefore health risk, or whether fitness level predicts mortality independently from activity pattern.[29,30] In a recent meta-analysis, Williams[29] compared the dose–response relationships between leisure-time physical activity and

fitness from published reports and their association with cardiovascular disease endpoints. The analysis included a remarkable 1,325,000 person-years of follow-up.

The results of the Williams meta-analysis[29] are summarized in Figure 13-2. Relative risks are plotted as a function of the cumulative percentages of the samples when ranked from least fit or active to most fit or active. In combining study results, a weighted average of the relative risks from the physical activity and fitness cohorts was computed at every 5th percentile between 5 and 100%. As illustrated in Figure 13-2, the risks of CHD decrease linearly with increasing percentiles of physical activity. This is contrasted by the fitness cohorts, in which a sharp drop in risk occurs before the 25th percentile of the fitness distribution. This suggests that the largest benefits in terms of CHD morbidity occur by the most unfit becoming moderately fit, confirming the observations of previous studies in both asymptomatic and clinically referred populations.[3,6,13,14] Perhaps more importantly, the precipitous drop in risk before the 25th percentile of the fitness distribution results in fitness being a more powerful predictor of CHD risk than physical activity. Stated differently, at all percentiles greater than the 25th, the relative risk reduction is greater for fitness

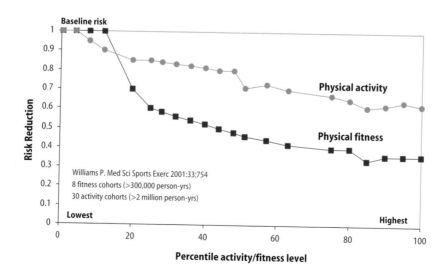

Figure 13-2. Degree of risk reduction in coronary heart disease or other cardiovascular diseases from 8 physical fitness and 30 physical activity cohorts, from the meta-analysis of Williams.[29]

than physical activity. Williams[29] interpreted these findings to mean that formulating activity recommendations on the basis of fitness studies may inappropriately demote the status of cardiorespiratory fitness as a risk factor while exaggerating the public health benefits of moderate amounts of physical activity.

It is important to note that dozens of studies over the last three decades have reported that *both* higher physical fitness levels *and* greater amounts of physical activity have an inverse association with the incidence of cardiovascular disease and all-cause mortality. Answering the question regarding whether fitness or activity more strongly predicts outcomes is a difficult undertaking, complicated by the fact that the two measures are related (with correlation coefficients ranging in the order of 0.30 to 0.60), and because fitness also has a strong genetic component, in addition to the fact that fitness may be influenced by subclinical disease and other factors. Even with large, prospective analyses addressing both fitness and activity measures in the same population, a complete answer to this issue will remain elusive. Physical activity develops physical fitness, although the magnitude of the response to an exercise stimulus is likely genetically determined. Nevertheless, activity is likely required to develop and maintain a fitness level that is consistent with good health. This scientific question should not be a distraction from the important public health message that sedentary individuals should become more physically active.

Resistance Training

Traditionally, exercise programs have emphasized aerobic lower extremity exercise. This was particularly true for individuals with cardiovascular disease, among whom training benefits were generally thought to occur only through dynamic exercise. Resistance exercise was generally limited to athletes attempting to improve performance. In addition, for many years resistance exercise was considered potentially dangerous for individuals who had existing cardiovascular disease. However, an increasing amount of recent research has demonstrated that resistance training not only improves both muscular strength and cardiovascular endurance,

but it also has positive influences on existing conditions such as hypertension, hyperlipidemia, obesity, and diabetes.[31] One of the most important effects of resistance training is its influence on bone health. Numerous cross-sectional and longitudinal studies have observed higher bone mineral density at multiple sites after resistance training. For these reasons, many governing bodies, including the AHA, ACSM, American Association of Cardiovascular and Pulmonary Rehabilitation, and the Surgeon General's Report on Physical Activity and Health, now consider resistance training an integral component of a fitness or rehabilitation program.[1-4,6]

Resistance exercise should complement, rather than replace, an aerobic conditioning program. Gains in muscular strength and endurance as well as benefits related to bone health and metabolism can occur by either static (isometric) or dynamic (isotonic or isokinetic) exercises. Dynamic exercises are generally recommended for healthy adults and patients in rehabilitation programs, both because they mimic activities of daily living and because they are associated with lower degrees of hemodynamic stress. Resistance training should be performed at a moderate-to-slow speed, should be rhythmical, and with a normal breathing pattern throughout the movement. Patients with cardiovascular disease should in particular avoid heavy resistance or isometric exercises, which can cause a dramatic increase in both systolic and diastolic pressures, particularly during the Valsalva maneuver.

Guidelines suggest that one set of 8 to 12 repetitions of 8 to 10 exercises that condition the major muscle groups, performed at least 2 days/week, is the recommended minimum to develop and maintain the benefits of resistance exercise. Patients with cardiovascular disease should begin a program using relatively lighter weights with higher repetitions (e.g. ≈15) and progress the resistance gradually as strength increases. Studies have shown that there is little additional benefit in terms of muscular strength and endurance from performing multiple sets. Thus, multiple sets should be limited in patients with cardiovascular disease. Resistance training can be reasonably included as a supplement to an aerobic session, or performed on a day separate from an aerobic session.

Physiologic Benefits of Exercise Training

Regular exercise increases work capacity; hundreds of studies have been performed cross-sectionally that document higher maximal oxygen uptake (VO_2max) values among active versus sedentary individuals, or between groups after a period of training. The magnitude of improvement in VO_2max with training varies widely, usually ranging from 10% to 25%, but increases as large as 50% have been reported. The degree of change in exercise capacity depends primarily on initial state of fitness and intensity of training. Training increases exercise capacity by increasing both maximal cardiac output and the ability to extract oxygen from the blood. The physiologic benefits of a training program can be classified as *morphologic*, *hemodynamic*, and *metabolic* (Table 13-5). Many animal studies have demonstrated significant morphologic changes with training, including myocardial hypertrophy with improved myocardial function, increases in coronary artery size, and increases in the myocardial capillary-to-fiber ratio. However, such changes have been difficult to demonstrate in humans.[32] The major morphologic outcome of a training program in humans is probably an increase in cardiac size; however, this adaptation appears to occur mainly in younger, healthy subjects, and is an unlikely outcome among individuals beyond the age of 40 or in patients with heart disease. However, significant hemodynamic changes have been well

TABLE 13-5. Physiologic adaptations to physical training in humans

Hemodynamic adaptations
Increased cardiac output
Increased blood volume
Increased end-diastolic volume
Increased stroke volume
Reduced heart rate for any submaximal workload

Metabolic adaptations
Increased mitochondrial volume and number
Greater muscle glycogen stores
Enhanced fat utilization
Enhanced lactate removal
Increased enzymes for aerobic metabolism
Increased maximal oxygen uptake

Morphologic adaptations
Myocardial hypertrophy (likely only in younger individuals)

TABLE 13-6. Changes in risk factors influenced by exercise training

Decrease in blood pressure
Increase in high-density lipoprotein cholesterol level
Reduction in plasma inflammatory risk markers (C-reactive protein, homocysteine)
Augmented weight reduction efforts
Psychological effects:
    Less depression
    Reduced anxiety
Improved glucose tolerance
Improved fitness level

documented among patients with heart disease after training. These include reductions in heart rate at rest and any matched submaximal workload, which is beneficial in that it results in a reduction in myocardial oxygen demand during activities of daily living. Other hemodynamic changes that have been demonstrated after training include reductions in blood pressure, increases in blood volume, and increases in maximal oxygen uptake. The most important physiologic benefits of training among patients with heart disease occur in the skeletal muscle. The metabolic capacity of the skeletal muscle is enhanced through increases in mitochondrial volume and number, capillary density, and oxidative enzyme content. These adaptations enhance perfusion and the efficiency of oxygen extraction.

An additional important influence of training is a favorable influence on the cardiovascular risk profile (Table 13-6). While this may include such things as reductions in blood pressure, reductions in body weight, reductions in total cholesterol and LDL, and an increase in HDL, recent studies suggest that a particularly potent influence of regular exercise is an improvement in insulin sensitivity. Recent studies also suggest that programs of regular exercise have favorable effects on plasma concentrations of inflammatory risk markers (C-reactive protein, homocysteine). As mentioned above, the condition of being sedentary has a profound effect on cardiovascular morbidity and mortality, so becoming more physically active lowers cardiac risk. It is also important to note that while the effect of exercise on any single risk factor may generally be small, the overall effect of continued, regular exercise on overall cardiovascular risk, when combined with other lifestyle modifications such as proper nutrition, smoking cessation, and medication use, can be dramatic.

Newer Concepts Regarding Physiologic Benefits of Exercise Training

A longstanding and attractive hypothesis is the concept that exercise training can reverse or retard the progression of atherosclerosis. The observation that regression of atherosclerosis occurred in animal studies dating back to the 1950s continues to stimulate interest in the effects of exercise on the coronary vasculature in humans. While this idea was largely rejected during the 1970s and 1980s, several notable studies were performed during the 1990s indicating that exercise training, when combined with multidisciplinary risk management, can improve myocardial perfusion.[33–35] This has been demonstrated indirectly using nuclear imaging[33] and directly by angiography.[34,35] Because most of these studies involved multidisciplinary risk reduction (e.g. diet, smoking cessation, stress management, and pharmacologic management of risk factors, including statin therapy) in addition to exercise training, it is not possible to determine the independent effects of exercise training.

There is also debate regarding the mechanism by which the apparent improvement in myocardial perfusion might occur following training. It is generally considered unlikely that changes in coronary blood flow during exercise in animals would apply to humans. Three mechanisms could potentially explain an improvement in perfusion after training: (1) direct regression of atherosclerotic lesions; (2) formation of collateral vessels; or (3) a change in the dynamics of epicardial flow via flow-mediated or endogenous stimuli of the vessel. While there has been evidence of small but significant improvements in lumen diameter after intensive exercise and risk reduction programs in patients with CAD, no evidence exists that collateral vessel formation occurs after training in humans. Interestingly, although changes in lumen diameter following these intervention programs are quite small, they are associated with considerable reductions in hospital admissions for cardiac reasons.[35] This suggests that patients in the intervention groups may achieve greater plaque stabil-

ity, without large changes in the coronary artery lumen.

In terms of the third mechanism, that is, changes in epicardial flow dynamics after training, a significant amount of recent research has demonstrated that training improves endothelial dysfunction, thus permitting enhanced peripheral and coronary blood flow in response to exercise. This represents a paradigm shift in the pathophysiology of CAD. The last decade has brought an awareness that the luminal diameter of epicardial vessels changes rapidly in response to mechanical (flow-related) and endogenous or pharmacological stimuli. Hambrecht et al.[36] studied the effects of exercise training in patients with reduced ventricular function and reported that leg blood flow during acetylcholine infusion was enhanced compared to controls. The improvement after training was attributed to an increase in endothelium-dependent vasodilation with an increase in basal nitric oxide formation. In a subsequent study, these investigators demonstrated an improvement in endothelium-dependent vasodilation in epicardial vessels as well as resistance vessels in patients with CAD. After 4 weeks of exercise training, there was a 29% increase in coronary artery flow reserve in comparison to the non-exercise control group.[37]

These findings have been confirmed by other groups,[38–40] and suggest an important role of endothelial dysfunction contributing to inadequate blood flow in patients with cardiovascular disease. Exercise training appears to have a profound effect on the vasodilatory properties of the vasculature. Further exploration into the effects of exercise training on the dynamic behavior of the endothelium is an important target area for future research in both patients with and without existing cardiovascular disease.

Summary

An impressive body of scientific evidence has accumulated over several decades documenting the importance of physical fitness and physical activity in reducing the risk for cardiovascular and all-cause morbidity and mortality. This evidence has met the scientific test of replication. Even modest amounts of activity, such as the minimal recommendations put forth by major health organizations (30 minutes/day of moderate activity, or ≈1000 kcal/week) are associated with 30–40% reductions in morbidity and mortality. Likewise, relatively small improvements in fitness level (e.g. 1-MET) can have dramatic effects on health outcomes (10–25% reductions in cardiovascular and all-cause mortality). The greatest potential for benefit has been consistently shown to occur among the least fit or least active individuals in a given population. Stated differently, sedentary or unfit individuals appear to benefit the most from initiating an exercise program.

While an individual's fitness level is in part genetically determined, all sedentary individuals can benefit from increasing their physical activity pattern, and activity is likely required to develop and maintain an activity level that is consistent with good health. Exercise capacity typically increases after a training program by 10–25%, depending on the initial state of fitness and the type of training program. A combination of central (cardiac) and peripheral (skeletal muscle) adaptations account for this increase. Health outcome benefits resulting from greater activity levels result in part from favorable changes in cardiovascular risk factors, including its effect on the condition of being sedentary or unfit itself. It is now appreciated that many similar benefits occur through a program of resistance exercise.

A sedentary lifestyle and lack of physical fitness are major precursors for cardiovascular disease. Western societies have become more sedentary in the last two decades, a circumstance that has contributed to marked increases in obesity, diabetes, and other conditions. The multitude of studies on the health benefits of physical activity performed over the last three decades should encourage healthcare providers to recognize physical activity as part of the standard treatment paradigm for patients with and without cardiovascular disease.

References

1. American College of Sports Medicine Position Stand. The recommended quantity and quality of exercise for developing and maintaining cardiorespiratory and muscular fitness, and flexibility in healthy adults. Med Sci Sports Exerc 1998;30:975–991.
2. Fletcher GF, Balady G, Amsterdam EA, et al. Exercise standards for testing and training: A statement for healthcare professionals from the American Heart Association. Circulation 2001;104:1694–1740.
3. Pate RR, Pratt MP, Blair SN, et al. Physical activity and public health: A recommendation from the Centers for Disease Control and Prevention and the American College of Sports Medicine. JAMA 1995; 273:402–407.
4. American College of Sports Medicine. Guidelines for Exercise Testing and Prescription, 6th edn. Philadelphia: Lippincott; 2000.
5. Giannuzzi P, Mezzani A, Saner H, et al. Physical activity for primary and secondary prevention. Position paper of the working group on cardiac rehabilitation and exercise physiology of the European society of cardiology. Eur J Cardiovasc Prev Rehabil 2003;10:319–327.
6. US Public Health Service, Office of the Surgeon General: Physical Activity and Health: A Report of the Surgeon General. Atlanta, US Department of Health and Human Services, Centers for Disease Control and Prevention, National Center for Chronic Disease Prevention and Health Promotion; 1996.
7. O'Conner GT, Buring JE, Yusaf S, et al. An overview of randomized trials of rehabilitation with exercise after myocardial infarction. Circulation 1989;80: 234–244.
8. Oldridge NB, Guyatt GH, Fischer ME, et al. Cardiac rehabilitation with exercise after myocardial infarction. JAMA 1988;260:945–950.
9. Taylor RS, Brown A, Ebrahim S, et al. Exercise-based rehabilitation for patients with coronary heart disease: Systematic review and meta-analysis of randomized controlled trials. Am J Med 2004; 116:682–692.
10. Smart N, Marwick TH. Exercise training for patients with heart failure: A systematic review of factors that improve mortality and morbidity. Am J Med 2004;116:693–706.
11. Exercise training meta-analysis of trials in patients with chronic heart failure (ExTraMATCH). BMJ 2004;328:189–195.
12. Damush TM, Stewart AL, Mills KM, et al. Prevalence and correlates of physician recommendations to exercise among older adults. J Gerontol A Biol Sci Med Sci 1999;54:M423–M427.
13. Myers JN, Prakash M, Froelicher VF, et al. Exercise capacity and mortality among men referred for exercise testing. N Engl J Med 2002;346:793–801.
14. Blair SN, Kohl HW III, Paffenbarger RS, et al. Physical fitness and all-cause mortality: A prospective study of healthy men and women. JAMA 1989; 262:2395–2401.

15. Roger VL, Jacobsen SJ, Pellikka PA, et al. Prognostic value of treadmill exercise testing: A population-based study in Olmsted County, Minnesota. Circulation 1998;98:2836–2841.

16. Goraya TY, Jacobsen SJ, Pellikka PA, et al. Prognostic value of treadmill exercise testing in elderly persons. Ann Intern Med 2000;132:862–870.

17. Snader CE, Marwick TH, Pashkow FJ, et al. Importance of estimated functional capacity as a predictor of all-cause mortality among patients referred for exercise thallium single-photon emission computed tomography: report of 3,400 patients from a single center. J Am Coll Cardiol 1997;30: 641–648.

18. Mora S, Redberg RF, Cui Y, et al. Ability of exercise testing to predict cardiovascular and all-cause death in asymptomatic women. A 20-year follow-up of the Lipid Research Clinics Prevalence Study. JAMA 2003;290:1600–1607.

19. Gulati M, Pandey DK, Arnsdorf MF, et al. Exercise capacity and the risk of death in women. The St James Women Take Heart Project Circulation 2003; 108:1554–1559.

20. Myers J. Beyond ST-segment displacement: newer diagnostic and prognostic markers from the exercise test. Am J Med Sports 2003;5:332–336.

21. Kannel WB, Wilson P, Blair SN. Epidemiological assessment of the role of physical activity and fitness in development of cardiovascular disease. Am Heart J 1985;109:876–885.

22. Ekelund LG, Haskell WL, Johnson JL, et al. Physical fitness as a predictor of cardiovascular mortality in asymptomatic North American men: The Lipid Research Clinics Mortality Followup Study. N Engl J Med 1988;319:1379–1384.

23. Booth FW, Gordon SE, Carlson CJ, et al. Waging war on modern chronic disease: Primary prevention through exercise biology. J Appl Physiol 2000;88: 774–787.

24. Paffenbarger RS, Hyde RT, Wing AL, et al. The association of changes in physical-activity level and other lifestyle characteristics with mortality among men. N Engl J Med 1993;328:538–545.

25. Blair SN, Kohl HW, Barlow CE, et al. Changes in physical fitness and all-cause mortality. A prospective study of health and unhealthy men. JAMA 1995;273:1093–1098.

26. Paffenbarger RS, Hyde RT, Wing AL, et al. Some interrelations of physical activity, physiological fitness, health, and longevity. In: Bouchard C, Shephard RJ, Stephens T, eds. Physical Activity, Fitness, and Health. Champaign, IL: Human Kinetics; 1994:119–133.

27. Kohl HW. Physical activity and cardiovascular disease: Evidence for a dose response. Med Sci Sports Exerc 2001;33(Suppl):S472–S483.

28. Lee IM, Paffenbarger RS. Do physical activity and physical fitness avert premature mortality? Exerc Sport Sci Rev 1996;24:135–172.

29. Williams PT. Physical fitness and activity as separate heart disease risk factors: a meta-analysis. Med Sci Sports Exerc 2001;33:754–761.

30. Blair SN, Jackson AS. Physical fitness and activity as separate heart disease risk factors: A meta-analysis. Med Sci Sports Exerc 2001;33:754–761.

31. Graves JE, Franklin BA. Resistance Training for Health and Rehabilitation. Champaign, IL: Human Kinetics; 2001.

32. Froelicher VF, Myers J. Exercise and the Heart, 4th edn. Philadelphia: WB Saunders; 2000.

33. Schuler G, Hambrecht R, Schlierf G, et al. Myocardial perfusion and regression of coronary artery disease in patients on a regimen of intensive physical exercise and low fat diet. J Am Coll Cardiol 1992;19:34–42.

34. Hambrecht R, Niebauer J, Marburger C, et al. Various intensities of leisure time physical activity in patients with coronary artery disease: Effects on cardiorespiratory fitness and progression of coronary atherosclerotic lesions. J Am Coll Cardiol 1993; 22:468–477.

35. Haskell WL, Alderman EL, Fair JM, et al. Effects of intensive multiple risk factor reduction on coronary atherosclerosis and clinical cardiac events in men and women with coronary artery disease: The Stanford Coronary Risk Intervention project (SCRIP). Circulation 1994;89:975–990.

36. Hambrecht R, Wolf A, Gielen S, et al. Effect of exercise on coronary endothelial function in patients with coronary artery disease. New Engl J Med 2000; 342:454–460.

37. Hambrecht R, Fiehen E, Weigl C, et al. Regular physical exercise corrects endothelial dysfunction and improves exercise capacity in patients with chronic heart failure. Circulation 1998;98:2709–2715.

38. Edwards DG, Schofield RS, Lennon SL, et al. Effect of exercise training on endothelial function in men with coronary artery disease. Am J Cardiol 2004;93: 617–620.

39. Gokce N, Vita JA, Bader DS, et al. Effect of exercise on upper and lower extremity endothelial function in patients with coronary artery disease. Am J Cardiol 2002;90:124–127.

40. Moyna NM, Thompson PD. The effect of physical activity on endothelial function in man. Acta Physiol Scand 2004;180:113–123.

14
Exercise Testing in Coronary Heart Disease

Stamatis Adamopoulos, Katerina Fountoulaki, and John T. Parissis

Introduction – General Overview of Exercise Testing Procedure

Coronary artery disease (CAD) is a chronic disorder with a natural history that spans multiple decades. In each affected individual, the disease can go over to a number of well-defined clinical phases: asymptomatic, stable angina, progressive angina, unstable angina, and acute myocardial infarction. Therefore, the approach to diagnosis and risk stratification of the coronary disease patient varies according to the phase of the disease in which the patient presents.

Exercise testing is a well-established procedure in the diagnosis of CAD and has been in widespread clinical use for many decades. Overall, the sensitivity and specificity of exercise testing for diagnosing CAD are about 63% and 74%, respectively.[1] Moreover, appropriate application of exercise testing requires consideration of Bayesian principles, according to which the predictive accuracy of the test is defined not only by its sensitivity and specificity but also by the prevalence of disease in the population studied. Table 14-1 is a modification of the review of Diamond and Forrester, and provides a reasonable estimation of the pretest probability of CAD based on clinical grounds.[2] The value of stress testing is greatest when the pretest likelihood is intermediate because the result of the test will probably have the greatest impact on the posttest probability of CAD, and therefore on clinical decision-making.

Exercise testing is generally a safe procedure. The risk is determined by the clinical characteristics of the patient referred for the procedure. In a nonselected patient population, the mortality is less than 0.01% whereas morbidity is less than 0.05%.[3] Good clinical judgment is therefore required to determine which patient can safely undergo an exercise test. Absolute and relative contraindications to exercise testing are summarized in Table 14-2.[1,4] Exercise testing should be performed under the supervision of an appropriately trained physician, and equipment, medications, and trained personnel to provide advanced cardiac life support must be readily available.

The electrocardiogram (ECG), heart rate, and blood pressure should be monitored carefully and recorded during each stage of exercise and during chest pain or ST-segment abnormalities. Exercise testing is commonly terminated when patients reach a defined percentage of predicted maximum heart rate. However, there are a number of other standard indications to terminate a test, listed in Table 14-3, whose application significantly reduces the risk.[4]

Interpretation of the exercise test includes exercise capacity (duration and metabolic equivalents), and clinical, hemodynamic, and electrocardiographic response. The most commonly used definition for a positive exercise test result, from an ECG standpoint, is the greater than or equal to 1 mm of horizontal or downsloping ST-segment depression or elevation for at least 60 to 80 milliseconds after the end of the QRS complex.[5] The occurrence of chest discomfort consistent with angina is important, particularly if it forces termination of the test. Abnormalities in exercise capacity, systolic blood pressure response to exercise, and heart rate response to exercise are also important findings.

TABLE 14-1. Pretest probability of coronary artery disease by age, gender, and symptoms*

Age (y)	Gender	Typical/Definite angina pectoris	Atypical/Probable angina pectoris	Nonanginal chest pain	Asymptomatic
30–39	Men	Intermediate	Intermediate	Low	Very low
	Women	Intermediate	Very low	Very low	Very low
40–49	Men	High	Intermediate	Intermediate	Low
	Women	Intermediate	Low	Very low	Very low
50–59	Men	High	Intermediate	Intermediate	Low
	Women	Intermediate	Intermediate	Low	Very low
60–69	Men	High	Intermediate	Intermediate	Low
	Women	High	Intermediate	Intermediate	Low

*No data exist for patients <30 or >69 years, but it can be assumed that prevalence of CAD increases with age. In a few cases, patients with ages at the extremes of the decades listed may have probabilities slightly outside the high or low range. High indicates >90%; intermediate, 10–90%; low, <10%; and very low, <5% probability.

TABLE 14-2. Contraindications to exercise testing

Absolute
Acute myocardial infarction (within 2 days)
High-risk unstable angina*
Uncontrolled cardiac arrhythmias causing symptoms or hemodynamic compromise
Symptomatic severe aortic stenosis
Uncontrolled symptomatic heart failure
Acute pulmonary embolus or pulmonary infarction
Acute myocarditis or pericarditis
Acute aortic dissection

Relative†
Left main coronary stenosis
Moderate stenotic valvular heart disease
Electrolyte abnormalities
Severe arterial hypertension‡
Tachyarrhythmias or bradyarrhythmias
Hypertrophic cardiomyopathy and other forms of outflow tract obstruction
Mental or physical impairment leading to inability to exercise adequately
High-degree atrioventricular block

*ACC/AHA Guidelines for the Management of Patients with Unstable Angina/Non-ST Segment Elevation Myocardial Infarction.
†Relative contraindications can be superseded if the benefits of exercise outweigh the risks.
‡In the absence of definitive evidence, the committee suggests systolic blood pressure of 200 mmHg and/or diastolic blood pressure of >110 mmHg.
Source: Modified from Fletcher et al.[4]

TABLE 14-3. Indications for terminating exercise testing

Absolute indications
Drop in systolic blood pressure of >10 mmHg from baseline blood pressure despite an increase in workload, when accompanied by other evidence of ischemia
Moderate to severe angina
Increasing nervous system symptoms (e.g. ataxia, dizziness, or near-syncope)
Signs of poor perfusion (cyanosis or pallor)
Technical difficulties in monitoring ECG or systolic blood pressure
Subject's desire to stop
Sustained ventricular tachycardia
ST elevation (≥1.0 mm) in leads without diagnostic Q waves (other than V1 or aVR)

Relative indications
Drop in systolic blood pressure of (≥10 mmHg from baseline blood pressure despite an increase in workload, in the absence of other evidence of ischemia
ST or QRS changes such as excessive ST depression (>2 mm of horizontal or downsloping ST-segment depression) or marked axis shift
Arrhythmias other than sustained ventricular tachycardia, including multifocal PVCs, triplets of PVCs, supraventricular tachycardia, heart block, or bradyarrhythmias
Fatigue, shortness of breath, wheezing, leg cramps, or claudication
Development of bundle branch block or IVCD that cannot be distinguished from ventricular tachycardia
Increasing chest pain
Hypertensive response*

*In the absence of definitive evidence, the committee suggests systolic blood pressure of >250 mmHg and/or a diastolic blood pressure of >115 mmHg.
ECG indicates electrocardiogram; PVCs, premature ventricular contractions; ICD, implantable cardioverter-defibrillator discharge; and IVCD, intraventricular conduction delay.
Source: Modified from Fletcher et al.[4]

Both treadmill and cycle ergometer devices are available for exercise testing. Although cycle ergometers are generally less expensive, smaller and produce less motion of the upper body than treadmills, the fatigue of the quadriceps muscles in patients who are not experienced cyclists is a major limitation, because subjects usually stop before reaching their maximum oxygen uptake. Consequently, treadmills are much more commonly used for exercise testing.[1]

Imaging Modalities of Exercise Testing in CAD

In recent years, the role of stress testing in the detection and risk assessment of CAD has changed considerably. The development of myocardial imaging modalities has significantly improved the diagnostic abilities in this area of clinical evaluation.

However, there is relatively little evidence comparing the cost-effectiveness ratios of treadmill exercise testing with more expensive imaging procedures. Compared with the treadmill exercise test, the cost of stress echocardiography is at least 2.1 times higher whereas the cost of stress single-photon emission computed tomographic (SPECT) myocardial imaging is 5.7 times higher. The lower cost of the treadmill exercise test does not necessarily translate into a lower overall cost of patient management, as the total cost of further testing and interventions may be higher when the initial exercise test is less accurate than the novel, more sophisticated procedures.[1]

Stress Myocardial Perfusion Imaging

Exercise perfusion imaging appears to be superior to exercise ECG alone in detecting CAD, in identifying multivessel disease, in localizing diseased vessels, and in determining the extent of ischemic and infarcted myocardium. Perfusion imaging is also useful for detecting myocardial viability in patients with left ventricular dysfunction, either regional or global, with or without Q waves, and provides important information with regard to risk stratification and therapeutic strategies.[6] Stress myocardial imaging is particularly valuable in the diagnosis of CAD in patients with abnormal resting ECG and those in whom ST-segment

responses cannot be interpreted accurately, such as patients with left ventricular hypertrophy, those with left bundle branch block or pre-excitation syndrome, and those receiving digitalis. Stress myocardial perfusion scintigraphy should not be used as a screening test in patients with low pretest probability of CAD, because the majority of abnormal tests will yield false-positive results.[7]

Given that the results with thallium-201 are comparable to those obtained with ^{99m}Tc-sestamibi or ^{99m}Tc-tetrofosmin, these agents can, generally, be used interchangeably for the diagnosis of CAD.[6]

For patients who are unable to exercise, especially the elderly and those with peripheral vascular disease, pulmonary disease, arthritis, or a previous stroke, pharmacological vasodilator stress with dipyridamole or adenosine may be used.

Stress Echocardiography

Stress echocardiography is the combination of two-dimensional echocardiography with a physical, pharmacological, or electrical stress. The diagnostic endpoint for the detection of myocardial ischemia is a stress-induced worsening of function in a region contracting normally at rest, whereas the stress echo sign of viability is a stress-induced improvement of function in a region that is abnormal at rest.[8]

Numerous studies have shown that stress echocardiography can detect CAD with an accuracy that is similar to that of stress myocardial perfusion imaging and superior to exercise ECG alone. Stress echocardiography is also useful in localizing and quantifying ischemic myocardium and provides important prognostic information in patients with known or suspected CAD.

Exercise stress echocardiography can be performed using a traditional treadmill or bicycle ergometry. The use of pharmacological agents minimizes factors that make the ultrasonic examination difficult during exercise, including hyperventilation, tachycardia, and excessive chest wall movement. The most well-studied and clinically available method is dobutamine stress echocardiography. Dobutamine increases heart rate and myocardial contractility and produces diagnostic changes in regional wall motion and systolic wall thickening as ischemia develops. Low-dose dobutamine infusion (5–10 µg/kg/min) is also valuable for assessing contractile reserve in hypokinetic or akinetic regions at rest as a means of identifying viable myocardium that may improve functionally after revascularization.[9] Atropine increases the accuracy of dobutamine stress echocardiography in patients with inadequate heart rate responses, especially those taking beta-blockers and those in whom second-degree heart block develops at higher atrial rates.

Recent developments proven to increase the accuracy of stress echocardiography include harmonic imaging and use of contrast agents. Moreover, Doppler tissue imaging, which allows quantification of intramural myocardial velocities, permits a more direct measure of myocardial function during stress, and may provide objective, quantitative evidence of stress-induced ischemia during echocardiography.

Stress Echocardiography Versus Nuclear Perfusion Imaging

Several studies have compared stress echocardiography with nuclear perfusion imaging. Overall, the sensitivity and specificity of the two techniques are comparable and range between 70% and 80%. Moreover, the negative predictive value for cardiac events (death, nonfatal myocardial infarction, and revascularization) of both techniques is greater than 90%. However, stress echocardiography may have a few advantages when compared with radionuclide imaging. First, echocardiography is a real time examination, allowing instantaneous imaging rather than averaging the image over several minutes. Second, echocardiography provides a more complete assessment of left ventricular wall motion. Moreover, echocardiography has no environmental impact and no biohazards for the patient and the physician, and lastly, the overall cost of echocardiography is lower than that of radionuclide imaging.[10]

Stress Magnetic Resonance Imaging

Stress magnetic resonance imaging (MRI) is useful for the diagnosis of CAD in patients unsuitable for dobutamine echocardiography.[11] Pharmacological stress is preferred to physiologic exercise to prevent motion artifacts within the MR imager. Several protocols using adenosine as a pharmacological stressor are being applied. One approach is to perform both stress and resting myocardial perfusion MRI to obtain perfusion reserve measurements.[12] An alternative approach is to assess stress myocardial perfusion only and detect areas of nonviable myocardium using delayed gadolinium-enhanced MRI.[13]

There are sparse data regarding the prognostic value of stress MRI. Outcome studies following normal stress MRI show a low event rate[11,14] whereas demonstration of inducible ischemia on dobutamine/atropine MRI is associated with higher risk for myocardial infarction or cardiac death at 20 months of follow-up.[15] Dipyridamole stress MRI has 85% agreement with T1-201 scintigraphy in detection of CAD and a correlation of 0,86 in sizing perfusion defects.[16]

Disadvantages of stress MRI include the inability to image patients with metal devices, the difficulty to image in the setting of irregular heart rhythm and the need for prolonged breath-holding.

Exercise Testing for Diagnosis and Risk Assessment of CAD

Exercise Testing in Asymptomatic Individuals Without Known CAD

The use of exercise testing for diagnosis of CAD in asymptomatic individuals is a controversial topic. The rationale of screening is the early detection of a disease that is the leading cause of death worldwide in the hope that treatment may prolong life or improve its quality and reduce the costs of treating acute events. Unfortunately, the accuracy of exercise testing in asymptomatic individuals has never been defined and probably never will be, because it is unethical to perform coronary angiography on them. Furthermore, more important than identifying CAD is to predict the outcome of the disease. Traditionally, the most important endpoint of screening is the prediction of myocardial infarction and death. Angina is less important as an endpoint as intervention can be postponed until its onset without this being harmful for the patient. In general, the relative risk of a subsequent event is increased in patients with a positive exercise test result, although the absolute risk of a cardiac event in asymptomatic patients remains only 1–2% per year, even if ST changes are associated with risk factors.[17] A positive exercise test result is more predictive of later presentation of angina than of occurrence of a major event. Moreover, most patients with subsequent cardiovascular death have a negative test result, because the sensitivity for detecting subsequent cardiovascular death is low. For these reasons, several studies have suggested evaluation of other data complementary to the presence of greater than 1 mm ST-segment depression in order to increase the predictive value of the exercise data alone. These include the ST/heart rate slope, the development of ischemia at low workload, risk factors, and the results of stress imaging tests. Impaired breathing as the only reason for exercise test termination in apparently healthy men (aged 40–59) has been recently associated with higher long-term CAD, pulmonary and total mortality.

The question is therefore whom to screen. Screening programs in the general population have the limitation that severe CAD in asymptomatic people is extremely rare. False-positive results may lead to unnecessary, expensive, and potentially hazardous additional testing, negative psychological implications, and serious consequences in work and insurance matters. In that respect, the recent US Preventive Services Task Force statement states that "false positive tests are common among asymptomatic adults, especially women, and may lead to unnecessary diagnostic testing, over treatment and labeling". For these reasons, the use of exercise testing in healthy asymptomatic patients has not been routinely recommended.[18] On the other hand, there are strong believers in the clinical and prognostic usefulness of exercise testing for screening healthy, asymptomatic subjects (men > 40 and women > 50 years of age) every 5 years, along with risk factor assessment based on the following rationales: (a) incremental risk ratios for the synergistic combination of the standard exercise test and more than one risk factors, (b) promotion of other more expensive diagnostic modalities, without the availability of the exercise test, for screening, (c) incentive to abandon physical inactivity and enhance exercise capacity with corresponding improvement in survival rates and decline in healthcare costs.

On the basis of prognostic evaluation, asymptomatic men older than 40–45 years with one or more risk factors may obtain useful prognostic information from exercise testing. The greater the pretest probability (i.e. the number of risk

factors), the more likely the patient will profit from screening. For these purposes, risk factors should be strictly defined: hypercholesterolemia as total cholesterol greater than 240 mg/dL, hypertension as systolic blood pressure greater than 140 mmHg or diastolic blood pressure greater than 90 mmHg, smoking, diabetes mellitus, and history of heart attack or sudden cardiac death in a first-degree relative less than 60 years old. The importance of more intensive risk factor management of persons with diabetes has been increasingly recognized. In asymptomatic diabetic persons, the likelihood of cardiovascular disease is increased if at least one of the following is present: age older than 35 years, type 2 diabetes of greater than 10 years' duration, type 1 diabetes of greater than 15 years' duration, any additional atherosclerotic risk factor for CAD, presence of microvascular disease (proliferative retinopathy or nephropathy, including microalbuminuria), peripheral vascular disease, or autonomic neuropathy.[1]

Other patient groups who are at increased risk of CAD but often asymptomatic despite the presence of this disease include patients with diabetes and peripheral vascular disease, chronic renal failure, and previous cardiac transplantation. Although these patients are more likely to have established CAD that may require intervention, functional testing is often nondiagnostic. Stress imaging tests seem to be of more value for risk stratification in these patients.

People whose occupation may affect public safety (i.e. airline pilots, professional drivers, firefighters) are often requested for statutory reasons to undergo periodic exercise testing for assessment of exercise capacity and prognostic evaluation of possible CAD. There are, however, sparse data to justify such an approach.

In patients with a history of cardiac disease who are about to begin a fitness program, exercise testing is recommended in order to stratify the risk. The risk of sudden death in patients with cardiac disease during supervised exercise has been estimated at 1 per 784,000 hours, and is higher than that in the general population. Similarly, patients with diabetes mellitus and arterial hypertension may benefit from exercise testing before a fitness program as a means of adjusting their training prescription. In asymptomatic patients without known cardiac disease, the absolute risk of a major cardiac event during exercise is small. However, cardiac arrest is more likely to occur during exercise than at rest, and this association is much greater in sedentary than in active persons. For this reason, exercise testing of asymptomatic men older than 45 years and women older than 55 years can be considered (especially if sedentary) if an exercise program more vigorous than walking is to be started.

Exercise Testing in Patients with Symptoms or a Prior History of CAD

Generally, patients with suspected or known CAD and new or changing symptoms that suggest ischemia should undergo exercise testing to assess the risk of future cardiac events, unless cardiac catheterization is indicated. The probability that the coronary disease of a given patient will progress to a higher risk state depends on multiple factors related to the underlying atherosclerotic process. The pathophysiologic model in which most major cardiac events occur is microscopic ruptures of vulnerable atherosclerotic plaques. However, most vulnerable plaques appear angiographically insignificant before rupture. Thus, the ability of stress testing of any type to detect vulnerable atheroscletotic lesions is limited by the lesser effect of these lesions on coronary blood flow and may explain the acute coronary events that occasionally occur after a negative treadmill test.

The choice of initial stress testing method should be based on evaluation of the patient's resting ECG, the patient's physical ability to exercise, and local expertise and technology. In patients with a normal resting ECG who are not taking digoxin, the exercise test should be the standard initial mode of stress testing used for risk assessment. Patients with widespread resting ST depression (greater than or equal to 1 mm) or patients with complete left bundle branch block, an intraventricular conduction defect with a QRS duration greater than 120 ms, ventricular paced rhythm, or pre-excitation should usually be tested with an imaging modality. In these patients, exercise testing may be still a useful prognostic tool but cannot be used to identify ischemia. Patients who cannot exercise because of physical limitations (e.g. arthritis, amputations, severe peripheral vascular disease, severe chronic obstructive pulmonary disease, or general debility) should undergo pharmacological stress testing in combination with imaging.

One of the most consistent prognostic markers of exercise testing is maximum exercise capacity. Exercise capacity is influenced primarily by the extent of resting left ventricular dysfunction and the amount of further left ventricular dysfunction induced by exercise, but is also affected by age, general physical conditioning, co-morbidities, and psychological state (especially the presence of depression). Several parameters can be used as markers of exercise capacity including maximum exercise duration, maximum MET level achieved, maximum workload achieved, maximum heart rate, chronotropic incompetence, and double product. The translation of exercise duration or workload into METs (oxygen uptake expressed in multiples of basal oxygen uptake, 3.5 O_2 mL/kg per minute) has the advantage of providing a common measure of performance regardless of the type of exercise test or protocol used.[1] Another group of prognostic exercise testing markers relates to exercise-induced ischemia and include exercise-induced ST-segment depression or ST-segment elevation (in leads without pathological Q waves and not in aVR), and exercise-induced angina. Other less powerful prognostic ST variables are the number of leads with significant ST-segment depression, the configuration of the exercise-induced ST depression (downsloping, horizontal, upsloping), and the duration of ST deviation into the recovery phase of the test. A number of studies have demonstrated the prognostic importance of other parameters from the exercise test, including chronotropic incompetence, abnormal heart rate recovery, and delayed systolic blood pressure response after exercise testing, though their use in risk stratification of symptomatic patients is not yet well established. Several investigators have attempted to incorporate multiple exercise variables into a prognostic tool. The most widely used is the Duke treadmill score, which applies to patients with known or suspected CAD, without prior revascularization or recent myocardial infarction, who undergo exercise testing before coronary angiography.

The post-exercise test risk assessment assists in management decisions that seem more appropriate when based on expected outcomes. The major management step addressed by exercise testing is whether to go on with additional testing which might reveal the need for revascularization. In patients who are classified as low risk on the basis of clinical and exercise testing information, there is no compelling evidence that an imaging modality adds significant new prognostic information to a standard exercise test. On the other hand, in patients with intermediate-risk treadmill score, myocardial perfusion imaging appears to be of value for further risk stratification. Patients with an intermediate-risk treadmill score and normal or near-normal exercise myocardial perfusion images and normal cardiac size are at low risk for future cardiac death and can be managed medically. Finally, patients with a high-risk exercise test result should usually be referred for cardiac catheterization.

Exercise Testing in Patients with Acute Coronary Syndromes

Acute coronary syndromes (i.e. unstable angina and non-ST-elevation myocardial infarction) represent an acute phase in the natural history of chronic CAD, which may either progress to myocardial infarction and death or return to the chronic stable phase of CAD. Patients with unstable angina are separated into low-, intermediate-, or high-risk groups on the basis of history and physical examination, 12-lead ECG, and serum cardiac markers. Low-risk patients can be treated on an outpatient basis, intermediate-risk patients can be treated in a monitored hospital bed, and high-risk patients are typically admitted to an intensive care unit. Little evidence exists regarding the safety of early exercise testing in unstable angina. One review of this topic found three studies including 632 patients with stabilized unstable angina who had a 0.5% death or myocardial infarction rate within 24 hours of their exercise test.[19]

Generally, exercise testing appears useful and safe in the evaluation of low-risk patients (normal or unchanged ECG during an episode of chest discomfort and normal cardiac markers) with unstable angina on an outpatient basis. In this group of patients, testing can be performed when patients have been free of symptoms of active ischemia or heart failure for a minimum of 8 to 12 hours. Intermediate-risk patients can be tested after 2 to 3 days, although carefully selected patients can be evaluated earlier. In general, as in stable angina, the exercise treadmill should be the standard mode of stress testing in patients with a normal resting ECG who are not taking digitalis.[1]

The Research on Instability in Coronary Artery Disease (RISC) study group examined the use of predischarge symptom-limited bicycle exercise testing in 740 men admitted with unstable angina or non-Q-wave myocardial infarction and found that the major independent predictors of 1-year infarction-free survival in multivariable regression analysis were the number of leads with ischemic ST-segment depression and peak exercise workload achieved.[20] Moreover, the Fragmin During Instability in Coronary Artery Disease (FRISC) study found in 766 unstable angina patients who had both a troponin T level test and a predischarge exercise test that the combination of a positive troponin T and exercise-induced ST depression stratified patients into groups with a risk of death or myocardial infarction that ranged from 1% to 20%.[21] Important exercise variables include not only ischemic parameters such as ST depression and chest pain but also parameters that reflect cardiac workload.

There is a growing body of evidence concerning the role of early exercise testing in emergency department chest pain centers. The rationale for its use in this setting is to provide rapid and efficient risk stratification and management for chest pain patients who possibly have acute coronary disease. Several studies have demonstrated that exercise testing improves the efficiency of management of low-risk and carefully selected intermediate-risk patients and may lower costs without compromising safety. However, exercise testing in emergency department chest pain centers should only be performed after the exclusion of high-risk features or other indications for hospital admission, and only as part of a carefully constructed management protocol.[19]

Exercise Testing after Myocardial Infarction

Over the past decade treatment strategies for the patients with acute myocardial infarction have dramatically changed. Shorter duration of hospitalization, widespread use of thrombolytic agents and coronary revascularization, and increased use of beta-adrenergic blockers and angiotensin-converting enzyme inhibitors have led to significant improvement in the prognosis of post-infarction patients, especially in those who have been treated with reperfusion. Therefore, the patient population presently eligible for predischarge exercise testing in clinical trials differs substantially from less selected historical populations. Their low cardiac event rate significantly reduces the predictive accuracy of early exercise testing. The available evidence on the ability of exercise testing to assess the cardiac risk in patients who have not received reperfusion therapy is limited. Although their mortality rates are lower than in patients treated in the prethrombolytic era because of therapeutic advances and revascularization, their absolute event rates are higher than in patients who have received thrombolysis. Moreover, patients who have not undergone coronary revascularization and are unable to perform an exercise test because of either clinical instability or disabling co-morbidities have the worst prognosis.

The exercise protocols after myocardial infarction can be either submaximal or symptom-limited. Submaximal protocols have a predetermined endpoint, defined as a peak heart rate of 120 beats/min, or 70% of the predicted maximum heart rate, or a peak MET level of 5. Symptom-limited tests are designed to continue until the patient demonstrates signs or symptoms that necessitate termination of exercise. The most commonly used treadmill protocols are the modified Bruce, the modified Naughton, and the standard Bruce. Timing of predischarge exercise tests in the relevant literature ranges from 5 to 26 days after infarction. Some studies have evaluated symptom-limited protocols at 4 to 7 days after myocardial infarction and demonstrated that they have the potential to be more useful in activity prescription before discharge, though their additive prognostic value has not yet been established. Postdischarge tests have been performed early (14 to 21 days), at 6 weeks, and at 6 months after infarction.[1] Exercise testing after myocardial infarction appears to be safe, though the majority of the safety data refer to exercise tests performed more than 7 days after myocardial infarction.

Exercise test predictors of adverse outcome in the post-infarction patient include ischemic ST-segment depression greater than or equal to 1 mm, especially if accompanied by symptoms, at a low level of exercise, or in the presence of controlled heart failure, functional capacity less than 5 METs, and inadequate blood pressure response (peak systolic blood pressure less than 110 mmHg in patients with Q-wave infarcts or less than 30 mmHg increase from resting level).

Exercise testing after myocardial infarction is useful for counseling patients about domestic, occupational, and recreational activities that can be safely performed after discharge from the hospital. Generally, functional capacity in METs derived from the exercise test can be used to estimate tolerance for specific activities. Moreover, the exercise test is an important tool in cardiac rehabilitation for the development of the exercise prescription, risk stratification, and determination of the level of monitoring required during the exercise program and the evaluation of the patient's response during the various phases of the training program.

Practically, according to the ACC/AHA Practice Guidelines for patients who do not present clinical indications of high risk at predischarge (i.e. hypotension, congestive heart failure, recurrent chest pain), two strategies for performing exercise testing can be used. One is a symptom-limited exercise test at 14 to 21 days. If the patient is on digoxin therapy or if the baseline ECG precludes accurate interpretation of ST-segment changes (e.g. left bundle branch block, pre-excitation syndrome, left ventricular hypertrophy), then an initial exercise imaging study could be performed. The results of exercise testing should be stratified to determine the need for additional invasive or exercise perfusion studies. Another strategy is to perform a submaximal exercise test at 4 to 7 days after myocardial infarction or just before hospital discharge. If the exercise test studies are negative, a second symptom-limited exercise test could be repeated at 3 to 6 weeks for patients undergoing vigorous activity during leisure time activities, at work, or exercise training as part of cardiac rehabilitation. The extent of reversible ischemia on the exercise imaging study should be considered before proceeding to cardiac catheterization. A small area contiguous to the infarct zone may not necessarily require catheterization.[22]

Exercise Testing Before and after Revascularization

Patients who are planned to undergo revascularization, and especially those who are asymptomatic, should have documented ischemic or viable myocardium.[5] This most commonly requires a more sensitive test than exercise ECG, particularly in the setting of one-vessel disease and when the culprit vessel supplies the posterior wall. However, documentation of pre-procedure exercise capacity may be of value.

With regard to the early phase after revascularization, the goal of an exercise test is to evaluate the immediate result, whereas in the late phase the goal of an exercise test is to assist in evaluation and treatment of patients as well as in guiding rehabilitation programs and return-to-work decisions.[1]

After coronary artery bypass graft surgery (CABG), the exercise ECG has a number of limitations. In symptomatic patients, exercise testing may be useful in distinguishing between cardiac and noncardiac causes of recurrent chest pain after surgery. However, the fact that resting ECG abnormalities are common together with the need to document not only the presence of ischemia but also its site and extent favor the use of stress imaging tests in this group of patients, although there are sparse data regarding the frequency of testing. Exercise testing in asymptomatic patients with successful coronary bypass grafting is not predictive of subsequent events when the test is performed within the first few years after the surgery. The test certainly provides more useful information when the likelihood of progression of CAD is enhanced (i.e. 5 to 10 years after CABG, in the presence of typical angina, diabetes mellitus, hemodialysis, or immunosuppressive therapy).

After percutaneous coronary intervention (PCI) the main concern is to investigate for restenosis. However, symptom status is an unreliable index to development of restenosis, as many patients complain of noncardiac pain after angioplasty whereas others experience silent ischemia. Silent restenosis is a frequent clinical manifestation, with 25% of asymptomatic patients presenting features of ischemia on exercise testing.

The clinical event of restenosis after PCI reflects a complex underlying pathophysiology. Because residual plaque is responsible for a significant proportion of restenosis, several researchers have reported success in performing exercise testing early after PCI (i.e. within 1 to 3 days). The presence of ischemia in these tests is predictive of restenosis. Moreover, the use of an exercise test early after PCI

may facilitate earlier return to work and daily activities. However, the safety of this approach has not been established and exercise when unstable plaque exists may lead to vessel occlusion.

The rationale of performing exercise testing later (i.e. 3 to 6 months) after PCI is to identify – rather than predict – restenosis. There are two main approaches regarding this issue: (a) routine testing, because restenosis is a frequent problem and worsens prognosis and (b) selective evaluation in high-risk patients, because the prognostic benefit of controlling silent ischemia needs to be proved.[1] Whichever policy is followed, the sensitivity of exercise ECG to investigate restenosis ranges from 40% to 55%, and is significantly less than that obtainable with SPECT or exercise echocardiography. The low sensitivity of exercise testing probably reflects the high prevalence of one-vessel disease in this population.

In conclusion, the lower sensitivity of exercise testing compared to imaging techniques and its inability to document localization of ischemia limits its value in patient management before and after revascularization. Despite the different modalities of exercise testing in this context, there are not enough data to establish a particular testing regimen after revascularization.

Exercise Testing in Special Groups

Women

Cardiovascular disease is one of the leading causes of death in women, exceeding mortality due to breast cancer by a factor of 11. However, the probability of CAD in women is most commonly in the low to intermediate probability range, especially in premenopausal women, and the investigation of CAD in women presents difficulties that are not experienced in the identification of the disease in men. These difficulties reflect gender differences in exercise physiology, coronary physiology, and prevalence of CAD.

The diagnostic accuracy of exercise-induced ST depression for obstructive CAD is less in women than in men, which reflects the lower prevalence of severe CAD and the inability of most women to exercise to maximum aerobic capacity. Moreover, women tend to have a greater release of catecholamines during exercise, which could lead to coronary vasoconstriction and abnormal ECG results. False-positive results have been reported to be more common during menses or preovulation and in postmenopausal women on isolated estrogen replacement therapy. The accuracy of exercise testing in women may be enhanced by attention to parameters other than the level of ST depression. The ST/heart rate relation seems to be of value but not yet in widespread application. Avoidance of evaluating ST depression in the inferior leads and identification of test positivity based on persistent changes enhance the predictive value of a positive test but may compromise the predictive value of a negative test.

Concerns about false-positive ST-segment responses may be addressed by careful evaluation of posttest probability and selective use of stress imaging tests before the patient proceeds to coronary angiography. Currently, there are insufficient data to justify routine use of stress imaging tests as the initial approach for diagnosing CAD in women.

Elderly

There is limited evidence for the use of exercise testing for diagnostic and prognostic assessment of CAD in patients older than 65 years. The prevalence of CAD increases with advancing age and therefore, from a Bayesian standpoint, the higher prevalence and greater severity of CAD in this special group increase the sensitivity of testing with a slight reduction in specificity.

Exercise testing is not contraindicated in the elderly, but it certainly poses several difficulties. Maximal aerobic capacity declines by 8–10% per decade in sedentary persons, with an approximate 50% reduction in exercise capacity between ages 30 and 80 years.[23] Muscle weakness or deconditioning often compromises exercise capacity, and therefore the decision about an exercise or pharmacological stress test is more important than in younger patients. For patients with coordination or gait problems, a bicycle exercise test may be an attractive alternative to a treadmill exercise test, although unfamiliarity is a common limitation in elderly patients. If treadmill exercise is used, physicians have to select more gradual protocols and attention must be paid to the mechanical hazards of exercise in elderly patients.

Interpretation of exercise testing in the elderly differs slightly from that in younger patients. Resting ECG abnormalities may compromise diagnostic accuracy of the exercise ECG. False-positive results may reflect the presence of left ventricular hypertrophy caused by valvular disease or hypertension, as well as conduction disturbances. Moreover, elderly patients may need to grasp the handrails for support, reducing the validity of treadmill time for estimating METs. ST depression in asymptomatic elderly patients is not associated with high event rate and therefore the predictive accuracy of these data may be enhanced by other exercise features and a stepwise approach combined with stress imaging tests.

Pharmacological stress perfusion imaging with magnetic resonance imaging (MRI) compares favorably with other methods and is performed in some centers, particularly for patients who present limitations for other imaging methods. In these patients MRI offers accurate evaluation of left ventricular function. Novel techniques are likely to lead to further improvements in MRI as a tool for stress testing.

Conclusion

Exercise test modalities are essential tools for the diagnosis and evaluation of disease severity in patients with suspected coronary artery disease, for the risk stratification and determination of prognosis in patients with known coronary artery disease, and finally, for the evaluation of efficacy of various medications and/or interventional procedures in patients being treated for coronary artery disease.

References

1. Gibbons RJ, Balady GJ, Bricker JT, et al. ACC/AHA 2002 guideline update for exercise testing. Summary article: A report of the American College of Cardiology/American Heart Association Task Force on Practice Guidelines (Committee to Update the 1997 Exercise Testing Guidelines). J Am Coll Cardiol 2002;40:1531.
2. Diamond GA, Forrester JS. Analysis of probability as an aid in the clinical diagnosis of coronary-artery disease. N Engl J Med 1979;300:1350–1358.

3. Stuart RJ Jr, Ellestad MH. National survey of exercise stress testing facilities. Chest 1980;77:94–97.

4. Fletcher GF, Balady G, Froelicher VF, Hartley LH, Haskell WL, Pollock ML. Exercise standards: a statement for healthcare professionals from the American Heart Association Writing Group: special report. Circulation 1995;91:580–615.

5. Eagle KA, Guyton RA, Davidoff R, et al. ACC/AHA guidelines for coronary artery bypass graft surgery: a report of the American College of Cardiology/American Heart Association Task Force Practice Guidelines (Committee to Revise the 1991 Guidelines Coronary Artery Bypass Graft Surgery). American College Cardiology/American Heart Association. J Am Coll Cardiol 1999;34:1262–1347.

6. Beller GA, Zaret BL. Contributions of nuclear cardiology to diagnosis and prognosis of patients with coronary artery disease. Circulation 2000;101:1465–1478.

7. Ritchie JL, Bateman TM, Bonow RO, et al. Guidelines for clinical use of cardiac radionuclide imaging: report of the American College of Cardiology/American Heart Association Task Force on Assessment of Diagnostic and Therapeutic Cardiovascular Procedures (Committee on Radionuclide Imaging), developed in collaboration with the American Society of Nuclear Cardiology. J Am Coll Cardiol 1995;25:521–547.

8. Picano E. Stress echocardiography. Expert Rev Cardiovasc Ther 2004;2(1):77–88.

9. Bax JJ, Poldermans D, Elhendy A, et al. Improvement of left ventricular ejection fraction, heart failure symptoms, and prognosis after revascularization in patients with chronic coronary artery disease and viable myocardium detected by dobutamine stress echocardiography. J Am Coll Cardiol 1999;34:163–169.

10. Tak T, Gutierrez R. Comparing stress testing methods. Available techniques and their use in CAD evaluation. Postgrad Med 2004;115(6):61–70.

11. Hundley WG, Hamilton CA, Thomas MS, et al. Utility of fast cine magnetic resonance imaging and display for the detection of myocardial ischemia in patients not well suited for second harmonic stress echocardiography. Circulation 1999;100:1697–1702.

12. Al-Saadi N, Nagel E, Gross M, et al. Noninvasive detection of myocardial ischemia from perfusion reserve based on cardiovascular magnetic resonance. Circulation 2000;101:1379–1383.

13. Schwitter J, Nanz D, Kneifel S, et al. Assessment of myocardial perfusion in coronary artery disease by magnetic resonance: a comparison with positron emission tomography and coronary angiography. Circulation 2001;103:2230–2235.

14. Kuijpers D, Ho KY, van Dijkman PR, Vliegenthart R, Oudkerk M. Dobutamine cardiovascular magnetic resonance for the detection of myocardial ischemia with the use of myocardial tagging. Circulation 2003;107:1592–1597.

15. Hundley WG, Morgan TM, Neagle CM, Hamilton CA, Rerkpattanapipat P, Link KM. Magnetic resonance imaging determination of cardiac prognosis. Circulation 2002;106:2328–2333.

16. Lauerma K, Virtanen KS, Sipila LM, Hekali P, Aronen HJ. Multislice MRI in assessment of myocardial perfusion in patients with single-vessel proximal left anterior descending coronary artery disease before and after revascularization. Circulation 1997;96:2859–2867.

17. Rautaharju PM, Prineas RJ, Eifler WJ, et al. Prognostic value of exercise electrocardiogram in men at high risk of future coronary heart disease: Multiple Risk Factor Intervention Trial experience. J Am Coll Cardiol 1986;8:1–10.

18. Smith SC Jr, Greenland P, Grundy SM. AHA Conference Proceedings: Prevention Conference V: Beyond secondary prevention: identifying the high-risk patient for primary prevention: executive summary. Circulation 2000;101:111–116.

19. Stein RA, Chaitman BR, Balady GJ, et al. Safety and utility exercise testing in emergency room chest pain centers: an advisory from the Committee on Exercise, Rehabilitation, and Prevention, Council on Clinical Cardiology, American Heart Association. Circulation 2000;102:1463–1467.

20. Nyman I, Larsson H, Areskog M, Areskog NH, Wallentin L, for the RISC Study Group. The predictive value of silent ischemia at an exercise test before discharge after an episode of unstable coronary artery disease. Am Heart J 1992;123:324–331.

21. Lindahl B, Andren B, Ohlsson J, Venge P, Wallentin L, for the FRISK Study Group. Risk stratification in unstable coronary artery disease: additive value of troponin T determinations and pre-discharge exercise tests. Eur Heart J 1997;18:762–770.

22. Ryan TJ, Antman EM, Brooks NH, et al. 1999 update: ACC/AHA guidelines for the management of patients with acute myocardial infarction: executive summary and recommendations: a report of the American College of Cardiology/American Heart Association Task Force on Practice Guidelines (Committee on Management of Acute Myocardial Infarction). Circulation 1999;100:1016–1030.

23. Rosen MJ, Sorkin JD, Goldberg AP, Hagberg JM, Katzel LI. Predictors of age-associated decline in maximal aerobic capacity: a comparison of four statistical models. J Appl Physiol 1998;84:2163–2170.

15
Cardiopulmonary Exercise Testing in Chronic Heart Failure

Alain Cohen-Solal, Florence Beauvais, and Jean Yves Tabet

Cardiopulmonary exercise testing (CPX) is being increasingly used in patients with chronic heart failure (CHF) for diagnostic and prognostic purposes. It provides major insights regarding the degree of functional impairment, the prognosis, and the effect of treatment. Despite the availability of simple and rapid gas analyzers, the general belief is that the procedure is complex, which is not the case. Peak oxygen uptake (peak VO_2) is generally the only variable used to evaluate exercise capacity and prognosis. However, CPX provides a lot of information besides peak VO_2.

Contraindications to CPX in CHF

Some conditions remain contraindications to exercise testing in CHF: very recent myocardial infarction, unstable angina, severe ventricular arrhythmias, symptomatic hypotension, and mobile intracardiac thrombus. Caution is warranted if there is severe pulmonary hypertension, aortic stenosis, or hypertrophic cardiomyopathy, although exercise testing is increasingly being used in these conditions. Left bundle branch block remains a contraindication unless coronarography is known to be normal. Heart failure per se clearly is no longer a contraindication but CPX has little value when done very recently after an acute decompensation or prolonged bedrest.

Protocols

The test can be carried out on a bicycle ergometer or treadmill. A treadmill has the advantage of more closely mimicking the conditions of exercise in real life. CHF patients often stop exercising on the treadmill because of dyspnea whereas on a bicycle, even if the main reported symptom is dyspnea, patients generally stop exercising because of leg fatigue. Peak achieved workrate is generally greater on a treadmill in CHF patients as in normal subjects, by about 10–15% (Figure 15-1).[1] On the other hand, ECG and ventilatory artifacts are more important on a treadmill. The increase in workrate is less linear on a treadmill and workload, depending on body weight, slope and speed, is more difficult to quantify than on a bicycle.

On a treadmill, the Bruce protocol allows achievement of the highest workload and VO_2. However, it is poorly tolerated in patients with severe CHF. Other protocols are more often used (standard or modified Naughton protocol, for example). Other protocols are specially designed for patients with a cardiac pacemaker. Others, finally, are designed to have similar VO_2 increments on a bicycle or treadmill.

On a bicycle, small workload increments of about 10 watts/minute are generally used. Increments of 20 or 30 watts are generally less well tolerated. Ramp protocols are also used where resistance is progressively increased over one minute. The duration of exercise should generally be around 10 minutes, whatever the exercise capacity of the patient (although this has been mainly validated in normal subjects). Peak VO_2 is generally underestimated with shorter protocols; on the other hand, it can also be lower with very long protocols because of boredom, especially

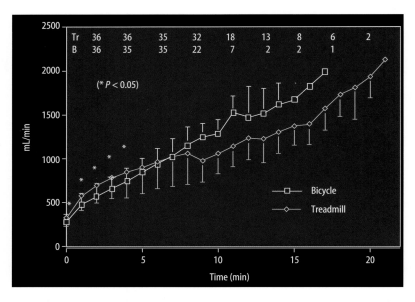

FIGURE 15-1. Comparison of peak VO_2 obtained during bicycle and treadmill exercise in the same subjects with heart failure. Peak VO_2 is always greater by about 10% on the treadmill. (From Page et al.[1] © 1994 by the American College of Chest Physicans. Reprinted with permission.)

when a mouthpiece is used. One has, however, always to remember that in CHF, the kinetics of VO_2 increase are reduced compared to normal subjects and, therefore, a steady state is never attained at the end of a stage of less than 3 minutes even with a 10 W/min protocol.

Other ergometers or exercise protocols are less often used and have a different finality.

– Arm exercise in patients who cannot walk or cycle; workrate is lower, ventilation higher, and this kind of exercise is painful for the arms.
– Constant workrate protocols have a different finality. They allow calculation of the kinetics of VO_2 increase at the beginning of exercise, which has been related to the increase in cardiac output. They are also the preferred protocol when hemodynamic or echocardiographic measurements are to be made during the test. This should also be in theory the method to determine the level of physical training in a rehabilitation endurance program. When workrate is set below the anaerobic threshold (AT), VO_2, VCO_2, VE and lactate plateau during the constant workrate exercise; in contrast, when workrate is situated above the level corresponding to the AT, there is a drift in VO_2 and

also in VCO_2 and VE. It is generally believed that the level of training, at least at the beginning, should be set around the AT and then progressively increased. Nowadays, the level of training is determined after a graded test, but whether the results are really similar to that obtained after constant workrate exercise is not known.

Equipment

Various commercial systems are available that differ in their methodology of measurement of O_2 and CO_2 concentrations and in their analysis software. The important point is to have a breath-by-breath measurement. However, for a better display of the curves, one generally use a moving average of the breath-by-breath values. It is, however, important to have data every 10–20 seconds. Because of the short duration of exercise in CHF, a 30-second interval of measurement appears too long.

Gas is sampled through a facial mask or a mouthpiece. A mouthpiece (with a nose-clip) is the equipment of reference because of the lack of leaks, especially at high levels of ventilation. However, it is uncomfortable for the patient, stressful, and generates hypersalivation. Face masks are better tolerated but it is often difficult to rule out leaks at high levels of exercise.

Calibration of the System

This is a very important part of the test. It should be done before each test and does not take more than one minute. The two main causes of errors in CPX results are errors in calibration and leaks.

Analysis of the resting phase is important and already provides some insights. It is necessary to wait 3–4 minutes of resting while gas exchange is measured to ensure stability. Baseline VO_2 should be between 3 and 5 mL/min/kg (but lower values may be found in patients with severe heart failure), the respiratory exchange ratio (RER) below 0.90, and ventilation quiet. Ventilatory oscillations can be observed at this stage; this is the consequence of a periodic way of breathing and is always associated with severe circulatory failure and/or pulmonary hypertension. The mechanism of this profile is not exactly known but seems to

be mainly related to the very low kinetics of oxygen transport.[2] It tends to diminish or disappear during the increase in workrate.

Evolution of Oxygen Uptake

VO_2 increases linearly with workrate, but the kinetics of this response decrease with the severity of heart failure. Schematically, the increment of VO_2 is about 10–11 mL O_2/min/watt during a 10 watts/min protocol in normal subjects. In patients with severe CHF, the VO_2/W slope may be decreased to 7 or 8 (Figure 15-2).[3] This is the reason why it is mandatory to measure VO_2 in CHF patients and not to derive it from peak workrate, based on various formulae established in normal subjects in whom the slope is relatively constant. The decrease in the slope is probably related to an altered kinetics of cardiac output increase and/or peripheral oxygen extraction.

In patients undergoing submaximal graded exercise, the VO_2/W slope provides some insights: a normal slope suggests a noncardiac cause to

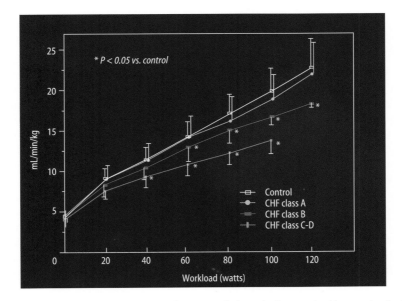

FIGURE 15-2. Relation between workrate and VO_2 increase during a graded exercise in normal subjects and patients with heart failure (10 watts/min increase protocol). In normal subjects, the slope of the VO_2/W relationship is between 10 and 12 mL O_2 per watt. It decreases with the severity of heart failure. If peak VO_2 was estimated from peak workrate in a C–D Weber class patient, the actual peak VO_2 would have been overestimated by nearly 50%.

stopping exercise, a decreased slope suggests circulatory failure. However, at the individual level, this slope exhibits a high variability, limiting its use. Various studies have suggested its prognostic role.[4]

Peak Exercise VO_2

Contrary to what is observed in athletes or fit subjects, what is measured at the end of exercise in a CHF patient is not a plateau of VO_2max. Therefore, one has to be sure, before interpreting the value of peak VO_2, that the test has been maximal or submaximal and can be considered valid. This is difficult a posteriori. Patients generally stop exercising because of fatigue, less often because of dyspnea (at least on a bicycle). Tests stopped for other reasons (chest pain, ischemia, decrease in blood presssure, arrhythmias) should not be considered for the assessment of peak VO_2. It is important to stimulate the patient during the test. A high RER value, greater than 1.1, and a peak heart rate close to the maximal predicted heart rate suggest that the exercise test was valid.

Peak VO_2 is usually measured at the end of the test. Results are given in mL/min or in mL/min/kg. Because this kind of indexation has limitations in obese or lean subjects, peak VO_2 should probably be indexed by predicted values in order to take into account the effect of age, sex, and previous level of fitness. A peak VO_2 of 18 mL/min/kg may correspond to a normal value for a 70-year-old woman. Conversely, a value of 25 mL/min/kg may represent a severe limitation to exercise in a 25-year-old former athlete.

Unfortunately, no table is perfect. One generally uses reference values given by Jones[5] or by Wasserman's group.[6] Other groups have suggested that indexing peak VO_2 by lean body weight is more accurate.[7]

A normal value of VO_2max for a normal, non-regularly exercising man is about 30–40 mL/min/kg. It is slightly lower in women because of a lower non-fat mass. VO_2max decreases with age. Training may increase peak VO_2 by 20–30%.

Peak VO_2 may allow classification of the patient into one of the four exertional classes described by Weber et al.[8]

The Anaerobic Threshold

The anaerobic threshold is a still debated concept. It represents the time when there is, in theory, a transition from an aerobic to an anaerobic metabolism during exercise. It can be detected noninvasively during CPX by analysis of the ventilatory curves.[9] At the time of the anaerobic threshold, VCO_2 increases along with an increased production resulting from the buffering of lactates by bicarbonates in the blood. When VCO_2 is plotted versus VO_2, an increase in the slope represents the AT. Other methods of determination are probably more accurate in CHF patients. For example, the analysis of the ventilatory equivalent curves is easier in practice. VE/VO_2 decreases at the beginning of exercise, then plateaus and increases at the level of the AT. The VE/VCO_2 curve also decreases at the beginning of exercise, then also plateaus, but increases only when VE increases disproportionately compared with VCO_2, at the point called the respiratory compensation point (RCP). At this time, VE increases disproportionately to VCO_2 because ventilation is driven by both an increase in CO_2 production and decrease in pH in the blood, as buffering of lactate by bicarbonates becomes insufficient. One can also detect the AT by analysis of the end-tidal pressure ($PETO_2$ and $PETCO_2$) curves; at the AT level, $PETO_2$ increases and $PETCO_2$ decreases. In general, it is better not to rely on a single curve to assess the AT.

In normal subjects, the AT occurs at about 50% of peak VO_2. It can be delayed by training, and in athletes it may be observed not before 90% of peak VO_2. In CHF patients, the AT is generally decreased for various reasons: low peripheral cardiac output, impaired utilization of O_2 by the muscles, deconditioning. In theory, the AT is observed at less than 50% of peak VO_2 but can occur later when exercise is submaximal.

The AT may be difficult to detect in patients with severe heart failure,[10] mainly in the presence of oscillations. The AT is independent of the patient's motivation. A normal AT with a low peak VO_2 suggests submaximal exercise. Because of problems of determination, the AT has never supplanted the peak VO_2 as a marker of functional capacity or prognosis in CHF patients.

Kinetics of VO_2 Increase at the Beginning of Exercise

In the first 30 seconds of a constant workrate exercise, it has been suggested by the group of Wasserman[11] that the kinetics of VO_2 increase are solely related to the increase in pulmonary blood flow, and thus to cardiac output. In heart failure, the kinetics of VO_2 increase are decreased. However, this parameter is seldom used because of poor repeatability and the need for a constant workrate exercise. Groups have indeed shown that the kinetics of VO_2 increase are more related to cardiac output than to peak VO_2.

Kinetics of VO_2 Recovery after Exercise

At recovery, VO_2 decreases exponentially after a graded exercise. The half-time of VO_2 recovery ($T_{1/2}$) has been shown to be 60–80 seconds in normal subjects after graded exercise. The kinetics of VO_2 are prolonged with the severity of heart failure. Patients with a peak VO_2 less than 10–12 mL/min/kg may need 3 minutes to decrease their VO_2 by 50%. This is probably related to the slow kinetics of reconstitution of the energetic stores after exercise. This VO_2-off kinetics has the advantage of being poorly influenced by the level of exercise; therefore, in submaximal exercise (at least when >50% of VO_2max), the VO_2-off kinetics can be used to analyze the degree of impairment of circulatory function.[12] A normal VO_2-off with a low peak VO_2 suggests submaximal exercise. Various groups have also shown that the half-time of VO_2 recovery has prognostic value.[13,14]

The Cleveland Clinic Group has promoted the heart rate recovery kinetics after exercise as a prognostic factor in patients with CAD.[15] However, the prognostic value of this variable has not been assessed in patients with heart failure.

The VE/VCO_2 Slope

The VE/VCO_2 slope has emerged in the recent years as a very popular parameter in patients with CHF.[16] During exercise, VE and VCO_2 are linearly related until the RCP, where VE increases disproportionately to VCO_2. The slope of this relationship, before the RCP, reflects the increase in the chemoreceptors gain that triggers ventilation in response to changes in the partial pressure of CO_2 (PCO_2) in the blood. The VE/VCO_2 slope has been related to increased pulmonary dead space, to the decrease of pulmonary blood flow, and to the activation of ergoreceptors originating from the muscle.

Whatever the exact mechanism of the VE/VCO_2 increase, it appears that this slope is increased in CHF and has prognostic value. Normal values are between 20 and 30; in CHF values can reach 80. The VE/VCO_2 is improved by training and by treatment. Its prognostic value has been compared to that in peak VO_2 in various studies. In some of them, the VE/VCO_2 slope appeared to better predict prognosis than peak VO_2. There are two situations in which the VE/VCO_2 slope may indeed have an advantage over peak VO_2 for predicting outcome: (1) in submaximal exercise; (2) in patients on beta-blocker therapy, where prognosis improves with treatment whereas peak VO_2 generally remains unchanged or increases only slightly and the VE/VCO_2 slope is decreased.[17]

There is still controversy on whether the VE/VCO_2 slope should be calculated across the overall data or only until the RCP[18]: using all points seems to increase the prognostic value.[19]

Other Parameters

Another slope, the *oxygen uptake efficiency slope*, the slope relating linearly VO_2 and the logarithm of VE during exercise, is another interesting parameter that can be used when exercise is submaximal.[20] It is decreased in heart failure.

The *oxygen pulse* is VO_2 divided by heart rate. It equals stroke volume times arteriovenous oxygen (AVO_2) difference. The peak value and the profile of the O_2 pulse during exercise thus mirrors the responses of both parameters. It has been suggested that the O_2 pulse is a good surrogate of stroke volume changes during exercise. This is probably not correct; indeed, during exercise, stroke volume changes are generally mild, both in normal subjects and in patients with heart failure: 30% is a maximum. On the other hand, the AVO_2 difference increases more; in athletes, it can

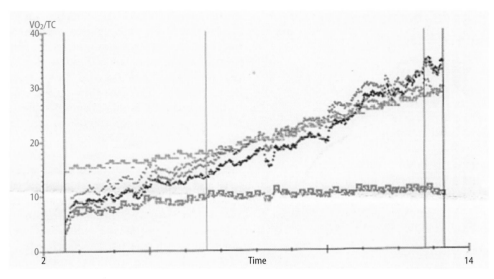

FIGURE 15-3. Plateauing of oxygen pulse in heart failure. In this patient, the oxygen pulse (red squares) plateaus, which means a continuous decrease in stroke volume during exercise. The other curves are heart rate in blue, VO_2 in green, VCO_2 in red, and ventilation in black.

increase 4-fold. In CHF, AVO_2 difference is already enlarged at rest and therefore cannot increase much, but it does so at least as much as stroke volume. A plateauing of the O_2 pulse (or a decrease) during exercise suggests a decrease in stroke volume as AVO_2 difference increases throughout exercise (Figure 15-3). A low peak O_2 pulse is generally associated with a poor prognosis but its predictive value is less than peak VO_2.

Other Abnormalities That May Be Observed During a CPX Test in CHF

– Ventilatory oscillations: this kind of periodic breathing (Figure 15-4) is mainly observed in severe heart failure. They are often associated with Cheyne–Stokes dyspnea during the night. They tend to decrease with the increase in load

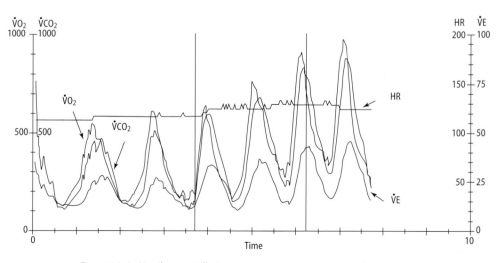

FIGURE 15-4. Ventilatory oscillations at rest in a patient with severe heart failure.

during exercise and reappear at recovery. Their meaning is still debated.[21] They always have a poor prognostic value. They also complicate the determination of the AT.

– A rebound or a continuous increase in VO_2 despite cessation of exercise is found in some patients with severe heart failure, while at the same time heart rate and VE decrease (Figure 15-5). This profile generally represents a marked slowing of blood velocity; it can also be related to a sudden decrease in peripheral vasoconstriction with the end of exercise. Studies have shown that this profile is associated with a rebound of stroke volume at recovery.

– It has long been known that it is important to analyze the blood pressure response during exercise. A decrease or a poor increase in blood pressure during exercise is generally associated with a poor cardiac output response. As in patients with CAD, it has been shown that the peak blood pressure value also has prognostic value in CHF patients.[22] When the blood pressure response is excessive, one may suspect that the cause of heart failure is hypertension. When the blood pressure response is poor whereas peak VO_2 is preserved or only mildly decreased, one may suspect that the preservation of a correct circulatory response is mainly due to a good peripheral

adaptation despite a poor cardiac output increase.

– Various studies have evaluated the value of invasive hemodynamic measurements during exercise in patients with CHF.[23,24] In these studies, two parameters have always emerged as being very predictive of outcome, with a potency greater than peak VO_2: the peak value of stroke work or of cardiac power. Stroke work is the product of stroke volume and mean blood pressure; cardiac power is the product of cardiac output and mean blood pressure. Interestingly, it may be possible to calculate or estimate these variables noninvasively:

  ◦ One method is to measure cardiac output at peak exercise noninvasively by techniques of rebreathing of the CO_2 or of acetylene.[25]
  ◦ A second method is to approach the value of peak cardiac power by the circulatory power, an index obtained by multiplying peak VO_2 by peak systolic blood pressure. This equals peak cardiac power times peak AVO_2 difference.[14]
  ◦ Various studies have shown that these two measurements have a very good prognostic value, at least equal to that of peak VO_2.

– In summary, the blood pressure response should always be considered besides peak VO_2 value.

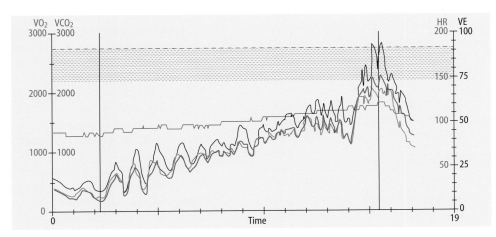

FIGURE 15-5. Typical pattern of exercise response in a patient with severe heart failure. Peak VO_2 is low and VO_2 decreases slowly at recovery with a rebound after stopping exercise. There are ventilatory oscillations at rest and during the first part of exercise.

Indications

The indications for CPX in CHF patients are many. However, the method needs good equipment, knowledge of the physiology of exercise, and a patient able to exercise. Therefore, these tests are less often performed in very elderly CHF patients, who are each year more frequent.

1. CPX is necessary to objectively assess the functional impairment of the patient. Patients often report poor limitation of exercise capacity when they have themselves limited their activities. However, exercise capacity may be maintained even in cases of severe heart failure and this has implications for therapy. One can classify the patient's response according to the Weber classification into one of four classes (Table 15-1), but this classification does not replace the evaluation of the patient's symptoms. Submaximal exercise capacity is not synonymous with either symptoms during daily life or quality of life.

2. CPX makes it possible to relate functional limitation to cardiac or pulmonary factors. Various criteria aid in distinguishing between a respiratory or a cardiac limitation of exercise (Table 15-2). The problem, however, is not so easy in patients with coexisting cardiac and pulmonary diseases.

3. The main indication of CPX is to assess prognosis. Various studies in the last 15 years have shown that peak VO_2 is probably the best prognostic factor in CHF among all the other variables obtained by biology, hemodynamics, or echocardiography (Figure 15-6). One of the reason for this is that peak VO_2 integrates the cardiac reserve while most of the other measurements are made at rest and may overlook the ability of the heart to respond to a stress.

The problem now is: which criteria? which cut-off?

a. Peak VO_2 remains the better parameter for assessment so long as the exercise really has been conducted until exhaustion. In theory,

TABLE 15-2. Parameters enabling distinction between a respiratory or a cardiac cause in case of exertional dyspnea

	Cardiac	Pulmonary
Peak VO_2	Reduced	Reduced
AT	Early	Normal
O_2 pulse	Early plateau	Normal
VO_2/Workrate	Reduced	Normal
Heart rate response	Variable	Normal or increased
Ventilatory reserve	Normal	Reduced
PaO_2	Normal	Reduced
SaO_2	Normal, unchanged	Decreased
AVO_2 difference	Normal	Decreased
Respiratory rate	Increased	Excessive
Vd/Vt	Normal, reduced	Constant

AT: aerobic threshold.
PaO_2: arterial oxygen pressure.
SaO_2: arterial oxygen saturation.
AVO_2: arteriovenous oxygen difference.
Vd/Vt: ration dead space / tidal volume.

it is better to index peak VO_2 by predicted values using formulae from Wasserman or Jones. However, this indexation is of value mainly in very young or old patients, or in obese or lean patients. For male patients between 20 and 60 years, its superiority over peak VO_2 indexed by body weight is not obvious.[26] In our opinion, it is valuable to give results expressed both in mL/min indexed by body weight and by predicted values. Other authors have also proposed indexing peak VO_2 to lean body weight.

b. The cut-off is not easy to determine. Following the pioneering work of Mancini[27] and other studies, it has appeared that:
  – A peak VO_2 less than 10 mL/min/kg is always associated with a very poor prognosis. If possible, these patients should be put on a transplant list.
  – A peak VO_2 >18 mL/min/kg is generally associated with a good outcome at one year. In these patients, survival without transplantation is better than after transplantation.
  – The cut-off value of 14 mL/min/kg has been retained as the cut-off value to predict transplantation because in Mancini's study, outcome at one year was similar to that in transplanted patients. However, since 1991, survival after transplantation and with medical therapy has

TABLE 15-1. Weber's classification of exercise capacity

Weber class	Peak VO_2	AT	Functional capacity
A	>20 mL/min/kg	>14	Mild/absent
B	16–20	11–14	Mild/moderate
C	10–15	8–11	Moderate/severe
D	<10	<8	Severe

AT: aerobic threshold.

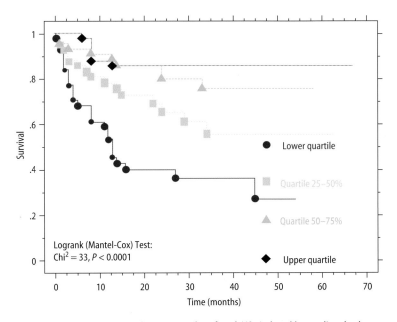

FIGURE 15-6. Survival according to quartiles of peak VO_2 indexed by predicted values.

improved, and indicating transplantation on only one value of peak VO_2 is dangerous. In practice, there is a gray zone around 14 mL/min/kg where other parameters, from CPX or from other techniques, should be taken into account. The VE/VCO_2 slope, the circulatory power, can be used here.

– Another major problem comes from the fact that most of the patients are (or should be) treated by beta-blockers. Beta-blockers dramatically improve prognosis whereas they have only a mild effect on peak VO_2. Whether the prognostic value of peak VO_2 is maintained in patients with beta-blockers has been questioned. It has clearly decreased and the above cut-offs are no longer valid. Various studies suggest that these cut-offs should be decreased by at least 2 mL/min/kg.[28] This means that the outcome of a patient with a peak VO_2 of 11–12 mL/min/kg on beta-blockers may not be worse than that of another patient not on beta-blockers with a peak VO_2 of 14 mL/min/kg. Clearly, further studies are necessary to define more precisely the cut-offs of peak VO_2 in patients on beta-blockers.

– In these patients, the VE/VCO_2 slope may have, according to some authors, a better prognostic value than peak VO_2.[29] The cut-offs are less well defined.

– We have recently shown that the circulatory power outperformed peak VO_2 in these patients.[14]

– The prognostic value of serial changes in peak VO_2 has also been suggested.

– Physical training may increase peak VO_2 by 20–30%. Whether this improvement has the same prognostic implications that after medical therapy targeting mainly the heart remains to be shown.

4. The role of CPX in valvular disease is currently not well defined.

a. In mitral stenosis, there is no relationship between valve area or gradient and peak VO_2. CPX may be useful to assess functional capacity and assess heart rate increase, especially in atrial fibrillation.

b. In aortic stenosis, CPX also allows objective assessment of symptoms. ST-segment decrease, low peak VO_2, and abnormal blood pressure increase may reflect a severe aortic stenosis. In general, coupling exercise with Doppler echocardiography provides the best insights.

c. The role of CPX in mitral regurgitation is not well defined.

5. Exercise testing now has a major role in establishing the prognosis of patients with hypertrophic cardiomyopathy. Besides peak VO$_2$, it is important to determine the blood pressure response. A decrease or a plateauing of blood pressure is associated with a poor prognosis.

6. After heart transplantation, CPX is often useful to appreciate functional capacity and prescribe cardiac rehabilitation. It also makes it possible to follow the normalization with time of the heart rate response. In patients with ventricular assistance, CPX may help in determining the best time to wean the patient from assistance.

7. CPX is also useful in patients who have a cardiac pacemaker. In chronotropic incompetence or sick sinus syndrome, exercise capacity is decreased and ventilation increased. CPX is very useful when symptoms persist or appear after implantation. In biventricular stimulation, CPX enables assessment of the improvement in exercise capacity with the optimization of the stimulation parameters.

In conclusion, CPX now has an important place in the evaluation of the patient with heart failure. It allows assessment of objectively functional impairment, the overall circulatory response to exercise, and prognosis. It is likely that we do not use, currently, all the information provided by CPX in these patients.

References

1. Page E, Cohen-Solal A, Jondeau G, et al. Comparison of treadmill and bicycle exercise in patients with chronic heart failure. Chest 1994;106:1002–1006.
2. Francis DP, Davies LC, Piepoli M, Rauchhaus M, Ponikowski P, Coats AJ. Origin of oscillatory kinetics of respiratory gas exchange in chronic heart failure. Circulation. 1999;100:1065–1070.
3. Cohen-Solal A, Chabernaud J, Gourgon R. Comparison of oxygen uptake during bicycle exercise in patients with chronic heart failure and in normal subjects. J Am Coll Cardiol 1990;16:80–85.
4. Koike A, Itoh H, Kato M, et al. Prognostic power of ventilatory responses during submaximal exercise in patients with chronic heart disease. Chest 2002;121:1581–1588.
5. Jones N, Makrides L, Hitchcock C, McCartney N. Normal standards for an incremental progressive cycle ergometer test. Am Rev Respir Dis 1985; 131:700–708.
6. Wasserman K, Hansen J, Sue D, Whipp B. Normal values. In: Wasserman K, Hansen J, Sue D, Whipp B, eds. Principles of Exercise Testing and Interpretation. Philadelphia: Lea & Febiger; 1987:72–85.
7. Osman AF, Mehra MR, Lavie CJ, Nunez E, Milani RV. The incremental prognostic importance of body fat adjusted peak oxygen consumption in chronic heart failure. J Am Coll Cardiol 2000;36:2126–2131.
8. Weber K, Kinasewitz G, Janicki J, Fishman A. Oxygen utilisation and ventilation during exercise in patients with chronic cardiac failure. Circulation 1982;65:1213–1223.
9. Wasserman K, Whipp B, Koyal S, Beaver W. Anaerobic threshold and respiratory gas exchange during exercise. J Appl Physiol 1973;35:236–243.
10. Cohen-Solal A, Benessiano J, Himbert D, Paillole C, Gourgon R. Ventilatory threshold during exercise in patients with mild to moderate chronic heart failure: determination, relation with lactate threshold and reproducibility. Int J Cardiol 1991;30:321–327.
11. Wasserman K. New concepts in assessing cardiovascular function. Circulation 1988;78:1060–1071.
12. Cohen-Solal A, Laperche T, Morvan D, Geneves M, Caviezel B, Gourgon R. Prolonged kinetics of recovery of oxygen consumption and ventilatory variables after maximal graded exercise in patients with chronic heart failure. Analysis with gas exchange and NMR spectroscopy study. Circulation 1995; 91:2924–2932.
13. de Groote P, Millaire A, Decoulx E, Nugue O, Guimier P, Ducloux G. Kinetics of oxygen consumption during and after exercise in patients with dilated cardiomyopathy. New markers of exercise intolerance with clinical implications. J Am Coll Cardiol 1996;28:168–175.
14. Cohen-Solal A, Tabet J, Logeart D, Bourgoin P, Tokmakova M, Dahan M. A non-invasively determined surrogate of cardiac power ("circulatory power") at peak exercise is a powerful prognostic factor in chronic heart failure. Eur Heart J 2002;23:806–814.
15. Cole CR, Blackstone EH, Pashkow FJ, Snader CE, Lauer MS. Heart-rate recovery immediately after exercise as a predictor of mortality. N Engl J Med 1999;341:1351–1357.
16. Metra M, Dei Cas L, Panina G, Visioli O. Exercise hyperventilation chronic congestive heart failure, and its relation to functional capacity and hemodynamics. Am J Cardiol 1992;70:622–628.

17. Agostoni P, Guazzi M, Bussotti M, De Vita S, Palermo P. Carvedilol reduces the inappropriate increase of ventilation during exercise in heart failure patients. Chest 2002;122:2062–2067.

18. Arena R, Humphrey R, Peberdy MA. Prognostic ability of VE/VCO$_2$ slope calculations using different exercise test time intervals in subjects with heart failure. Eur J Cardiovasc Prev Rehabil 2003; 10:463–468.

19. Tabet JY, Beauvais F, Thabut G, Tartiere JM, Logeart D, Cohen-Solal A. A critical appraisal of the prognostic value of the VE/VCO$_2$ slope in chronic heart failure. Eur J Cardiovasc Prev Rehabil 2003;10: 267–272.

20. Baba R, Nagashima M, Goto M, et al. Oxygen uptake efficiency slope: a new index of cardiorespiratory functional reserve derived from the relation between oxygen uptake and minute ventilation during incremental exercise. J Am Coll Cardiol 1996;28:1567–1572.

21. Ben-Dov I, Sietsema KE, Casaburi R, Wasserman K. Evidence that circulatory oscillations accompany ventilatory oscillations during exercise in patients with heart failure. Am Rev Respir Dis 1992; 145:776–781.

22. Osada N, Chaitman B, Miller L, et al. Cardioplumonary exercise testing identifies low risk patients with heart failure and severely impaired exercise capacity considered for heart transplantation. J Am Coll Cardiol 1998;31:577–582.

23. Metra M, Faggiano P, D'Aloia A, et al. Use of cardiopulmonary exercise testing with hemodynamic monitoring in the prognostic assessment of ambulatory patients with chronic heart failure. J Am Coll Cardiol 1999;33:943–950.

24. Roul G, Moulichon M, Bareiss P, et al. Prognostic factors of chronic heart failure in NYHA class II or III: value of invasive exercise haemodynamic data. Eur Heart J 1995;16:1387–1398.

25. Williams SG, Cooke GA, Wright DJ, et al. Peak exercise cardiac power output; a direct indicator of cardiac function strongly predictive of prognosis in chronic heart failure. Eur Heart J 2001;22:1496–1503.

26. Aaronson KD, Mancini DM. Is percentage of predicted maximal exercise oxygen consumption a better predictor of survival than peak exercise oxygen consumption for patients with severe heart failure? J Heart Lung Transplant 1995;14:981–989.

27. Mancini D, Eisen H, Kussmaul W, Mull R, Edmunds L, Wilson J. Value of peak exercise oxygen consumption for optimal timing of cardiac transplantation in ambulatory patients. Circulation 1991;83: 778–786.

28. Zugck C, Haunstetter A, Kruger C, et al. Impact of beta-blocker treatment on the prognostic value of currently used risk predictors in congestive heart failure. J Am Coll Cardiol 2002;39:1615–1622.

29. Corra U, Mezzani A, Bosimini E, et al. Limited predictive value of cardiopulmonary exercise indices in patients with moderate chronic heart failure treated with carvedilol. Am Heart J 2004;147:553–560.

16
Exercise Testing in Valvular Heart Disease

Christa Gohlke-Bärwolf

Introduction: Exercise Testing in Patients with Valvular Heart Disease

Exercise testing (ET) has been the cornerstone in the diagnosis and prognostic evaluation of coronary artery disease (see Chapter 14).[1,2] Even in apparently healthy men exercise testing provides important prognostic informations.[3] Although ET was recently recommended in the management of asymptomatic patients with valvular heart disease (VHD),[4,5] this recommendation is based on a small database. In the Euro Heart Survey on Valvular Heart Disease of the European Society of Cardiology, exercise testing was used in less than 8% of 5001 patients, evaluated in hospital or as an outpatient in 27 European countries.[6] The reasons for performing exercise testing in these patients are listed in Table 16-1.

There are several explanations for the infrequent use of exercise testing in patients with VHD. Previously exercise testing was used to diagnose coronary artery disease also in adult patients with VHD, particularly in patients with aortic stenosis. But because of the occurrence of false-positive tests among adult patients with VHD this is considered a class III indication in the ACC/AHA Recommendations for exercise testing for the diagnosis of coronary artery disease (CAD) in patients with VHD.[1,7] Nonetheless ET is still used for this purpose as shown in Table 16-1. The incidence of false-positive tests in these patients is attributed to left ventricular hypertrophy (LVH) and/or repolarization disturbances at rest. Yet many patients with moderate–severe valve lesions may have a normal ECG and no severe LVH. In these patients the production of severe ST-segment depression (>2 mm) most likely indicates a pathological reaction which requires further diagnosis, even if it may not indicate associated CAD.

A further reason for the infrequent use of ET in patients with VHD is the fact that until recently patients with valvular heart disease were operated on only after severe symptoms had occurred, typically NYHA class III or IV; thus in this stage of the disease there is no need for further exercise testing to induce symptoms or hemodynamic alterations. The treatment in these patients is unanimously agreed upon and consists of valve surgery.

In the 2002 update of the AHA guidelines, assessment of functional capacity and symptomatic responses was considered a class I recommendation only in patients with aortic insufficiency and a history of equivocal symptoms.[1]

Yet exercise testing can also be of value in patients with atypical symptoms in other types of valve disease, particularly in the elderly in whom the symptomatic status is difficult to assess because of inactivity.

With the widespread availability of Doppler echocardiography, increasingly *asymptomatic or mildly symptomatic* patients are being diagnosed for whom exercise testing has become important to assess functional capacity objectively, and to determine if symptoms occur during exercise and if pathological hemodynamic responses (e.g. inadequate blood pressure increase) appear during exercise. This information is of importance

TABLE 16-1. Reasons for performing exercise testing (in 70% bicycle exercise tests) in 8% of all patients with VHD

Reason	
Detection of coronary artery disease	61.0%
Assessment of functional capacity in patients with no or equivocal symptoms	49.1%
Prior to allowing strenuous exercise	13.1%
Prognostic evaluation in the presence of left ventricular dysfunction	12.1%
Routine basis	22.9%

Source: Lung, 2003.[6] With permission from Oxford University Press and European Society of Cardiology.

in the decision on medical or surgical therapy and for advice concerning exercise and leisure time activities (Table 16-2).

The occurrence of hypotension during exercise testing in asymptomatic patients with VHD is also an important indicator of hemodynamic impairment. It is not specific for patients with valvular heart disease, since it has been described in patients with CAD[8,9] and in hypertrophic obstructive cardiomyopathy.[10–12]

Further Indications for Exercise Testing

Exercise testing has gained an increasing role during follow-up of patients with VHD, particularly in patients with aortic stenosis (Table 16-2). Exercise testing is also of importance concerning recommendations for vocational and recreational activities and sports. During follow-up, detection of newly occurring STT wave changes, blood pressure abnormalities, or angina pectoris may be a sign of newly developing coronary artery disease.

After valve interventions or valve surgery, exercise testing is helpful to assess the results, to determine the level and type of exercise program during rehabilitation, advise on vocational and leisure time activity, for preoperative assessment before noncardiac surgery, and as a research tool

TABLE 16-2. Value of exercise testing in patients with VHD

To assess objective functional capacity
To assess atypical symptoms
Production of prior unnoticed symptoms
To induce pathological hemodynamic responses:
– inadequate blood pressure rise or a fall in blood pressure
– inadequate heart rate response (tachycardic or bradycardic)
– marked STT wave changes (>2 mm)
– severe arrhythmias

in long-term follow-up.[13] That exercise testing can provide valuable information in patients with valvular heart disease, especially in those whose symptoms are difficult to assess was acknowledged in the new ACC/AHA guidelines 2006.[53]

Baseline Information to Be Obtained Prior to Exercise Testing

All patients should undergo a careful clinical evaluation including history with emphasis on the usual daily activity level, physical examination, and ECG. In patients with evidence of VHD on clinical examination, an echocardiogram should be performed prior to exercise testing (Table 16-3).

The level of activity or exercise that is associated with normal hemodynamics without symptoms is a guide for further medical management, training and leisure time activities, and for the decision about surgery.

The rating of perceived exertion[14] and the "talk test" (ability to conduct a "small talk" conversation during exercise) are valuable assessments of the intensity of exertion.

Special Test Requirements

The supervising physician should be experienced in exercising high-risk patients, knowing the warning signs of possible problems and following them accordingly.

The test should be started with a low workload, and increased in low workload steps.

The test should be terminated if there is inadequate blood pressure augmentation, slowing of heart rate, or other significant arrhythmias, if symptoms occur, and if there is more than 2 mm ST depression.[1]

TABLE 16-3. Baseline information to be obtained during exercise testing

Heart rate and rhythm
Blood pressure
Symptoms
ST-segment changes
Exercise capacity adjusted for age
Rating of perceived exertion such as the Borg scale[14] or "talk test"
In certain patients Doppler echocardiography to determine:
– valve gradients
– pulmonary pressures

Type of Exercise Testing

In Anglo-Saxon countries exercise testing in patients with VHD has been performed predominantly using a treadmill,[15–17] whereas in European countries it is mostly performed as bicycle ergometry,[18–22] in either supine or upright position. With treadmill exercise only post-exercise imaging is available. Bicycle exercise, particularly in the supine position, has marked advantages concerning the quality of ECG monitoring, blood pressure measurement, and safety aspects for the patient, particularly for the elderly.

Stress Doppler echocardiography has recently been employed for the evaluation of patients with VHD. In treadmill exercise testing only post-exercise imaging is available, which may influence the results markedly, for example measuring Doppler gradients after exercise. It may also lead to false-negative results concerning exercise-induced wall motion abnormalities, which may have resolved rapidly after exercise. In contrast, Doppler gradients and pulmonary artery pressure can be measured continuously during exercise with bicycle ergometry, especially in the supine position.

In patients with unexplained symptoms and apparently only moderate mitral stenosis determination of valve gradients and pulmonary artery pressure assessed from the tricuspid regurgitant jet during exercise is very helpful.[23,24] In these patients determination of exercise hemodynamics during supine bicycle ergometry can also elucidate the causes of symptoms.[21,22]

Exercise Testing in Patients with Aortic Stenosis (AS)

Since the first description of effort syncope by Gallaverdin in 1933 and the reports of sudden death associated with it, exercise has been considered dangerous in patients with significant AS and thus, exercise testing has been discouraged and considered contraindicated by many experts until recently (see above).

Symptomatic Patients with Significant AS

In these patients the indication for aortic valve replacement is unanimously agreed upon; there-fore further evaluation with ET is neither necessary nor indicated.[4]

Asymptomatic Patients with AS

Exercise testing has been used for many years to assess severity, progression, and indications for intervention in children with aortic stenosis.[25–27]

In adult patients with aortic stenosis exercise testing was performed in only 5.7% of asymptomatic patients in the Euro Heart Survey representing the present clinical practice in Europe.[6]

In adults the first prospective prognostic study in asymptomatic patients with moderate AS[16] indicates that ET in asymptomatic or mildly symptomatic patients with AS is not a risky procedure, provided it is performed under expert supervision with appropriate attention to test requirements and criteria for discontinuation of the test.

Three studies in adults with moderate to severe aortic stenosis (valve areas of 0.5 to 1.5 cm^2, mean gradients of 18 to 64 mmHg) have shown that with the appropriate precautions, exercise testing can be safely performed in patients with aortic stenosis.[16,17,18]

Results of Exercise Testing

ET in AS has greatly enhanced our understanding of the pathophysiology and hemodynamic consequences of AS.

Even in asymptomatic patients exercise tolerance is reduced and systemic and LV hemodynamics are impaired in a significant number of patients.

Inadequate blood pressure increase during exercise has been demonstrated in 80% of symptomatic patients with significant AS[28] and about 10% of asymptomatic patients.[16]

Hypotension or inadequate blood pressure increase has been defined as:

1. blood pressure at maximal exercise less than at rest
2. an increase of less than 20 mmHg
3. a drop to values below the resting value.[1,29]

The mechanism for hypotension or inadequate blood pressure response in patients with AS is not clear. Studies in patients with hypertrophic cardiomyopathy indicate that hypotension occurs due to severe hemodynamic left ventricular impairment during exercise.

Due to abnormal baseline ECG, LVH, and impaired coronary reserve, the predictive value for coronary artery disease in AS is limited.[1]

Pharmacological stress testing has been suggested for this purpose.[30] A definite role for these tests has not yet been established.

Complications of Exercise Testing in AS

A review of case reports on adverse events associated with ET shows that most are from the pre echo-Doppler era and that inadequate pretest diagnosis and test performance with ignorance about premonitory signs have contributed to the complications.[19,20]

The experience of ET in symptomatic patients with AS from Scandinavia,[18,19,31] the studies by Otto et al.,[15,16] Das et al.,[17] and our own experience indicated no serious complications in asymptomatic or mildly symptomatic patients with AS. The total published database for complications during exercise testing in patients with severe AS however is still small.

Since ET uncovers functional and hemodynamic impairment that may be associated with severe AS even in clinically asymptomatic patients, unexpected hypotension, severe rhythm disturbances, and signs of ischemia can occur. Therefore the physician performing the test should have a high level of suspicion that these events can occur and be prepared to stop the test and deal with these complications. But even if complications at a given exercise level occur in the exercise laboratory, the patient is better served than if they occurred during daily activities.

Exercise Testing for Risk Stratification in Asymptomatic Patients

The excellent early results of aortic valve surgery in symptomatic patients with AS and some late deterioration of LV function in those patients with impaired LV function preoperatively have led to suggestions to operate earlier in patients with AS, and also in those without symptoms.[32] Yet prognostic studies by Pellikka et al.[33] and Otto et al.[16] have shown that as long as symptoms are absent, prognosis is good in the short term.

Exercise Testing to Predict Occurrence of Symptoms in Asymptomatic Patients with Severe AS and Sudden Death

The role of exercise testing for induction of symptoms was recently evaluated. During treadmill exercise testing 37% of asymptomatic patients developed limiting symptoms (breathlessness, chest tightness, and dizziness). These were independent predictors of symptom onset within 1 year. The positive predictive accuracy for exercise-induced symptoms was 79% for patients aged under 70 without significant limitations in daily life.[17]

In the study by Pellikka et al.,[33] sudden death occurred only in those patients who had developed symptoms at least 3 months prior to the occurrence of sudden death or in patients who had been operated upon. In a recent study by Pellikka et al. in 2005,[34] only 1% of patients suffered sudden death per year without identified symptoms prior to death. Medical follow-up was limited in 50% of patients. These patients exhibited a broad range of ages, aortic valve areas, and aortic valve flow velocities. Clinical and echocardiographic parameters in this study did not identify these patients. Amato et al.[35] have shown that exercise testing in asymptomatic patients with severe AS identifies those patients at higher risk for sudden death; 6 of 66 patients died during follow-up. All had an abnormal exercise test (development of angina pectoris or significant ST-segment depression) in the presence of severe AS with a valve area of less than $0.6\,cm^2$.

These exercise parameters (Table 16-4) are of prognostic importance whereby the implications

TABLE 16-4. Criteria for an abnormal exercise ECG in patients with severe aortic stenosis

1. Development of symptoms of dyspnea, angina pectoris, syncope, or near syncope
2. Rise in systolic blood pressure during exercise of less than 20 mmHg
3. Inability to reach 80% of the normal level of exercise tolerance according to age and gender-adjusted levels
4. More than 2 mm horizontal or downsloping ST-segment depression during exercise in comparison to baseline levels, which are not attributable to causes other than severe AS
5. Complex ventricular arrhythmias (ventricular tachycardia, more than four PVCs in a row)

PVC, premature ventricular contraction.
Source: Iung, 2002.[5] With permission from Oxford University Press and European Society of Cardiology.

of an abnormal exercise test for the indication for surgery are strongest for the occurrence of symptoms and abnormal blood pressure responses.

In contrast, patients with normal functional aerobic capacity and normal circulatory response to exercise have a good short- and median-term prognosis even in the presence of significant AS.

Thus exercise testing allows risk stratification and identification of those patients in whom the severity of AS is already associated with silent impairment of hemodynamics, LV dysfunction and symptoms which may appear only during exercise testing. These patients can benefit from surgery. The results of exercise testing are also important concerning the recommendations for vocational and recreational activities and sports.[36,37]

Pharmacological Stress Testing in AS

In Patients with Normal Left Ventricular Function

Consideration can also be given to stress echocardiography in these patients, yet there is no conclusive evidence for its value in asymptomatic patients. In patients with AS and normal left ventricular function, valve compliance during dobutamine stress echocardiography predicted the occurrence of symptoms better than resting measures of AS.[38]

In Patients with Impaired Left Ventricular Function

In patients with low gradient AS and impaired left ventricular function, stress echocardiography with dobutamine allows evaluation of valve hemodynamics and contractile reserve and is of prognostic value for operative risk stratification and long-term outcome. The hemodynamic response to dobutamine allows the differentiation between patients with true severe AS, with contractile reserve, who have an acceptable operative risk and patients with relative AS with intrinsic impairment of myocardial contractility who have a high operative mortality. When stroke volume and pressure gradient increase with dobutamine, and aortic valve area decreases or remains unchanged, true severe AS is present. In patients in whom valve area increases with a rise in stroke volume, relative AS is present. In patients without a change in hemodynamics, severe intrinsic impairment of myocardial contractility is present.[39]

Conclusions

The role of exercise testing in patients with AS has evolved. Exercise testing has become an important method for risk assessment in asymptomatic adult patients with significant AS. It should be included in the decision process for surgery and during clinical follow-up of patients.

Exercise Testing in Patients with Aortic Insufficiency (AI)

Patients with AI are markedly less prevalent than patients with AS, representing only 13.3% of all valve lesions in the Euro Heart Survey on VHD.[6] Patients with AI can remain asymptomatic for many years and exercise capacity is usually maintained until late in the course of the disease. Indications for surgery have been defined on the basis of symptoms, impaired left ventricular ejection fraction at rest, and enlarged left ventricular size.[4,5] Since LV dysfunction may occur silently, exercise testing is a reasonable way to identify those patients with severe AI who may develop symptoms and asymptomatic LV dysfunction during exercise. However, studies proving this correlation are lacking. LV ejection fraction response to exercise has been evaluated as a predictor of symptomatic deterioration or LV dysfunction. A positive correlation was identified by Borer et al. in 1998.[40] Yet this could not be demonstrated in other studies.[41,42] The exercise ejection fraction and the change in ejection fraction from rest to exercise are often abnormal in patients with severe AI,[43] even in asymptomatic patients. However, these have not been proven to have independent prognostic value. In one small study the left ventricular response to exercise was used to monitor the response of asymptomatic patients to medical therapy.[44] The indication for exercise testing in patients with AI according to the AHA/ACC is depicted in Table 16-5.

TABLE 16-5. Recommendations for exercise testing in chronic aortic insufficiency

Indication	Class
1. Assessment of functional capacity and symptomatic responses in patients with a history of equivocal symptoms	I
2. Evaluation of symptoms and functional capacity before participation in athletic activities	IIa
3. Prognosis assessment before aortic valve replacement in patients with LV dysfunction	IIa
4. Exercise hemodynamic measurements to determine the effect of AI on LV function	IIb
5. Exercise radionuclide angiography for assessing LV function in symptomatic or asymptomatic patients	IIb
6. Exercise echocardiography or dobutamine stress echocardiography for assessing LV function in asymptomatic and symptomatic patients	III

Source: Bonow et al., 1998.[4] © 1998 American Heart Association Inc. Reprinted with permission.

Although not recommended in the AHA guidelines for the management of patients with VHD[4] (see above) or on exercise testing,[1] the author feels that during clinical follow-up of asymptomatic patients with severe AI with preserved systolic function, serial exercise testing is helpful to objectively assess functional capacity and symptomatic responses. A decrease in exercise tolerance and VO$_2$max, the appearance of marked ST-segment depression, a reduction in heart rate response to each workload, or symptom development on serial exercise testing might be of prognostic value in addition to the resting ejection fraction and end-systolic diameter of the left ventricle. These pathological exercise parameters, particularly new occurrence of symptoms with exercise, should lead to further investigations – such as coronary angiography – and consideration of surgery. But prospective studies to confirm this are lacking.

Exercise Testing in Patients with Mitral Stenosis (MS)

Increasing numbers of asymptomatic patients with severe MS are being diagnosed with echo-Doppler. Due to the long duration of their disease these patients have slowly adjusted to their restrictions and frequently do not report symptoms or nonspecific symptoms like fatigue. This is particularly the case in elderly patients. In these patients exercise testing is of clinical value. Induction of dyspnea during exercise, excessive heart rate responses to a relatively low level of exercise, and excessive exercise-induced pulmonary hypertension are important parameters, which indicate the need for better medical management or interventional therapy (balloon valvuloplasty or surgery). In patients with only moderate mitral stenosis and unexplained symptoms, determination of valve gradients and pulmonary artery pressure assessed from the tricuspid regurgitant jet during bicycle exercise is very helpful.[23]

Patients with significant mitral stenosis may have an excessive increase in heart rate during exercise, particularly when atrial fibrillation is present. As stroke volume cannot be increased, the usual increase in cardiac output is less and may eventually fall during exercise, frequently accompanied by exercise-induced hypotension. The increase in heart rate and right ventricular pressure results in an increase in right ventricular myocardial oxygen demand. In patients with mitral stenosis, chest discomfort and ST-segment depression during exercise may occur either due to coronary artery disease or secondary to pulmonary hypertension. The shortening of diastole associated with tachycardia and the increase in pulmonary blood flow associated with exercise increase left atrial pressure and may cause pulmonary congestion and dyspnea.

The value of treadmill stress exercise echocardiography in patients with mitral stenosis with and without significant mitral insufficiency was shown by Lev et al. in 2004.[45] Despite marked differences in mitral valve area between patients with predominantly MS or MR (mitral regurgitation), systolic pulmonary artery pressures were similar both at rest and during peak exercise (Table 16-6).

This demonstrates that patients with combined lesions may become more symptomatic than each lesion by itself would imply. In these patients direct measurement of hemodynamics with right heart catheterization during exercise is of great value in determining the significance of the combined lesion and the indication for surgery.[21,22]

TABLE 16-6. Echocardiographic parameters at rest and during peak exercise

Parameter	Predominantly MS ($n = 24$)	Predominantly MR ($n = 24$)	P value
Baseline			
Mean mitral gradient (mmHg)	10.2 ± 4.8	7.0 ± 3.1	0.008
Peak mitral gradient (mmHg)	20 ± 7	15 ± 6	0.02
Mitral valve area (cm²)	1.1 ± 0.3	2.1 ± 0.6	<0.0001
Tricuspid regurgitation systolic gradient (mmHg)	37 ± 11	37 ± 13	1
Degree of MR	0.9 ± 0.5	2.1 ± 0.4	<0.0001
Peak exercise			
Mean mitral gradient (mmHg)	25 ± 14	17 ± 9	0.04
Peak mitral gradient (mmHg)	42 ± 18	30 ± 12	0.01
Tricuspid regurgitation systolic gradient (mmHg)	60 ± 16	55 ± 13	0.8

Source: Lev et al., 2004.[45] © 2004 Elsevier. Reprinted with permission.

Exercise Testing in Patients with Mitral Regurgitation (MR)

Mitral regurgitation has become the second most common valve lesion after aortic stenosis. Mitral regurgitation was present in 31.5% of patients in the Euro Heart Survey on VHD.[6] Since these patients are increasingly diagnosed echocardiographically, exercise testing has gained an important role in management of MR.

Exercise testing in patients with severe MR is helpful to identify those clinically asymptomatic patients with impaired exercise tolerance, pathological hemodynamic responses, and the occurrence of symptoms during exercise. To determine the degree of MR and pulmonary artery pressures during exercise, bicycle ergometry with Doppler echocardiography has been of increasing importance. Because resting ejection fraction is a poor guide to ventricular function in patients with mitral regurgitation, combinations of exercise testing and assessment of left ventricular function may be of value in documenting occult dysfunction and influence further medical or surgical management.[46] In patients with mitral valve prolapse but without regurgitation at rest, exercise-induced MR has been associated

with the subsequent development of progressive MR, congestive heart failure, and syncope.[47] Concomitant Doppler imaging during exercise may demonstrate severe MR in patients with symptoms out of proportion to mild MR observed on the resting echocardiogram. Exercise-induced increases in MR are also of prognostic importance in patients with ischemic heart disease.[48–50]

Exercise Testing in Patients after Valve Surgery

Valve surgery usually leads to a marked improvement in symptoms as evidenced by a decrease in the NYHA class and an increase in exercise tolerance. The degree of improvement depends on the preoperative symptom status, degree of left ventricular impairment, presence of pulmonary hypertension, and the type of valve disease present.

In patients who are asymptomatic prior to surgery a documentation of improvement is frequently only possible by comparing the pre- and postoperative exercise tolerance. Thus with exercise testing postoperatively improvements in exercise parameters can be evaluated. At present, only 7.4% of patients after valve surgery patients undergo exercise testing in representative hospitals in Europe.[6]

Exercise Hemodynamics (see Chapter 20)

After valve intervention or valve surgery in most patients symptomatic and hemodynamic improvement occurs both at rest and during exercise. Particularly in patients with aortic stenosis and impaired left ventricular function preoperatively, a marked decrease in pulmonary capillary wedge pressure and an increase in ejection fraction after surgery can be demonstrated.[21,22] Patients after mitral valve replacement have a markedly lower exercise tolerance (Figure 16-1), and only 40–60% of patients have normal hemodynamics at rest and only 25% during exercise (Figure 16-2).[21,22] Abnormal rest and exercise hemodynamics may persist for 6 to 12 months after surgery[21,22,51] (Figure 16-3).

The objective assessment of these patients by exercise testing, with determination of

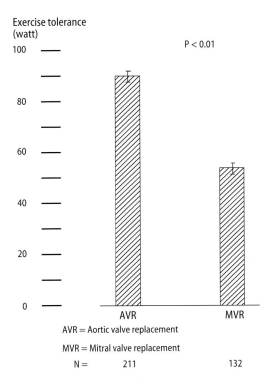

FIGURE 16-1. Patients after aortic valve replacement have better exercise performance than patients after mitral valve replacement. (From Gohlke-Bärwolf et al.[21] © 1992 ICR Publishers Ltd. Reprinted with permission.)

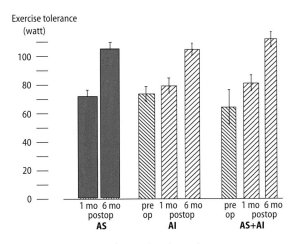

FIGURE 16-2. Patients after aortic valve replacement can expect significant improvement in exercise tolerance regardless of preoperative valve lesion. (AS = aortic stenosis; AI = aortic insufficiency; Pre = preoperative; postop = postoperative; mo = month; OP = operation.) (From Gohlke-Bärwolf et al.[21] © 1992 ICR Publishers Ltd. Reprinted with permission.)

pulmonary pressures during stress echocardiography or invasive hemodynamic measurement, can be of help in the postoperative management of these patients, regarding medical therapy, determination of rehabilitative measures, and advice on vocational and recreational activities.[21,22]

The results of exercise testing prior to and after mitral valve repair and mitral valve replacement are not unanimous. While marked symptomatic and functional improvement after both aortic and mitral valve replacement was demonstrated postoperatively by Gohlke-Bärwolf et al.[21,22] and Kim et al.[52] this could not be shown after mitral valve replacement. Even after mitral valve repair no change in peak VO$_2$ was demonstrated in spite of an improvement in NYHA class, exercise duration, and echocardiographic parameters. We found a constant improvement in exercise tolerance between the first and sixth months after surgery, in comparison to preoperatively, in

all valve lesions, although there was a marked difference between patients with mitral and aortic valve replacement. In patients with AS who were candidates for surgery no preoperative exercise testing was performed (Figure 16-3).

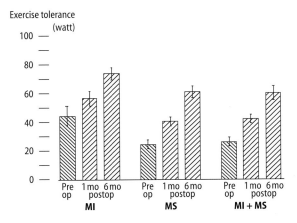

FIGURE 16-3. Patients with pure mitral insufficiency (usually degenerative lesion) can expect higher exercise tolerance after valve replacement than patients after mitral stenosis or combined usually rheumatic lesions. However, the "relative" improvement is at least as great in patients with rheumatic valvular disease. (MI = mitral insufficiency; MS = mitral stenosis; Pre = preoperative; postop = postoperative; mo = month; OP = operation.) (From Gohlke-Bärwolf et al.[21] © 1992 ICR Publishers Ltd. Reprinted with permission.)

Summary

Exercise testing is of great value in patients with valvular heart disease. It has an important role in eliciting symptoms in asymptomatic patients (which can influence the decision for surgery), in evaluating atypical symptoms and assessing true exercise capacity, and is of prognostic importance in patients with aortic stenosis; this applies also to patients with mitral insufficiency due both to mitral valve prolapse and to coronary artery disease (ischemic mitral insufficiency). After valve interventions or valve surgery, the response to medical and surgical therapy can be evaluated. An exercise test is advised prior to starting an exercise training program, to assess its safety but also to evaluate the medical management. The determination of the patient's exercise capacity affords an objective measurement of the degree of overall cardiac impairment or improvement after valve surgery. At present, exercise testing is underused in clinical practice.

References

1. Gibbons RJ, Balady RJ, Bricker JT, et al. ACC/AHA 2002 guideline update for exercise testing: summary article: a report of the ACC/AHA Task Force on Practice Guidelines (Committee to Update the 1997 Exercise Testing Guidelines). J Am Coll Cardiol 2002;40:1531–1540.
2. Gohlke H, Samek L, Betz P, Roskamm H. Exercise testing provides additional prognostic information in angiographically defined subgroups of patients with coronary artery disease. Circulation 1983;68: 979–985.
3. Bodegard J, Erikssen G, Bjørnholt JV, Gjesdal K, Liestøl K, Erikssen J. Reasons for terminating an exercise test provide independent prognostic information. 2014 apparently healthy men followed for 26 years. Eur Heart J 2005;26:1394–1401.
4. Bonow RO, Carabello B, de Leon AC Jr, et al. ACC/AHA Guidelines for the Management of Patients With Valvular Heart Disease: a report of the American College of Cardiology/American Heart Association Task Force on Practice Guidelines (Committee on Management of Patients With Valvular Heart Disease). J Am Coll Cardiol 1998;32:1486–1588.
5. Iung B, Gohlke-Bärwolf C, Tornos P, et al. Recommendations on the management of the asympto-matic patient with valvular heart disease. Eur Heart J 2002;23:1253–1266.
6. Iung B, Baron G, Butchart EG, et al. A prospective survey of patients with valvular heart disease in Europe: The Euro Heart Survey on Valvular Heart Disease. Eur Heart J 2003;24:1231–1243.
7. Gibbons RJ, Beasley JW, Bricker JT, et al. ACC/AHA guidelines for exercise testing: a report of the American College of Cardiology/American Heart Association Task Force on Practice Guidelines (Committee on Exercise Testing). J Am Coll Cardiol 1997;30:260–315.
8. Dubach P, Froelicher VF, Klein J, Oakes D, Grover-McKay M, Friis R. Exercise-induced hypotension in a male population: criteria, causes and prognosis. Circulation 1988;78:1380–1387.
9. Gibbons RJ, Hu DC, Clements IP, Mankin HT, Zinsmeister AR, Brown ML. Anatomic and functional significance of hypotensive response during supine exercise radionuclide ventriculography. Am J Cardiol 1987;60:1–4.
10. Ciampi Q, Betocchi S, Lombardi R, et al. Hemodynamic determinants of exercise-induced abnormal blood pressure response in hypertrophic cardiomyopathy. J Am Coll Cardiol 2002;40:278–284.
11. Olivotto I, Maron BJ, Montereggi A, Mazzuoli F, Dolara A, Cecchi F. Prognostic value of systemic blood pressure response during exercise in a community-based patient population with hypertrophic cardiomyopathy. J Am Coll Cardiol 1999;33:2044–2051.
12. Kim JJ, Lee CW, Park SW, et al. Improvement in exercise capacity and exercise blood pressure response after transcoronary alcohol ablation therapy of septal hypertrophy in hypertrophic cardiomyopathy. Am J Cardiol 1999;83:1120–1123.
13. Butchart EG, Gohlke-Bärwolf C, Antunes MJ, et al. Recommendations for the management of patients after heart valve surgery. Eur Heart J 2005;26(22): 2463–2471.
14. Borg GA. Psychophysical basis of perceived exertion. Med Sci Sports 1982;14:377–381.
15. Otto CM, Pearlman AS, Kraft CD, Miyake-Hull CY, Burwash IG, Gardner CJ. Physiology changes with maximal exercise in asymptomatic valvular aortic stenosis assessed by Doppler echocardiography. J Am Coll Cardiol 1992;20:1160–1167.
16. Otto CM, Burwash IG, Legget ME, et al. Prospective study of asymptomatic valvular aortic stenosis. Clinical, echocardiographic, and exercise predictors of outcome. Circulation 1997;95:2262–2270.
17. Das P, Rimington H, Chambers J. Exercise testing to stratify risk in aortic stenosis. Eur Heart J 2005;26:1309–1313.

18. Areskog NH. Exercise testing in the evaluation of patients with valvular aortic stenosis. Clin Physiol 1984;4:201–208.
19. Atterhög J-H, Jonsson B, Samualsson R. Exercise testing: A prospective study of complication rates. Am Heart J 1979;98:572–579.
20. Atwood JE, Kawanishi S, Myers J, Froelicher VF. Exercise testing in patients with aortic stenosis. Chest 1988;93:1083–1087.
21. Gohlke-Bärwolf C, Gohlke H, Samek L, et al. Exercise tolerance and working capacity after valve replacement. J Heart Valve Dis 1992;1:189–195.
22. Gohlke-Barwolf C, Roskamm H. Ergebnisse des Herzklappenersatzes. Prognose – Arbeits-und Leistungsfähigkeit – Berufliche Wiedereingliederung. Versicherungsmedizin 1992;44:163–168.
23. Aviles RJ, Nishimura RA, Pellikka PA, Andree KM, Holmes DR Jr. Utility of stress Doppler echocardiography in patients undergoing percutaneous mitral balloon valvotomy. J Am Soc Echocard 2001;14: 676–681.
24. Armstrong WF, Zoghbi WA. Stress echocardiography: current methodology and clinical applications. J Am Coll Cardiol 2005;45:1739–1747.
25. Halloran KH. The telemetered exercise electrocardiogram in congenital aortic stenosis. Pediatrics 1971;47:31–39.
26. Chandramouli B, Ehmke DA, Lauer RM. Exercise induced electrocardiographic changes in children with congenital aortic stenosis. J Pediatr 1975;87: 725–730.
27. James FW, Schwartz DC, Kaplan S, Spilkin SP. Exercise electrocardiogram, blood pressure, and working capacity in young patients with valvular or discrete subvalvular aortic stenosis. Am J Cardiol 1982;50:769–775.
28. Nylander E, Ekman I, Marklund T, Sinnerstad B, Karlsson E, Wranne B. Severe aortic stenosis in elderly patients. Br Heart J 1986;55:480–487.
29. Fletcher GF, Balady GJ, Amsterdam EA, et al. Exercise standards for testing and training: a statement for healthcare professionals from the American Heart Association. Circulation 2001;104: 1694–1740.
30. Maffei S, Baroni M, Terrazzi M, et al. Preoperative assessment of coronary artery disease in aortic stenosis: a dipyridamole echocardiographic study. Ann Thorac Surg 1998;65:397–402.
31. Linderholm H, Osterman G, Teien D. Detection of coronary artery disease by means of exercise ECG in patients with aortic stenosis. Acta Med Scand 1985;218:181–188.
32. Lund O, Magnussen K, Knudsen M, Pilegaard H, Nielsen TT, Albrechtsen OK. The potential for normal long term survival and morbidity rates after valve replacement for aortic stenosis. J Heart Valve Dis 1996;5:258–267.
33. Pellikka AP, Nishimura AR, Bailey KR, Tajik AJ. The natural history of adults with asymptomatic, hemodynamically significant aortic stenosis. J Am Coll Cardiol 1990;15:1012–1017.
34. Pellikka AP, Sarano ME, Nishimura RA, et al. Outcome of 622 adults with asymptomatic, hemodynamically significant aortic stenosis during prolonged follow-up. Circulation 2005;111:3290–3295.
35. Amato MC, Moffa PJ, Werner KE, Ramires JA. Treatment decision in asymptomatic aortic valve stenosis: role of exercise testing. Heart 2001;86:381–386.
36. Bonow RO, Cheitlin MD, Crawford MH, Douglas PS. Task Force 3: valvular heart disease. J Am Coll Cardiol 2005;45:1334–1340.
37. Pelliccia A, Fagard R, Bjornstad HH, et al. for the Study Group of Sports Cardiology of the Working Group of Cardiac Rehabilitation and Exercise Physiology; Working Group of Myocardial and Pericardial Diseases of the European Society of Cardiology. Recommendations for competitive sports participation in athletes with cardiovascular disease: a consensus document from the Study Group of Sports Cardiology of the Working Group of Cardiac Rehabilitation and Exercise Physiology and the Working Group of Myocardial and Pericardial Diseases of the European Society of Cardiology. Eur Heart J 2005;26:1422–1445.
38. Das P, Rimington H, Smeeton N, Chambers J. Determinants of symptoms and exercise capacity in aortic stenosis: a comparison of resting haemodynamics and valve compliance during dobutamine stress. Eur Heart J 2003;24:1254–1263.
39. Monin JL, Quere JP, Monchi M, Petit H, et al. Low-gradient aortic stenosis: operative risk stratification and predictors for long-term outcome: a multicenter study using dobutamine stress hemodynamics. Circulation 2003;108:319–324.
40. Borer JS, Hochreiter C, Herrold EM, et al. Prediction of indications for valve replacement among asymptomatic or minimally symptomatic patients with chronic aortic regurgitation and normal left ventricular performance. Circulation 1998;97:525–534.
41. Greenberg B, Massie B, Thomas D, et al. Association between the exercise ejection fraction response and systolic wall stress in patients with chronic aortic insufficiency. Circulation 1985;71:458–465.
42. Shen WF, Roubin GS, Choong CYP, et al. Evaluation of relationship between myocardial contractile state and left ventricular function in patients with aortic regurgitation. Circulation 1985;71:31–38.
43. Kawanishi DT, McKay CR, Chandraratna PA, et al. Cardiovascular response to dynamic exercise

in patients with chronic symptomatic mild-to-moderate and severe aortic regurgitation. Circulation 1986;73:62–72.

44. Schön HR, Dorn R, Barthel P, Schömig A. Effects of 12 months quinapril therapy in asymptomatic patients with chronic aortic regurgitation. J Heart Valve Dis 1994;3:500–509.

45. Lev EI, Sagie A, Vaturi M, Sela N, et al. Value of exercise echocardiography in rheumatic mitral stenosis with and without significant mitral regurgitation. Am J Cardiol 2004;93:1060–1063.

46. Hochreiter C, Borer JS. Exercise testing in patients with aortic and mitral valve disease: current applications. Cardiovasc Clin 1983;13:291–300.

47. Stoddard MF, Prince CR, Dillon S, Longaker RA, Morris GT, Liddell NE. Exercise induced mitral regurgitation is a predictor of morbid events in subjects with mitral valve prolapse. J Am Coll Cardiol 1995;25:693–699.

48. Lancellotti P, Lebrun F, Piérard LA. Determinants of exercise-induced changes in mitral regurgitation in patients with coronary artery disease and left ventricular dysfunction. J Am Coll Cardiol 2003;42: 1921–1928.

49. Lancelotti P, Troisfontaines P, Toussaint AC, et al. Prognostic importance of exercise-induced changes in mitral regurgitation in patients with chronic ischemic left ventricular dysfunction. Circulation 2003;108:1713–1717.

50. Lancellotti P, Gerard PL, Pierard LA. Long-term outcome of patients with heart failure and dynamic functional mitral regurgitation. Eur Heart J 2005; 26:1528–1532.

51. Bettinardi O, Bertolotti G, Baiardi P, et al. Can anxiety and depression influence the six-minute walking test performance in post-surgical heart valve patients? A pilot study. Monaldi Arch Chest Dis 2004;62:154–161.

52. Kim HJ, Ahn SJ, Park SW, et al. Cardiopulmonary exercise testing before and one year after mitral valve repair for severe mitral regurgitation. Am J Cardiol 2004;93:1187–1189.

53. Bonow RO, Carabello BA, Chatterjee K, et al. ACC/AHA guidelines for the management of patients with valvular heart disease: a report of the American College of Cardiology/American Heart Association Task Force on Practice Guidelines. J Am Coll Cardiol 2006;48(3e):1–148.

Section III
Exercise Training in Heart Disease

Main Messages

Chapter 17: Exercise Training in Coronary Heart Disease

Exercise training provides a wide range of cardio-protective benefits both for the healthy population and for the coronary patient. Over the years physical training has remained the cornerstone of comprehensive cardiac rehabilitation worldwide. In this chapter the numerous effects of exercise training are described and the risks of training are mentioned. New knowledge on the cellular level, i.e. endothelial function, is included. Thus, the rationale for the use of exercise training components in cardiovascular prevention and rehabilitation remains convincing and unaltered. The chapter concludes with recommendations for prescribing physical activity and maintaining physical fitness in patients with coronary artery disease.

Chapter 18: Exercise Training in Diabetes Mellitus: An Efficient but Underused Therapeutic Option in the Prevention and Treatment of Coronary Artery Disease

Diabetes mellitus is one of the major risk factors for coronary artery disease. The disease progresses faster in diabetic patients and is associated with a worse prognosis. Although bypass surgery or percutaneous interventions with stent implantation provide quick symptomatic relief for patients with stable coronary artery disease it has no substantial prognostic benefit, except in patients with a significant stenosis of the left main stem or proximal left coronary artery.

A multifactorial intervention including dietary measures, blood glucose control, antihypertensive treatment, and regular physical exercise does have a positive influence on the modifiable risk factors, and improves cardiovascular fitness and angina-free exercise tolerance.

As shown by the United Kingdom Prospective Diabetes Study (UKPDS) and others it is of utmost importance to keep HbA1c levels <6.0% and LDL cholesterol levels <2.5 mmol/L (100 mg/dl) in order to reduce the incidence of cardiovascular events. Since the incidence of diabetes mellitus correlates inversely with the degree of physical activity, regular physical exercise (e.g. 30 min/day of aerobic exercise at a moderate intensity) can cut the risk for impaired glucose tolerance by half and the diabetes risk by up to three-quarters.

Endurance training is recommended for everybody including patients with stable coronary artery disease. Energy consumption should ideally be between 1000 and 2000 kcal/week, which corresponds to 3–5 hours of submaximal endurance training per week. This has been shown to lead to increased exercise performance; it also improves the cardiovascular risk profile, reduces the cardiovascular complication rate, improves myocardial perfusion, and slows the progression of coronary artery disease. Furthermore, endothelial function improves in patients with diabetes mellitus type 2 after 6 months of an intensive program of secondary prevention focusing on daily aerobic exercise training.

Exercise training is an effective therapeutic method which is largely underused and under-prescribed. In order to reduce the risk of atherosclerosis or to attenuate the progression of the disease, awareness on the part of physicians and patients has to increase so that this effective "drug" is incorporated into the daily life of patients.

Chapter 19: Exercise Training in Heart Failure

The upcoming epidemic of chronic heart failure (CHF) is inevitable in an aging society. The prevalence of CHF increases with age and reaches 10% among individuals >75 years. Disease-associated morbidity and disability are especially high among elderly CHF patients who account for more than three-quarters of all CHF-related hospital admissions. As a consequence, adjunctive therapeutic interventions are necessary aimed at improving exercise capacity and sustaining patients' ability to maintain an independent life.

Before initiating an exercise-based intervention in a CHF patient several important contraindications need to be ruled out: Cardiac decompensation in the previous 3 months, progressive worsening of exercise tolerance or dyspnea at rest or on exertion over the previous 3–5 days, myocardial ischemia during low-intensity exercise (<2 METs, <50 W), uncontrolled diabetes, acute systemic illness or fever, recent embolism, thrombophlebitis, active pericarditis or myocarditis, myocardial infarction within the previous 3 weeks, and new onset atrial fibrillation.

Before enrolling patients with CHF into a training program they should be in a stable condition without clinical evidence of fluid overload. A typical patient evaluation should be performed by an experienced cardiologist and involves: medical history, clinical examination, a resting ECG, a symptom-limited ergometry, and echocardiography. Other supplementary options are: Holter ECG, 24-hour blood pressure measurements, stress echocardiography, chest x-ray, and, in a few cases, evaluation of left ventricular filling pressures with a Swan – Ganz-catheter under stress conditions. If the clinical status of a patient is unclear and previous examinations/tests are lacking, invasive diagnostic measures should be undertaken in order to clarify the situation. It should be underlined that patients included in training studies have to be on optimized medical therapy and in a stable clinical condition for at least 4 weeks before the initiation of the training program.

Although the prescribed training programs vary widely with regard to exercise type and intensity it is generally recommended to *start low and go slow:* One should start with a workload of 50% of peak oxygen uptake for 5–10 minutes. When well tolerated, first the training duration per session, then the number of sessions per day should be increased. Finally, workload may gradually be increased to 70% of peak oxygen uptake.

While exercise interventions in CHF require a certain amount of enthusiasm and perseverance on the physician's side they are clinically highly rewarding: Exercise capacity may be increased by 20–30% and meta-analyses indicate a 35% reduction in all-cause mortality and a 28% reduction in hospitalization.

Chapter 20: Exercise Training in Valvular Heart Disease

Asymptomatic or mildly symptomatic patients with valvular heart disease are usually not included in medically supervised exercise training programs as part of the conservative management. However, physical conditioning and individually tailored exercise training are advisable for most patients after valve replacement, taking into account left ventricular function, previous level of training, the type of valve replaced, pulmonary hypertension, and heart rate. The general circulatory responses to exercise are of benefit to most of these patients, and could contribute to an overall improvement in the quality of life.

Chapter 21: The Role of Sports in Preventive Cardiology

There is wide documentation that physical activity reduces cardiovascular morbidity and mortality. The effect is more pronounced on increasing activity; it also has to be regular. In addition to the effect on classical risk factors, a positive effect on endothelial function also has been demonstrated. A similar effect is demonstrated by increasing fitness, and also when the effect of fitness on cardiovascular risk factors is corrected for. However, physical activity is more important, and the effect of fitness probably is induced by physical activity.

The risk of physical activity is by far outweighed by the benefit. Thus, the risk of sudden death is four times higher in persons not exercising than in those who exercise regularly. However, in young athletes the risk of sudden death is increased compared to sedentary persons of the same age, and the prevention of sudden death in this population also is an aspect of preventive cardiology. Myocarditis only accounts for 10% of deaths, but nevertheless physical training and competitions during febrile illness should be discouraged. Hypertrophic cardiomyopathy is the most important cause of sudden death in this population, and in most cases can be detected by ECG at rest. According to the European recommendations from 2005, a clinical examination and a standard ECG are sufficient in screening of competitive athletes aged 12–35 years. Exercise ECG should be done in male athletes above 35 years and female athletes above 40 years with a high risk of coronary disease before recommending participation in sports competitions.

There are no clear data on the harmful long-term cardiac effects of athletic training, and there is clear evidence of increased longevity in athletes provided physical training is continued.

Thus the message is clear that unless physical activity is regular and persistent it has no documented effect on the prevention of cardiovascular disease. Therefore, sports activity as a lifestyle has great potential as a tool in preventive cardiology. Involvement in sports for children and adolescents may be important in this regard. Whereas there is good evidence that fitness in the young is a good predictor of cardiovascular health later in life, the data on physical activity are less solid.

However, one can state that sports in the young can have a positive effect on cardiovascular morbidity and mortality. One of the increasing problems in this regard is juvenile obesity. This is also a sociocultural problem, as also is the lack of participation in sports and exercise in adolescents, which particularly affects female immigrants.

Thus there is good evidence to promote organized sports, which should be supported by families, community agencies, and schools.

Chapter 22: Advising Patients with Cardiac Disease and after Cardiac Interventions about Sports Activities

Physical exercise is often classified as dynamic and static. Dynamic exercise is usually advised in heart patients, but static exercise has been shown to be less hazardous than previously thought.

Competitive sports can be advised in several heart disorders, but in some cases must be discouraged. Due to pressure from athletic organizations, the media, sponsors, and the athlete's own ambitions and finances, the athlete often has a considerable motivation to carry on the activity, and recommendations are needed in order to give correct medical advice. In 1994 the American Bethesda Guidelines were published, and in 2005 Recommendations from the European Society of Cardiology were published. Grown up congenital heart disease patients benefit from regular exercise, and patients with ASD and VSD have no limitations in athletic activity 3 months after closure provided the ECG and echocardiogram are normal. In mild aortic and mitral regurgitation also all sports are allowed. This also is the case in well-controlled mild hypertension without additional risk factors and 3 months after successful ablation of paroxysmal supraventricular tachycardia.

In cardiomyopathies, however, competitive sports are not generally recommended, and in myocarditis competitions should be stopped for 6 months. In competitive athletes without symptoms and a low-risk profile, exercise testing is not routinely recommended in males below 35 years and females below 45 years.

Recreational sports generally can be advised in heart patients. In heart failure, reduction of mortality has been demonstrated by physical training.

(see Chapter 19) Generally, previous favorite sports should be encouraged, but in certain conditions there should be taken some precautions. Thus contact sports should not be recommended in patients on warfarin treatment, in patients with Marfan syndrome, and after valve prosthesis.

Sports in which there is a risk of falls should not be advised because of the risk of syncopal attacks. Scuba diving should be discouraged in recreational divers with decompression sickness with patent foramen ovale (PFO), in professional divers closure of the PFO should be performed.

17
Exercise Training in Coronary Heart Disease

Helmut Gohlke

Historical Perspective

Regular physical exercise and a high exercise capacity have been hallmarks of health and vitality for millennia and were associated with a distinct survival advantage in a hostile environment. In the modern civilized environment it is usually not the external enemy who is to be defeated. One of the enemies of survival is lack of physical activity and the resulting decreased physical fitness: both emerge once again as enemies of survival, this time in an all too friendly and comfortable environment.

Systematic studies on the benefit of physical activity in the modern world in healthy persons were conducted in the 1950s. Since the Framingham Study it has been well known that people who are physically active in their free time have a better long-term survival rate and a reduced age-adjusted rate of myocardial infarction and cardiovascular death than those who are less fit and less active. This is true for men and women.[1-4] Most of the knowledge on risks and benefits of habitual exercise and exercise training is derived from observational studies in persons or populations without known heart disease.

Because of the high prevalence of coronary artery disease (CAD) in these populations it is likely that many of these people had asymptomatic atherosclerotic disease. It is therefore also likely that even in a normal population those with asymptomatic atherosclerotic disease are those who benefit most from exercise. Therefore, the knowledge on the effects of exercise gained in a "normal" population can probably also be applied to stable patients with CAD. There is a large number of potentially beneficial effects of regular physical activity which could have prognostic implications, the most important of which are listed in Table 17-1.

Effects of Training on Heart Rate and Blood Pressure Response to Exercise

There is a number of mechanisms by which endurance exercise training may improve myocardial oxygen supply and thereby result in an antiischemic effect.

Exercise training reduces myocardial work at a given (submaximal) exercise level. This effect is achieved by improved adaptation of the peripheral circulation. A comparable external work can be achieved with a lower heart rate and blood pressure, thereby reducing myocardial oxygen demands and coronary blood flow requirements in myocardial areas with a potentially critical perfusion deficit. As myocardial perfusion is related to the length of the diastole, the time for perfusion of the myocardium decreases with increasing heart rate. Thus, exercise training improves the economy of the heart work and facilitates myocardial perfusion in patients with coronary artery stenoses.

A lower heart rate and a lower systolic blood pressure during exercise is a usual though somewhat transient phenomenon after exercise training in normal persons as well as in patients with CAD. To maintain this training effect exercise has

TABLE 17-1. Potentially prognostic beneficial effects of regular physical activity in patients with coronary artery disease

Maintenance and improvement of total exercise capacity
Improvement of symptom-free exercise capacity
Decrease of LDL cholesterol
Increase of HDL cholesterol
decrease of triglycerides
Increase of fibrinolytic activity
Decrease of blood viscosity
Decrease of body weight
Decrease of arterial blood pressure
Decrease of catecholamine levels
Increase of fibrillation threshold
Improvement of endothelial function
Increase of the number of circulating endothelial progenitor cells
Stress reduction
Improvement of quality of life

to be incorporated into the daily routine – like medication.

Many studies have shown that the symptomatic improvement as a consequence of exercise training is primarily due to a reduction in the rate–pressure product at submaximal workloads with no change in the rate–pressure product at the onset of angina.[5]

Exercise Training and Ischemia

Later reports also demonstrated an increase in the rate–pressure product at the onset of angina as well as a reduction in the ischemic response measured as angina or ST-segment depression, at a given rate–pressure product, suggesting that exercise training improves myocardial oxygen delivery.

Ehsani and coworkers in a non-randomized study examined whether an intense endurance exercise training program over 12 months could decrease ST-segment depression at a given rate–pressure product in patients with coronary artery disease. They also evaluated the course of the beginning and the extent of ischemic ST-segment depression during exercise. Interestingly ST-segment depression was regularly elicited during the training session, apparently without adverse events. Maximum oxygen uptake capacity increased by 38% after training. The extent of ischemic ST-segment depression

at a given heart rate–pressure product decreased and 0.1 mV ST-segment depression occurred at a 22% higher double product compared to before the training sessions.[6] These findings indicate that training in dedicated patients, if sufficiently intense and prolonged, can result in a reduction of myocardial ischemia at the same or a higher double product, suggesting enhanced myocardial perfusion as the cause for this improvement.

In the randomized Heidelberg exercise study, assessment of physical work capacity was performed during maximal, symptom-limited treadmill testing without cardiac medication. In the intervention group, patients significantly increased their physical work capacity, and levels achieved were well above both those reached at baseline and those seen in patients receiving usual care. Despite an increase in physical work capacity of 28%, myocardial oxygen consumption (estimated by the rate–pressure product) remained essentially unchanged. Improved angiographic collateralization or regression of coronary atherosclerosis that might be a reason for less ischemia could not be demonstrated, despite the intensive exercise training program. However, there was a significant trend for decreased progression after one[7] and six years of rather intense exercise,[8] particularly in those patients who attended more sessions of the structured training program.

In the randomized study of Belardinelli et al., after myocardial infarction there was greater improvement in residual scintigraphic perfusion defects in the exercise group compared to the usual care group.[9] The training effect therefore may vary in different patient populations and may also depend on the intensity of the exercise program. Ehsani's exercise program was probably somewhat more intense than that of the Heidelberg group.

The question whether ischemia should be avoided during endurance training in stable patients is not completely resolved at present. The studies of Ehsani et al.[6] suggest that in selected patients significant ST-segment depression can be tolerated without adverse effects. However, for safety reasons it is usually recommended to avoid ischemia during endurance training to minimize risks and maximize benefits. In patients with symptoms suggesting instability, exercise is not recommended until the phase of instability has resolved.[10]

Exercise Training and Left Ventricular Function

The influence of exercise training on left ventricular (LV) function is an important issue, because left ventricular function is one important determinant of prognosis.

Increased metabolic capacity and improved mechanical performance of the myocardium are well-recognized effects of endurance exercise training.[11]

To evaluate whether prolonged, intense exercise training can improve left ventricular function, Ehsani et al. studied 25 patients, 52 ($\pm$2) years old with coronary artery disease and mildly impaired LV function (ejection fraction 53%).[6] They compared these to 14 patients with comparable maximal exercise capacities and ejection fractions who did not undergo an exercise training program. The exercise group completed a 12-month program of very intense endurance exercise training of progressively increasing intensity, frequency, and duration. During the last 3 months the patients were running an average of 18 miles (29 km) per week, or doing an equivalent amount of exercise on a cycle ergometer. This is almost equivalent to a training volume for healthy persons preparing for a half-marathon run. Maximal attainable VO$_2$ increased by 37% ($P < 0.001$). Of the 10 patients with effort angina, five became asymptomatic, three experienced less angina, and two were unchanged after training. Ejection fraction did not change during maximal supine exercise before training (52 $\pm$ 3%), but after training it increased during exercise to 58 ($\pm$3%; $P < 0.01$), despite a higher rate–pressure product during maximal exercise, providing some evidence for an improvement in contractile state after training – or also for improved perfusion with less ischemic impairment of myocardial function during exercise. In patients who did not participate in training the ejection fraction response to exercise was unchanged after 12 months.

Exercise Capacity and Cardiovascular Morbidity

Not only the history given by the patient but also the measured exercise capacity is an important prognostic factor in persons as well as in patients with cardiovascular disease (see Chapter 13). Also patients with an angiographically defined extent of coronary artery disease and left ventricular (dys)function can be stratified according to their exercise performance into high- and low-risk subgroups. The total exercise performance is more important for the occurrence of cardiovascular events than the ST-segment response during exercise.[12] The maximal cardiac output achieved during exercise was able to differentiate low-risk from high-risk groups; for example, patients with three-vessel disease and normal or only mildly impaired LV function who reached a cardiac output of more than 13 L/min during exercise had a 5-year survival rate of 92% whereas patients who reached a cardiac output of less than 10 L/min had a significant lower 5-year survival rate of only 73%.[12,13]

Exercise capacity is also a marker for overall prognosis in patients with suspected cardiovascular disease but without angiographically defined coronary disease. This applies to patients referred for cardiac evaluation[14] but also to a population-based sample. In a finnish population a difference of one MET in exercise performance correlated with a 17–29% decrease in nonfatal and a 28–51% reduction in fatal cardiac events.[15] This observational study – like many before it – demonstrates an association between exercise capacity or exercise volume and overall event rate or mortality but not necessarily a causal relation. Therefore conclusions on the beneficial effects of exercise in terms of prognosis are based on category B evidence.

Habitual Exercise and Cardiovascular Disease

More than 40 observational studies give a clear message of an inverse dose–response relation between the volume of physical activity and all-cause mortality rates in asymptomatic younger and older men and women. The majority of these studies refer to subjects without definite CAD. But because of the gradual development of cardiovascular disease it can be assumed that many of these individuals had asymptomatic atherosclerotic disease and the conclusions derived from these studies are also applicable to patients with stable coronary artery disease.

In studies of male Harvard college alumni, the risk of death became progressively lower as physical activity levels increased from an expenditure of 500 to 3500 kcal/week (2.1 to 14.7 kJ/week). There was a 24% reduction in cardiovascular mortality in subjects whose energy expenditure was 2000 kcal/week (8.4 kJ/week). Alumni who were initially inactive and later increased their activity levels demonstrated significantly reduced cardiovascular risk compared with those remaining inactive.[3] The data regarding exercise intensity are less clear than those addressing total dose.

Regular activity of moderate intensity (4 to 7 kcal/min; 17 to 29 kJ/min) reduces cardiovascular mortality in men and women in a broad age range of social strata, ethnic origin, and age.[16,17] More intense activity is more strongly associated with lower cardiovascular mortality than is less intense activity.[18,19]

A threshold of intensity is probably required to achieve benefit. Although this threshold cannot be defined from available information, much of the exercise described in published reports that is associated with good health is at least moderate in intensity, such as brisk walking ($\sim$5 km/h); complete bedrest of three weeks as the extreme form of inactivity has a profound negative impact on physical work capacity similar to that of three decades of aging, as a recent longitudinal follow-up study suggested.[20,21] This emphasizes the importance of even low levels of exercise to at least maintain the physical work capacity at a constant level. The age-related decline in aerobic power among five middle-aged men occurring over 30 years could be completely reversed by a more intense 6-month endurance training program. However, no subject achieved the same VO_2max attained after intensive training as young men. The improved aerobic power after training was primarily the result of peripheral adaptation, with no effective improvement in maximal oxygen delivery.

Thus, it seems that the benefits of exercise occur already at moderate intensity; the total amount of activity is more important for health than the performance of high-intensity exercise. For patients in a cardiac rehabilitation program it has to be considered that the somewhat greater benefits from vigorous exercise are counterbalanced by more orthopedic injuries and higher dropout rates in structured programs, particularly in patients who have not been active for years or decades.[10]

Minimal adherence to current physical activity guidelines, which results in an energy expenditure of about 1000 kcal per week (= 4200 kJ per week), which is equivalent to 3.5 hours (i.e. half an hour per day) of walking of moderate intensity per week, is associated with a significant 20–30% reduction in risk of all-cause mortality. For each 90 minutes of brisk walking (5 km/h) per week (about 360 kcal or 1512 kJ) the coronary risk is reduced by 15%.[2,17,22] The risk of stroke in older people is also diminished by physical activity.[23] Due to limited data, it is also unclear whether vigorous-intensity activity confers additional benefit beyond its contribution to volume of physical activity when compared with moderate-intensity activity.[24] The relationship between exercise volume and relative improvement of prognosis is similar in persons with and without cardiovascular disease although at a different risk level.

Meta-Analyses on Exercise Training in Patients with CAD

Meta-analyses of studies evaluating the effects on prognosis of exercise-based cardiac rehabilitation in patients after myocardial infarction strongly suggest a beneficial effect of exercise training on mortality rates.[25,26] A more recent and comprehensive meta-analysis identified 51 randomized controlled trials of exercise-based cardiac rehabilitation.[27] This review adds more than 4000 patients to the prior, widely cited meta-analyses of cardiac rehabilitation.[25,26] All studies were published before January 1, 1999, and included 8440 patients who were primarily middle-aged, low-risk men. Patients were included if they had suffered a myocardial infarction, had undergone coronary artery bypass grafting or percutaneous transluminal coronary angioplasty, had angina pectoris, or had CAD identified by angiography. Supervised exercise training in these programs was generally of 2 to 6 months' duration followed by unsupervised exercise. The mean follow-up was 2.4 years. Results were analyzed according to whether the cardiac rehabilitation program consisted of exercise only or also included psychosocial and/or educational interventions. Total mortality was reduced by 27% ($P < 0.05$) with the exercise-only intervention and 13% ($P = NS$) with comprehensive rehabilitation. Cardiac mortality was reduced by 31% ($P < 0.05$) and 26% ($P < 0.05$) for the exercise-only and comprehensive programs, respectively. Neither the exercise-only program nor the comprehensive intervention significantly reduced the rate of nonfatal myocardial infarction or sudden cardiac death.[27] The meta-analysis confirms that exercise-based cardiac rehabilitation reduces cardiac mortality but does not reduce the risk of recurrent myocardial infarction. In contrast to the prior analyses, however, these recent results suggest that the exercise component is a critical aspect of the rehabilitation process. The reduction in death without a reduction in nonfatal reinfarction raises the possibility that exercise training enhanced electrical stability and reduced ventricular fibrillation[28] or reduced myocardial damage directly or via other factors such as ischemic preconditioning.[29]

Many of the studies in this meta-analysis preceded most of the present treatments for CAD patients, including widespread use of aggressive lipid management, use of beta-adrenergic blockers, and angiotensin-converting enzymes, primary angioplasty or acute thrombolytic therapy in the acute phase, and aggressive revascularization after the acute event.

Newer Randomized Studies

However, there is increasing evidence from randomized studies in patients with established coronary artery disease that exercise training not only improves factors that correlate with prognosis like several risk factors as well as exercise capacity and maximal O_2 consumption but that it also improves prognosis itself.

Two more recent randomized studies examined the effect of cardiac rehabilitation on morbidity and mortality: Belardinelli and coworkers[3] randomized 118 consecutive patients after percutaneous coronary intervention into an exercise group which underwent a 6-month exercise training program of moderate intensity (three times a week at 60% of peak VO_2) and a control group. During a follow-up time of 33 months, trained patients had fewer events (12% vs. 32%; $P < 0.01$) and a lower hospital readmission rate (19 vs. 46%; $P < 0.02$) than patients in the usual care group.

These findings of decreased morbidity as a consequence of exercise training in patients with CAD were corroborated by a more recent randomized study. Hambrecht and coworkers randomized 101 patients with stable CAD and documented exercise-induced ischemia to undergo either a 12-month exercise training program or a percutaneous coronary intervention (PCI) followed by usual care.[30] All patients had an angiographically documented stenosis suitable for PCI. Within the exercise training program patients exercised during the first 2 weeks in the hospital six times per day for 10 minutes on a bicycle ergometer at 70% of the symptom-limited maximal heart rate. Before discharge from the hospital the target heart rate for home training was determined by a maximal symptom-limited ergospirometry. The target heart rate was defined as 70% of the maximal heart rate during this symptom-limited exercise test. Patients were asked to exercise on their bicycle ergometer close to the target heart rate for 20 minutes per day and to participate in one 60-minute group training session of aerobic exercise per week. If a caloric expense of 600 kcal/h during this exercise intensity is assumed this would amount to an equivalent of 1800–2000 kcal/week, an exercise volume that was shown by the Heidelberg/Leipzig group in previous studies to have a beneficial effect on fitness and progression of coronary atherosclerosis.[7,8]

Patients in the exercise training group had a higher event-free survival rate than patients who underwent PCI.[30] Although both PCI and exercise training were equally effective in improving symptom-free exercise tolerance and the Canadian Cardiovascular Society angina class the exercise training group in addition had a higher exercise capacity and maximal oxygen uptake after 12 months (i.e. was functionally superior to the group treated by PCI).

The overall cardiovascular event rate was significantly lower in the exercise group than in the PCI group as a consequence of complications associated with the procedure and as a consequence of more frequent repeat coronary angiographies in patients undergoing PCI.[30]

Although the number of patients randomized in these two studies is small, the results are in agreement with the extensive epidemiologic and observational database and suggest, indeed, that there is a causal relationship between exercise training and prognosis after PCI.

Risks of Exercise Training

Despite its beneficial effects, exercise is associated with an increased risk of acute cardiac events. Although many factors affect the risk of exercise, two of the most important risk indicators in patients with CAD are age, and intensity of exercise. Screening procedures can be used that identify individuals at increased risk for an exercise-related cardiac event. These are patients who are generally at increased risk of sudden death: in particular patients with severely impaired LV function or ischemia at low levels of exercise. The results of studies reporting the risks of sudden cardiac arrest during exercise training indicate that this risk is low even during vigorous exercise.

In a supervised setting there was 1 event during 65,000 to 130,000 hours of exercise. These studies strongly suggest that the incidence of sudden cardiac arrest across a variety of activities, with the exception of jogging, is similar to that expected by chance alone. In subjects with heart disease, jogging seems to be associated with a greater incidence of sudden cardiac arrest compared with other activities. This is probably related to exercise intensity. Jogging at even the slowest pace may generate a VO_2 that exceeds 80% of the maximum for many untrained individuals.

Exercise and Myocardial Infarction

Exercise can be a potent trigger of myocardial infarction (MI), which is seven times more likely to occur than sudden cardiac death. It can be assumed that this increased risk is confined to persons with pre-existing coronary artery disease. Approximately 4–20% of MIs occur during or soon after exertion.[31-33] Physical exertion at a level >6 METs has been reported within 1 hour of acute MI in 4–7% of patients. However, the adjusted relative risk has been found to be greater in persons who do not regularly participate in physical activity.[31,32] Among sedentary individuals, the relative risk of MI during exercise was 107 times that of baseline, whereas among individuals who regularly exercise 5 times per week, the relative risk of infarction during exercise is only 2.4 times greater than that of baseline.[31] This inverse relationship between regular physical activity and MI is of clinical importance because a person's functional capacity must be considered when recommending the intensity of an exercise endurance program. The least active subjects are at greatest risk for MI during exercise; both leisure-time physical activity and cardiorespiratory fitness have a strong inverse relationship with the risk of acute MI during exercise.[1]

Mechanisms Promoting Cardiovascular Protection by Exercise

Regular physical activity is associated with favorable modification of cardiovascular risk factors such as hypercholesterolemia, hypertension, diabetes, and obesity. Additional aspects are listed in Table 17-1.

Exercise Effects on Lipids and Weight

Serum lipids have a profound influence on the development of atherosclerosis. Exercise can modify the level of various lipid subfractions and also of total body weight.

In the Heidelberg study total cholesterol decreased by 10% ($P < 0.001$), and triglycerides by 24% ($P < 0.001$); high-density lipoproteins increased by 3% ($P = NS$).[7] The changes in the lipid profile are quantitatively moderate; however, in addition to the total reduction there is a shift with exercise from the smaller more atherogenic LDL particles to the larger, less atherogenic particles rather than a marked reduction in the LDL cholesterol content.[34]

Lipid levels also influence endothelial function in a reversible manner, depending on the actual lipid level, particularly after meals.

We all spend the majority of our lives in the postprandial state, and the changes in metabolism seen during the hours after meal ingestion are likely to play an important role in the atherosclerotic disease process. Postprandial lipoproteins and their remnants can probably directly infiltrate the arterial wall and accumulate in atheromatous plaques. In particular, the atherogenic lipoprotein phenotype of small, dense, low-density lipoprotein (LDL) and a low level of high-density lipoprotein (HDL) have an unfavorable influence.[35]

Additional non-lipid metabolic changes occur in the postprandial state: *systemic inflammation* is increased and endothelial function is impaired postprandially, with some correlation to the postprandial triglyceride increase. As endothelial dysfunction and inflammation are central to atherogenic progression, it is likely that these daily, transient postprandial changes influence the long-term risk of vascular disease.

The beneficial effects of exercise on a variety of lipid and lipoprotein variables are seen most clearly in short-term studies with a large amount of high-intensity exercise. Kraus and coworkers[34] examined a total of 111 sedentary, overweight men and women with mild-to-moderate dyslipidemia. They were randomly assigned to participate for 6 months in a control group or for approximately 8 months in one of three exercise groups: high-amount–high-intensity exercise, the caloric equivalent of jogging 20 miles (32 km) per week at 65–80% of peak oxygen consumption; low-amount–high-intensity exercise, the equivalent of jogging 12 miles (19.2 km) per week at 65–80% of peak oxygen consumption; or low-amount–moderate-intensity exercise, the equivalent of walking 12 miles (19.2 km) per week at 40–55% of peak oxygen consumption.

Higher amounts of exercise resulted in greater improvements than did lower amounts of exercise. But even lower amount of exercise had better responses than the control group. The improvements were related to the amount of activity and not to the intensity of exercise or improvement in fitness.[34]

In a recent study a single 90-minute treadmill exercise activity in the afternoon decreased fasting triglyceride the next morning and post-prandial triglyceride concentrations by 25% in lean and obese subjects about 16–18 hours after the exercise session. Obese subjects started at a higher level of triglycerides but had a similar relative reduction.[35]

The effect of exercise on weight is usually overestimated by patients. In patients participating in the Heidelberg intervention trial[7] aiming to increase exercise and to improve their diet according to the AHA recommendations phase 3, body weight decreased by 5% after 12 months ($P < 0.001$).

In a program of 6 months of endurance training, on average, only a 4% decline in body weight (100 vs. 96 kg) and a decrease in body mass index by 1.1 (29.1 vs. 28.0) were observed, with no change in percent body fat. These observations suggest that the increased energy expenditures of training were accompanied by a concomitant increase in caloric intake, underscoring the importance of dietary prescription as an adjunct to physical exercise if weight loss is a desired outcome.[21]

The mechanisms mediating the atheroprotective effects of exercise, however, are not clearly defined, although multiple possible mediators have been suggested, including various physiological adaptations, altered autonomic function, and metabolic adjustments (see Table 17-1).

Exercise, Endothelial Function, and Endothelial Progenitor Cells (EPCs)

One of the major favorable effects of exercise is the improvement of endothelial dysfunction. Endothelial dysfunction is a precursor of clinically significant atherosclerotic disease and is an indicator for an increased cardiovascular event rate.[36,37] The endothelium is one of the largest organs of the body and there is some evidence that the endothelium of different parts of the arterial system responds in similar manner to the exposure to conventional risk factors. Different attempts have been made to correct the impaired endothelium-dependent vasodilatation. In recent years it has become apparent that exercise affects the functional activity of the vascular endothelium: Whereas normal coronary arteries dilate, atherosclerotic coronary arteries often exhibit a paradoxical vasoconstriction in response to exercise-induced flow or acetylcholine, thereby causing critical ischemia even in moderate epicardial stenosis.

Hambrecht et al. evaluated the effects of exercise on endothelial function in a randomized training study. Patients in the training group exercised in hospital under the supervision of a physician three times daily for 10 minutes on a rowing ergometer and three times daily for 10 minutes on a bicycle ergometer (in addition to 5 minutes for warming up and 5 minutes for cooling down) for 4 weeks. Workloads were adjusted so that patients did not experience chest pain and did not show any signs of ischemia in the ECG during exercise.

Patients assigned to the control group continued their sedentary lifestyle, resumed treatment with their individually tailored cardiac medication, and were supervised by their private physicians. Hambrecht and coworkers could show that chronic intermittent bouts of exercise training, associated with increases of flow and shear stress in the vasculature, improve coronary endothelial function by increasing coronary blood flow reserve and by reducing pathological vasoconstriction.[38]

Endothelium-derived NO is the main mediator of improved endothelial function and exerts a multitude of anti-atherosclerotic functions. Acting on the endothelial cell itself, NO inhibits endothelial cell apoptosis, suppresses inflammatory activation, and increases the activity of oxygen radical-scavenging enzymes.

Furthermore NO inhibits platelet aggregation via luminal release from the endothelium and also inhibits vascular smooth muscle cell proliferation and promotion of positive arterial remodeling via abluminal release.

Studies using cultured endothelial cells and animal experiments suggest that increases in endothelial NO synthase (eNOS) expression and protein phosphorylation are possible mechanisms. The authors could also delineate the mechanism in a randomized study harvesting thoracica interna arteries during open heart surgery after a preceding training period of 4 weeks: exercise training in stable CAD leads to an improved agonist-mediated endothelium-dependent vasodilatory capacity.[39]

From the same group Adams and coworkers[40] found that regular exercise limited the arterial content of angiotensin type I receptors and enhanced expression of angiotensin type II receptors. They also found that arterial production of reactive oxygen species was significantly reduced by exercise training. In total, these effects produced an improvement in endothelial function. These data provide tangible evidence that exercise training has a direct impact on the vascular wall.

Recent evidence has shown that vascular function not only depends on cells that reside within the vessel wall but also appears to be significantly modulated by circulating cells derived from the bone marrow. A specific subset of these stem cells – endothelial progenitor cells (EPCs) – has been shown to enhance angiogenesis, promote vascular repair, improve endothelial function, inhibit atherosclerosis, and increase ventricular function after myocardial infarction. Although myocardial infarction and bypass surgery acutely increase the circulating numbers, accumulation of vascular risk factors appears to reduce these bone marrow-derived cells, which suggests that vascular health and repair processes after injury require increased numbers of this potentially beneficial population of cells. Laufs and coworkers could show that patients with coronary artery disease display increasing numbers of circulating EPCs in response to physical training, suggesting that EPCs, which appear important for maintaining endothelial integrity and crucial for neovascularization of ischemic tissue, can be increased in numbers by physical training.[41]

These results help to explain why the beneficial effects of regular physical activity cannot be accounted for solely by reduction of the conventional risk factors, because the association with reduced mortality is independent of other coronary risk factors. Thus these results give support to the view that physical inactivity is an independent risk factor and that physical activity in itself has a favorable influence on prognosis.

Recommendations for Physical Activity in Patients with Coronary Artery Disease

Given the high prognostic value of exercise capacity relative to other markers of risk in observational and recent randomized studies, clinicians should advise and encourage patients with coronary disease to increase their exercise volume and improve their exercise capacity.

TABLE 17-2. Risk classification for exercise training. Class B: Presence of known, stable coronary heart disease with low risk for complications with vigorous exercise, but slightly greater than for apparently healthy individuals

This classification includes individuals with any of the following diagnoses:

1. *CAD (MI, CABG, PCI, angina pectoris, abnormal exercise test, and abnormal coronary angiograms) whose condition is stable and who have the clinical characteristics outlined below*

Clinical characteristics (must include all of the following):
a. New York Heart Association class I or II
b. Exercise capacity ≥6 METs
c. No evidence of congestive heart failure
d. No evidence of myocardial ischemia or angina at rest or on the exercise test at or below 6 METs
e. Appropriate rise in systolic blood pressure during exercise
f. Absence of sustained or non-sustained ventricular tachycardia at rest or with exercise
g. Ability to satisfactorily self-monitor intensity of activity

2. *Exercise test abnormalities that do not meet any of the high-risk criteria outlined in class C (see Table 17-3)*

Activity guidelines: Activity should be individualized, with exercise prescription provided by qualified individuals and approved by primary healthcare provider.

Supervision required: Medical supervision during initial prescription session is desirable.

Supervision by appropriate trained nonmedical personnel for other exercise sessions should occur until the individual understands how to monitor his or her activity.

Medical personnel should be trained and certified in Advanced Cardiac Life Support. A cardioverter/defibrillator should be available if a training session is largely confined to coronary patients.

Nonmedical personnel should be trained and certified in Basic Life Support (which includes cardiopulmonary resuscitation including cardiac defibrillation).

ECG and blood pressure monitoring: Useful during the early prescription phase of training, usually 6 to 12 sessions.

Source: Modified from Fletcher et al., 2001.[10]

TABLE 17-3. Risk classification for exercise training. Class C: Those at moderate-to-high risk for cardiac complications during exercise and/or unable to self-regulate activity or to understand recommended activity level

This classification includes individuals with the following diagnoses:
1. *CAD with the following clinical characteristics (any of the following):*
   a. New York Heart Association class III or IV
   b. Exercise test results:
      Exercise capacity <6 METs
      Angina or ischemic ST depression at a workload <6 METs
      Fall in systolic blood pressure below resting levels during exercise
      Non-sustained ventricular tachycardia with exercise
   c. Previous episode of primary cardiac arrest (i.e. cardiac arrest that did not occur in the presence of an acute myocardial infarction or during a cardiac procedure)
   d. A medical problem that the physician believes may be life-threatening

2. *Complex ventricular arrhythmias not well controlled*

Activity guidelines: Activity should be individualized, with exercise prescription provided by qualified individuals and approved by primary healthcare provider.

Supervision: Medical supervision during all exercise sessions until safety is established.

ECG and blood pressure monitoring: Continuous during exercise sessions until safety is established, usually about 12 sessions.

*Class C patients who have successfully completed a series of supervised exercise sessions may be reclassified to class B providing that the safety of exercise at the prescribed intensity is satisfactorily established by appropriate medical personnel and that the patient has demonstrated the ability to self-monitor.

Source: Modified from Fletcher et al., 2001.[10]

When advising the patient about physical activity early after myocardial infarction or after bypass surgery, risk classification is important to delineate the intensity of the recommended activity. Patients with established or suspected coronary artery disease will usually be in the risk category B (Table 17-2) or C (Table 17-3). It should be decided whether medical supervision is advisable during exercise training sessions before starting with a structured exercise program (Tables 17-2 and 17-3).

Improving exercise tolerance and increasing habitual physical activity requires much more attention and effort from physicians, and at least as much as is given to the improvement of other major risk factors. Of course, the maintenance of a higher habitual exercise level is much more difficult than for example prescribing a lipid-lowering medication but the benefits are probably similar, more immediate and result in an improvement in the quality of life.

The available evidence strongly suggests that for patients with coronary artery disease the benefits of regular exercise greatly exceed the risks – if patients exercise prudently. When starting with exercise training in patients with CAD, a few general rules should be followed.

In unsupervised training sessions, a "small talk" conversation should still be possible ("talk test"). This helps to ensure that the exercise intensity is below the anaerobic threshold.

Patients should begin at a more moderate intensity, shorter duration, and lower frequency than the ultimate goal. A moderate activity is in the range of 40–60% of maximal O_2 uptake or 55–70% of the age-adjusted maximal heart rate. The heart rate range for moderate activity in different age groups is shown in Figure 17-1. Most patients will be on a beta-blocker, which tends to decrease the heart range in a variable manner. Success should be assessed and reinforcement provided regularly. Gradual increases in activity are not only safer for sedentary patients with CAD, but short-term successes may increase

the patient's self-efficacy for being physically active.[10]

The guidelines for secondary prevention of coronary disease for patients in a chronic and stable phase suggest that physical activities of moderate intensity 4–5 times per week for 30–45 minutes are desirable.[42,43] This adds up to an exercise volume of 2 hours to almost 4 hours with a kcal expenditure between 900 and 1700 kcal/week. Endurance activities like walking, jogging, or bicycling are preferable; however, particularly in the elderly, improvement of the strength of the thigh muscles and of the shoulder girdle is important to prevent falls.[44] Detailed recommendations for resistance training in patients with CAD have been published recently.[44a]

The intensity of the endurance activity should be in the moderate range.

It is important to consider the age-adjusted exercise capacity and heart rate to avoid overexertion and not to endanger persons who have been rather inactive for long periods of time. The corresponding heart rates in different intensities of activities in various age groups are given in Table 17-4.

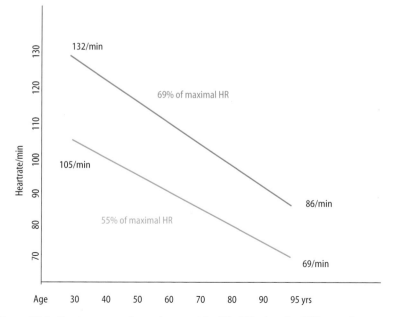

FIGURE 17-1. Heart rate range for moderate activity (55–69% of maximal HR) according to age.

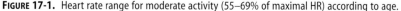

TABLE 17-4. Relative intensity of comparable activities in different age groups

| Relative intensity | Relative and absolute (METs) intensity of comparable activities in different age groups of healthy adults, Endurance-type activity | | | | | | | | Strength-Type Exerc./Rel. Intensity* |
	Young (20–39 years) METs	HR-range	Middle-aged (40–64 years) METs	HR range	Elderly (65–79 years) METs	HR range	Old (80+ years) METs	HR range	Max. voluntary contraction, %
Very light	<2.4	63–67	<2.0	55–63	<1.6	49–54	<1.0	46–49	<30
Light	2.4–4.7	63–103	2.0–3.9	55–97	1.6–3.1	49–84	1.1–1.9	46–76	30–49
Moderate	4.8–7.1	100–132	4.0–5.9	86–124	3.2–4.7	78–107	2.0–2.9	72–97	50–69
Hard	7.2–10.1	127–170	6.0–8.4	109–160	4.8–6.7	99–138	3.0–4.2	92–125	70–84
Very hard	≥10.2	163–191	≥8.5	140–180	≥6.8	127–155	≥4.25	118–140	≥85
Max.‡	12.0		10.0		8.0		5.0		100

*Based on 8 to 12 repetitions for persons <50–60 years old and 10 to 15 repetitions for persons aged ≥50–60 years.
Borg rating of Relative Perceived Exertion (RPE), 6–20 scale.
Max. values are mean values achieved during max. exercise by healthy adults. Absolute intensity values are approximate mean values for men. Mean values for women are ~1 to 2 METs lower than those for men.
Source: Adapted from Fletcher et al. 2001.[10]

More activity in daily life, such as walking during work breaks, using stairs instead of elevators, and gardening, are advantageous. Any physical activity over and above everyday activities can be considered favorable.

Already light to moderate regular physical activity reduces the risk for acute coronary events in people who do not perform intense physical activity. The difference in free time activities was able to explain for example the differences in coronary event rates between Northern Ireland and France.[45]

Summary

Improvement of exercise capacity is of great importance for the coronary patient in terms of improvement of the cardiac risk profile, the quality of life, and prognosis. A structured endurance training program after myocardial infarction should only be started after risk stratification. The baseline exercise intensity that can be achieved without symptoms and without objective signs of ischemia should be defined, if necessary, including stress echocardiogram or exercise hemodynamics.

The risk classification for exercise training is a valuable guideline to identify patients who will

clearly benefit and those who are at greatly increased risk for adverse events during exercise. The latter will need closer monitoring, particularly during the initial training sessions until stability has been shown.

Similarly, patients who are unlikely to benefit from an exercise program or patients who are endangered by exercise have to be identified and supervised closely or in individual cases even be excluded; corrective actions – if feasible – should be undertaken to decrease the risk. Patients with heart failure should be free of congestion before an exercise program is started. Heart failure patients benefit particularly from a tailored exercise program (see Chapter 19).

Thus, in conclusion, there are very few patients with CAD who cannot participate in an individually adapted exercise training program.

References

1. Lakka TA, Venalainen JM, Rauramaa R, et al. Relation of leisure-time physical activity and cardiorespiratory fitness to the risk of acute myocardial infarction. N Engl J Med 1994;330: 1549–1554.
2. Manson JAE, Hu FB, Rich-Edwards JW, et al. A prospective study of walking as compared with vigorous exercise in the prevention of coronary

heart disease in women. N Engl J Med 1999;341: 650–658.

3. Paffenbarger RS, Hyde RT, Wing AL, Hsieh C-C. Physical activity, all cause mortality and longevity of college alumni. N Engl J Med 1986;314:605–613.

4. Sandvik L, Erikssen J, Thaulow E, Erikssen G, Mundal R, Rodahl K. Physical fitness as a predictor of mortality among healthy, middle-aged Norwegian men. N Engl J Med 1993;328:533–537.

5. Thompson et al., AHA Scientific Statements. Exercise and physical activity in the prevention and treatment of atherosclerotic cardiovascular disease. Circulation 2003;107:3109–3116.

6. Ehsani AA, Heath GW, Hagberg JM, Sobel BE, Holloszy JO. Effects of 12 months of intense exercise training on ischemic ST-segment depression in patients with coronary artery disease. Circulation 1981;64:1116–1124.

7. Schuler G, Hambrecht R, Schlierf G, et al. Regular physical exercise and low fat diet: effects on progression of coronary artery disease. Circulation 1992;86:1–11.

8. Niebauer J, Hambrecht R, Velich T, et al. Attenuated progression of coronary artery disease after 6 years of multifactorial risk intervention – role of physical exercise. Circulation 1997;96:2534–2541.

9. Belardinelli R, Paolini I, Cianci G, Piva R, Georgiou D, Purcaro A. Exercise training intervention after coronary angioplasty: the ETICA trial. J Am Coll Cardiol 2001;37:1891–1900.

10. Fletcher GF, Balady GJ, Amsterdam EA, et al. Exercise standards for testing and training: a statement for healthcare professionals from the American Heart Association. Circulation 2001;104:1694–1740.

11. Shephard RJ, Balady GJ. Exercise as cardiovascular therapy. Circulation 1999;99:963–972.

12. Gohlke H, Samek L, Betz P, Roskamm H. Exercise testing provides additional prognostic information in angiographically defined subgroups of patients with coronary heart disease. Circulation 1983;68:979–985.

13. Gohlke H, Betz P, Roskamm H. Improved risk stratification in patients with coronary artery disease. Application of a survival function using continuous exercise and angiographic variables. Eur Heart J 1988;9:427–434.

14. Myers J, Prakash M, Froelicher V, Do D, Partington S, Atwood JE. Exercise capacity and mortality among men referred for exercise testing. N Engl J Med 2002;346:793–801.

15. Laukkanen JA, Kurl S, Salonen R, Rauramaa R, Salonen JT. The predictive value of cardiorespiratory fitness for cardiovascular events in men

with various risk profiles: a prospective population-based cohort study. Eur Heart J 2004;25:1428–1437.

16. National Institutes of Health. Clinical guidelines on the identification, evaluation, and treatment of overweight and obesity in adults: the evidence report. Obes Res 1998;6 (Suppl):51S–209S.

17. Hakim AA, Petrovitch H, Burchfiel CM, et al. Effects of walking on mortality among nonsmoking retired men. N Engl J Med 1998;338:94–99.

18. Bijnen FC, Caspersen CJ, Feskens EJ, et al. Physical activity and 10-year mortality from cardiovascular diseases and all causes: the Zutphen Elderly Study. Arch Intern Med 1998;158:1499–1505.

19. Lee IM, Hsieh CC, Paffenbarger RS Jr. Exercise intensity and longevity in men: the Harvard Alumni Health Study. JAMA 1995;273:1179–1184.

20. McGuire DK, Levine BD, Williamson JW, et al. A 30-year follow-up of the Dallas Bed Rest and Training Study: I. Effect of age on the cardiovascular response to exercise. Circulation 2001;104:1350–1357.

21. McGuire DK, Levine BD, Williamson JW, et al. A 30-year follow-up of the Dallas Bed Rest and Training Study: II. Effect of age on cardiovascular adaptation to exercise training. Circulation 2001;104:1358–1366.

22. Hakim AA, Curb JD, Petrovitch H, et al. Effects of walking on coronary heart disease in elderly men – the Honolulu Heart Program. Circulation 1999;100:9–13.

23. Agnarsson U, Thorgeirsson G, Sigvaldason H, Sigfusson N. Effects of leisure-time physical activity and ventilatory function on risk for stroke in men: The Reykjavik Study. Ann Intern Med 1999; 130:987–990.

24. Lee I-M, Skerrett PJ. Physical activity and all-cause mortality – what is the dose-response relation? Med Sci Sports Exerc 2001;33(Suppl):S459–471.

25. O'Connor GT, Buring JE, Yusuf S, et al. An overview of randomized trials of rehabilitation with exercise after myocardial infarction. Circulation 1989;80:234–244.

26. Oldridge NB, Guyatt GH, fischer ME, et al. Cardiac rehabilitation after myocardial infarction: combined experience of randomized clinical trials. JAMA 1988;260:945–950.

27. Jolliffe JA, Rees K, Taylor RS, et al. Exercise-based rehabilitation for coronary heart disease. Cochrane Database Syst Rev 2001;(1):CD001800.

28. Billman GE. Aerobic exercise conditioning: a non-pharmacological antiarrhythmic intervention. J Appl Physiol 2002;92:446–454.

29. Hamilton KL, Powers SK, Sugiura T, et al. Short-term exercise training can improve myocardial

tolerance to I/R without elevation in heatshock proteins. Am J Physiol Heart Circ Physiol 2001;281: H1346–H1352.

30. Hambrecht R, Walther C, Möbius-Winkler S, et al. Percutaneous coronary angioplasty compared with exercise training in patients with stable coronary artery disease – a randomized trial. Circulation 2004;109:1371–1378.

31. Mittleman MA, Maclure M, Tofler GH, et al. Triggering of acute myocardial infarction by heavy physical exertion: protection against triggering by regular exertion: Determinants of Myocardial Infarction Onset Study Investigators. N Engl J Med 1993;329:1677–1683.

32. Willich SN, Lewis M, Lowel H, et al. Physical exertion as a trigger of acute myocardial infarction: Triggers and Mechanisms of Myocardial Infarction Study Group. N Engl J Med 1993;329: 1684–1690.

33. Tofler GH, Muller JE, Stone PH, et al. Modifiers of timing and possible triggers of acute myocardial infarction in the Thrombolysis in Myocardial Infarction Phase II (TIMI II) Study Group. J Am Coll Cardiol 1992;20:1049–1055.

34. Kraus WE, Houmard JA, Duscha BD, et al. Effects of the amount and intensity of exercise on plasma lipoproteins. N Engl J Med 2002;347:1483–1492.

35. Gill JMR, Al-Mamari A, Ferrell WR, et al. Effects of prior moderate exercise on postprandial metabolism and vascular function in lean and centrally obese men. J Am Coll Cardiol 2004;44:2375–2382.

36. Schächinger V, Britten MB, Zeiher AM. Prognostic impact of coronary vasodilator dysfunction on adverse long-term outcome of coronary heart disease. Circulation 2000;101:1899–1906.

37. Suwaidi JA, Hamasaki S, Higano ST, Nishimura RA, Holmes DR, Lerman A. Long-term follow-up of patients with mild CAD and endothelial dysfunction. Circulation 2000;101:1002–1006.

38. Hambrecht R, Gielen S, Linke A, et al. Effect of exercise on coronary endothelial function in patients with coronary artery disease. N Engl J Med 2000;342:454–460.

39. Hambrecht R, Adams V, Erbs S, et al. Regular physical activity improves endothelial function in patients with coronary artery disease by increasing phosphorylation of endothelial nitric oxide synthase. Circulation 2003;107:3152–3158.

40. Adams V, Linke A, Kränkel N, et al. Impact of regular physical activity on the NAD(P)H oxidase and angiotensin receptor system in patients with coronary artery disease. Circulation 2005;111:555–562.

41. Laufs U, Werner N, Link A, et al. Physical training increases endothelial progenitor cells, inhibits neointima formation, and enhances angiogenesis. Circulation 2004;109:220–226.

42. Gohlke H, Kübler W, Mathes P, et al. für die Deutsche Gesellschaft für Kardiologie – Herz-Kreislaufforschung. Empfehlungen zur umfassenden Risikoverringerung für Patienten mit koronarer Herzerkrankung, Gefäßerkrankungen und Diabetes. Z Kardiol 2001;90:148–149.

43. Smith SC Jr, Greenland P, Grundy SM. AHA Conference Proceedings. Prevention Conference V: beyond secondary prevention: identifying the high-risk patient for primary prevention: executive summary. American Heart Association. Circulation 2000;101:111–116.

44. Tinetti ME. Preventing falls in elderly persons. N Engl J Med 2003;348:42–49.

44a. Bjarnason-Wehrens B, Mayer-Berger W, Meister ER, Baum K, Hambrecht R, Gielen S. Recommendations for resistance exercise in cardiac rehabilitation: recommendation of the German Federation for Cardiovascular Prevention and Rehabilitation. Eur J Cardiovasc Prev Rehabil 2004;11:352–361.

45. Wagner A, Simon C, Evans A, et al. on behalf of the PRIME Study Group. Physical Activity and Coronary Event Incidence in Northern Ireland and France: The Prospective Epidemiological Study of Myocardial Infarction (PRIME). Circulation 2002;105:2247–2252.

18

Exercise Training in Diabetes Mellitus: An Efficient but Underused Therapeutic Option in the Prevention and Treatment of Coronary Artery Disease

Josef Niebauer

Diabetes mellitus type 2 is one of the most common diseases in industrialized countries and is one of the main risk factors for the development of micro- and macrovascular diseases. Vascular complications are causes of death in up to 80% of these patients and 75% of deaths are due to coronary artery disease.[1,2]

Although exercise training should be part of the treatment regimen in patients with diabetes according to national and international guidelines, it is only integrated into the daily routine by a minority of patients. This ought to change, since only a multifactorial risk intervention which includes exercise training has the potential to treat the underlying causes of both diabetes and coronary artery disease (Figure 18-1).[3]

Physical Exercise

The incidence of diabetes mellitus correlates inversely with the degree of physical activity.[4] Regular aerobic exercise of 30 min/day at a moderate intensity can cut the risk for impaired glucose tolerance by half and the diabetes risk by up to three-quarters.[5–7]

Although there is no direct proof that endothelial dysfunction leads to atherosclerosis, it has been shown that endothelial dysfunction is associated with increased cardiovascular mortality.[8] Endothelial dysfunction is found when the endothelium has been damaged. This occurs as a result of smoking, hyperglycemia, hyperlipidemia, and hypertension. It can be improved by intensive physical exercise not only in normoglycemic patients but also in patients with diabetes mellitus and coronary artery disease.[6,9] In diabetics, however, this effect is not yet found after 4 weeks but only after a prolonged training period of 6 months. This delayed improvement in diabetic patients, as compared to normoglycemic patients, may be due to the rather diffuse atherosclerotic process that occurs in diabetes throughout the coronary tree with little normally functioning endothelium left to release nitric oxide (NO) and to react with a vasodilatory stimulus such as acetylcholine (Figure 18-2).

A meta-analysis showed that normoglycemic patients with coronary artery disease[10] benefited from endurance training as part of a rehabilitation program, with a reduction in mortality of 31%. This prognostic effect of physical exercise, especially for diabetic patients, has been demonstrated in several studies[4,11] (see Table 18-1) and includes a marked reduction in both the risk of developing coronary artery disease and the rate of cardiac mortality.[12] To obtain these benefits, energy consumption due to physical exercise training should ideally be between 1000 and 2000 kcal/week, which corresponds to 3–5 hours of submaximal endurance training per week.[13]

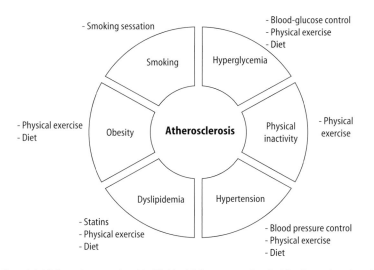

FIGURE 18-1. Multifactorial risk factor intervention: Modifiable risk factors associated with atherosclerosis and their respective treatment options.

Exercise Training Combined with Blood Glucose Control

The importance of early diagnosis and subsequent therapy of diabetes has been highlighted by the United Kingdom Prospective Diabetes Study (UKPDS). The results showed that it is necessary to keep HbA1c levels <6.0 mmol/L in order to reduce the incidence of cardiovascular events.[14] These data were confirmed by a study of Hu et al.

in 84,941 nurses where it could be demonstrated in a subgroup with a low-risk profile (body mass index <25, healthy diet, >30 minutes of physical exercise per day, non-smokers, less than half a unit of alcohol drink per day) that the incidence of diabetes mellitus type 2 was significantly lower than for the rest of the nurses.[13] It was also shown that 91% of the cases of newly developed diabetes could have been prevented by a lifestyle similar to that of the subgroup of nurses with a low-risk profile.

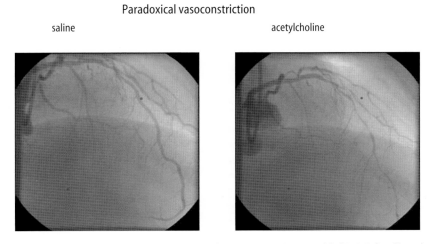

FIGURE 18-2. The left panel shows the left coronary artery without focal stenoses. When acetylcholine is infused into the vessel as shown in the right panel, in healthy vessels vasodilatation would occur, whereas in diabetes paradoxical vasoconstriction occurs due to extensive damage to the endothelium.

TABLE 18-1. Therapeutic strategies and their effects on diabetes mellitus

Author/study	Treatment	Result
Turner et al.[14]	Blood glucose control	Reduction of cardiovascular complication rate
UKPDS 38[21]	Blood glucose control	Reduction of risk for micro- and macrovascular complications
Gaede et al.[17]	Multifactorial	50% reduction of cardiovascular complications
Hu et al.[5]	Diet, physical activity	Prevention of diabetes through a healthier lifestyle
Hu et al.[13]	Physical activity	Risk reduction for developing diabetes (50%)
Tanasescu et al.[12]	Physical activity	Risk reduction for CAD (33%) and mortality (40%)
Wei et al.[7]	Physical fitness	Risk reduction for developing diabetes by 25%
Hu et al.[13]	Physical activity	Risk reduction for CV events inversely proportional to increasing physical activity
Batty et al.[11]	Physical activity	Risk reduction for CV events depending on running speed and leisure-time activity
Wei et al.[23]	Physical activity	Reduction of mortality through exercise by 50%
HPS[24]	Statins	Reduction of cardiovascular disease by 33%
4-S[25]	Statins	Risk reduction for CV events and mortality
CARE[26]	Statins	Reduction of cardiovascular events by 5.2%

CAD = coronary heart disease; CV = cardiovascular.

Tuomilehto et al.[15] studied 522 overweight patients with impaired glucose tolerance to assess the impact of dietary counseling and the recommendation to exercise regularly on the incidence of type 2 diabetes mellitus. After 4 years the incidence of newly developed diabetes was significantly lower in the intervention group (11%) than in the control group (23%).

Another study compared the effect of a healthy lifestyle on the occurrence of diabetes with that of metformin.[16] After an average of 2.8 years it was shown that a healthy lifestyle could prevent diabetes mellitus type 2 more effectively (58%) than metformin (31%).

The STENO-2 study investigated the influence of standard care with an intensified treatment approach that included behavioral changes which aimed at weight reduction, increased physical activity, and intensified pharmacological therapy on type 2 diabetic patients with micro-albuminuria.[17] After an average study period of 7.8 years intensified therapy was able to reduce cardiovascular and microvascular events by 50% (Table 18.1).[17]

In the studies mentioned, physical training was only recommended but not conducted under close supervision.[17] Future studies must show whether increased exercise compliance due to group exercise sessions or supervision of home exercise with the help of telemedicine can urther augment these beneficial effects. Our own data show that not only in-hospital but also ambulatory group training in addition to daily home exercise can further improve the risk factor profile.[18]

Although it is beyond the scope of this chapter, it ought to be mentioned how important lipid control is and that statin therapy has to be part of the regimen, regardless of patients' cholesterol levels, due to its pleiotropic effects, which are associated with a mortality benefit. Although risk factors for normoglycemic patients with coronary artery disease such as dyslipoproteinemia, hypertension, and obesity can be treated successfully with intensified physical exercise and an individually adapted diet, only lipid control has been convincingly shown to reduce cardiovascular mortality.[19,20]

Conclusion

For patients with stable coronary artery disease an intensive multifactorial risk factor intervention is a feasible intervention strategy. It increases exercise performance, improves the cardiovascular risk factor profile, myocardial perfusion, and endothelial function and has been shown to be associated with improved morbidity and mortality in epidemiologic studies. Although exercise training is inexpensive, ubiquitously available, and extremely effective, it remains underused and underprescribed. Awareness of physicians and patients has to increase to help include this effective "drug" into the daily life of as many patients as possible.

References

1. Turner RC, Millns H, Neil HA, et al. Risk factors for coronary artery disease in non-insulin dependent diabetes mellitus: United Kingdom Prospective Diabetes Study (UKPDS: 23). BMJ 1998;316:823–828.
2. Webster MWI, Scott RS. What cardiologists need to know about diabetes. Lancet 1997;350:23–28.

3. Aronson D, Rayfield EJ, Cheselro JH. Mechanisms determining course and outcome of diabetic patients who have acute myocardial infarction. Ann Intern Med 1997;126:296–306.

4. Helmrich SP, Ragland DR, Leung RW, Paffenbarger RS Jr. Physical activity and reduced occurrence of non-insulin-dependent diabetes mellitus. N Engl J Med 1991;325:147–152.

5. Hu FB, Manson JE, Stampfer MJ, et al. Diet, lifestyle, and the risk of type 2 diabetes mellitus in women. N Engl J Med 2001;345:790–797.

6. Sixt SPT, Halfwassen U, Diederich KW, Schuler G, Niebauer J. 6 months multifactorial intervention with focus on exercise training in patients with diabetes mellitus type 2 and coronary artery disease improves cardiovascular risk factor profile and endothelial dysfunction. Circulation 2004; abstract.

7. Wei M, Gibbons LW, Mitchell TL, Kampert JB, Lee CD, Blair SN. The association between cardiorespiratory fitness and impaired fasting glucose and type 2 diabetes mellitus in men. Ann Intern Med 1999;130:89–96.

8. Schachinger V, Britten MB, Zeiher AM. Prognostic impact of coronary vasodilator dysfunction on adverse long-term outcome of coronary heart disease. Circulation 2000;101:1899–1906.

9. Hambrecht R, Wolf A, Gielen S, et al. Effect of exercise on coronary endothelial function in patients with coronary artery disease. N Engl J Med 2000; 342:454–460.

10. Jolliffe JA, Rees K, Taylor RS, Thompson D, Oldridge N, Ebrahim S. Exercise-based rehabilitation for coronary heart disease. Cochrane Database Syst Rev. 2000:CD001800.

11. Batty GD, Shipley MJ, Marmot M, Smith GD. Physical activity and cause-specific mortality in men with type 2 diabetes/impaired glucose tolerance: evidence from the Whitehall study. Diabet Med 2002;19:580–588.

12. Tanasescu M, Leitzmann MF, Rimm EB, Hu FB. Physical activity in relation to cardiovascular disease and total mortality among men with type 2 diabetes. Circulation 2003;107:2435–2439.

13. Hu FB, Stampfer MJ, Solomon C, Liu S, Colditz GA, Speizer FE, Willett WC, Manson JE. Physical activity and risk for cardiovascular events in diabetic women. Ann Intern Med 2001;134:96–105.

14. Turner R, Cull C, Holman R. United Kingdom Prospective Diabetes Study 17: a 9-year update of a randomised, controlled trial on the effect of improved metabolic control on complications in NIDDM. Ann Intern Med 1996;124:136–145.

15. Tuomilehto J, Lindstrom J, Eriksson JG, et al. Prevention of type 2 diabetes mellitus by changes in lifestyle among subjects with impaired glucose tolerance. N Engl J Med 2001;344:1343–1350.

16. Diabetes Prevention Program Research Group. Reduction in the incidence of type 2 diabetes with lifestyle intervention or metformin. N Engl J Med 2002;346:393–403.

17. Gaede P, Vedel P, Larsen N, Jensen GV, Parving HH, Pedersen O. Multifactorial intervention and cardiovascular disease in patients with type 2 diabetes. N Engl J Med 2003;348:383–393.

18. Peschel TSS, Beitz F, Tarnok A, Schuler G, Niebauer J. High- but not low-intensity exercise training reduces expression of adhesion molecules on mononuclear cells in both diabetic and non-diabetic patients with coronary artery disease. Circulation 2004; abstract.

19. Laakso M, Lehto S, Penttilä I, Pyörälä K. Lipids and lipoproteins predicting coronary heart disease mortality and morbidity in patients with non-insulin-dependent diabetes. Circulation 1993;88: 1421–1430.

20. Syvänna M, Taskinen MR. Lipids and lipoproteins as coronary risk factor in non-insulin-dependent diabetes mellitus. Lancet 1997;350:20–23.

21. Tight blood pressure control and risk of macrovascular and microvascular complications in type 2 diabetes: UKPDS 38. UK Prospective Diabetes Study Group. BMJ 1998;317:703–713.

22. Hu FB, Sigal RJ, Rich-Edwards JW, Colditz GA, Solomon CG, Willett WC, Speizer FE, Manson JE. Walking compared with vigorous physical activity and risk of type 2 diabetes in women: a prospective study. JAMA 1999;282:1433–1439.

23. Wei M, Gibbons LW, Kampert JB, Nichaman MZ, Blair SN. Low cardiorespiratory fitness and physical inactivity as predictors of mortality in men with type 2 diabetes. Ann Intern Med 2000;132: 605–611.

24. Collins R, Armitage J, Parish S, Sleigh P, Peto R; Heart Protection Study Collaborative Group. MRC/BHF Heart Protection Study of cholesterol-lowering with simvastatin in 5963 people with diabetes: a randomised placebo-controlled trial. Lancet 2003;361:2005–2016.

25. Standberg TE, Pyorala K, Cook TJ, Wilhelmsen L, Faergeman O, Thorgeirsson G, Pedersen TR, Kjekshus J; 4S Group. Mortality and incidence of cancer during 10-year follow-up of the Scandinavian Simvastatin Survival Study (4S). Lancet 2004; 364:771–777.

26. Sacks FM, Pfeffer MA, Moye LA, Rouleau JL, Rutherford JD, Cole TG, Brown L, Warnica JW, Arnold JM, Wun CC, Davis BR, Braunwald E. The effect of pravastatin on coronary events after myocardial infarction in patients with average cholesterol levels. Cholesterol and Recurrent Events Trial investigators. N Engl J Med 1996;335: 1001–1009.

19
Exercise Training in Heart Failure

Stephen Gielen, Josef Niebauer, and Rainer Hambrecht

We are all on a trajectory to heart disease. It's called age. (J.N. Cohn, University of Minneapolis, at the Annual Scientific Meeting of the Heart Failure Society of America, Toronto, Canada, 2004)

Heart Failure in an Aging Society

Two fundamental factors determine the growing prevalence of heart failure in the Western hemisphere: average life expectancy and age-adjusted incidence of chronic heart failure (CHF).

Since the 1840s the average maximum life expectancy has been increasing at a constant rate of 3 months per year with no change in sight.[1] In most industrialized societies the age group over 65 years is the fastest growing proportion.

It is exactly in this age group that CHF is most prevalent: 6.6% of all women and 6.8% of all men between 65 and 74 years are affected by CHF in the US. This number climbs to nearly 10% above 75 years of age (Figure 19-1).[2]

The combined impact of the aging population and the age distribution of CHF has caused an epidemic growth in disease numbers. In the 22 years between 1979 and 2001 hospital discharges for CHF rose by 164% and today 79% of all hospitalized patients are older than 65 years.[2] Elderly patients with CHF pose a special task for cardiac rehabilitation because of the overlap of age-related and disease-associated impairment of exercise tolerance.

Training in Heart Failure – from Fear to Favor

Until the late 1980s chronic heart failure was widely regarded as a classical contraindication for exercise-based rehabilitation approaches in guidelines and clinical practice alike. Progressive immobilization was recommended for CHF patients with exercise intolerance as routine therapy to prevent any hemodynamic overload on the diseased left ventricle. It was assumed that patients with extensive myocardial damage and severely depressed left ventricular function had an excessive risk for exercise-related morbidity and mortality. However, this concept was shattered two decades ago by the lack of any clear relation between left ventricular ejection fraction and exercise capacity[3] – a finding which led to the novel concept that peripheral factors might significantly contribute to the pathogenesis of exercise intolerance. This paradigm shift inspired a new generation of clinical researchers to objectively assess the clinical and hemodynamic effects of exercise in CHF patients.

The results of a whole series of prospective randomized training studies which unanimously confirmed an improvement in peak oxygen uptake by 12–21% (+1.2 to +5.7 L/min/m^2) with no exercise-associated additional morbidity or mortality being reported (Table 19-1). As a result exercise training is now recommended in national and international guidelines for the treatment of patients with chronic heart failure.

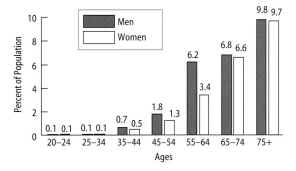

FIGURE 19-1. Prevalence of chronic heart failure by age and sex according to NHANES III (1988–1994) according to the American Heart Association.[2] Red bars represent men, white bars women. (Reproduced with permission, Heart Disease and Stroke Statistics-2005 Update, © 2004, American Heart Association.)

In this chapter both basic principles of exercise physiology in health and disease and the practical aspects of initiating a training program in CHF patients (including patient selection, training methods, and adaptation of individual training intensities) will be addressed. Finally, clinical results and prognostic implications of training interventions in CHF will be discussed.

The Time Course of Training Adaptations

The physiological response to exercise follows a well-established pattern in both health and disease. The concept of the *supercompensation cycle*[4] is based on the idea that a training stimulus disturbs the stability of the organism and induces physiological adaptations or training effects. This primary stimulus is called *overload*. An overload is characterized as physical exercise which demands more than the normal physical work capability of the organism and leads to a temporarily reduced muscular function resulting in fatigue.

The overload phase is followed by *restoration*, which implies that regenerative mechanisms restore the exercise capacity to pretraining levels. The time course of the restoration is different for different organ functions: Typically, heart rate, ventilation, neurohormonal levels, and body temperature return to normal within minutes or hours, while it may take days to fill up carbohydrate stores and to repair muscular damage.

The hallmark of the training cycle is the *adaptation* phase, in which the tissue and organ

TABLE 19-1. Effects of exercise training on peak oxygen consumption: results of randomized trials

Author	n	Duration	Etiology	VO_2max (L/min/m²)	ΔVO_2max (L/min/m²)
Coats 1990[42]	11	8 weeks	ICM	13.5	+3.2
Jette 1991[43]	15	4 weeks	post-MI	12.2	+3.6
Coats 1992[44]	17	8 weeks	ICM	13.2	+2.4
Belardinelli 1995[45]	55	8 weeks	DCM	15.0	+1.2
Kiilavuori 1995[46]	20	12 weeks	DCM/ICM	20.7	+2.2
Kiilavuori 1996[19]	27	24 weeks	DCM/ICM	19.3	+2.4
Keteyian 1996[47]	40	24 weeks	DCM/ICM	16.0	+2.5
Meyer 1997[48]	18	3 weeks	DCM/ICM	12.2	+2.4
Dubach 1997[49]	25	8 weeks	post-MI	19.4	+5.7
Belardinelli 1999[50]	99	2 years	DCM/ICM	15.7	+4.2
Hambrecht 2000[20]	73	24 weeks	DCM/ICM	18.2	+4.8
McKelvie 2002[51]	181	12 weeks	DCM/ICM	14.0	+1.4
Gianuzzi 2003[7]	89	24 weeks	DCM/ICM	13.8	+2.4
Niebauer 2005[52]	30	8 weeks	DCM/ICM	25.3	+2.7

DCM, dilative cardiomyopathy; ICM, ischemic cardiomyopathy; Post-MI, after myocardial infarction.

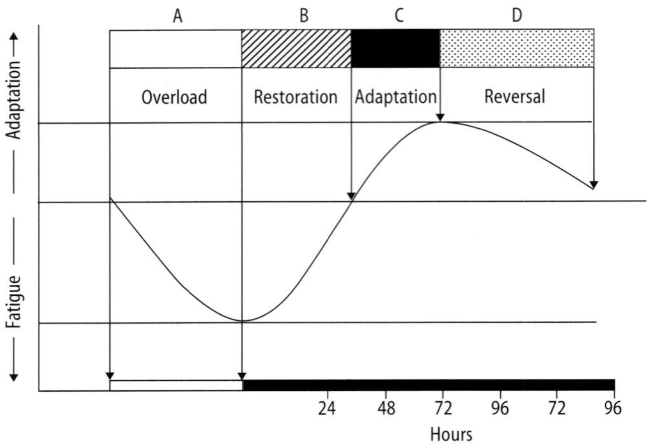

FIGURE 19-2. The primary training stimulus is termed "overload" (A) because it exceeds the organism's current work capacity, resulting in temporary fatigue. During restoration, organs return to pretraining levels (B). Training adaptation occurs as a supercompensation due to structural changes and adaptations (C). A reversal of previously gained adaptations is possible once training is stopped (D). (Reprinted with permission from Moyna.[4])

damages are *supercompensated*. The physiological changes in this phase include increases in skeletal muscle mass, strength, mitochondrial density, key aerobic enzyme activity, and fuel storage capacity. The cardiovascular system adapts to exercise by increasing capillary density in the exercised muscle, increased blood volume, increased left ventricular end-diastolic volume, and maximal stroke volume. Thereby each training cycle produces a higher fitness level which allows for greater workload and training benefits in the subsequent training sessions. Once regular training is stopped, the adaptations are gradually lost as a result of disuse – a phase termed *reversal* (Figure 19-2).

Differences in Physical Responses to Exercise in Health and Disease

While the basic pattern of the supercompensation system is valid in both health and disease some important differences should be noted:

1. In the presence of cardiovascular disease exercise capacity is limited. As a result, lower than normal levels of physical exertion result in fatigue and in the temporary reduction of organ function during the overload phase.

2. A patient with cardiovascular disease will need more time to regenerate following an overload, which implies that the supercompensation cycle is prolonged.

3. As a result of peripheral intrinsic alterations associated with certain forms of cardiovascular disease (i.e. chronic heart failure), the ability of the skeletal muscle to respond to an overload by muscle hypertrophy and improved oxidative energy metabolism may be impaired.

Why are these aspects important in cardiovascular rehabilitation? As indicated in Figure 19-3, training effectiveness critically depends on an optimal timing and dose of exercise. Ideally, a training session should be performed at the height of the adaptation phase. At this time the individual has the best physical preconditions to tolerate a second overload (Figure 19-3A). When training sessions are timed too late the training adaptations may already be lost (Figure 19-3B), when timed too early the individual may still be in the restoration phase so that a second overload could have detrimental effects and lead to further loss of function (Figure 19-3C).

The most important factors determining physiological adaptation and magnitude of improvements in exercise performance include age, intensity, duration and frequency of exercise, genetic background, and pretraining fitness levels. It has to be kept in mind that the gains in physical capacity achieved during prolonged training programs are greatest following initiation of the exercise program.

The molecular mechanisms involved in mediating beneficial training effects are discussed in detail in Chapter 12. Suffice it to say that

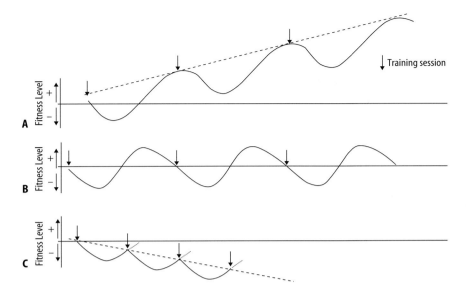

FIGURE 19-3. Fitness improvements are greatest when training sessions coincide with the peak of the adaptation phase (A). If timed later no significant gains in fitness are to be expected; if timed too early training sessions will result in worsening of function (C). (Reprinted with permission from Moyna.[4])

endurance training partially reverses the intrinsic pathologic alterations in skeletal muscle metabolism and catabolism, improves ventilatory function, reduces autonomic and neurohormonal activation, attenuates local and possibly systemic inflammatory activation, and improves endothelial dysfunction resulting in reduced afterload and higher stroke volume.

Patient Selection for Exercise Training in CHF

Patients with CHF have higher morbidity and mortality rates as compared to most other forms of heart disease (especially stable coronary artery disease). Therefore, current guidelines stratify CHF patients as a high-risk group for training interventions. As indicated above this implies a more detailed diagnostic evaluation before initiation of exercise training which includes echocardiography and a 12-lead ergometry.

What are the potential risks of exercise training for CHF patients? The most widespread fear has long been the adverse effect of exercise training on

left ventricular remodeling after a myocardial infarction. In a single non-controlled clinical study, Jugdutt et al. reported a negative influence of training on left ventricular (LV) performance in post-infarct patients.[5] However, several prospective randomized clinical trials have since shown that training favorably affects LV geometry and function.[6,7] The second major concern was a *proarrhythmogenic adverse effect* of training. However, meta-analyses of controlled training trials did not substantiate this concern: There were 56 adverse events in the 622 CHF patients in training programs and 75 adverse events in the 575 subjects in the control group ($P = 0.60$).[8] On a pathophysiological basis the reductions in neurohormonal activation and circulating catecholamines in training patients should beneficially affect the incidence of malignant arrhythmias. However, systematic studies in this area are still missing.

Indications for Exercise Training in CHF

Today, exercise-based cardiac rehabilitation is officially recommended by current ESC and

AHA guidelines as an adjunctive therapy for patients with stable CHF, without any cardiac decompensation in the preceding 3 months, and with uptitrated guideline-oriented pharmacological therapy.[9,10] While most training studies recruited primarily patients in NYHA class II, subgroup analysis shows that patients in more advanced CHF (NYHA class III) benefit equally from the training intervention.[11,12]

Contraindications for Exercise Training in CHF

Any patient who wants to start regular physical training in the presence of CHF has to pass two lists of contraindications, the first for *exercise testing*, the second for *exercise training*. Contraindications for exercise testing apply because a maximal exercise test (ergometry, treadmill, or spiroergometry) is required to calculate the correct training heart rate (Table 19-2, A).

Contraindications for exercise training are less well defined. However, it is generally agreed that patients may not have any cardiac decompensation in the preceding 3 months or any acute systemic illness (Table 19-2, B). In addition to the list of clear contraindications, clinical situations in which there is an increased risk for training therapy are listed in Table 19-3. While the conditions described do not prohibit exercise they should be resolved whenever possible prior to the initiation of training interventions (e.g. by implantation of an internal cardioverter/defibrillator in complex ventricular arrhythmias, especially in ischemic cardiomyopathy).

In prospectively conducted exercise training studies in stable CHF patients, adverse events are surprisingly low, with post-exercise hypotension, atrial or ventricular arrhythmias, and worsening heart failure symptoms being the most common complications.

Although the risk to patients with ventricular arrhythmias during training interventions has never been prospectively evaluated, most studies have excluded patients with evidence of ventricular arrhythmias (≥Lown IV during Holter ECG).

Vigorous uncontrolled exercise may precipitate cardiac decompensation in CHF patients. However, there are no reports of an increased rate of pulmonary edema in long-term submaximal training trials in stable CHF patients. In patients with stable compensated chronic heart failure (CHF) no additional risk of maximal exercise testing has been reported with no major complications reported in one study of 1286 bicycle ergometer tests.[13]

Risk Stratification and Patient Screening

The American Heart Association (AHA) and the American College of Sports Medicine (ACSM) have published detailed guidelines on exercise

TABLE 19-3. Increased risk for exercise training

<1.8 kg increase in body mass over the previous 1–3 days
Concurrent continuous or intermittent dobutamine therapy
Decrease in systolic blood pressure with exercise
NYHA functional class IV
Complex ventricular arrhythmia at rest or appearing with exertion
Supine resting heart rate >100 beats/min
Preexisting co-morbidities limiting exercise tolerance

TABLE 19-2. Contraindications to exercise testing (A) and exercise training (B)

A. *Contraindications to exercise testing (according to AHA guidelines[53])*
Acute myocardial infarction <2 days
Unstable angina with recent rest pain
Untreated life-threatening cardiac arrhythmias
Uncompensated congestive heart failure
Uncontrolled hypertension
Advanced atrioventricular block
Acute myocarditis and pericarditis
Symptomatic aortic stenosis
Severe hypertrophic obstructive cardiomyopathy
Acute systemic illness
B. *Contraindications to exercise training*
Cardiac decompensation in the previous 3 months
Progressive worsening of exercise tolerance or dyspnea at rest or on exertion over previous 3–5 days
Significant ischemia during low-intensity exercise (<2 METs, <50 W)
Uncontrolled diabetes
Acute systemic illness or fever
Recent embolism
Thrombophlebitis
Active pericarditis or myocarditis
Myocardial infarction within the previous 3 weeks
New onset atrial fibrillation

TABLE 19-4. Risk stratification according to the recommendations of the AHA

AHA classification	NYHA class	Exercise capacity	Clinical characteristic	ECG monitoring
A. Apparently healthy			Men <45 years Women < 55years Without symptoms, no major risk factors, normal exercise stress test	No supervision or monitoring required
B. Stable cardiovascular disease with low risk for vigorous exercise but unable to self-regulate activity	I–II	>6 METs >1.4 W/kg body weight	Free of ischemia or angina at rest or on the exercise stress test Stable CHF (EF ≥ 30%). No ventricular arrhythmias	Monitored and supervised only during prescribed sessions (6–12 sessions). Light resistance training may be included in comprehensive rehabilitation programs
C. Moderate-to-high risk for cardiac complications during exercise	III	<6 METs <1.4 W/kg body weight	No ability to self-monitor exercise Pathologic response to exercise test (drop in BP, signs of ischemia etc.), nsVT during exercise	Continuous ECG monitoring during rehabilitation until safety is established. Medical supervision during all exercise sessions until safety is established
D. Unstable patients. Physical activity for training contraindicated	III–IV	<6 METs <1.4 W/kg body weight	Unstable angina Uncompensated heart failure Uncontrollable arrythmias	No physical activity recommended for conditioning purposes Attention should be directed to restoring patient to class C or higher

in clinical populations and encourage risk stratification of patients prior to initiating an exercise training program.[14] A widely used risk assessment scheme was proposed by the AHA (Table 19-4).[15] The majority of CHF patients will be classified as class B or C. Medical supervision including ECG monitoring is necessary until the clinical safety of the training program is established.

Before enrolment in a training program, a patient with CHF should be in a stable condition without clinical evidence of fluid overload. A typical patient evaluation should be performed by an experienced cardiologist and involves: medical history, clinical examination, a resting ECG, a symptom-limited ergometry, and echocardiography. Other supplementary options are: Holter ECG, 24-hour blood pressure measurements, stress echocardiography, chest x-ray, and, in a few cases, evaluation of left ventricular filling pressures with a Swan–Ganz catheter under stress conditions. If the clinical status of a patient is unclear and previous examinations/tests are lacking, invasive diagnostic measures should be undertaken in order to clarify the situation (Figure 19-4).

A thorough medical examination must also be carried out in order to exclude patients who have cardiovascular and/or orthopedic mus-

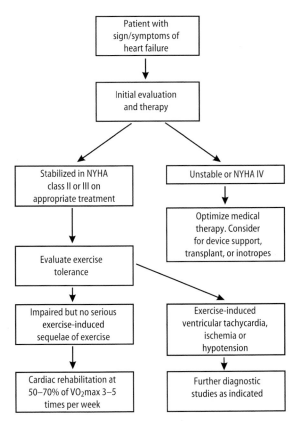

FIGURE 19-4. Clinical evaluation of CHF patients prior to the enrolment into a training program according to current guidelines. (Adapted from Braith.[54])

culoskeletal contraindications. Muscle atrophy – which may occur as a result of aging, long-term bed confinement, sedentary lifestyle or glucocorticoid therapy – must be evaluated and recorded.

It should be underlined that patients included in training studies have to be on optimized medical therapy and in stable clinical condition for at least 4 weeks before the initiation of the training program. It is recommended that patients should be uptitrated according to current guidelines on standard heart failure medication (especially ACE inhibitors and beta-blockers) prior to training. Training interventions in CHF are based on aerobic steady-state exercise sessions at 50–80% of the peak oxygen uptake for 15–30 min 3–5 times per week. In highly symptomatic patients with very low symptom-free exercise tolerance (<75 W) shorter training sessions at low intensity (50% of VO_2max) may be required. When patients tolerate this regimen well, first the session duration should be prolonged, then training intensity can be increased.

Selection of the Optimal Training Protocol

Training protocols vary in a number of variables:

- Exercise level: aerobic versus anaerobic.
- Exercise type: endurance versus resistance.
- Exercise application: systemic versus regional.
- Exercise method: continuous versus intermittent.
- Exercise control: supervised versus non-supervised.

Exercise Level: Aerobic Versus Anaerobic

Most of the training protocols to date are derived from classical protocols used in patients with coronary artery disease. Individual training intensities are fixed at 70–80% of peak oxygen consumption or chronotropic reserve. Exercise training at these conventional workloads, however, may be unsuitable for severely affected

CHF patients whose initial functional exercise capacity is very low. Moreover, intermittent exercise at workloads >70% of peak VO_2 exposes the heart to periodically elevated LV filling pressures. Based on small exercise trials, some authors hypothesized that the elevated LV filling pressures induce further LV dilation.[5] However, large trials in ischemic patients with LV dysfunction did not reveal any deleterious effect of exercise on LV volume, function, or wall thickness.[6,7,16] Nevertheless, aerobic exercise training at low workloads (≤50% of peak aerobic capacity) appears to be a promising approach to physical training in patients with severely compromised LV function because exercising at low workloads does increase peak aerobic capacity and vascular flow capacity of the lower limb while exposing the left ventricle to lower wall stress than that associated with conventional workloads.[17-19]

Exercise Type: Endurance Versus Resistance

Endurance training leads to a reduction in afterload with a decrease in systemic resistance at rest and at maximal exertion as well as to a small improvement in LV ejection fraction.[20] Similar data for resistance training in CHF patients do not exist. Aerobic endurance training thus still forms the basis of training therapies for CHF patients. Critical appraisal of (predominantly) isometric resistance training (hand-grip training, stress time >3 min) is based on older studies that found a drastic rise in afterload along with an acute reduction in cardiac output[21] and an increase in the severity of mitral regurgitation.[22] In contrast to these findings, 2 × 10 repetition leg-press exercises at 70% of maximal capacity or interval training do not cause a clinically relevant decrease in ejection fraction/increase in systolic blood pressure.[23,24] By shortening the isometric and lengthening the isotonic exercise phase, it is possible to avoid hemodynamic strain. Pure resistance training in CHF patients leads to an increase in muscular strength. There is, however, no accompanying increase in maximal O_2 uptake.[25] It is only by combining resistance and endurance training that the important prognostic marker VO₂max can be improved.[26]

Experimental studies with animals have shown that resistance training leads to enhanced local expression of insulin-like growth factor I (IGF-I). It may therefore be possible that supplementary, individually adapted resistance training of specific extremities positively influences the catabolic breakdown of muscle tissue which is often associated with congestive heart failure. Specific data relating to this area still lacking.

To summarize, patients in risk groups B and C (compare Table 19-4) may benefit from a resistance training program with short stress phases (maximal capacity 10 repetitions) at <60% MVC, interrupted by phases of muscle relaxation, without causing hemodynamic deterioration. As a supplementary training modality, resistance training can complement, but not replace, the well-established aerobic endurance training.

Exercise Application: Systemic Versus Regional

Segmental training has been proved to be effective in CHF patients in improving muscle force and functional status.[27,28] The low hemodynamic burden on the myocardium makes segmental exercise suitable in particular for selected patients in NYHA class IV, who are often unable to engage in sufficient whole body exercise. Nevertheless, no study to date has specifically compared the long-term effects of different modes and levels of exercise training in CHF with regard to functional work capacity and LV function.

Exercise Method: Continuous Versus Intermittent

Limited information is available for isometric training or interval training with short bouts of stimuli on peripheral muscles. First results from Meyer et al.[29] demonstrated that interval training permits more intense exercise stimuli on peripheral muscles with minimal cardiac strain as compared with hemodynamic response during ergometry.

Derived from controlled training studies, exercise is usually recommended for 20 to 60 minutes on 3 to 5 days per week. The lower and upper cut-off level regarding frequency and duration of exercise sessions, however, is not known.

Exercise Control: Supervised Versus Non-supervised

There are no convincing data that home-based exercise training is less safe than strictly supervised exercise training. Experience from controlled trials of physical training in Europe demonstrated higher symptomatic benefit after combined home- and hospital-based training programs than in the hospital-based only programs, which may reflect improved patient compliance with the former protocol.[30] However, it is currently recommended to initiate a training program in heart failure patients only under supervised conditions. Home-based training can be started as soon as the safety of the training protocol has been established and the patient is acquainted with the safety precautions associated with exercise (i.e. control of training pulse).

Initiation of Training Therapy and Progression of Training Intensity

In most training intervention trials, a minimal symptom-free exercise tolerance of 25 W is required for the initiation of the training program. In patients with very low exercise tolerance (<50 W), training is started with several short training sessions of 5 (−10) minutes per day at 50% of peak oxygen uptake. At higher baseline exercise capacities the initial training session duration can be 10–15 minutes. An adequate warm-up and cool-down period consisting of stretching or aerobic exercise at a very low intensity is also recommended.

As the training adaptations progress, first training duration, then training intensity are gradually increased aiming at 20 min of exercise at 60–70% of VO₂max for 5 days per week (Figure 19-5).

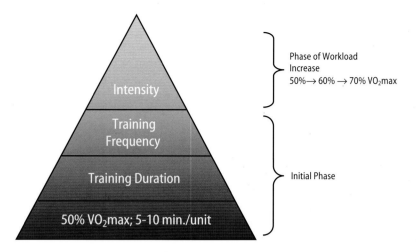

FIGURE 19-5. The training pyramid illustrates the gradual increase in training duration, frequency, and intensity which occurs at the beginning of a training program in CHF patients.

Clinical Effects of Exercise in Chronic Heart Failure

Prognostic and Symptomatic Effects

The results of the ExTraMATCH meta-analysis of the ESC with a total of 801 CHF patients documented a significant reduction of total mortality by 35% (odds ratio 0.65; CI 0.46–0.92, $P = 0.015$), and of hospitalization by 28% (odds ratio 0.72; CI 0.56–0.93, $P = 0.018$).[11]

With regard to symptomatic benefit a recent meta-analysis of randomized controlled trials by the European Heart Failure Training Group revealed an improvement of peak VO_2 by up to 2 mL/kg/min with a range of +14 to +31% increase versus control patients. Although modest in absolute terms, this increase of about 20% translates into a considerably better quality of life for most patients.

Cardiac function is not worsened by exercise training; indeed, a small but significant improvement of ejection fraction and reduction in cardiomegaly was observed in one prospective randomized trial.[20] Based on this trial, improved endothelium-dependent vasodilation[31] with reduced total peripheral resistance – both at rest and at peak exercise – is a major contributing factor to the increase in ejection fraction (Figure 19-6). The improvement of endothelium-dependent vasodilation is not limited to the trained limb but is a systemic training effect if the muscle mass involved is large enough to elicit increases in cardiac output during exercise sessions.[32] However, beneficial adaptations of the respiratory, neurohormonal, and autonomic system are also involved.

Interactions with Medication

Current guidelines require patients to be uptitrated on a combination therapy of ACE inhibitors, beta-blockers, diuretics, spironolactone, and digitalis according to clinical status. The question naturally arises how these medications might affect training response in CHF patients. This concern is especially related to beta-blocker therapy as it affects the heart rate response to exercise.

According to a small, non-randomized French study in patients with stable CHF, the effect of exercise training as measured by ergospirometry was not influenced by the presence or absence of beta-blocker treatment.[33] This holds true despite lower training heart rates among patients under beta-blockade. However, patients should be uptitrated to their optimal individual beta-blocker dose prior to the initiation of the training program.

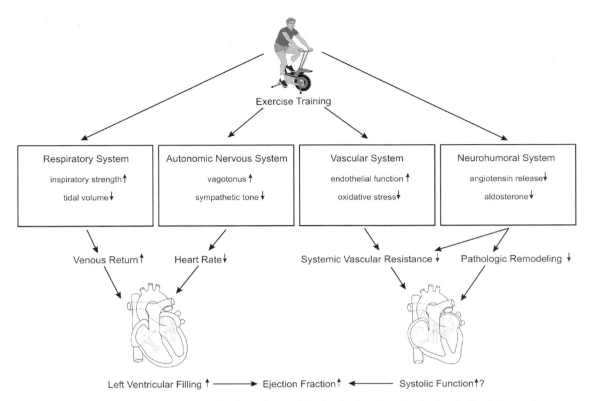

FIGURE 19-6. Effects of exercise training on cardiac dimensions and ejection fraction. Note that ejection fraction is improved as a consequence of reduced afterload and improved preload rather than by intrinsic myocardial effects.

Special Patient Subgroups

Patients with ICDs

The evidence that cardiac mortality is reduced in CHF by implantation of internal cardioverters/defibrillators (ICDs) is mounting, fuelled by prospective randomized trials such as the MADIT-II and the COMPANION study. While biventricular pacing was associated with symptomatic improvement, the biventricular ICD group benefited from a reduced rate of sudden cardiac deaths resulting in lower cardiac mortality.

Rehabilitation institutions have long been reluctant to offer training programs to CHF patients with ICDs. The major concerns were based on the notion that ICD patients represent a high-risk subgroup for ventricular arrhythmias, and that most rehabilitation facilities lack the equipment, personnel, and expertise to treat patients effectively after a shock delivery. As a consequence, only specialized institutions have evaluated training post ICD implantation. In these small studies, however, training appears to be both safe and feasible.[34,35] Certain safety concerns remain and should be addressed.

Risk of Training-Related Shock Delivery and Device Failure

In a single-center non-randomized follow-up study, the rate of ICD malfunction was reported to be 10.2% ($n = 12$ patients), requiring reoperation in 3 and reprogramming in 9 patients.[36] While no exercise-related shocks were observed in this study, Vanhees reported that 3 out of 95 patients experienced adequate shocks for ventricular tachycardia (VT) during exercise. These patients terminated the training program. In addition, one patient had several shocks the day after training. Two additional patients had asymptomatic VTs terminated with overdrive pacing – one during exercise testing, one during a training session.[35]

Risk of Inadequate Shocks During Exercise-Induced Supraventricular Tachycardias

Inadequate ICD discharges triggered by supraventricular tachyarrhythmias are well recognized in ICD patients[37] and may induce life-threatening ventricular arrhythmias in individual patients.[38,39] In the recent Vanhees study[35] inadequate defibrillator discharge during an exercise session occurred in one patient but did not result in any proarrhythmic complications. Other studies did not observe any training session-related inadequate ICD discharges.

Special Recommendations for Training Interventions in ICD Patients

- While no excess mortality was observed in the non-randomized observational ICD training studies, close cooperation is needed between rehabilitation centers and electrophysiologists to determine the optimal training heart rate for the patient, so that he remains below the threshold for VT detection. In patients with atrial fibrillation optimal pharmacological rate control should be established prior to initiating a training program.
- Maximal exercise testing in an institution with ICD support should be performed prior to the training intervention to rule out exercise-induced ventricular arrhythmias.
- Given the relatively high ICD malfunction rate of 10.2% in one study, it seems prudent to check the ICD function after the first 2–4 weeks of training therapy.

Elderly Patients

In addition to having heart failure, elderly people often suffer from disability caused by mental depression, low aerobic fitness levels, low skeletal muscle mass, and presence of orthopedic co-morbidities. Despite these factors, the elderly benefit equally from cardiac rehabilitation, but from a lower baseline.

Evidence Base for Beneficial Training Effects in the Elderly

Despite the demographic changes and the high proportion of elderly people among patients hos-pitalized for CHF, systematic studies comparing training effectiveness between younger and older CHF patients are still scarce. In a meta-analysis of 14 training studies, Piepoli identified only 14 out of 134 patients (10%) >70 years of age.[40] In this minor subgroup, clinical symptoms were significantly improved after training; however, peak oxygen uptake was unchanged. A recent observational study in 17 CHF patients between 61 and 91 years, on the other hand, 6 months of exercise training resulted in a 23% increase in VO_2max.[41]

While clearly more studies are needed to compare the symptomatic effectiveness of training between younger and older CHF patients, Piepoli recently presented a large mortality meta-analysis of CHF training studies. A total of 117 patients ≥60 years were included, of whom 52 were randomized to exercise training.[11] No difference in mortality reduction by training was found between younger and older CHF patients (hazard ratio 0.64 ≥60 years and 0.65 <60 years, $P = 0.74$). This is remarkable since age itself is the best predictor of death.

Recommendations for Exercise Training in Elderly CHF Patients

- When initiating aerobic exercise the exercise intensity should be carefully weighted against a higher risk of injuries with higher workloads. Even workloads as low as 60–65% of the maximal heart rate have documented effects on exercise capacity. To avoid orthopedic injuries ergometer training is preferably to walking or jogging.
- To antagonize the loss of muscle mass endurance exercises are often supplemented with moderate-intensity resistance training (e.g. elastic bands) with 8–10 set repetitions at 40–60% of the 1-repetition maximum.
- The aim of exercise-based rehabilitation in the elderly is the improvement of locomotor coordination, endurance, and muscle force so that patients are able to perform the physical duties of their daily life. Therefore, the primary goal is prevention of disease-associated disability and hospitalization, and maintenance of independent living.

Future Perspectives of Training Interventions in Heart Failure

The reliability of practical recommendations is always related to the soundness of the study database. Three areas can be identified where there is clearly a need for further trials:

1. While meta-analyses indicate a prognostic benefit of training in CHF patients the final randomized mortality study is still pending. It has recently been started in the US (HF-ACTION study: *Heart Failure – A Controlled Trial Investigating Outcomes of exercise traiNing*) and will finally settle the debate about the training-related mortality reduction in patients with CHF.

2. There is still uncertainty on the issue whether exercise training can safely be initiated on an outpatient basis. The vast majority of training studies in CHF started the training program in hospital with close monitoring of training sessions by experienced staff. While this is clearly optimal therapy it would exclude thousands of patients from the benefits of training interventions if in-hospital training was required for all patients. Future studies need to identify subgroups in whom it is safe to offer monitored training sessions without concomitant hospitalization.

3. Resistance training is being increasingly employed in CHF patients in clinical practice. However, the database for such modifications of established aerobic training programs is not sound. While meta-analysis clearly indicates a prognostic benefit of endurance training for CHF, similar data are lacking for resistance exercise. Large-scale randomized studies comparing aerobic, resistance, and combined training programs in CHF are still pending.

The majority of people involved in cardiac rehabilitation share a practical, "hands-on" approach to training interventions and may tend to modify training programs based on personal experience rather than clinical studies. Without doubting the value of experience, we have to remember that training interventions in CHF must be regarded in the same way as powerful medications with a need for optimal dosing, consideration of side-effects, and close clinical follow-up by an experienced cardiologist. We are therefore well advised to demand the same level of evidence for training interventions as for pharmaceuticals. Such a way of proceeding will not only assure the optimal benefit and safety for the patient but provide the best chances to receive adequate funding in times of shrinking healthcare resources.

References

1. Oeppen J, Vaupel JW. Demography. Broken limits to life expectancy. Science 2002;296(5570):1029–1031.
2. American Heart Association. Heart Disease and Stroke Statistics – 2004 Statistical Update. Dallas: American Heart Association; 2004.
3. Franciosa JA, Park M, Levine TB. Lack of correlation between exercise capacity and indexes of resting left ventricular performance in heart failure. Am J Cardiol 1981;47:33–39.
4. Moyna NM. Principles of exercise training for physicians. In: Thompson PD, ed. Exercise and Sports Cardiology. New York: McGraw-Hill; 2001:110–123.
5. Jugdutt BI, Michorowski BL, Kappagoda CT. Exercise training after anterior Q wave myocardial infarction: Importance of regional left ventricular function and topography. J Am Coll Cardiol 1988;12:362–372.
6. Dubach P, Myers J, Dziekan G, et al. Effect of exercise training on myocardial remodeling in patients with reduced left ventricular function after myocardial infarction. Circulation 1997;95:2060–2067.
7. Giannuzzi P, Temporelli PL, Corra U, Tavazzi L. Antiremodeling effect of long-term exercise training in patients with stable chronic heart failure: results of the Exercise in Left Ventricular Dysfunction and Chronic Heart Failure (ELVD-CHF) Trial. Circulation 2003;108(5):554–559.
8. Smart N, Marwick TH. Exercise training for patients with heart failure: A systematic review of factors that improve mortality and morbidity. Am J Med 2004;116(10):714–716.
9. Task force for the diagnosis and treatment of heart failure. Guidelines for the diagnosis and treatment of chronic heart failure. Eur Heart J 2001; 22:1527–1560.
10. Hunt SA, Baker DW, Chin MH, et al. Evaluation and management of heart failure in the adult. Report of the American College of Cardiology/American Heart Association Task Force on Practice

Guidelines (Committee to Revise the 1995 Guidelines for the Evaluation and Management of Heart Failure). American College of Cardiology Web Site 2001.

11. Piepoli MF, Davos C, Francis DP, Coats AJ. Exercise training meta-analysis of trials in patients with chronic heart failure (ExTraMATCH). BMJ 2004; 328(7433):189.

12. Erbs S, Linke A, Gielen S, et al. Exercise training in patients with severe chronic heart failure: impact on left ventricular performance and cardiac size. A retrospective analysis of the Leipzig Heart Failure Training Trial. Eur J Cardiovasc Prev Rehabil 2003;10(5):336–344.

13. Tristani FE, Hughes CV, Archibald DG, Sheldahl LM, Cohn JN, Fletcher R. Safety of graded symptom-limited exercise testing in patients with congestive heart failure. Circulation 1987;76(6):VI54–VI58.

14. American College of Sports Medicine (ACSM) (eds) Guidelines for Exercise Testing and Prescription. Baltimore: Williams & Wilkins; 1995.

15. Fletcher GF, Balady G, Froelicher VF, Hartley LH, Haskell WL, Pollock ML. Exercise standards. A statement for healthcare professionals from the American Heart Association. Writing Group. Circulation 1995;91(2):580–615.

16. Giannuzzi P, Temporelli P, Corrà U, Gattone M, Giordano P, Tavazzi L. Attenuation of unfavorable remodeling by exercise training in postinfarction patients with left ventricular dysfunction. Results of the Exercise in Left Ventricular Dysfunction (ELVD) Trial. Circulation 1997;96:1790–1797.

17. Demopoulos L, Bijou R, Fergus I, Jones M, Strom J, LeJementel TH. Exercise training in patients with severe congestive heart failure: Enhancing peak aerobic capacity while minimizing the increase in ventricular wall stress. J Am Coll Cardiol 1997;29:597–603.

18. Belardinelli R, Georgiou D, Scocco V, Barstow T, Purcaro A. Low intensity exercise training in patients with chronic heart failure. J Am Coll Cardiol 1995;26:975–82.

19. Kiilavuori K, Sovijärvi A, Näveri H, Ikonen T, Leinonen H. Effect of physical training on exercise capacity and gas exchange in patients with chronic heart failure. Chest 1996;110:985–991.

20. Hambrecht R, Gielen S, Linke A, et al. Effects of exercise training on left ventricular function and peripheral resistance in patients with chronic heart failure. A randomised trial. JAMA 2000;283: 3095–3101.

21. Elkayam U, Roth A, Weber L, et al. Isometric exercise in patients with chronic advanced heart failure: hemodynamic and neurohumoral evaluation. Circulation 1985;72:975–981.

22. Keren G, Katz S, Gage J, Strom J, Sonnenblick EH, LeJemtel TH. Effect of isometric exercise on cardiac performance and mitral regurgitation in patients with severe congestive heart failure. Am Heart J 1989;118(5):973–979.

23. McKelvie RS, McCartney N, Tomlinson CW, Bauer R, MacDougall JD. Comparison of hemodynamic responses to cycling and resistance exercise in congestive heart failure secondary to ischemic cardiomyopathy. Am J Cardiol 1995;76:977–979.

24. Meyer K, Hajric R, Westbrook S, et al. Hemodynamic response during leg press exercise in patients with chronic heart failure. Am J Cardiol 1999; 83(11):1537–1543.

25. Pu CT, Johnson MT, Forman DE, et al. Randomized trial of progressive resistance training to counteract the myopathy of chronic heart failure. J Appl Physiol 2001;90:2341–2350.

26. Maiorana A, O'Driscoll G, Cheetham C, et al. Combined aerobic and resistance exercise training improves functional capacity and strength in CHF. J Appl Physiol 2000;88:1565–1570.

27. Magnusson G, Gordon A, Kaijser L, et al. High intensity knee extensor training in patients with chronic heart failure. Eur Heart J 1996;17:1048–1055.

28. Koch M, Douard H, Brouset JP. The benefit of graded physical exercise in chronic heart failure. Chest 1998;101(5):231S–235S.

29. Meyer K, Samek L, Schwaibold M, et al. Physical response to different modes of interval exercise in patients with chronic heart failure – application to exercise training. Eur Heart J 1996;17:1040–1047.

30. Piepoli M, Flather M, Coats AJS. Overview of studies of exercise training in chronic heart failure: the need for a prospective randomized multicentre European trial. Eur Heart J 1998;19:830–841.

31. Hambrecht R, Fiehn E, Weigl C, et al. Regular physical exercise corrects endothelial dysfunction and improves exercise capacity in patients with chronic heart failure. Circulation 1998;98:2709–2715.

32. Linke A, Schoene N, Gielen S, et al. Endothelial dysfunction in patients with chronic heart failure: systemic effects of lower-limb exercise training. J Am Coll Cardiol 2001;37:392–397.

33. Curnier D, Galinier M, Pathak A, et al. Rehabilitation of patients with congestive heart failure with or without beta-blockade therapy. J Card Fail 2001;7(3):241–248.

34. Vanhees L, Schepers D, Heidbuchel H, Defoor J, Fagard R. Exercise performance and training in patients with implantable cardioverter-defibrillators and coronary heart disease. Am J Cardiol 2001; 87(6):712–715.

35. Vanhees L, Kornaat M, Defoor J, et al. Effect of exercise training in patients with an implantable cardioverter defibrillator. Eur Heart J 2004;25(13): 1120–1126.

36. Kamke W, Dovifat C, Schranz M, Behrens S, Moesenthin J, Voller H. Cardiac rehabilitation in patients with implantable defibrillators. Feasibility and complications. Z Kardiol 2003;92(10):869–875.

37. Barold HS, Newby KH, Tomassoni G, Kearney M, Brandon J, Natale A. Prospective evaluation of new and old criteria to discriminate between supraventricular and ventricular tachycardia in implantable defibrillators. Pacing Clin Electrophysiol 1998; 21(7):1347–1355.

38. Cohen TJ, Chien WW, Lurie KG, et al. Implantable cardioverter defibrillator proarrhythmia: case report and review of the literature. Pacing Clin Electrophysiol 1991;14(9):1326–1329.

39. Kou WH, Kirsh MM, Stirling MC, Kadish AH, Orringer CE, Morady F. Provocation of ventricular tachycardia by an automatic implantable cardioverter defibrillator. Am Heart J 1990;120(1):208–210.

40. European Heart Failure Training Group. Experience from controlled trials of physical training in chronic heart failure. Protocol and patient factors in effectiveness in the improvement in exercise tolerance. European Heart Failure Training Group. Eur Heart J 1998;19(3):466–475.

41. Vaitkevicius PV, Ebersold C, Haydar Z, et al. The utility of exercise training to improve functional capacity of elderly heart failure patients. Circulation 1997;96(Suppl I).

42. Coats AJS, Adamopoulos S, Meyer TE, Conway J, Sleight P. Effects of physical training in chronic heart failure. Lancet 1990;335:63–66.

43. Jette M, Heller R, Landry F, Blümchen G. Randomized 4-week exercise program in patients with impaired left ventricular function. Circulation 1991;84:1561–1567.

44. Coats AJS, Adamopoulos S, Radaelli A, et al. Controlled trial of physical training in chronic heart failure: Exercise performance, hemodynamics, ventilation, and autonomic function. Circulation 1992;85:2119–131.

45. Belardinelli R, Georgiou D, Cianci G, Berman N, Ginzton L, Purcaro A. Exercise training improves left ventricular diastolic filling in patients with dilated cardiomyopathy. Circulation 1995;91:2775–2784.

46. Kiilavuori K, Toivonen L, Näveri H, Leinonen H. Reversal of autonomic derangements by physical training in chronic heart failure assessed by heart rate variability. Eur Heart J 1995;16:490–495.

47. Keteyian SJ, Levine AB, Brawner CA, et al. Exercise training in patients with heart failure. Ann Intern Med 1996;124:1051–1057.

48. Meyer K, Schwaibold M, Westbrook S, et al. Effects of exercise training and activity restriction on 6-minute walking test performance in patients with chronic heart failure. Am Heart J 1997;133: 447–453.

49. Dubach P, Myers J, Dzienkan G, et al. Effect of high intensity exercise training on central hemodynamic response to exercise in men with reduced left ventricular function. J Am Coll Cardiol 1997;29: 1591–1598.

50. Belardinelli R, Georgiou D, Cianci G, Purcaro A. Randomized, controlled trial of long-term moderate exercise training in chronic heart failure. Circulation 1999;99:1173–1182.

51. McKelvie RS, Teo KK, Roberts R, et al. Effects of exercise training in patients with heart failure: the Exercise Rehabilitation Trial (EXERT). Am Heart J 2002;144(1):23–30.

52. Niebauer J, Clark A, Webb-Peploe KM, Coats AJS. Exercise training in chronic heart failure: Effects on pro-inflammatory markers. Eur J Heart Fail 2005;7:189–193.

53. Gibbons RJ, Balady GJ, Bricker JT, et al. ACC/AHA 2002 guideline update for exercise testing: A report of the American College of Cardiology/American Heart Association Task Force on Practice Guidelines (Committee on Exercise Testing). American College of Cardiology Web Site 2002.

54. Braith R. Exercise for chronic heart failure and heart transplant patients. In: Thompson PD, ed. Exercise and Sports Cardiology. New York: McGraw-Hill; 2001:317–353.

20
Exercise Training in Valvular Heart Disease

Christa Gohlke-Bärwolf

Introduction

Exercise training is the core component of cardiac rehabilitation in patients with coronary artery disease (CAD) and the positive effects have been studied extensively (see Chapter 17).[1-5] Markedly less information is available concerning the results of exercise training in patients with valvular heart disease (VHD). This is mainly due to the fact that patients with native VHD have rarely been considered candidates for exercise training. In the guidelines on the management of patients with VHD no comments are made on this topic in patients with native VHD or after valve surgery.[6] In the new recommendation by the working group on valvular heart disease of the European Society of Cardiology suggestions for exercise training after valve surgery are outlined.[7]

As long as patients are asymptomatic or mildly symptomatic with VHD they are usually not included in medically supervised exercise training programs as part of the conservative management. Therefore experience in patients with VHD and exercise training is limited.

Recommendations for exercise training in athletes with asymptomatic VHD have been dealt with by Pelliccia et al.[8] and Bonow et al.[9]

Until recently patients came to the attention of cardiologists after development of symptoms. At this point training was usually not an option, because symptomatic patients need valve surgery or valve interventions. Thus also in these patients little experience with exercise training is available.

In patients with asymptomatic significant mitral stenosis, exercise training may acutely increase heart rate, particularly in patients with atrial fibrillation, and thus cause symptoms acutely. Studies on chronic exercise training in these patients are not available.

In women with documented mitral valve prolapse, a 12-week aerobic exercise program improved symptoms and functional capacity. Compared with the control group, the exercise group showed a significant decrease in anxiety, as well as increases in general well-being, functional capacity, and a decline in symptoms such as chest pain, fatigue, dizziness, and mood swings.[10] Thus a supervised program may be recommended for these patients. Contraindications for exercise training are present in patients with a history of syncope, documented to be arrhythmogenic in origin, family history of sudden death associated with mitral valve prolapse, repetitive forms of sustained and non-sustained supraventricular arrhythmias, particularly if exaggerated by exercise, and severe mitral regurgitation.

In asymptomatic patients with severe aortic stenosis, careful evaluation with exercise testing is required before embarking on a training program. Exercise training is not an option, if during exercise testing a pathological response occurs (see Chapter 16). These patients require surgery, unless contraindications exist. Whether exercise training may be helpful or harmful in aggravating left ventricular hypertrophy in these patients has not been studied.

In patients with aortic regurgitation, dynamic exercise acutely increases heart rate, which shortens diastole and the time available for aortic regurgitation. Yet bradycardia, induced in the chronic state of exercise training, prolongs diastole and may increase aortic regurgitation, and may theoretically aggravate left ventricular dysfunction. There are no studies examining the long-term effects of endurance training in aortic regurgitation.

In patients with severe symptoms, exercise training is usually not possible or feasible prior to surgery, although one could argue that a specially designed exercise training program, similar to programs used in patients with heart failure, might be of value prior to surgery to counteract the deconditioning that is usually present at the time of operation. But studies concerning this topic are not available.

Thus medically supervised exercise training was mainly started in the postoperative or post-interventional period as part of the management after valve surgery or valve interventions.

Exercise Training in Patients after Valve Surgery

Many studies in patients after bypass surgery have demonstrated the positive effects of exercise training.[2,3,11–16] There is also convincing evidence from a randomized study by Belardinelli et al.[17] on the positive effects of exercise training in patients after interventional revascularization (PCI) (see Chapter 17).

The known positive effects of exercise training on cardiovascular fitness, such as an improvement in general circulatory response to exercise with reduced heart rate and blood pressure, greater exercise tolerance, and attenuated progression of coronary artery disease,[18] make a physical training program for patients after valve replacement particularly advisable since there are still patients who present for valve surgery after years of severe restriction of physical activity. This applies especially to elderly patients. Cardiorespiratory fitness is further impaired by surgical trauma, the effects of cardiopulmonary bypass, postoperative anemia, and inactivity, with the result that patients recovering from successful cardiac surgery can be in a markedly reduced state of cardiorespiratory fitness. Improving this is one of the major goals of exercise training.

The most recent developments in valve surgery with excellent results in reconstructive surgical techniques have led to recommendations to operate at an earlier stage of the disease, even in the asymptomatic state.[19] This applies particularly to younger patients in generally good condition, who wish to exercise and return to work early after surgery.

The effect of exercise training in patients after valve replacement has been examined in only a few studies[20–23] (Table 20-1, Figure 20-1). A consistent increase in exercise capacity of between 25% and 38% was demonstrated without serious risks. In a small study in patients after mitral valve replacement, slight hemolysis occurred, without serious valve dysfunction.[22]

TABLE 20-1. Studies of cardiac rehabilitation following heart valve surgery

Study	No. of patients	Outcomes in comparison to controls
Sire 1987[20]	44	Work capacity increased by 38% at 6 months after surgery
Habel-Verge et al. 1987[22]	10	Work capacity increased by 25% after 8 weeks of exercise training
Jairath et al. 1995[23]	29	Peak VO$_2$ increased by 25%, after 3 months. There was no difference to controls, but more than 50% in the control group exercised
Newell et al. 1980[21]	24	Controlled, but non-randomized study of exercise training revealed improvements in cardiorespiratory fitness 12 and 24 weeks after surgery in the trained group

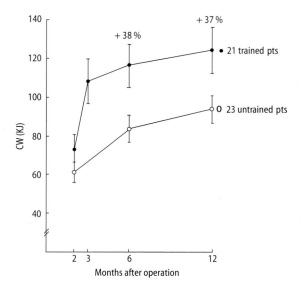

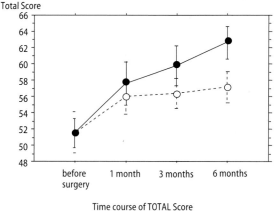

FIGURE 20-3. Changes in quality of life. (From Ueshima et al.[25])

FIGURE 20-1. Physical training and occupational rehabilitation after aortic valve replacement (AVR); cardiac work (CN). (From Sire.[20] © 1987 European Society of Cardiology. Reprinted with perimission.)

In a recent study by Vanhees et al.,[24] it was shown that patients who had valve surgery had a similar improvement after physical training as other cardiac patients (relative increase in peak VO_2 of 25.9% as compared to patients after bypass surgery) (Figure 20-2).

With exercise training improvements in quality of life were also documented in patients after valve surgery[25] (Figure 20-3).

Complications of Exercise Training

Studies evaluating the specific determinants of complications in patients after valve surgery are not available. Yet Vanhees et al.[24] studied the

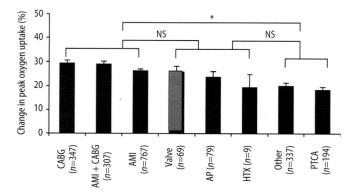

Comparison of training effects for peak VO_2 (F=7.76; $P<0.001$) in patients with various cardiac pathologies, expressed as relative change. The Tukey test was used for post-hoc comparisons, $P<0.05$. Data are presented as mean ±SEM. CABG, coronary artery bypass grafting; AMI, myocardial infarction; Valve, artificial valve implantation; AP, angina pectoris; HTX, heart transplantation; PTCA, percutaneous transluminal coronary angioplasty. *Significantly different; NS, not significantly different.

FIGURE 20-2. Comparison of training effects for peak VO_2. (From Vanhees et al.[24] © 2004 Lippincott Williams & Wilkins. Reprinted with permission.)

predictors of complications requiring resuscitation during exercise training in 1909 patients with various cardiac diseases, including 69 patients with valvular heart disease. One resuscitation per 29,214 patient hours of exercise occurred during exercise in hospital versus 1 resuscitation per 16,533 patient hours of exercise at the local sports club during the phase III rehabilitation. The intake of anti-arrhythmics (odds ratio 5.5; CI = 1.95–15.51; $P < 0.001$) and the presence of significant ($\geq 1\,mm$) ST-segment depression during baseline exercise testing (odds ratio 1.6; CI = 1.21–2.06; $P < 0.001$) were positively associated with severe complications requiring resuscitation.

Exercise Haemodynamics after Valve Surgery

The hemodynamic improvement after valve surgery depends on preoperative degree of impairment and the valve lesion. In patients with aortic stenosis and impaired left ventricular function preoperatively, hemodynamics improve significantly at rest and during exercise after valve surgery. In contrast, patients after mitral valve replacement have a markedly lower exercise tolerance; only 40–60% of patients have normal hemodynamics at rest and only 25% during exercise. In patients with mitral stenosis, pulmonary capillary wedge pressure falls significantly after surgery as well as pulmonary hypertension. The degree of pulmonary hypertension preoperatively and the speed of postoperative regression of pulmonary hypertension is of importance for further management, including exercise training.[26–28]

Besides symptomatic and hemodynamic improvement, several other factors need to be taken into account to determine the type and intensity of exercise training, including the degree of regression of left ventricular hypertrophy and improvement in left ventricular function following correction of the various valve lesions.

Evaluation for Exercise Training

Prior to inclusion in an exercise program all patients should undergo an exercise test (see Chapter 16). A submaximal exercise test can be performed after completion of early mobilization and climbing two flights of stairs without symptoms, usually 2 weeks after surgery. A symptom-limited (maximal exercise) test can be performed after 3 to 4 weeks.

Aortic Valve Surgery

Patients with pure aortic stenosis and normal ventricular function, those with aortic insufficiency and preserved left ventricular function pre- and postoperatively and an uncomplicated postoperative course can be expected to be candidates for exercise training postoperatively. This can usually be demonstrated by submaximal exercise testing at 2 weeks and a symptom-limited maximal exercise test 4 weeks after surgery.

Mitral Valve Surgery

Patients with isolated mitral valve insufficiency preoperatively due to mitral valve prolapse, especially if they have undergone mitral valve reconstruction, with an uncomplicated postoperative course, can be included in an exercise program early.

Patients with mitral stenosis or a combined mitral valve lesion usually have a low exercise tolerance pre- and postoperatively. In addition, the residual gradient across the valve and the marked increase in gradient with rising heart rate make an exercise program for these patients particularly challenging. Before conditioning begins, the heart rate needs to be controlled by medication, preferably beta-blockers, both at rest and during exercise. This is particularly important for patients with atrial fibrillation. If possible, atrial fibrillation should be converted to sinus rhythm. A program specifically designed for these patients, including walking, callisthenics, gymnastics and low level bicycle ergometry with special consideration of the heart rate achieved, appears to be of particular benefit. These patients could follow the training groups for heart failure patients.

Additional factors to be taken into account when making recommendations concerning exercise and recreational activity in patients following valve replacement include previous level of training, age, weight, and postoperative functional status assessed by exercise testing, echocardiography, and Holter monitoring for arrhythmias.

As a simple guide to determine the optimal training level, the results of the exercise test and, in some cases, the exercise hemodynamics are very useful. The level of activity or exercise that is still associated with normal hemodynamics can be taken as a guide for leisure-time activities. If hemodynamics are not available, a rating of perceived exertion such as the Borg scale[29] or the so-called "talk test" are valuable measurements of the intensity of exertion. The "talk test" refers to that level of exertion at which the patient can still hold a "small talk" conversation.

Type of Exercise

Dynamic, aerobic type of exercise like walking, jogging, and cycling is preferable to isometric exercise. However, in elderly patients who present with problems of muscle weakness, high-intensity strength training to improve muscle strength and coordination has been shown to be of benefit.[30,31] Swimming is associated with an energy requirement equivalent to 100–150 watts, as far as the response of heart rate, norepinephrine (noradrenaline), and lactate levels are concerned.[32] Patients should be informed about the amount of energy expenditure associated with different types of exercise and advised about the activities suitable for them.

Recommendations

Exercise prescription should include advice on aerobic and resistance training and should specify intensity, duration, frequency, and modality.

For aerobic exercise:

- Intensity (50–80% of exercise capacity)
- Heart rate guided: <130 beats/min
- Duration 20 to 60 minutes
- Frequency 3 to 5 times/week
- Modality: walking, cycling, treadmill, stair, climbing, arm ergometry.

For resistance exercise:

- Intensity: 5 repetitions for strength training, 8–15 repetitions for endurance training
- Duration: 1–3 sets of 6–10 different upper and lower body exercise (20–30 minutes)
- Frequency 2–3 times/week
- Modality: elastic bands, cuff weights, free weights, weight machines.

Start of Training

Training can be started at low intensity (heart rate approximately <100 beats/min) after 2 weeks in patients with aortic valve replacement or mitral valve repair and normal left ventricular function. In patients with mitral valve replacement and those with impaired left ventricular function, the start of training may need to be delayed until the third week, increasing slowly thereafter. In an over-anxious or over-competitive patient, a commercially available heart rate monitor during exercise training at home can be helpful to direct the exercise intensity.

Swimming can be started when the sternal wound is completely healed and the sternum is stable (usually after 2–3 months), providing that it does not cause pain or rhythm disturbances. Several factors influence the time interval from the operation after which an exercise training program can be started and the type of training that is possible. These factors are outlined in Table 20-2.

TABLE 20-2. Factors influencing exercise recommendations after valve replacement

Age of patient
Weight
Previous level of training
Type of cardiac disease and valve replaced
Postoperative functional status, determined by:
    clinical assessment
    results of exercise testing
    hemodynamic status
Echocardiographically determined left ventricular function and size
Arrhythmias identified by Holter monitoring

Source: Modified from Gohlke-Bärwolf et al. 1992.[26]

Conclusion

Exercise training as part of a multidisciplinary rehabilitation program is beneficial and advisable for all patients after valve surgery. Exercise leads to improvement of functional capacity, enhanced muscular endurance, strength, and flexibility, and contributes to overall lowering of cardiovascular risk. Physical conditioning and individually tailored exercise training are advisable for most patients after valve replacement, taking into account left ventricular function, previous level of training, the type of valve replaced, pulmonary hypertension, and heart rate. The general circulatory responses to exercise, like decreased heart rate and blood pressure at a given exercise load, and increased exercise tolerance, are of benefit to most of these patients, and could enable them to participate more fully in social activities and live a more active and productive life. This leads to an overall improvement in the quality of life for these patients.

References

1. O'Connor GT, Buring JE, Yusuf S, et al. An overview of randomized trials of rehabilitation with exercise after myocardial infarction. Circulation 1989; 80:234–244.
2. Fletcher GF, Balady GJ, Amsterdam EA, et al. Exercise standards for testing and training: a statement for healthcare professionals from the American Heart Association. Circulation 2001;104:1694–1740.
3. Pollock ML, Franklin BA, Balady GJ, et al. AHA Science Advisory. Resistance exercise in individuals with and without cardiovascular disease: benefits, rationale, safety, and prescription: An advisory from the Committee on Exercise, Rehabilitation, and Prevention, Council on Clinical Cardiology, American Heart Association; Position paper endorsed by the American College of Sports Medicine. Circulation 2000;101:828–833.
4. Vanhees L, McGee HM, Dugmore LD, Schepers D, van Daele P. CARINEX Working Group: CAdiac Rehabilitation INformation EXchange. A representative study of cardiac rehabilitation activities in European Union Member States: the CARINEX survey. J Cardiopulm Rehabil 2002;22:264–272.
5. Cottin Y, Cambou JP, Casillas JM, Ferrieres J, Cantet C, Danchin N. Specific profile and referral bias of rehabilitated patients after an acute coronary syndrome. J Cardiopulm Rehabil 2004;24:38–44.
6. Bonow RO, Carabello B, de Leon AC Jr, et al. ACC/AHA Guidelines for the Management of Patients with Valvular Heart Disease: a report of the American College of Cardiology/American Heart Association Task Force on Practice Guidelines (Committee on Management of Patients With Valvular Heart Disease). J Am Coll Cardiol 1998; 32:1486–1588.
7. Butchart EG, Gohlke-Bärwolf C, Antunes MJ, et al. Recommendations for the management of patients after heart valve surgery. Eur Heart J 2005; 26(22):2463–2471.
8. Pelliccia A, Fagard R, Bjornstad HH, et al. for the Working Group of Myocardial and Pericardial Diseases of the European Society of Cardiology. Recommendations for competitive sports participation in athletes with cardiovascular disease: a consensus document from the Study Group of Sports Cardiology of the Working Group of Cardiac Rehabilitation and Exercise Physiology and the Working Group of Myocardial and Pericardial Diseases of the European Society of Cardiology. Eur Heart J 2005; 26:1422–1445.
9. Bonow RO, Cheitlin MD, Crawford MH, Douglas PS. Task Force 3: valvular heart disease. J Am Coll Cardiol 2005;45:1334–1340.
10. Scordo KA. Effects of aerobic exercise training on symptomatic women with mitral valve prolapse. Am J Cardiol 1991;67:863–868.
11. Belardinelli R, Georgiou D, Cianci G, et al. Randomized, controlled trial of long-term moderate exercise training in chronic heart failure: effects on functional capacity, quality of life, and clinical outcome. Circulation 1999;99:1173–1182.
12. Wright DK, Williams SG, Riley R, Marshall P, Tan LB. Is early, low level, short term exercise cardiac rehabilitation following coronary bypass surgery beneficial? A randomised controlled trial. Heart 2002;88:83–84.
13. Balady GJ, Ades PA, Comoss P, et al. Core components of cardiac rehabilitation/secondary prevention programs: A statement for healthcare professionals from the American Heart Association and the American Association of Cardiovascular and Pulmonary Rehabilitation Writing Group. Circulation 2000;102:1069–1073.
14. Fox KF, Nuttall M, Wood DA, et al. A cardiac prevention and rehabilitation program for all patients at first presentation with coronary artery disease. Heart 2001;85:533–538.
15. Task force of the Working Group on Cardiac Rehabilitation of the European Society of Cardiology 1992. Long-term comprehensive care of cardiac patients – recommendations by the Working Group

on Rehabilitation of the ESC, Cardiac Rehabilitation: Definition and Goals. Eur Heart J 1992; 13(Suppl C):1–2.

16. Giannuzzi P, Saner H, Björnstad H, et al. Secondary prevention through cardiac rehabilitation: position paper of the Working Group on Cardiac Rehabilitation and Exercise Physiology of the European Society of Cardiology. Eur Heart J 2003;24: 1273–1278.

17. Belardinelli R, Paolini I, Cianci G, Piva R, Georgiou D, Purcaro A. Exercise training intervention after coronary angioplasty: the ETICA trial. J Am Coll Cardiol 2001;37:1891–1900.

18. Hambrecht R, Gielen S, Linke A, et al. Effects of exercise training on left ventricular function and peripheral resistance in patients with chronic heart failure: a randomized trial. JAMA 2000;283:3095–3101.

19. Iung B, Gohlke-Bärwolf C, Tornos P, et al. Recommendations on the management of the asymptomatic patient with valvular heart disease. Eur Heart J 2002;23:1253–1266.

20. Sire S. Physical training and occupational rehabilitation after aortic valve replacement. Eur Heart J 1987;8:1215–1220.

21. Newell JP, Kappagoda CT, Stoker JB, Deverall PB, Watson DA, Linden RJ. Physical training after heart valve replacement. Br Heart J 1980;44:638–649.

22. Habel-Verge C, Landry F, Desaulnier D, et al. L'entrainement physique après un remplacement valvulaire mitral. Can Med Ass J 1987;136:142–147.

23. Jairath N, Salerno T, Chapman J, et al. The effect of moderate exercise training on oxygen uptake post-aortic/mitral valve surgery. J Cardiopulm Rehabil 1995;15:424–430.

24. Vanhees L, Stevens AN, Schepers D, et al. Determinants of the effects of physical training and of the complications requiring resuscitation during exercise in patients with cardiovascular disease. Eur J Cardiovasc Prev Rehabil 2004;11:304–312.

25. Ueshima K, Kamata J, Kobayashi N, et al. Effects of exercise training after open heart surgery on quality of life and exercise tolerance in patients with mitral regurgitation or aortic regurgitation. Jpn Heart J 2004;45:789–797.

26. Gohlke-Barwolf C, Gohlke H, Samek L, et al. Exercise tolerance and working capacity after valve replacement. J Heart Valve Dis 1992;1:189–195.

27. Führer U, Both G, Fischer K, et al. Sozialanamnestische und hämodynamische Untersuchungen 4 bis 6 Jahre nach prothetischem Klappenersatz. Z Kardiol 1977;66:251–256.

28. Mattern H, Wisshirchen KJ, Fricke G, Bernard A. Belastbarkeit und berufliche Wiedereingliederung nach prothetischem Klappenersatz in Abhängigkeit von der postoperativen H Z Kardiol 1979;68: 36–40.

29. Borg GA. Psychophysical basis of perceived exertion. Med Sci Sports 1982;14:377–381.

30. Fiatarone MA, Marks EC, Ryan ND, Meredith CN, Lipsitz LA, Evans WJ. High-intensity strength training in nonagenarians. Effects on skeletal muscle. JAMA 1990;263:3029–3034.

31. Lunel C, Laurent M, Corbineau H, et al. Return to work after cardiac valvular surgery. Retrospective study of a series of 105 patients. Arch Mal Coeur Vaiss 2003;96:15–22.

32. Samek L, Lehmann M, Keul J, Roskamm H. Rückwirkungen leichter Schwimmbelastungen bei KHK-Patienten und gesunden Kontrollpersonen auf Kreislaufgrößen, Katecholamine und Laktatspiegel. In: Rieckert H, ed. Sportmedizin – Kursbestimmung. Heidelberg: Springer-Verlag; 1987: 912–915.

21
The Role of Sports in Preventive Cardiology

Hans H. Bjørnstad, Tor H. Bjørnstad, and Yngvar Ommundsen

Sports Activity and Cardiovascular Disease

Sport and Physical Activity as Preventive Tools Against Cardiovascular Disease

There are a large number of studies demonstrating that physical activity reduces cardiovascular morbidity and mortality. Some studies are on physical activity during work, some on leisure-time activity and some on a combination of the two.

Regarding physical activity at work, the study of Morris from 1953 of bus drivers versus conductors in London was one of the first. The best-known studies on leisure-time physical activity are the studies of Pfaffenbarger in Harvard alumni[1] and the so-called MRFIT study from Minneapolis by Leon; there have been similar findings in a recent study from Finland.[2] According to Pfaffenbarger, there is an increasing protective effect with increasing intensity of training, but at very high intensities the effect of an increase is marginal. It also has been shown that the activity has to be sustained over time; thus seasonal activity is not protective.[3] This message also should be considered for sports activity, which needs to be regular to be protective. That sports activity is protective was also shown by Pfaffenbarger et al.,[1] but not more than heavy exercise. The effect of physical activity on endothelial function also has been demonstrated by Hambrecht et al.,[4] who also showed an effect on endothelial progenitor cells. Increased endothelial function also has been demonstrated in top athletes.[5] Mea-surement of the physical activity is important in such studies, and is also a source of bias. Therefore the effect of physical activity probably is stronger than that measured in most studies. Furthermore, a tendency to a stronger effect in the best studies has been shown by Froelicher.[4a]

The Impact of Fitness on Cardiovascular Diseases

Physical fitness can be measured easily and exactly, and has been shown to have a negative correlation to coronary heart disease. However, there is also a negative correlation between increasing fitness and risk factors like hypertension and hypercholesterolemia. Intervention by physical training has been shown to reduce these risk factors in studies at the Cooper Clinic in Dallas. If these confounders are corrected for, physical inactivity doubles the risk of coronary disease. In highly trained Norwegian skiers, a risk reduction of 4.8 was found compared to the least fit group in the study. In the same study, the quartile with the highest fitness had a relative risk of cardiovascular death of 0.4 compared to the quartile with poorest fitness.[5] Large studies from the US also show a double risk in persons with low exercise capacity compared to those with a high exercise capacity.[6] Still it may be questioned whether the training or the high fitness per se is protective. This is addressed in a study by Hein et al.,[7] where indirect O_2 consumption was measured and physical activity monitored. The conclusion was that physical activity is protective irrespective of the fitness level.

Cardiovascular Risk of Exercise

The data are varying, but according to a study by Thompson et al. there is one death per 400,000 jogging hours.[8] Most deaths occur in those aged above 40 years, as in a study on squash players, [8a] and in many cases there are many coronary risk factors. On the other side, physical activity protects against sudden death during exercise, and this benefit by far outweighs the risk. Thus the risk of sudden death during exercise is six times higher in persons never exercising compared to regular exercisers, and the total risk of sudden death four times higher in persons never exercising.[9]

Role of Sports in Prevention of Cardiovascular Disease

There are many studies showing reduced mortality in training when following rehabilitation programs. However, there are no specific studies on sports participation in secondary prevention. Still, sport is a useful tool in the maintenance of physical activity. Play and sports in school children now outweigh walking to school as a source of physical activity. In fact one study[10] showed no effect of walking to school on total physical activity in primary school children, demonstrating the dominant effect of play and sports in this regard. In Nordic athletes an active lifestyle is maintained after the active career both in an old[11] and in our own study done recently. The effect of sports on the level of exercise in the community and thereby as a preventive tool on cardiovascular disease will be dealt with separately.

Preventive Cardiology in Athletes

Sudden Death in Athletes

In athletes below 35 years, hypertrophic cardiomyopathy is the most important cause of sudden death according to Maron et al.[12] (Figure 21-1). However, according to Italian data,[13] right ventricular dysplasia is the most important cause. Myocarditis accounts for only about 10% of deaths, but an increase of ventricular dilatation and of antibodies in autoimmune myocarditis has been shown. Therefore, training and competition during febrile infectious disease should be discouraged. According to the European recommendations for screening of athletes, a clinical examination and a standard ECG should be taken in competitive athletes.[14]

In athletes above 35 years, ischemic heart disease is the most important cause of sudden death. According to the European recommendations, exercise ECG should be done in high-risk individuals (males above 35 and females above 40).[15]

Long-Term Effect of Athletic Activity on the Heart

The athlete's heart was first described more than 100 years ago by Henschen, and was then looked upon as pathological. Later there was wide agreement that it is a normal phenomenon, and a harmonious increase in heart size is seen in top athletes.[16] However, this has been questioned in editorials in the *European Heart Journal*, and the need for long-term follow-up studies has been stated. [16a,16b]

ECG

The most typical findings in athletes are sinus bradycardia, increased voltage, and precordial ST elevations.[17] In a 15-year follow-up of elite endurance athletes who had all ended their active careers, we found regression of ST elevations and Sokolow index, while heart rate was not significantly reduced except during night hours (Figure 21-2).

Rhythm Disorders

In some follow-up studies there were a few cases of atrial fibrillation, though not reaching significance; but a significantly increased prevalence of atrial fibrillation in veteran athletes and in a middle-aged sports population has been demonstrated. However, these results are not necessarily applicable to previous top athletes. In our study of Norwegian top endurance athletes, no cases of atrial fibrillation were found at 15-year follow-up. In a 3-year follow-up on continuously active endurance athletes. We found

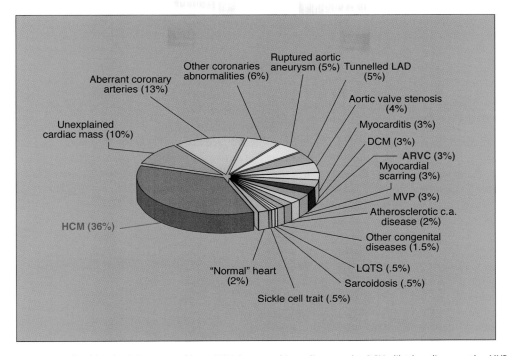

FIGURE 21-1. Causes of sudden death in young athletes. HCM, hypertrophic cardiomyopathy; DCM, dilatd cardiomyopathy; MVP, mitral valvular prolapse; ARVC, arrhythmogenic right ventricular cardiomyopathy; LQTS, Long QT Syndrome; LAD, left anterior descending coronary artery. (After Maron et al.[12]).

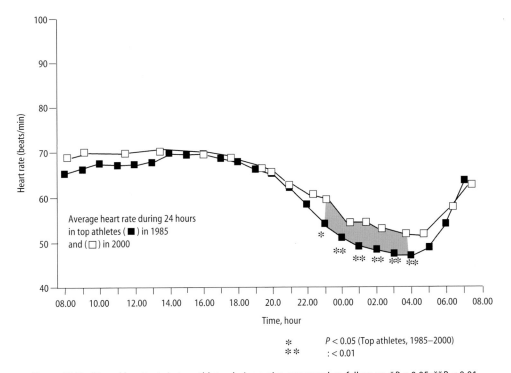

FIGURE 21-2. Diurnal heart rate in top athletes during active career and on follow-up. *$P < 0.05$; **$P < 0.01$.

regression of pauses up to 3.1 seconds[18] in athletes after their stopping active careers, and also regression off season[19] has been shown. In our study, this regression occurred during the night, when heart rate was also increased (Figure 21-2).

Left Ventricular Hypertrophy

Left ventricular mass tends to decrease when athletic activity is stopped; this has also been shown in short-term detraining.[20] However, in Norwegian top endurance athletes we only found a minor reduction, probably due to continued training despite stopping participation in major competitions. Also x-ray studies have shown high or unchanged heart volume in previous Nordic top endurance athletes who were also performing some training.[21] We found that relative wall thickness tended to decrease in endurance athletes after their active career; this has also been shown in relation to seasonal detraining of cyclists.[21a] An increased relative wall thickness was found in a study on veteran cyclists by Miki, but these were still performing intensive training and therefore represent a different population than ex-athletes.

We found no reduction of left ventricular volume on detraining, which is in accordance[21b] with the conclusion of Dickhut that a relatively small amount of training can maintain an increased heart volume. However, when training is stopped, a raised heart volume is reduced according to a study by Pelliccia.[21c]

Diastolic Function

In a study on veteran cyclists, reduced diastolic function was found. However, this has not been confirmed by other investigators, who found it to be improved or unchanged. Animal studies have also shown that training reduces the age-induced decline of diastolic function. We also found normal diastolic function, assessed by mitral flow and tissue Doppler, in ex-athletes, in accordance with most other investigators.

Cardiovascular Mortality

Reduced mortality has been demonstrated in athletes who continue training,[1,10] but unchanged or

increased mortality in those who stop athletic activity, who also may have an unhealthy lifestyle. Reduced coronary risk factors and diabetes also have been demonstrated in previous top athletes who continue training.[22] Reduced blood pressure also has been shown in previous top athletes still training and in veteran athletes.[23] While increased heart size is usually an indicator of reduced longevity, this is not the case in highly trained individuals.[5] Comparing different groups of athletes, the biggest reduction of mortality is found in endurance athletes, which may be due to a more active lifestyle after the end of their active careers.

Summary on Preventive Cardiology in Athletes

As there is an increased risk of sudden death during intense athletic activity, a screening including standard ECG should be done in young top athletes in order to prevent sudden death. In middle-aged athletes with a high cardiovascular risk profile, exercise ECG should be performed. There is no evidence of a long-term deleterious effect on the heart due to athletic activity, but there are some data that the prevalence of atrial fibrillation is increased in master athletes. Previous athletes generally have increased life expectancy, reduced cardiovascular risk factors, and a higher level of physical activity. This is most prominent in endurance athletes. Increased life expectancy is limited to those who continue some physical training.

Promoting Enhanced Physical Activity (PA) and Sport in Preventive Cardiology – the Challenge for Youth Sport

Organized sports participation comprises a huge part of young people's total involvement in physical activity and exercise activities.[23] Involvement in sports for children and adolescents becomes particularly important in preventive cardiology given that health-enhancing physical activity patterns in adults and older age are established in young age.[24] There is, however, recent evidence that physical fitness in youth rather than physical activity by itself is related to a healthy cardiovascular disease (CVD) risk profile later in life.[25] Further, the evidence that activity in young age provides protection from CVD in adulthood is weak.[26] Nevertheless, behavioral scientists argue that a focus on the behavior of physical activity is more appropriate for health behavior change and maintenance into adulthood than the outcome of fitness.

A review on the prevalence of physical activity (PA) and sedentary behaviors shows that many young people are active, but this declines with age.[27] Even though it is not possible to determine objectively whether there has been a decline in physical activity in recent years in young people, a substantial number are not sufficiently active for health benefits. Furthermore, current trends in juvenile obesity are a cause for concern, in that data on energy intake and body mass indirectly suggest that young people have reduced their energy expenditure.[28]

Determinants of young people's involvement in sports and physical activity are complex. First, gender and social-cultural factors influence sports involvement. For example, the level of sedentariness with increasing age seems greater among girls and among those from less resourceful backgrounds.[29] Among psychological factors, enjoyment is particularly important and is consistently associated with participation in sport and PA. Other important determining factors comprise feelings of competence, control, autonomy, self-efficacy, positive attitudes to PA and sport including perceived benefits and decreased barriers to sport and PA, and having personal goals that focus on effort and improvement.[30] In terms of social and environmental factors, there is substantial evidence that family and peer modeling and support correlate with sport and PA levels of young people. Further, access to appropriate environments can enhance their participation.[30] A full understanding can only be achieved through studying the interplay of psychological, social, and environmental factors.

Several contexts are candidates for interventions to enhance young people's involvement in sport and PA. These include families, schools (including physical education programs), and communities. Physical education in schools cannot alone generate lifelong interest in physical activity and sport, although recent research suggests that physical education classes may stimulate leisure-time sport interest.[31] Thus, family level interventions and community level agencies and sports clubs should be regarded as important intervention targets. Clearly coaches, and community youth organizations have the potential to positively influence and reinforce young people's sport attitudes and behaviors by being able to offer a variety of stimulating, challenging, and enjoyable sport and physical activity experiences. Moreover, it would seem important also to facilitate opportunities for young people to organize their own sport and physical activities in ways that fit in with their own culture and preferences.

Summary

There is much evidence that physical activity reduces the risk of cardiovascular disease, and more so with increasing level of exercise, including sports activity. The small cardiovascular risk of sports activity is by far outweighed by the benefit, but this risk can be reduced by appropriate screening measures. There is no evidence that athletic activity at young age has deleterious long-term effects on the heart, and athletes who continue an active lifestyle have increased longevity. However, it is a clear message that unless physical activity is regular it has no documented effect on prevention of cardiovascular disease. Hence, in order to sustain physical activity throughout life, it is important to help stimulate physical activity in youth. Organized sport may play an important role in generating a health-enhancing physically active lifestyle, provided young people's interest in physical activity and sport are maintained in younger years. Feelings of competence and enjoyment, social support, and suitable sport offerings and physical environments suitable for activity exploration seem to be decisive factors in young people's sport and physical activity motivation. Families, community agencies, and schools have an important role to play in developing and sustaining interest and participation in sports for young people.

References

1. Paffenbarger RS, Wing AL, Hyde RT. Physical activity as an index of heart attack risk in college alumni. J Epidemiol 1978;108:161–175.
2. Barengo N, Hu G, Lakka TA, Pekkarinen H, Nissinen A, Tuomilehto J. Low physical activity as a predictor of total and cardiovascular disease in middle-aged men end women in Finland. Eur Heart J 2004;24:2204–2211.
3. Magnus K, Matroos A, Stracke J. Walking, cycling, or gardening, with or without seasonal interruption, in relation to acute coronary events. Am J Epidemiol 1979;110(6):724–733.
4. Hambrecht R, Wolf A, Gielen S, et al. Effects of exercise on coronary endothelial function in patients with coronary artery disease. N Engl J Med 2000;342:454–460.
4a. Froelicher V, Myers J. Exercise and the Heart, 4th ed. Philadelphia: Saunders; 2000.
5. Sandvik L, Erikssen J, Thaulow E, Erikssen G, Mundal R, Rodal K. Physical fitness as a predictor of mortality among healthy, middle-aged Norwegian men. N Engl J Med 1993;328:533–537.
6. Blair N, Kohl HK, Paffenberger RS, Clarck DG, Cooper H, Gibbons LW. Physical fitness and all-cause mortality. JAMA 1989;262:2395–2401.
7. Hein HO, Suadicani P, Gyntelberg F. Physical fitness or physical activity as a predictor of ischaemic heart disease? A 17-year follow-up in the Copenhagen male study. J Intern Med 1992; 232:471–479.
8. Thompson PD, Funk EJ, Carleton RA, Sturner WQ. Incidence of death during jogging in Rhode Island from 1975 through 1980. JAMA 1982;247:2535–2538.
8a. Northcote RJ, Flannigan C, Ballantyne D. Sudden death and vigorous exercise: a study of 60 deaths associated with squash. Br Heart J 1986;55:198–203.
9. Siscovick DS, Weiss NS, Fletcher RH, Lasky T. The incidence of primary cardiac arrest during vigorous exercise. N Engl J Med 1984;311:874–877.
10. Metcalf B, Voss L, Jeffery A, Perkins J, Wilkin T. Physical activity cost of the school run: impact on schoolchildren of being driven to school (Early Bird 22). BMJ 2004;329:832–833.
11. Karvonen MJ. Effects of vigorous exercise on the heart. Clin Physiol 1959;199–210.
12. Maron BJ, Epstein SE, Roberts WC. Causes of sudden death in competitive athletes. J Am Coll Cardiol 1986;7:204–214.
13. Corrado D, Basso C, Thiene G. Arrhythmogenic right ventricular cardiomyopathy: diagnosis, prognosis and treatment. Heart 2000;83:588–595.
14. Corrado D, Pelliccia A, Bjørnstad H, et al. Cardiovascular pre-participation screening of young competitive athletes for prevention of sudden death: proposal for a common European protocol. Eur Heart J 2005;26:516–524.
15. Pelliccia A, Fagard R, Bjørnstad H, et al. Recommendations for competitive sports participation in athletes with cardiovascular disease. Eur Heart J 2005;26:1422–1445.
16a. McCann GP, Muir DF, Hillis WS. Athletic left ventricular hypertrophy: long-term studies are required. Eur Heart J 2000;21:351–353.
16b. Coumel P. Atrial fibrillation: one more sporting inconvenience. Eur Heart J 2000;21:351–350.
16. Bjørnstad H, Smith G, Storstein L, Meen HD, Hals O. Electrocardiographic and echocardiographic findings in top athletes, athletic students and sedentary controls. Cardiology 1993;82:66–74.
17. Bjørnstad H, Storstein L, Meen HD, Hals O. Eelctrocardiographic findings in athletic students and sedentary controls. Cardiology 1991;79:290–305.
18. Bjørnstad H, Storstein L, Meen HD, Hals O. Ambulatory electrocardiographic findings in top athletes, athletic students and control subjects. Cardiology 1994;84:42–50.
19. Caru B, Righetti G, Bossi M, Gerosa C, Gazzotti G, Maranetto D. Limits of cardiac functional adaptation in "top level" resistance athletes. Ital Heart J 2001;2(Suppl):150–154.
20. Martin WH, Coyle EF, Bloomfield SA, Ehsani AA. Effects of physical deconditioning after intense endurance training on left ventricular dimensions and stroke volume. J Am Coll Cardiol 1986;7:982–989.
21. Pyörälä K, Karvonen MJ, Taskinen P, Takkunen J, Kyröseppä H, Peltokallio P. Cardiovascular studies on former endurance athletes. Am J Cardiol 1967;20:191–205.
21a. Fagard R, Aubert A, Lysens R, Staessen J, Vanhees L, Amery A. Noninvasive assessment of seasonal variations in cardiac structure and function in cyclists. Circulation 1983;67:989–1001.
21b. Dickhut HH, Reindell H, Lehmann M, Keul J. Ruckbildungs fahigkeit des sportherzens. Z Kardiol 1985;74(Suppl):135–143.
21c. Pellicia A, Maron BJ, DeLuca R, Di Paolo FM, Spataro A, Culasso F. Remodeling of left ventricular hypertrophy in elite athletes after long-term deconditioning. Circulation 2002;944–949.
22. Kujala UM, Kaprio J, Taimela S, Sarna S. Prevalence

of diabetes, hypertension and ischemic heart disease in former elite athletes. Metabolism 1994: 43:1255–1260.

23. Viljalmsson R, Kristjansdottir G. Gender differences in physical activity in older children and adolescents: the central role of organized sport. Social Sci Med 2003:56:363–374.

24. Stucky-Ropp R, DiLorenzo T. Determinants of exercise in children. Prev Med 1993;22:880–889.

25. Twisk JWR, Kemper HCG, Van Mechelen W. Prediction of cardiovascular disease risk factors later in life by physical activity and physical fitness in youth. General comments and conclusions. Int J Sports Med 2002;23(suppl):44–50.

26. Rowland. T. The role of physical activity and fitness in the prevention of adult cardiovascular disease. Prog Pediatr Cardiol 2001;12:199–203.

27. Cavill N, Biddle S, Sallis JF. Health enhancing physical activity for young people: statement of the United Kingdom expert consensus conference. Pediatr Exerc Sci 2001;13:12–25.

28. Craig S, Goldberg J, Dietz W. Psychosocial correlates of physical activity among fifth and eighth graders. Prev Med 1996;25:506–513.

29. Wold B, Hendry L. Social and environmental factors associated with physical activity in young people. In: Biddle S, Sallis J, Cavill N, eds. Young and Active. London: Health Education Authority; 1998:119–132.

30. Sallis J, Prochaska J, Taylor W. A review of correlates of physical activity of children and adolescents. Med Sci Sports Exerc 2000;32:963–975.

31. Hagger M, Chatzisarantis NLD, Culverhouse T, Biddle S. The processes by which perceived autonomy support in physical education promotes leisure-time physical activity intentions and behaviour. A trans-contextual model. J Ed Psych 2003;95:784–795.

22
Advising Patients with Cardiac Disease and after Cardiac Interventions about Sports Activities

Hans H. Bjørnstad, Asle Hirth, Saied Nadirpour, and Britt Undheim

Introduction

Cardiac rehabilitation increases fitness and quality of life and should therefore be offered to all patients after acute cardiac events and interventions. After a rehabilitation program of 4–8 weeks further physical activity is important, and usually previous sports can be taken up at some level. In most cases this will be recreational sports, but sometimes also recommendations for competitive sports are needed after a cardiac event or diagnosis of a cardiac disorder.

Classification of Sports

Exercise is usually classified into dynamic (isotonic) and static (isometric) and the intensity as low, moderate, or high. Running is typical dynamic exercise and leads to increased cardiac output, oxygen consumption, and systolic blood pressure, whereas diastolic blood pressure may fall due to decreased peripheral resistance. Static exercise leads to pressure overload with little influence on oxygen consumption and cardiac output. Traditionally, dynamic exercise is preferred in cardiac patients, but static exercise has been proved to be less dangerous then previously thought. Table 22-1 gives an overview of the most common sport activities and their classification.

Competitive Sports in Cardiac Diseases

Cardiovascular disease may induce an increased risk of sudden death or deterioration of disease on competitive athletic activity; therefore recommendations are important to provide careful directions for physicians and consultant cardiologists. By competitive athletes is meant individuals of young or adult age who are engaged in regular exercise training and participation in official sports competitions. The recommendations are particularly important in elite athletes due to the intense pressure they are exposed to by the media, athletic associations, and sponsors. Protecting the athlete's health is the paramount objective of the physician, and when the cardiovascular risk appears to be unreasonably high, the physician should be responsible for the final decision, with the aim to prevent adverse clinical events and/or reduce risk of disease progression.

The American guidelines were published in 1994.[2] In 2005 the European Society of Cardiology made new recommendations,[3] which are the basis for the following recommendations.

Grown up Congenital Heart Disease (GUCH)

Patients with congenital heart disease (CHD) reaching adulthood are a growing population.[4] Most of them require lifelong care. The hemodynamic situation of the patient with CHD varies considerably. This makes it impossible

TABLE 22-1. Classification of sports

	A. Low dynamic	B. Moderate dynamic	C. High dynamic
I. Low static	Archery	Table tennis	Badminton
	Bowling	Tennis (doubles)	Walking
	Cricket	Volleyball	Running (marathon)
	Golf	Baseball*	Cross-country skiing
	Riflery		(classic)
II. Moderate static	Auto racing* ⚡	Fencing	Basketball*
	Diving ⚡	Field events (jumping)	Biathlon
	Equestrian* ⚡	Figure skating*	Ice hockey*
	Motorcycling* ⚡	**Lacrosse***	Field hockey*
	Gymnastics* ⚡	Running (sprint)	Football*
	Karate/Judo*		Soccer*
	Sailing		Cross-country skiing
			(skating)
			Running (mid/long)
			Swimming
			Squash*
			Tennis (single)
			Team handball*
III. High static	Bobsledding* ⚡	Body building* ⚡	Boxing*
	Field events (throwing)	Downhill skiing* ⚡	Canoeing, Kayaking
	Luge* ⚡	Wrestling*	Cycling* ⚡
	Rock climbing* ⚡		**Decathlon**
	Water skiing* ⚡		Rowing
	Weight lifting*		Speed skating
	Windsurfing* ⚡		

Symbols: *Danger of bodily collision. ⚡ Increased risk if syncope occurs.
Source: Adapted and modified after Mitchell et al.[1]

to give recommendations that are valid in all cases. Nevertheless, studies suggests that GUCH patients benefit greatly from regular physical exercise and therefore only those patients who are likely to deteriorate as a consequence of regular physical exercise and/or those in whom exercise may trigger serious arrhythmias should be restricted from sport participation.

Shunts

Patients with closed or small atrial septal defect (ASD), ventricular septal defect (VSD), and persistent ductus arteriosus (PDA) with normal ECG and echocardiography have no exercise limitations. PDA with audible murmur and lesions with significant shunt need to be corrected and only low to moderate leisure sport activity is recommended until after catheter or surgical repair.

Tetralogy of Fallot (TOF)

Common hemodynamic alterations in TOF are abnormal right ventricular RV function, pulmonary valve insufficiency, and arrhythmia. Most patients have no exercise restrictions and will benefit from increased physical activity. If significant residual disease is present the patient is not allowed to participate in competitive sport.

Transposition of the Great Arteries (TGA)

Patients with TGA corrected by arterial switch can perform all kinds of exercise if significant pulmonary stenosis, aortic insufficiency, and ischemia on exercise ECG have been ruled out.

Coarctation of the Aorta (CoA)

If no signs of residual CoA or recoarctation, no hypertension, no associated aortic stenosis, and normal exercise blood pressure response are found, patients with CoA can perform all kinds of sports without limitations.

Complex Lesions

The majority of patients with more complex lesions will have some form of residual cardiac, pulmonary, or cerebral dysfunction. They have increased risk of arrhythmias and deterioration during heavy exercise, and only dynamic sport of low and moderate intensity and/or static sport of low intensity can be recommended. In this category would be patients with single ventricle, TGA corrected by Senning, Mustard or Rastelli operations, and Ebstein anomaly. Patients with Eisenmenger syndrome or secondary pulmonary hypertension should only do low-intensity leisure sport activity.

Marfan Syndrome

These patients are at increased risk of aortic dissection and sudden death during exercise and are not allowed to do any form of competitive sport. So long as patients avoid sports with the risk of bodily collision, low and moderate dynamic leisure sport activity can be performed.

Valvular Disease

Aortic Stenosis (AS)

Low–moderate dynamic and static sports are allowed in mild AS (mean gradient below 20 mmHg, area above $1.5\,cm^2$, normal left ventricular (LV) function at rest and exercise). Exercise echocardiography can help to evaluate the development of the aortic gradient during exercise. Low dynamic/low static sports are allowed in moderate stenosis (mean gradient 21–49 mmHg, area 1–$1.5\,cm^2$, and normal LV function at rest and exercise).

Aortic Regurgitation (AI)

All sports are allowed in mild AI with normal LV size and function at rest and exercise and no arrhythmias.

Mitral Stenosis (MS)

All sports except high dynamic and high static are allowed in mild MS (area >$1.5\,cm^2$, mean pressure <7 mmHg, pulmonary artery pressure below 35 mmHg).

Mitral Regurgitation (MI)

All sports are allowed in mild MI (regurgitation area <$4\,cm^2$, normal LV size and function, normal exercise testing, sinus rhythm). In atrial fibrillation and warfarin treatment, contact sports are not advised.

In moderate MI (regurgitation area 4–$8\,cm^2$, mild LV dilatation, normal LV function at rest and stress, no arrhythmias, no symptoms) low–moderate dynamic and low–moderate static sports are allowed.

Mitral or Aortic Artificial Valves

Recommendations are the same as for moderate MI.

In mild mitral regurgitation with atrial fibrillation and adequate anticoagulation, all sports except contact sports are advised.

Cardiomyopathies and Myocarditis

Cardiomyopathy is the most important cause of death in young athletes.

Hypertrophic cardiomyopathy (HCM) has a prevalence of 0.5% and accounts for 30% of sudden deaths (SD) in young athletes in the US.[5] When the diagnosis is certain, competitive sports generally are not recommended. A differentiation from physiological hypertrophy is crucial.[3]

However, low dynamic, low static sports may be allowed in athletes with a low risk profile according to history, physical examination, ECG, exercise testing (blood pressure response, optionally Doppler investigation of intraventricular gradient), and Holter monitoring. In some cases determination of the genotype also may be done. In these cases yearly follow-up should be carried out.

Dilated cardiomyopathy (DCM) is a far less common cause of SD in athletes. Sometimes differentiation from physiological hypertrophy with dilatation may be difficult. In these cases, tissue Doppler and exercise echocardiography may be helpful in the differentiation. Generally, ejection fraction (EF) in normal adaptation is above 50%

and there are no wall motion abnormalities. A family history of DCM strongly suggests this diagnosis.

In definite diagnosis of DCM, competitive sports generally are not recommended.

However, low–moderate dynamic and low static sports may be recommended in low-risk cases where there is no sudden death in relatives, no symptoms, EF > 40%, normal blood pressure response on exercise testing, and no complex ventricular arrhythmias (Holter monitoring should be done).

Right ventricular dysplasia (ARVD) is an important cause of SD in young athletes, particularly in Italy where many athletes with HCM have been ruled out by screening. The diagnosis may be difficult, but can be suspected from ECG: RBBB is common. Negative T waves are present in more than 40% and ventricular arrhythmias with LBBB pattern are common.

In definite cases of ARVD, athletic competitions are not recommended.

Myocarditis and Pericarditis

Myocarditis accounts for about 10% of SD in young athletes and should be assessed by standard clinical examination included viral serology (particularly enteroviruses), ECG, and echocardiography (including tissue Doppler). In active myocarditis, athletic competitions are not recommended. Six months after onset competitions may be resumed provided there are no symptoms, normal LV function, and no arrhythmias assessed by ECG, echocardiography, exercise ECG, and Holter monitoring. A new cardiological assessment should be done every 6 months.

Even if myocarditis is not the most common cause of SD, there are good reasons for caution on training and competitions during and immediately after infections. There are also experimental data suggesting that myocarditis is worsened by physical training.[6] Furthermore, there is some evidence that infections increase the risk of acute coronary episodes.

Pericarditis may be followed by a myocarditis and should preclude athletic activity in its active stage. The same examinations should be done as for myocarditis. In clinically isolated pericarditis, competitions may be resumed 3 months after clinical onset of disease, with the same investigations being done as in myocarditis before resumption. Cardiological control after 6 months is recommended.

Hypertension

Hypertension is defined as systolic blood pressure (BP) 140 mmHg or above and/or diastolic BP 90 mmHg or above, or patients on antihypertensive treatment. The prevalence is approximately 15%, 30%, and 55% in males aged 18–39 years, 40–59 years, and above 60 years. Corresponding numbers in females are 5%, 30%, and 65%. However, 25% of patients with hypertension by conventional measurements have a normal blood pressure on 24-hour monitoring.[7] According to a meta-analysis by Fagard and Amery,[8] exercise reduces systolic/diastolic blood pressure by 6/7 mmHg in borderline hypertensives and 10/8 mm in hypertensives.

Athletic competitions without any restrictions can be recommended in hypertensives with well-controlled mild hypertension without additional risk factors (dyslipidemia, smoking, abdominal obesity, family history of premature coronary disease).

All sports except high static, high dynamic sports can be recommended in well-controlled moderate hypertension or mild hypertension with one or two risk factors.

All sports except high static sports can be recommended in well-controlled severe hypertension without risk factors or well-controlled mild/moderate hypertension with three or more risk factors or target organ damage.

Low–moderate dynamic and low static sports are recommended in well-controlled hypertension with associated clinical conditions (cerebrovascular, coronary or peripheral artery disease, renal disease, retinopathy) or well-controlled severe hypertension with risk factors.[3]

Ischemic Heart Disease (IHD)

IHD accounts for most exercise-related sudden deaths in individuals above 35 years. Although the benefit of regular physical activity outweighs the risk, sports participation should be individually advised in patients with IHD.

Necessary investigations are history, resting and exercise ECG (and in some cases stress echocardiography), echocardiography, coronary angiography and Holter monitoring included a training session.

Low risk for exercise-induced cardiac events in patients with evidence of IHD is characterized by ejection fraction above 50%, normal exercise capacity, absence of exercise-induced ischemia at lower steps, absence of significant coronary stenosis (>70% of major coronary arteries or >50% of left main stem) and stable clinical condition. After an intervention outpatient rehabilitation should be completed before considering sports competitions.

Athletes with a high-risk profile (>5% global risk according to SCORE) should be evaluated by maximal exercise ECG. If this is negative, the risk of a major cardiac event during physical activity can be considered small. If there is a positive stress test, further diagnostic evaluation should be done to rule out coronary disease. In asymptomatic athletes with a low-risk profile, routine use of exercise testing is not recommended in men below 35 years and women below 45 years.

Myocardial ischemia also may be induced by other conditions than atherosclerosis:

– cocaine abuse[9]
– congenital coronary artery anomalies are associated with sudden death in young athletes, and are often not revealed by exercise testing
– in myocardial bridging, however, the risk is not high; the same probably is the case in syndrome X.

In spasm angina, the clinical course is unpredictable and competitive sports activity generally should be discouraged unless the condition has been asymptomatic for 1 year.

Arrhythmias

Sinus Bradycardia (≤30 beats/min and/or sinus pauses 3–3.5 s)

Athletes can participate in all sports if there are no symptoms and no cardiac disease.[10,11]

Atrioventricular (AV) Block

Individuals with AV block grade I and second-degree AV block type Wenckebach (Mobitz type I) can participate in all sports if there are no symptoms, no structural heart disease, and no progression of AV block during exercise.

Those with Mobitz type II or third-degree AV block can participate in low–moderate dynamic, and low–moderate static sports in the absence of symptoms, cardiac disease, ventricular arrhythmias during exercise, and if the resting heart rate is >40 beats/min.

Paroxysmal Supraventricular Tachycardia (AVNRT or WPW Syndrome and AVRT)

Catheter ablation is recommended.

Affected individuals can participate in all sports following successful catheter ablation after an asymptomatic period of more than 1 month, and no cardiac disease.

If ablation is not performed and AVNRT is sporadic without hemodynamic consequences, and without relation to exercise, individuals can participate in all sports, except those with increased risk (see Table 22-1).

WPW Syndrome and Atrial Fibrillation or Flutter

Catheter ablation is mandatory.

Participation in all sports is possible following successful catheter ablation after an asymptomatic period of more than 1 month, and if there is no cardiac disease.

Asymptomatic WPW Pattern (Pre-excitation Pattern) on ECG

Catheter ablation is recommended.

Asymptomatic athletes at low risk (normal hearts without inducible AF or AVRT) and not ablated can participate in all sports, except sports with increased risk (see Table 22-1).

Atrial Fibrillation (AF)

Paroxysmal AF: individuals can participate in all sports after 3 months without AF recurrence under rhythm control therapy in the absence of cardiac disease or WPW.

Permanent AF: a ventricular rate comparable to that of an appropriate sinus tachycardia during exercise should be guaranteed before returning to competitive sports.

Asymptomatic athletes with structural heart disease can participate in competitive sports as determined by the limitations of the cardiac abnormality.

Athletes who require anticoagulation therapy with warfarin should not participate in sports where there is a danger of bodily collision or trauma.

Atrial Flutter

Catheter ablation is mandatory.

Athletes can participate in all sports 3 months after successful ablation without recurrence of the arrhythmia and no cardiac disease or WPW.

Asymptomatic athletes with structural heart disease can participate in competitive sports as determined by the limitations of the cardiac abnormality 3 months after successful ablation without recurrence of arrhythmia.

Athletes not treated by catheter ablation should not return to full participation to all sports until they are free of arrhythmia recurrence for 6 months with or without drug therapy.

Ventricular Premature Beats (VPB)

Individuals can participate in all sports in the absence of cardiac disease, arrhythmogenic condition (cardiomyopathies, ischemic heart disease, and channelopathies), family history of sudden death, symptoms (syncope), worsening on exercise, and frequent and/or polymorphic VPBs and/or frequent couplets with short RR interval. Holter monitoring, exercise testing, and echocardiography is recommended in frequent VPBs.

Nonsustained Ventricular Tachycardia (NSVT), Slow Ventricular Tachycardia (Idioventricular Accelerated Rhythm), Fascicular VT, Right Ventricular Outflow Tachycardia (RVOT)

Athletes can participate in all sports, except those with increased risk (see Table 22-1), in the absence of cardiac disease, arrhythmogenic condition, family history of sudden death, symptoms

(syncope), relation with exercise, and multiple episodes of NSVT or VT over 24 hours and/or with short RR interval. Athletes with symptomatic fascicular tachycardia or RVOT who undergo catheter ablation can participate in competitive sports 3 months after successful ablation if asymptomatic and without recurrence of tachycardia.

Malignant Ventricular Tachycardias (Sustained VT, Polymorphic VT, Torsade de Pointes, and Ventricular Fibrillation)

All competitive sports are contraindicated.

An exception is represented by ventricular arrhythmias occurring in the context of acute and completely reversible conditions, such as myocarditis, commotio cordis, acute electrolytic depletion, when the cause has been resolved.

Arrhythmogenic Conditions (Long QT Syndrome, Brugada Syndrome)

All competitive sports are contraindicated.

Syncope

Neurocardiogenic: Athletes can participate in all sports, except those with increased risk.

Arrhythmic or primary cardiac: See specific cause.

Implanted Pacemaker

Patients can participate in low–moderate dynamic and low static sports, except those with risk of bodily collision, if there is normal heart rate increase during exercise, no significant arrhythmias and normal cardiac function.

Patients with specific heart disease can participate only in sports consistent with the limitations of the arrhythmia and the underlying heart disease.

Implantable Cardioverter Defibrillator (ICD)

Patients can participate in low–moderate dynamic and low static sports, except those with risk of bodily collision, if normal cardiac function, no malignant VTs and at least 6 months after the implantation or the last tachyarrhythmia intervention.[12]

Recreational Sports in Certain Groups of Patients

Heart failure

Exercise training is an important part of the treatment of heart failure patients, improving functional status and also reducing mortality.[13] Improvement by exercise training can be obtained after resynchronization therapy. Before starting an exercise training program, the condition should be stable and the fluid volume status should be controlled. Complete cardiological investigation is necessary, ensuring that there is no ischemia, which should be treated with revascularization. An exercise test is mandatory; if possible ergospirometric evaluation should be done. Anaerobic threshold is a good guideline for the level of training, particularly in atrial fibrillation where heart rate is not a reliable parameter of intensity. Previously, only dynamic exercise was advocated, but moderate isometric exercise has also turned out to be feasible and safe. Lactate measurement and (in sinus rhythm) pulse watch monitoring may be helpful. Competition sports usually are not advisable in heart failure.

Heart Transplant Patients

In order to regain a good functional status with good quality of life, physical training is crucial after heart transplantation, and participation in long distance races is possible.[14] However, it is controversial whether training modifies the reinnervation.[15] Also resistance exercise is beneficial for counteracting osteoporosis and skeletal muscle myopathy.[16] However, due to sympathetic denervation, hypotension during resistance exercise is a problem in about 25% of patients, particularly when lifting above the level of the heart. Therefore exercises improving venous return should be done (cool-down walk 2–5 min, alternate upper body and lower body exercises). In severe osteoporosis, resistance exercises should be done with care.

Children with Cardiac Diseases

Children under the age of 10 with diseases where the heart is involved should be allowed to perform physical activity without restrictions. A restrictive attitude in this age group is not necessary since the children will limit themselves. Many children with heart disease have impaired exercise capacity due to overprotection and lack of exercise experience. On the other hand, parents should know if their child has a cardiac disease that will need restrictions in adolescence or adult life in order to direct their hobbies or physical training towards non-competitive, moderate-intensity activities.[17] The most important ones have already been described above. In addition, children with cardiomyopathy or disorders leading to cardiomyopathy, children with arrhythmic disorders such as long QT syndrome, arrhythmic right ventricle dysplasia and Brugada syndrome, and children with suspected Marfan syndrome should be mentioned. Children with Kawasaki syndrome should be restricted from moderate- and high-intensity sport until 3 months after recovery from disease/disappearance of coronary abnormalities.

Heart Surgery

Following surgery, training can start after 2–4 weeks guided by a maximal exercise test 3–5 weeks after the operation. A rehabilitation program is recommended before return to competitive or leisure-time sports. The complete healing of the sternotomy usually takes 3 months, which has to be considered when taking up sports. Generally earlier sports can be resumed, but contact sports should be avoided in warfarin treatment and in artificial valves. If there are significant pericardial effusions, training should be postponed.

Endocarditis

Prophylaxis should be given according to standard rules. Sports should be discouraged during feverish illness.

Anticoagulation

Sports with risk of bodily collision (see Table 22-1) should be avoided.

Practical Advice on Sports in Cardiac Rehabilitation

Contact Sports (Table 22-1)

These should be avoided in patients on warfarin, with Marfan syndrome, valve prosthesis, and congenital heart disease and conduit.

Isometric Sports

Blood pressure may increase to 320/250 in weightlifters.[18] One study showed 311/184 with Valsalva, 198/175 without Valsalva.[19] Generally, isometric sports are not advised in patients with hypertension.

High-Risk Sports (Table 22-1)

Sports where there is a risk of falling down (climbing, parachuting) or being trapped (diving, swimming) should not be performed if there is a risk of syncope.

Swimming

Holter monitoring during swimming has shown increased arrhythmias in some patients. After open heart surgery, breast swimming can be started cautiously after 2 months, but may still cause some pain for 2 more months. It corresponds to an energy load of at least 75 W.

Scuba Diving

Non-randomized studies suggest an increased risk of decompression sickness (DCS) in patients with patent foramen ovale (PFO).[20] Those who experience DCS despite a safe diving profile should be screened for PFO by transesophageal echocardiography (TEE). If PFO is found, the recreational diver should give up his hobby. Professional divers should be offered catheter closure of the PFO. Diving can then be resumed after 3 months.

References

1. Mitchell JH, Haskell WL, Raven PB. Classification of sports. J Am Coll Cardiol 1994;24:864–866.
2. Maron BJ, Mitchell JH. 26th Bethesda Conference: Recommendations for determining eligibility for competition in athletes with cardiovascular abnormalities. J Am Coll Cardiol 1994;24:845–899.
3. Pelliccia A, Fagard R, Bjørnstad H. Eligibility for sports participation in athletes. Eur Heart J; Submitted.
4. Perloff JK, Warnes C. Congenital heart diseases in adults: a new cardiovascular speciality. Circulation 2001;84:1881–1890.
5. Maron BJ, Epstein SE, Roberts WC. Causes of sudden death in competitive athletes. Am J Cardiol 1986;7:204–214.
6. Hosenpud JD, Cambell SM, Niles NR, Lee J, Mendelsohn D, Hart MV. Exercise induces augmentation of cellular and humoral autoimmunity associated with increased cardiac dilatation in experimental autoimmune myocarditis. Cardiovasc Res 1987;21:217–222.
7. O'Brian E, Asmar R, Beilin L, et al. European Society of Hypertension. Recommendations for conventional, ambulatory and home blood pressure measurements. J Hypertens 2003;21:821–848.
8. Fagard R, Amery A. Physical exercise. In: Laragh JH, Brenner BM, eds. Hypertension: Pathophysiology, Diagnosis and Management, 2nd edn. New York: Raven Press; 1995:2669–2681.
9. Cregler LL. Substance abuse in sports: the impact of cocaine, alcohol, steroids, and other drugs on the heart. In: Williams RA, ed. The Athlete and Heart Disease. Philadelphia: Lippincott, Williams & Wilkins; 1999:131–153.
10. Bjørnstad H, Storstein L, Dyre Meen H, Hals O. Ambulatory electrocardiographic findings in top athletes, athletic students and control subjects. Cardiology 1994;84:42–45.
11. Caru B, Righetti G, Bossi M, Gerosa C, Gazzotti G, Maranetto D. Limits of cardiac functional adaptation in "top level" resistance athletes. Ital Heart J 2001;2(Suppl):150–154.
12. Vanhees L, Shepers D, Heidbuchel H, Defoor J, Fagard R. Exercise performance and training in patients with implantable cardioverter-defibrillators and coronary heart disease. Am J Cardiol 2001;87:712–715.
13. Piepoli MF, Davos C, Francis DP, Coats AJ; ExTraMATCH collaboration. Exercise training meta-analysis of trials in patients with chronic heart failure (ExTraMATCH). BMJ 2004;328 (7433):189.
14. Richard R, Verdier JC, Duvallet A, et al. Chronotropic competence in endurance trained heart transplant recipients: Heart rate is not a limiting factor for exercise capacity. J Am Coll Cardiol 1999;33:192–197.

15. Kobashigawa JA, Leaf DA, Lee N, et al. A controlled trial of exercise rehabilitation after heart transplantation. N Engl J Med 1999;340:272–277.

16. Braith RW, Limacher MC, Leggett SH, et al. Skeletal muscle strength in heart transplant recipients. J Heart Lung Transplant 1993;12:1018–1023.

17. Maron BJ, Chaitman BR, Ackerman M, et al. Recommendations for physical activity and recreational sports participation for young patients with genetic cardiovascular disease. Circulation 2004;109:2807–2816.

18. MacDougall JD, Tuxen D, Sale G, et al. Arterial blood pressure response to heavy resistance exercise. J Appl Physiol 1985;59:785–790.

19. Narloch JA, Branstater ME. Influence of breathing technique on arterial blood pressure during heavy weight lifting. Arch Phys Med Rehabil 1995;76:457–462.

20. Kerut EK, Norfleet WT, Plotnick GD, Giles TD. Patent foramen ovale: a review of associated conditions and the impact of physiological size. J Am Coll Cardiol 2001;38:613–623.

Section IV
Nutrition

Hippocrates' famous aphorism "we are what we eat" is more than ever pertinent at the present time. Indeed, strong scientific evidence has demonstrated that dietary patterns are important determinants of health status, especially concerning the cardiovascular system. However, nutrition must be considered not only as an energetic source, but must be integrated with its other components: culture, beliefs, tradition, and pleasure. This complexity explains why behavioral modifications in nutrition are so difficult to promote and sustain in people, often needing deep changes in ways of being and thinking. Moreover, as cardiovascular prevention is multifactorial, healthy food choices must often be combined with other behavioral modifications, such as smoking cessation or physical exercise, so our main task will be to help patients to cope with all these recommendations. For this purpose, this section will deal not only with the theoretical aspects, but also with the practical aspects of nutrition.

Main Messages

Chapter 23: Secondary Prevention of Coronary Heart Disease: Impact of Nutrition on the Risk of Fatal Complications and Importance of the Concept of Omega-3 Deficiency

In this chapter the role of nutrients in the prevention, occurrence, and treatment of cardiovascular disease (CVD), including heart failure, is described, as is the protective role of nutrients against sudden cardiac death.

Can adequate food habits protect against the development of the inflammatory component of CVD? Can it prevent plaque rupture? A recommendation for a "minimum" dietary program based upon the experiences from the Mediterranean diet studies concludes the chapter.

Chapter 24: Nutrition Counseling for Diabetic Patients

Nutritional counseling is a key component of cardiac prevention and rehabilitation and this is especially the case for the many diabetic patients among participants in cardiac rehabilitation programs.

This chapter gives a concise overview of the specific nutritional guidelines for patients with diabetes mellitus and concludes with useful practical recommendations on cooking, reading food labels, and eating out.

Chapter 25: Nutritional Counseling for Overweight Patients and Patients with Metabolic Syndrome

The global pandemic of overnutrition and the metabolic syndrome (MetS) calls for a structural change in programs for cardiovascular disease prevention and rehabilitation. Weight control has become increasingly important. Reducing energy intake is the cornerstone of weight management therapy and the key to successful weight management is to provide patients with a dietary regimen that results in long-term compliance.

This chapter states that the most effective therapeutic intervention in subjects with MetS is lifestyle changes, with the focus on modest weight reduction and regular leisure-time physical activities.

Chapter 26: Nutritional Counseling: Practical Models

The road from nutritional guidelines to practical application in the context of a comprehensive cardiac rehabilitation program is not an easy one for health workers and patients. This chapter aims at giving practical guidance based upon the long-standing experience of the team at the Bois-Gilbert Cardiac Rehabilitation Centre in France.

The chapter includes organizational issues and practical modalities and looks at nutritional counseling from the patient's perspective.

23

Secondary Prevention of Coronary Heart Disease: Impact of Nutrition on the Risk of Fatal Complications and Importance of the Concept of Omega-3 Deficiency

Michel de Lorgeril and Patricia Salen

Introduction

Active prevention of coronary heart disease (CHD) is usually started immediately after the first clinical manifestation of CHD. Secondary prevention should primarily focus on the risk of death. The two main causes of death in these patients are sudden cardiac death (SCD) and heart failure (HF), often resulting from myocardial ischemia and subsequent necrosis. In that context, it is crucial to understand that our populations are chronically and severely deficient in some major nutrients, in particular omega-3 fatty acids (n-3 PUFA). Actually, consumption of n-3 PUFA is inversely correlated with the risk of SCD, the main cause of death in CHD patients. On the other hand, the main mechanism underlying recurrent cardiac events is myocardial ischemia resulting from atherosclerotic plaque rupture or ulceration. Plaque rupture is usually the consequence of intraplaque inflammation in conjunction with a high lipid content of the lesion and high concentration of leukocytes and lipid peroxidation products. Thus, in patients with established CHD, the three main aims of the preventive strategy are (1) to prevent malignant ventricular arrhythmias and SCD, (2) to prevent the development of severe ventricular dysfunction and heart failure, and (3) to minimize the risk of plaque inflammation and ulceration. For that purpose, the adoption of a Mediterranean diet rich in omega-3 fatty acids seems to be the most effective strategy.

Dietary Prevention of Sudden Cardiac Death

Sudden cardiac death is usually defined as death from a cardiac cause occurring within one hour from the onset of symptoms.[1] In many studies, however, investigators used quite different definitions with a time frame of 3 hours or even 24 hours in the old World Health Organization definition. The magnitude of the problem is considerable as SCD is a very common, and often the first, manifestation of CHD, and it accounts for not less than 60% of cardiovascular mortality in developed countries.[1,2] In most cases, SCD occurs without prodromal symptoms and out of hospital. In fact, this mode of death is a major public health issue. Since up to 80% of SCD patients had CHD,[1] the epidemiology and potential preventive approaches in SCD should, in theory, parallel those of CHD. In other words, any treatment aimed at reducing CHD should reduce the incidence of SCD.

Fish, n-3 Fatty Acids, and SCD

The hypothesis that eating fish may protect against SCD is derived from the results of a secondary prevention trial, the Diet And Reinfarction Trial (DART), which showed a significant reduction in total and cardiovascular mortality (both by about 30%) in patients who had at least two servings of fatty fish per week.[3] The authors suggested that the protective effect of fish might be explained by a preventive action on ventricular fibrillation (VF), since no benefit was observed on the incidence of nonfatal acute myocardial infarction (AMI). This hypothesis was consistent with experimental evidence suggesting that n-3 polyunsaturated fatty acids (PUFA), the dominant fatty acids in fish oil and fatty fish, have an important effect on the occurrence of VF in the setting of myocardial ischemia and reperfusion in various animal models, both in vivo and in vitro.[4] In the same studies, it was also apparent that saturated fatty acids are proarrhythmic as compared to unsaturated fatty acids. Using an elegant in vivo model of SCD in dogs, Billman and co-workers demonstrated a striking reduction of VF after intravenous administration of pure n-3 PUFA, including both the long chain fatty acids present in fish oil and alpha-linolenic acid, their parent n-3 PUFA occurring in some vegetable oils.[4] These authors have found the mechanism of this protection to result from the electrophysiological effects of free n-3 PUFA when these are simply partitioned into the phospholipids of the sarcolemma without covalently bonding to any constituents of the cell membrane. After dietary intake, these fatty acids are preferentially incorporated into membrane phospholipids. It has also been shown that a very important pool of free (non-esterified) fatty acids exists in the normal myocardium and that the amount of n-3 PUFA in this pool is increased by supplementing the diet with n-3 PUFA. This illustrates the potential of diet to modify the structure and biochemical composition of cardiac cells. In ischemia, phospholipases and lipases quickly release new fatty acids from phospholipids, including n-3 fatty acids in higher amounts than the other fatty acids, thus further increasing the pool of free n-3 fatty acids that can exert an antiarrhythmic effect. It is important to remember that the lipoprotein lipase is particularly active following the consumption of n-3 PUFA. One hypothesis is that the presence of the free form of n-3 PUFA in the membrane of every cardiac muscle cell renders the myocardium more resistant to arrhythmias, probably by modulating the conduction of several membrane ion channels. So far, it seems that the very potent inhibitory effects of n-3 PUFA on the fast sodium current, I_{Na}, and the L-type calcium current, I_{CaL},[4] are the

major contributors to the antiarrhythmic actions of these fatty acids in ischemia. Briefly, n-3 PUFA act by shifting the steady-state inactivation potential to more negative values, as was also observed in other excitable tissues such as neurons.[4]

Another major aspect of that question is that most Western populations are severely deficient in omega-3 fatty acids from both the marine and terrestrial world. In the United States, experts from the American Heart Association claim that the average consumption of omega-3 fatty acids should be multiplied by 4 to attain the recommended intakes.[5] Intake of vegetable omega-3 should be doubled. The same trends are observed in European countries such as France. Chronic deficiency in omega-3 fatty acids probably explains at least partly the high prevalence of cardiac death (and SCD) in these countries.

Another important aspect of the implication of n-3 PUFA in SCD is their role in the metabolization of eicosanoids. In competition with n-6 PUFA, they are the precursors to a broad array of structurally diverse and potent bioactive lipids (including eicosanoids, prostaglandins, and thromboxanes), which are thought to play a role in the occurrence of VF during myocardial ischemia and reperfusion. These fatty acids (both n-6 PUFA and n-3 PUFA) also play a role in the development of vascular inflammation and atherosclerosis through the leukotriene pathway.[6]

Other clinical data show suppression (by more than 70%) of ventricular premature complexes in middle-aged patients with frequent ventricular extrasystoles randomly assigned to take either fish oil or placebo. Also, survivors of AMI and healthy men receiving fish oil were shown to improve their measurements of heart rate variability, suggesting other mechanisms by which n-3 PUFA may be antiarrhythmic.

Support for the hypothesis of a clinically significant antiarrhythmic effect of n-3 PUFA in the secondary prevention of CHD, as put forward in DART,[3] came from two randomized trials testing the effect of ethnic dietary patterns (instead of that a single food or nutrient), i.e. a Mediterranean type of diet and an Asian vegetarian diet, in the secondary prevention of CHD.[1,7] The two experimental diets included a high intake of essential alpha-linolenic acid, the main vegetable n-3 PUFA. Whereas the incidence of SCD was markedly reduced in both trials, the number of cases was small and the antiarrhythmic effect cannot be entirely attributed to alpha-linolenic acid as these experimental diets were also high in other nutrients with potential antiarrhythmic properties, including various antioxidants.

These findings were extended by the population-based case-control study conducted by Siscovick and colleagues on the intake of n-3 PUFA among patients with primary cardiac arrest, compared to that of age- and sex-matched controls.[8] These data confirm the very low consumption of n-3 PUFA in the Western populations (especially in comparison with the Japanese) and indicated that the intake of about 5 to 6 grams of n-3 PUFA per month (an amount provided by consuming fatty fish once or twice a week) was associated with a 50% reduction in the risk of cardiac arrest. In that study, the use of a biomarker, the red blood cell membrane level of n-3 PUFA, considerably enhanced the validity of the findings, which also were consistent with the results of many (but not all) cohort studies suggesting that consumption of one to two servings of fish per week is associated with a marked reduction in CHD mortality as compared to no fish intake. In most studies, however, the SCD endpoint is not reported.

In a large prospective study (more than 20,000 participants with a follow-up of 11 years), Albert et al. examined the specific point that fish has antiarrhythmic properties and may prevent SCD.[9] Again these investigators found a very low average consumption of n-3 PUFA. They found that the risk of SCD was 50% lower for men who consumed fish at least once a week than for those who had fish less than once a month. Interestingly, the consumption of fish was not related to non-sudden cardiac death, suggesting that the main protective effect of fish (or n-3 PUFA) is related to an effect on arrhythmia.

The GISSI-Prevenzione trial was aimed at helping in addressing the question of the health benefits of foods rich in n-3 PUFA (and also in vitamin E) and their pharmacological substitutes.[10] Patients ($n = 11,324$) surviving a recent AMI (<3 months) and having received the prior advice to come back to *a Mediterranean type of diet* were randomly assigned supplements of n-3 PUFA (0.8 g daily), vitamin E (300 mg daily), both, or neither (control) for 3.5 years. The primary efficacy endpoint was the combination of death and nonfatal AMI and stroke. Secondary analyses included overall mortality, cardiovascular (CV) mortality, and SCD. Treatment with n-3 PUFA significantly lowered the risk of the primary endpoint (the relative risk decreased by 15%). Secondary analyses provided a clearer profile of the clinical effects of n-3 PUFA. Overall mortality was reduced by 20% and CV mortality by 30%. However, it was the effect on SCD (45% lower) that accounted for most of the benefits seen in the primary combined endpoint and both overall and CV mortality. There was no difference across the treatment groups for nonfatal CV events, a result comparable to that of DART.[3] Thus, the results obtained in this randomized trial are consistent with previous controlled trials,[1] large-scale observational studies,[8,9] and experimental studies,[4] which together strongly support an effect of n-3 PUFA in relation to SCD.

Regarding the physiopathology, administering n-3 PUFA *intravenously* to patients with an ICD (implanted defibrillator) and at very high risk of SCD seems to provide these patients with an extraordinary degree of protection against malignant ventricular arrhythmias.[11] Recently, at the 2004 meeting of the European Society of Cardiology in Munich, Leaf and colleagues reported that the main protective effect of very long chain n-3 PUFA, eicosapentaenoic acid (EPA), and docosahexaenoic acid (DHA) probably results from the prevention of malignant arrhythmias. In fact, in the Fatty Acid Anti-Arrhythmia Trial (FAAT) conducted in more than 400 patients at high risk of SCD (and with ICDs), patients randomized to receive (double-blind protocol) a mix of 2.4 g of EPA + DHA had a 40% reduction of the risk of malignant ventricular arrhythmias as recorded by the ICD compared with those receiving the placebo.

Saturated Fatty Acids, Oleic Acid, *trans* Fatty Acids, and n-6 Fatty Acids

Regarding the other dietary fatty acids, animal experiments have clearly indicated that a diet rich in saturated fatty acids is associated with a high incidence of ischemia- and reperfusion-induced ventricular arrhythmia, whereas PUFAs of either the n-6 or n-3 family reduce that risk.[4] Large (but not all) epidemiological studies have shown consistent associations between the intake of saturated fatty acids and CHD mortality.[1] However, the SCD endpoint is usually not analyzed in these studies. In addition, a clear demonstration of a causal relationship between dietary saturated fatty acids and SCD would require the organization of a randomized trial, which is not ethically acceptable. Thus, besides the effect of saturated fatty acids on blood cholesterol levels, the exact mechanism(s) by which saturated fats increase CHD mortality remain unclear. If animal data, demonstrating a proarrhythmic effect of saturated fatty acids, are confirmed in humans, the first thing to do in order to prevent SCD in humans would be to drastically reduce the intake of saturated fats. In fact, this has been done in randomized dietary trials and, as expected, the rate of SCD decreased in the experimental groups.[1] However, as written above about the same trials,[1] the beneficial effect cannot be entirely attributed to the reduction of saturated fats, because other potentially antiarrhythmic dietary factors, including n-3 PUFA, were also modified in these trials.

In contrast with n-3 PUFA, few data have been published so far in humans regarding the effect of n-6 PUFA on the risk of SCD. Roberts et al. have reported that the percentage content of linoleic acid (the dominant n-6 PUFA in the diet) in adipose tissue (an indicator of long-term dietary intake) was inversely related to the risk of SCD, which was defined in that study as instantaneous death or death within 24 hours of the onset of symptoms.[1] This is in line with most animal data and may suggest that patients at risk of SCD may benefit from increasing their dietary intake of n-6 PUFA, in particular linoleic acid, in the same way as for n-3 PUFA. It should be mentioned, however, that n-3 PUFA were more effective on SCD than n-6 PUFA in most animal experiments.[4]

In addition, diets high in n-6 PUFA increase the linoleic acid content of lipoproteins and render them more susceptible to oxidation, which would be an argument against such diets because lipoprotein oxidation is a major step in the inflammatory process that renders atherosclerotic lesions unstable and prone to rupture.

Erosion and rupture of atherosclerotic lesions were shown to trigger CHD complications (see the section on plaque inflammation and rupture

below) and myocardial ischemia and to considerably enhance the risk of SCD. In fact, in the secondary prevention of CHD, diets high in n-6 PUFA failed to improve the overall prognosis of the patients. Also, in the Dayton study (the Los Angeles Veteran trial), a mixed primary and secondary prevention trial, in which the chief characteristic of the experimental diet was the substitution of n-6 PUFA for saturated fat, the number of SCDs was apparently lower in the experimental group than in the control group (18 vs. 27) but the number of deaths from other causes, in particular cancers, was higher in the experimental group (85 vs. 71), thus offsetting the potential protective effect of n-6 PUFA on SCD and resulting in no effect at all on mortality. Such negative effects were not reported with n-3 PUFA.

Thus, despite the beneficial effect of n-6 PUFA on lipoprotein levels, which could, in theory, reduce SCD in the long term by reducing the development of atherosclerosis, it seems preferable not to increase the consumption of n-6 PUFA beyond the amounts required to prevent deficiencies in the essential n-6 fatty acid, linoleic acid (approximately 4–6% of the total energy intake), which are found in the current average Western diet. As a substitute for saturated fat, the best choice is obviously to increase the intake of vegetable monounsaturated fat (oleic acid) in accordance with the Mediterranean diet pattern. If oleic acid has apparently no effect on the risk of SCD (at least by comparison with n-3 and n-6 PUFA), its effects on blood lipoprotein levels are similar to those of n-6 PUFA and it has the great advantage of protecting lipoproteins against oxidation.

Thus, the best fatty acid combination to prevent SCD (and the other complications of CHD) and, in other words, to cumulate antiarrhythmic, antioxidant, and hypolipidemic effects, would result from the adoption of a diet close to the Mediterranean diet pattern.

Finally, Roberts et al. reported no significant relationship between *trans* isomers of oleic and linoleic acids in adipose tissue and the risk of SCD whereas Lemaitre et al. found that cell membrane *trans* isomers of linoleic acid (but not of oleic acid) are associated with a large increase in the risk of primary cardiac arrest. As for the role of *trans* fatty acids on ventricular arrhythmias, it has not been investigated in experimental models.

Thus, although specific human data on the effect of saturated fatty acids on SCD are lacking, results of several trials suggest that it is important to reduce their intake in the secondary prevention of CHD. Despite a possible beneficial effect on the risk of SCD, increasing consumption of n-6 PUFA should not be recommended in clinical practice for patients with established CHD. Diets including low intakes in saturated fatty acid (as well as *trans* isomers of linoleic acid) and n-6 PUFA (but enough to provide the essential linoleic acid) and high intakes in n-3 PUFA and oleic acid (Mediterranean diet pattern) appear to be the best option to prevent both SCD and nonfatal AMI recurrence.[12]

Alcohol and SCD

The question of the effect of alcohol on heart and vessel diseases has been the subject of intense controversy in recent years. The consensus is now that moderate alcohol drinking is associated with reduced cardiovascular mortality, although the exact mechanism(s) by which alcohol is protective are still unclear. In experimental models, an ethanol preconditioning phenomenon[13] has been reported, suggesting that low dose ethanol drinking protects the myocardium against damages provoked by ischemia. In contrast, chronic heavy drinking has been incriminated in the occurrence of atrial as well as ventricular arrhythmias in humans, an effect called "the holiday heart" because it is often associated with binge drinking by healthy people, specifically during the weekend. Studies in animals have shown varying and apparently contradictory effects of alcohol on cardiac rhythm and conduction, depending on the animal species, the experimental model, and the dose of alcohol. If given acutely to non-alcoholic animals, ethanol may even have antiarrhythmic properties.

In humans, few studies have specifically investigated the effect of alcohol on SCD. The hyperadrenergic state resulting from binge drinking, as well as from withdrawal in alcoholics, seems to be the main mechanism by which alcohol induces arrhythmias in humans. In the British Regional Heart Study, the relative risk of SCD in heavy drinkers (>6 drinks per day) was twice as high as in occasional or light drinkers. However, the effect of binge drinking on SCD was more evident in

men with no pre-existing CHD than in those with established CHD. In contrast, in the Honolulu Heart Program, the risk of SCD among healthy middle-aged men was positively related to blood pressure, serum cholesterol, smoking, and left ventricular hypertrophy but inversely related to alcohol intake. In fact, the effect of moderate "social" drinking on the risk of SCD in non-alcoholic subjects has been addressed so far in only one study. Investigators of the Physicians' Health Study assessed whether light-to-moderate alcohol drinkers apparently free of CHD at baseline have a decreased risk of SCD.[14] After controlling for multiple confounders, men who consumed 2 to 4 drinks per week or 5 to 6 drinks per week at baseline had a significantly reduced risk of SCD (by 60–80%) compared with those who rarely or never consumed alcohol. Analyses were repeated after excluding deaths occurring during the first 4 years of follow-up (in order to exclude the possibility that some men who refrained from drinking at baseline did so because of early symptoms of heart diseases), and also using the updated measure of alcohol intake ascertained at year 7 to address potential misclassification in the baseline evaluation of alcohol drinking.[14] These secondary analyses basically provided the same results and confirmed the potential protective effect of moderate drinking on the risk of SCD. Despite limitations (the selected nature of the cohort, an exclusively male study group, no information on beverage type and drinking pattern), this study suggests that a significant part of the cardioprotective effect of moderate drinking is related to the prevention of SCD. Further research should be directed at understanding the mechanism(s) by which moderate alcohol drinking may prevent ventricular arrhythmias and SCD.

In practice, current state knowledge suggests that in CHD patients at risk of SCD, there is no reason not to allow moderate alcohol drinking. From a practical point of view, we advise one or two drinks per day, preferably wine, preferably during the evening meal, and never before driving a car or doing dangerous work.

Cholesterol Lowering and SCD

Another important issue at a time when so many people are taking cholesterol-lowering drugs with the hope to improve their life expectancy is whether cholesterol lowering might reduce the risk of SCD. According to recent data standardized to the 2000 US population,[2] of 719,456 cardiac deaths among adults aged >35 years, 63% were defined as sudden cardiac death (SCD). In that study, SCD was defined as death occurring out of the hospital or in the emergency room or as "dead on arrival" with an underlying cause of death reported as a cardiac disease. Among those aged 35 to 55, about 75% of cardiac deaths were SCD.[2]

Another question is: are we able to identify people at risk of SCD? In other words, are the traditional risk factors of CHD predictive of SCD? Several studies have recently tried to answer that question. For instance, in a prospective study in healthy men, investigators found that only C-reactive protein (CRP) was significantly associated with the risk of SCD whereas homocysteine and all lipid parameters, including total and LDL cholesterol levels, were not.[15] In another study investigating the determinants of SCD in women, diabetes and smoking conferred markedly elevated risk of SCD whereas hypercholesterolemia did not increase the risk of SCD.[16] Thus, it seems that high cholesterol level is not a risk factor for SCD while SCD appears to be the main cause of CHD death.

If these epidemiological data are true, the next obvious question is whether (or in which proportions) cholesterol lowering is able to reduce the risk of SCD and consequently the risk of CHD death. As the best cholesterol-lowering treatments are the statin drugs, it is important to look at the SCD data (and CHD mortality data) in the recently published statin trials. However, in most (recent as well as old) statin trials, there is curiously no data regarding the effect of statins on SCD. This suggests that, as expected from epidemiological data, statins had no significant effect on SCD. Given the importance of SCD as a cause of death in CHD patients, we can therefore suspect that the effect of cholesterol lowering by statins on CHD death was, at best, small. In fact, when carefully looking at the published trials, it appears that the effect of statins on mortality was either small or non significant. For instance, in HPS, PROSPER, ALLHAT-LLT, ASCOT-LLA, and ALLIANCE, the death rate ratios were 0.87(indicating a risk reduction of 13%), 0.97

(nonsignificant), 0.99 (nonsignificant), 0.87 (nonsignificant), and 0.92 (nonsignificant), respectively.[17–21] Furthermore, the effect of statins specifically in women has been recently analyzed using a meta-analysis of 13 studies retained in the Cochrane database.[22] The authors conclude that in both primary and secondary prevention, statins had no significant effect on mortality in women. Finally, in the most recent statin trials focusing on patients with acute CHD syndromes and early and intensive lipid lowering (MIRACL, PROVE-IT, A to Z Trial), the effects on mortality were again small or nonsignificant despite the recruitment of several thousand patients in these trials.[23,24] Thus, cholesterol lowering with statins does not appear to be a very effective way of reducing CHD mortality in our populations. This is not unexpected as the main cause of CHD death is SCD (up to 75% of cardiac deaths among people aged 35–55) and SCD is apparently not determined by lipid factors.

Diet and the Risk of Heart Failure Following AMI

The incidence of chronic heart failure (CHF), the common end-result of most cardiac diseases, is increasing steadily in many countries despite (and probably because of) considerable improvements in the acute and chronic treatment of CHD, which is nowadays the main cause of CHF in most countries.[25] In recent years, most research effort about CHF has been focused on drug treatment, and there has been little attention paid to non-pharmacological management. Some unidentified factors may indeed contribute to the rise in the prevalence of CHF and should be recognized and corrected if possible. For instance, CHF is now seen also as a metabolic problem with endocrine and immunological disturbances potentially contributing to the progression of the disease. In particular, the role of tumor necrosis factor (TNF) is discussed below. Only recently has it also been recognized that increased oxidative stress may contribute to the pathogenesis of CHF. The intimate link between diet and oxidative stress is obvious, knowing that the major antioxidant defenses of our body are derived from essential nutrients.

While it is generally considered that a high sodium diet is detrimental (and may result in acute decompensation of heart failure through a volume overload mechanism), little is known about other aspects of diet in CHF in terms of both general nutrition and micronutrients such as vitamins and minerals. In these patients, it is important not only to take care of the diagnosis and treatment of the CHF syndrome itself and the identification and aggressive management of traditional risk factors of CHD such as high blood pressure and diabetes (because they can aggravate the syndrome), but also to recognize and correct malnutrition and deficiencies in specific micronutrients.

The vital importance of micronutrients for health and the fact that several micronutrients have antioxidant properties are now fully recognized. These may be as direct antioxidants such as vitamins C and E or as components of antioxidant enzymes: superoxide dismutase or glutathione peroxidase. It is now widely believed (but still not causally demonstrated) that diet-derived antioxidants may play a role in the development (and thus in the prevention) of CHF. For instance, clinical and experimental studies have suggested that CHF may be associated with increased free radical formation and reduced antioxidant defenses and that vitamin C may improve endothelial function in patients with CHF. In the secondary prevention of CHD, in dietary trials in which the tested diet included high intakes of natural antioxidants, the incidence of new episodes of CHF was reduced in the experimental groups. Taken altogether, these data suggest (but do not demonstrate) that antioxidant nutrients may help prevent CHF in postinfarction patients.

Other nutrients, however, may also be involved in some cases of CHF. While deficiency in certain micronutrients, whatever the reason, can actually cause CHF and should be corrected (see below), it is important to understand that patients with CHF also have symptoms that can affect their food intake and result in deficiencies, for instance tiredness when strained, breathing difficulties, and gastrointestinal symptoms like nausea, loss of appetite, and early feeling of satiety. Drug therapy can lead to loss of appetite and excess urinary losses in case of diuretic use. All of these are mainly consequences, not causative factors, of

CHF. Thus the basic treatment of CHF should, in theory, improve these nutritional anomalies. However, since they can contribute to the development and severity of CHF, they should be recognized and corrected as early as possible.

Finally, it has been shown that up to 50% of patients with CHF are malnourished to some degree, and CHF is often associated with weight loss. There may be multiple etiologies to the weight loss, in particular lack of activity resulting in loss of muscle bulk and increased resting metabolic rate. There is also a shift towards catabolism with insulin resistance and increased catabolic relative to anabolic steroids. TNF, sometimes called cachectin (see above), is higher in many patients with CHF, which may explain weight loss in these patients. Interestingly, there is a positive correlation between TNF and markers of oxidative stress in the failing heart, suggesting a link between TNF and antioxidant defenses in CHF (the potential importance of TNF in CHF is discussed below in the section on dietary fatty acids and CHF). Finally, cardiac cachexia is a well-recognized complication of CHF, its prevalence increases as symptoms worsen, and it is an independent predictor of mortality in CHF patients. However, the pathophysiological alteration leading to cachexia remains unclear and at present, there is no specific treatment apart from the treatment of the basic illness and correction of the associated biological abnormalities.

Deficiency in Specific Micronutrients

As discussed above, an important practical point is that deficiencies in specific micronutrients can actually cause CHF, or at least aggravate it. The prevalence of these deficiencies among patients with CHF (and post-infarction patients) is unknown. Whether we should systematically search for them also remains unclear. In particular, we do not know whether the association of several borderline deficiencies that do not individually result in CHF may result in CHF, especially in the elderly. For certain authors, however, there is sufficient evidence to support a large-scale trial of dietary micronutrient supplementation in CHF.

There is no room here to fully explore the present knowledge in this field. Nonetheless, if we restrict our comments only to human data, things can be summarized as follows. Cases of hypocalcemia-induced cardiomyopathy (usually in children with a congenital cause for hypocalcemia) that can respond dramatically to calcium supplementation have been reported. Hypomagnesemia is often associated with a poor prognosis in CHF, and correction of the magnesium levels (in anorexia nervosa for instance) leads to an improvement in cardiac function. Low serum and high urinary zinc levels are found in CHF, possibly as a result of diuretic use, but there are no data regarding the clinical effect of zinc supplementation in that context. In a recent study, plasma copper was slightly higher and zinc slightly lower in CHF subjects than in healthy controls. As expected, dietary intakes were in the normal range and no significant relationship was found between dietary intakes and blood levels in the two groups. It is not possible to say whether these copper and zinc abnormalities may contribute to the development of CHF or are simply markers for the chronic inflammation known to be associated with CHF. Further studies are needed to address the point, since the implications for prevention are substantial.

Selenium deficiency has been identified as a major factor in the etiology of certain non-ischemic CHF syndromes, especially in low-selenium soil areas such as eastern China and West Africa. In Western countries, cases of congestive cardiomyopathy associated with low antioxidant nutrients (vitamins and trace elements) have been reported in malnourished HIV-infected patients and in subjects on chronic parenteral nutrition. Selenium deficiency is also a risk factor for peripartum cardiomyopathy. In China, an endemic cardiomyopathy called Keshan disease seems to be a direct consequence of selenium deficiency. Whereas the question of the mechanism by which selenium deficiency results in CHF remains open, recent data suggest that selenium may be involved in skeletal (and cardiac) muscle deconditioning (and in CHF symptoms such as fatigue and low exercise tolerance) rather than in left ventricular dysfunction. Actually, in the Keshan area, the selenium status coincides with the clinical severity rather than with the degree of left ventricular dysfunction as assessed by echocardiographic studies. When the selenium

levels of residents were raised to the typical levels in the non-endemic areas, the mortality rate declined significantly but clinically latent cases were still found and the echocardiographic prevalence of the disease remained high. What we learn from Keshan disease and other studies conducted elsewhere is therefore that in patients with a known cause of CHF, even a mild deficiency in selenium may influence the clinical severity of the disease (tolerance to exercise).

These data should serve as a strong incentive for the initiation of studies testing the effects of natural antioxidants on the clinical severity of CHF. In the meantime, however, physicians would be well advised to measure selenium in patients with an exercise inability disproportionate to their cardiac dysfunction.

Finally, low whole blood thiamine (vitamin B_1) levels have been documented in patients with CHF on loop diuretics and hospitalized elderly patients, and thiamine supplementation induced a significant improvement in cardiac function and symptoms.

Dietary Fatty Acids and Sodium Intake, Cytokines, LVH, and CHF

Beyond the well-known effect of high sodium intake on the clinical course of CHF (and the occurrence of acute episodes of decompensation), another important issue is the role of diet in the development of left ventricular hypertrophy (LVH), a major risk factor for CHF (and also SCD), as well as for cardiovascular and all-cause mortality and morbidity.

The cause of LVH is largely unknown. Whereas male gender, obesity, heredity, and insulin resistance may explain some of the variance in LVH, hypertension (HBP) is generally regarded as the primary culprit. Thus, the risks associated with LVH and HBP are intimately linked. Recent data also suggested that low dietary intake of polyunsaturated fatty acids and high intake of saturated fatty acids, as well as HBP and obesity, at age 50 predicted the prevalence of LVH 20 years later. Although the source of saturated fatty acids is usually animal fat, the source of unsaturated fatty acids in that specific Scandinavian population and at that time was less clear and there was no adjustment for other potential dietary confounders such as magnesium, potassium, calcium, and sodium. Thus this study did not provide conclusive data regarding the dietary lipid determinants of LVH. However, it does suggest that dietary fatty acids may be involved in the development of LVH and that this "diet–heart connection" may partly explain the harmful effect of animal saturated fatty acids on the heart.

Another "diet–heart connection" in the context of advanced CHF relates to the recent theory that CHF also is a low-grade chronic inflammatory disease with elevated circulating levels of cytokines and cytokine receptors that are otherwise independent predictors of mortality. High-dose ACE inhibition with enalapril, a treatment that reduces mechanical overload and shear stress (two stimuli for cytokine production in patients with CHF), was recently shown to decrease both cytokine bioactivity and left ventricular wall thickness. Finally, various anti-cytokine and immunomodulating agents were shown to have beneficial effect on heart function and clinical functional class in patients with advanced CHF, suggesting a causal relationship between high cytokine production and CHF. This also suggests that there is a potential for therapies altering cytokine production in CHF. In that regard, it has been shown that dietary supplementation with n-3 fatty acids (either fish oil or vegetable oil rich in n-3 fatty acid) reduces cytokine production at least in healthy volunteers. An inverse exponential relationship between leukocyte n-3 fatty acid content and cytokine production by these cells was found, most of the reduction in cytokine production being seen with eicosapentaenoic acid in cell membrane lower than 1%, a level obtained with rather moderate n-3 fatty acid supplementation. However, further studies are warranted to test whether (and at which dosage) dietary n-3 fatty acids might influence the clinical course of CHF through an anti-cytokine effect.

Sodium intake is the environmental factor that is currently most suspected of influencing blood pressure and the prevalence of HBP. However, the full damaging potential of high sodium intake for the heart (and also the kidney) seems to be largely independent of the pressor effect of sodium. Animal experiments and clinical studies have consistently shown that high sodium intake is a powerful and independent determinant of LVH and that such an arterial-pressure-independent effect of salt is not confined to the heart.

Whereas the long-term effect of a reduced sodium intake after a recent AMI is unknown, in particular on LVH, experts claim that even a 50 mmol reduction in the daily sodium intake would reduce the average systolic blood pressure by at least 5 mmHg (in patients aged over 50 years) and CHD mortality by about 16%. Thus, as regards the damaging effect of high sodium intake on the heart, and despite the lack of strong data showing the beneficial effect of reducing sodium intake in that specific group of patients, we believe that cardiologists should extend their dietary counseling about sodium not only to patients with HBP or CHF but also to all post-infarction patients.

Diet and the Prevention of Plaque Inflammation and Rupture

For several decades, the prevention of CHD (including the prevention of ischemic recurrence after a prior AMI) has focused on the reduction of the traditional risk factors: smoking, HBP, hypercholesterolemia. Priority was given to the prevention (or reversion) of vascular atherosclerotic stenosis. As discussed above, it has become clear in secondary prevention that it is of primary importance to prevent the fatal complications of CHD such as SCD. This does not mean, however, that we should not try slowing down the atherosclerotic process, and in particular plaque inflammation and rupture. Indeed, it is critical to prevent the occurrence of new episodes of myocardial ischemia whose repetition in a recently injured heart can precipitate SCD or CHF. Myocardial ischemia is usually the consequence of coronary occlusion caused by plaque rupture and subsequent thrombotic obstruction of the artery. Recent progress in the understanding of the cellular and biochemical pathogenesis of atherosclerosis suggests that, in addition to the traditional risk factors of CHD, there are other very important targets of therapy to prevent plaque inflammation and rupture. In this regard, the most important question is: how and why does plaque rupture occur?

CHD Is an Inflammatory Disease

Most investigators agree that atherosclerosis is a chronic low-grade inflammatory disease.[26] Pro-inflammatory factors (free radicals produced by cigarette smoking, hyperhomocysteinemia, diabetes, peroxidized lipids, hypertension, elevated and modified blood lipids) contribute to the injury to the vascular endothelium, which results in alterations of its antiatherosclerotic and antithrombotic properties. This is thought to be a major step in the initiation and formation of arterial fibrostenotic lesions. From a clinical point of view, however, an essential distinction should be made between unstable, lipid-rich and leukocyte-rich lesions and stable, acellular fibrotic lesions poor in lipids, as the propensity of these two types of lesion to rupture into the lumen of the artery, whatever the degree of stenosis and lumen obstruction, is totally different.

In 1987, we proposed that inflammation and leukocytes play a role in the onset of acute CHD events.[27] This has recently been confirmed. It is now accepted that one of the main mechanisms underlying the sudden onset of acute CHD syndromes, including unstable angina, myocardial infarction, and SCD, is the erosion or rupture of an atherosclerotic lesion, which triggers thrombotic complications and considerably enhances the risk of malignant ventricular arrhythmias. Leukocytes have been also implicated in the occurrence of ventricular arrhythmias in clinical and experimental settings, and they contribute to myocardial damage during both ischemia and reperfusion. Clinical and pathological studies showed the importance of inflammatory cells and immune mediators in the occurrence of acute CHD events and prospective epidemiological studies showed a strong and consistent association between acute CHD and systemic inflammation markers. A major challenge is to understand why there are macrophages and activated lymphocytes in atherosclerotic lesions and how they get there. Issues such as local inflammation, plaque rupture, and attendant acute CHD complications follow.

The Lipid Oxidation Theory of CHD

Steinberg et al. proposed in 1989 that oxidation of lipoproteins causes accelerated atherogenesis.[28]

Elevated plasma levels of low-density lipoproteins (LDL) are a major factor in CHD, and reduction of blood LDL levels (for instance by drugs) results in less CHD. However, the mechanism(s) behind the effect of high LDL levels is not fully understood. The concept that LDL oxidation is a key characteristic of unstable lesions is supported by many reports. Two processes have been proposed. First, when LDL particles become trapped in the artery wall, they undergo progressive oxidation and are internalized by macrophages, leading to the formation of typical atherosclerotic foam cells. Oxidized LDL is chemotactic for other immune and inflammatory cells and upregulates the expression of monocyte and endothelial cell genes involved in the inflammatory reaction. The inflammatory response itself can have a profound effect on LDL, creating a vicious circle of LDL oxidation, inflammation and further LDL oxidation. Second, oxidized LDL circulates in the plasma for a period sufficiently long to enter and accumulate in the arterial intima, suggesting that the entry of oxidized lipoproteins within the intima may be another mechanism of lesion inflammation, in particular in patients without hyperlipidemia. Elevated plasma levels of oxidized LDL are associated with CHD, and the plasma level of malondialdehyde-modified LDL is higher in patients with unstable CHD syndromes (usually associated with plaque rupture) than in patients with clinically stable CHD. In the accelerated form of CHD typical of post-transplantation patients, higher levels of lipid peroxidation and of oxidized LDL were found as compared to the stable form of CHD in non-transplanted patients. Reactive oxygen metabolites and oxidants influence thrombus formation, and platelet reactivity is significantly higher in transplanted patients than in non-transplanted CHD patients.

The oxidized LDL theory is not inconsistent with the well-established lipid-lowering treatment of CHD, as there is a positive correlation between plasma levels of LDL and markers of lipid peroxidation, and a low absolute LDL level results in reduced amounts of LDL available for oxidative modification. LDL levels can be lowered by drugs or by reducing saturated fats in the diet. Reduction of the oxidative susceptibility of LDL was reported when dietary fat was replaced with carbohydrates. Pharmacological/quantitative (lowering of cholesterol) and nutritional/qualitative (high antioxidant intake) approaches to the prevention of CHD are not mutually exclusive but additive and complementary. An alternative way to reduce LDL concentrations is to replace saturated fats with polyunsaturated fats in the diet. However, diets high in polyunsaturated fatty acids increase the polyunsaturated fatty acid content of LDL particles and render them more susceptible to oxidation (which would argue against use of such diets (see the section on SCD and n-6 PUFA above). In fact, in the secondary prevention of CHD, such diets failed to improve patient prognosis. In that context, the traditional Mediterranean diet, with low saturated fat and polyunsaturated fat intakes, appears to be the best option. Diets rich in oleic acid increase the resistance of LDL to oxidation independent of the antioxidant content and results in leukocyte inhibition. Thus, oleic acid-rich diets decrease the pro-inflammatory properties of oxidized LDL. Constituents of olive oil other than oleic acid may also inhibit LDL oxidation. Various components of the Mediterranean diet may also affect LDL oxidation. For instance, alpha-tocopherol or vitamin C, or a diet combining reduced fat, low-fat dairy products and a high intake of fruits and vegetables, was shown to favorably affect either LDL oxidation itself or/and the cellular consequences of LDL oxidation.

Finally, a significant correlation was found between certain dietary fatty acids and the fatty acid composition of human atherosclerotic plaques, which suggests that dietary fatty acids are rapidly incorporated into the plaques. This implies a direct influence of dietary fatty acids on plaque formation and the process of plaque rupture. It is conceivable that fatty acids that stimulate oxidation of LDL (n-6 PUFA) induce plaque rupture whereas those that inhibit LDL oxidation (oleic acid) inhibit leukocyte function (n-3 PUFA), or prevent "endothelial activation," and the expression of pro-inflammatory proteins (oleic acid and n-3 fatty acids) helps to pacify and stabilize the dangerous lesions. In this regard, it is noteworthy that moderate alcohol consumption, a well-known cardioprotective factor, was recently shown to be associated with low blood levels of systemic markers of inflammation, suggesting a new protective mechanism to explain the inverse relationship between alcohol and CHD rate. Similarly, the potential of dietary n-3 fatty acids to reduce the production of inflammatory cytokines by leukocytes (as discussed in the section on dietary fatty acids and CHF) should be underlined. As both dietary n-3 fatty acids and moderate alcohol consumption are major characteristics of the Mediterranean diet, it is not surprising to observe that this diet was associated with lower rate of new episodes of CHF in the Lyon Diet Heart Study.[12]

Thus, any dietary pattern combining a high intake of natural antioxidants, a low intake of saturated fatty acids, a high intake of oleic acid, a low intake of omega-6 fatty acids, and a high intake of omega-3 fatty acids would logically produce a highly cardioprotective effect. This is consistent with what we know about the *Mediterranean diet pattern*[29] and with the results of the Lyon Diet Heart Study and was recently confirmed by the GISSI investigators.

A Minimum Clinical Priority Dietary Program

Despite the increased evidence that dietary prevention is critical in the post-AMI patient, many physicians (and their patients) remain rather poorly informed about the potential of diet to reduce cardiac mortality, the risk of new CHD complications, and the need for recurrent hospitalization and investigation. There are many reasons for that, the main one probably being an insufficient knowledge of nutrition. For that reason (and knowing the resistance of many physicians to the idea that diet is important in CHD), we propose *a minimum dietary program* that every CHD patient, whatever his/her medical and familial environment, should know and follow. This minimum "Mediterranean" diet should include the following:

1. Reduced consumption of animal saturated fat (for instance, by totally excluding butter and cream from the daily diet and drastic reduction of fatty meat) and increased consumption of n-3 fatty acids through increased intakes of fatty fish (a minimum of about 200 g, twice a week). For patients who cannot eat fish (for any reason),

taking capsules of n-3 fatty acids (for instance, a mix of alpha-linolenic acid and long chain n-3 fatty acids) is the best alternative option. Very importantly, the patients (and their physicians) should be aware that n-3 fatty acid supplementation will be even more cardioprotective if associated with adequate dietary modifications discussed in the text above.

2. Increased intake of anti-inflammatory fatty acids (oleic acid and n-3 fatty acids) and decreased intake of pro-inflammatory fatty acids (n-6 fatty acids). The best way is to exclusively use olive oil and canola oil for cooking and salad dressing and canola oil-based margarine instead of butter and polyunsaturated oils and margarines. Patients should also systematically reject convenience food prepared with fats rich in saturated, polyunsaturated, and *trans* fatty acids.

3. Increased intake of natural antioxidants (vitamins and trace elements) and folates through increased consumption of fresh fruits and vegetables and tree nuts.

4. Moderate intake of alcoholic beverages (1 or 2 drinks per day), preferably wine, preferably during the evening meal, and never before driving or making a dangerous technical manipulation.

5. Reduction of sodium intake (below 100 mmol per day if possible) knowing that it is a very difficult task at the present time because of the high sodium content of many natural (including typical Mediterranean foods such as olives and cheeses) and convenience foods.

However, patients (and physicians) should keep in mind that an optimal (and individual) dietary prevention program should be managed under the guidance of a professional dietitian aware of the most recent scientific advances in the field.

References

1. de Lorgeril M, Salen P, Defaye P, et al. Dietary prevention of sudden cardiac death. Eur Heart J 2002;23:277–285.
2. Zheng ZJ, Croft JB, Giles WH, Mensah GA. Sudden cardiac death in the United States, 1989 to 1998. Circulation 2001;104:2158–2163.
3. Burr ML, Fehily AM, Gilbert JF, et al. Effects of changes in fat, fish, and fibre intakes on death and myocardial reinfarction: Diet And Reinfarction Trial (DART). Lancet 1989;ii:757–761.
4. Leaf A, Kang JX, Xiao YF, Billman GE. Clinical prevention of sudden cardiac death by n-3 polyunsaturated fatty acids and mechanism of prevention of arrhythmias by n-3 fish oils. Circulation 2003;107: 2646–2652.
5. Kris-Etherton PM, Shaffer Taylor D, Yu-Poth S, et al. Polyunsaturated fatty acids in the food chain in the United States. Am J Clin Nutr 2000;71(suppl): 179S–88S.
6. De Caterina A, Zampoli R. From asthma to atherosclerosis – 5-lipoxygenase, leukotrienes, and inflammation. N Engl J Med 2004;350:4–7.
7. de Lorgeril M, Renaud S, Mamelle N, et al. Mediterranean alpha-linolenic acid-rich diet in secondary prevention of coronary heart disease. Lancet 1994; 343:1454–1459.
8. Siscovick DS, Raghunathan TE, King I, et al. Dietary intake and cell membrane levels of long-chain n-3 polyunsaturated fatty acids and the risk of primary cardiac arrest. JAMA 1995;274:1363–1367.
9. Albert CM, Hennekens CH, O'Donnel CJ, et al. Fish consumption and the risk of sudden cardiac death. JAMA 1998;279:23–28.
10. GISSI-Prevenzione investigators. Dietary supplementation with n-3 polyunsaturated fatty acids and vitamin E after myocardial infarction: results of the GISSI-Prevenzione trial. Lancet 1999;354:447–455.
11. Schrepf R, Limmert T, Wever PC, et al. Immediate effects of n-3 fatty acid infusion on the induction of sustained ventricular tachycardia. Lancet 2004;363: 1441–1442.
12. de Lorgeril M, Salen P, Martin JL, et al. Mediterranean diet, traditional risk factors and the rate of cardiovascular complications after myocardial infarction. Final report of the Lyon Diet Heart Study. Circulation 1999;99:779–785.
13. Guiraud A, de Lorgeril M, Boucher F, et al. Cardioprotective effect of chronic low dose ethanol drinking. Insights into the concept of ethanol preconditioning. J Mol Cell Cardiol 2004;36:561–566.
14. Albert CM, Manson JE, Cook NR, et al. Moderate alcohol consumption and the risk of sudden cardiac death among US male physicians. Circulation 1999;100:944–950.
15. Albert CM, Ma J, Rifai N, et al. Prospective study of C-reactive protein, homocysteine, and plasma lipid levels as predictors of sudden cardiac death. Circulation 2002;105:2595–2599.
16. Albert CM, Chae CU, Grodstein F, et al. Prospective study of sudden cardiac death among women in the United States. Circulation 2003;107:2096–2101.
17. Heart Protection Study Collaborative Group. MRC: BHF heart protection Study of cholesterol lowering

with simvastatin in 20536 high-risk individuals: a randomised placebo-controlled trial. Lancet 2002; 360:7–22.

18. Shepherd J, et al. Pravastatin in elderly individuals at risk of vascular disease (PROSPER): a randomised controlled trial. Lancet 2002;360:1623–1630.

19. The ALLHAT Officers and Coordinators for the ALLHAT Collaborative Research Group. Major outcomes in moderately hypercholesterolemic, hypertensive patients randomized to pravastatin vs. usual care: the Antihypertensive and Lipid-Lowering Treatment to prevent Heart Attack Trial (ALLHAT-LLT). JAMA 2002;288:2998–3007.

20. Sever PS, Dahlof B, Poulter NR, et al. Prevention of coronary and stroke events with atorvastatin in hypertensive patients who have average or lower-than average cholesterol concentrations in the Anglo-Scandinavian Cardiac Outcomes Trial – Lipid Lowering Arm (ASCOT-LLA): a multicentre randomised controlled trial. Lancet 2003;361:1149–1158.

21. Koren MJ, Hunninghake DB; ALLIANCE Investigators. Clinical outcomes in managed-care patients with coronary heart disease treated aggressively in lipid-lowering diseases management clinics. The ALLIANCE Study. J Am Coll Cardiol 2004;44: 1772–1779.

22. Walsh JM, Pignone M. Drug treatment of hyperlipidemia in women. JAMA 2004;291:2243–2249.

23. Schwarz GG, Olsson AG, Ezekowitz MD. Effects of atorvastatin on early recurrent ischemic events in acute coronary syndromes. The MIRACL Study: a randomized controlled trial. JAMA 2001;285:1711–11718.

24. Cannon CP, Braunwald E, McCabe CH, et al. Intensive versus moderate lipid lowering with statins after acute coronary syndromes. N Engl J Med 2004;350:1495–1504.

25. Cowie MR, Mostred A, Wood DA, et al. The epidemiology of heart failure. Eur Heart J 1997;18:208–225.

26. Ross R. Atherosclerosis: an inflammatory disease. N Engl J Med 1999;340:115–126.

27. de Lorgeril M, Latour JG. Leukocytes, thrombosis and unstable angina. N Engl J Med 1987;316:1161.

28. Steinberg D, Parthasarathy S, Carew TE, et al. Beyond cholesterol: modifications of low-density lipoproteins that increase its atherogenicity. N Engl J Med 1989;320:915–924.

29. Kris-Etherton P, Eckel R, Howard B, St Jeor S, Bazzarre T. Lyon Diet Heart Study. Benefits of a Mediterranean-style, National Cholesterol Education Program/American Heart Association Step I Dietary Pattern on cardiovascular disease. Circulation 2001;103:1823–1825.

24
Nutrition Counseling for Diabetic Patients

Bénédicte Vergès-Patois and Bruno Vergès

Introduction

Diabetes mellitus is a common disease in the population and it is clearly recognized that patients with diabetes have an increased risk for coronary heart disease. Indeed, several studies have shown that diabetic subjects have a two to four times greater risk of developing and dying from coronary heart disease than non-diabetic persons.[1–3]

The estimated prevalence of diabetes among adults is, at present, situated between 8% and 10% in the United States and between 6% and 7% in Europe. Prevalence of diabetes in patients hospitalized for acute coronary event is between 38% and 45%.[4,5] Therefore, it is not surprising that the percentage of diabetic patients enrolled for cardiac rehabilitation after an acute coronary event is high.[6] Nutrition counseling is an integral component of diabetes management and is an important part of the comprehensive educational program, during cardiac rehabilitation, in diabetic patients.

Criteria for the Diagnosis of Diabetes

According to the WHO, the ADA (American Diabetes Association), the IDF (International Diabetes Federation), and the ALFEDIAM (Association de Langue Française pour l'Etude du DIAbète et des maladies Métaboliques),[7–10] the criteria for diagnosis are:

- fasting plasma glucose ≥126 mg/dL (7.0 mmol/L), on two occasions

- or, 2-hour post oral load (75 g) glucose ≥200 mg/dL (11.1 mmol/L)
- or, symptoms of diabetes (such as polyuria, polydipsia, weight loss) and casual plasma glucose level ≥200 mg/dL.

Two other glucose metabolism abnormalities exist: IGT (impaired glucose tolerance) and IFG (impaired fasting glucose). Both IGT and IFG are associated with increased cardiovascular risk.

Impaired glucose tolerance or IGT is defined by:

- 2-hour post oral load (75 g) glucose ≥140 mg/dL (7.8 mmol/L) and less than 200 mg/dL (11.1 mmol/L)[7–10]

Impaired fasting glucose or IFG is defined by:

- fasting plasma glucose ≥110 mg/dL (6.1 mmol/L) and less than 126 mg/dL (7.0 mmol/L) for the WHO, IDF, and ALFEDIAM recommendations[7,9,10]
- fasting plasma glucose ≥100 mg/dL (5.5 mmol/L) and less than 126 mg/dL (7.0 mmol/L) for the ADA recommendations.[8]

More recently, criteria for the diagnosis of a syndrome of insulin resistance close to type 2 diabetes, the metabolic syndrome, have been defined. According to the experts of the National Cholesterol Education Program (NCEP)-Adult Treatment Panel (ATP)-III, three of the following five items are needed for diagnosis of metabolic syndrome[11]:

- waist circumference >102 cm in men and >88 cm in women

- plasma triglycerides ≥150 mg/dL (1.7 mmol/L)
- HDL cholesterol <40 mg/dL (1.0 mmol/L) in men and <50 mg/dL (1.3 mmol/L) in women
- blood pressure ≥130/85 mmHg
- fasting blood glucose ≥110 mg/dL (6.1 mmol/L).

Nutrition counseling for patients with the metabolic syndrome is described in Chapter 25. As far as diabetes mellitus is concerned, three kinds of diabetes exist:

- Type 1 diabetes due to pancreatic beta-cell destruction leading to absolute insulin deficiency. The major cause of type 1 diabetes is autoimmune destruction of the beta-cells of the pancreas.
- Type 2 diabetes, due to the combination of insulin resistance and relative insulin deficiency. This form is the most frequent type of diabetes.
- Other specific types of diabetes, including diseases of the exocrine pancreas, endocrinopathies, acromegaly, Cushing's syndrome, drug- or chemically induced diabetes, genetic defects of the beta-cell, genetic defect in insulin action.

Nutrition Guidelines for Diabetes

The American Diabetes Association (ADA) and the ALFEDIAM have published nutrition guidelines for patients with diabetes that are summarized here.[11-13]

Energy Balance

Energy intake does not have to be modified in diabetic patients when their weight is normal. However, since obesity is frequent in patients with type 2 diabetes, weight loss is an important therapeutic objective in many type 2 diabetic patients. Indeed weight loss in subjects with type 2 diabetes is associated with decreased insulin resistance and improvement of glycemia, lipid profile, and blood pressure. A moderate decrease in caloric intake (500–1000 kcal/day) will result in slow but progressive weight loss. For most patients weight loss diets should supply at least 1000–1200 kcal/day for women and 1200–1600 kcal/day for men. In order to lose weight, fat is the most important nutrient to restrict. Physical activity is also an important

component of a comprehensive weight management program.

Carbohydrates

The recommended range of carbohydrate intake is 45–65% of total calories. Both the amount (grams) of carbohydrates and the type of carbohydrate in a food influence blood glucose levels. However, with regard to the glycemic effects of carbohydrates, the total amount of carbohydrate in meals or snacks is more important than the source or type. Monitoring total grams of carbohydrate, whether by use of exchanges or carbohydrate counting, remains a key strategy in achieving glycemic control. The use of the glycemic index (a measure of the glycemic effect of types of carbohydrate) can provide an additional benefit over that observed when total carbohydrate is considered alone. Low carbohydrate diets (restricting total carbohydrate to <130 g/day) are not recommended in the management of diabetes.

Carbohydrates are recommended in each meal of the day. Foods containing carbohydrates from whole grains, fruits, vegetables, and low-fat milk should be included in the diet. Like the general population, patients with diabetes are encouraged to consume fiber-containing foods (such as whole grains, fruits, and vegetables) because they provide vitamins, minerals, fiber, and other substances important for good health. However, there is no reason to advise people with diabetes to consume a greater amount of fiber than nondiabetic individuals.

As sucrose does not increase glycemia to a greater extent than isocaloric amounts of starch, sucrose and sucrose-containing foods do not need to be restricted by people with diabetes. However, they should be substituted for other carbohydrate sources in the diet. Non-nutritive sweeteners (saccharin, aspartame, acesulfame potassium and sucralose) are safe when consumed within acceptable daily intake levels.

Lipids

The recommended range of fat intake is 30–35% of total calories. One of the primary dietary fat goals in patients with diabetes is to limit saturated fat intake. Many studies have shown that diets low in saturated fat decrease plasma LDL cholesterol and reduce cardiovascular disease. Thus, it is recommended in patients with diabetes, as in the general population, to reduce dietary saturated fats less to than 10% of energy intake. In persons with plasma LDL cholesterol ≥100 mg/dL, the saturated fat intake should be reduced to less than 7%. Polyunsaturated fat intake should be 10% of energy intake. Among foods containing polyunsaturated fat, those containing n-3 polyunsaturated fatty acids (such as fish) are recommended, since they lower plasma triglycerides in type 2 diabetic patients and have been shown, in the general population, to have cardioprotective effects. Thus, two or three servings of fish per week are recommended in persons with diabetes. The consumption of monounsaturated fat should be between 10% and 20% of energy intake. Plant sources that are rich in monounsaturated fatty acids include vegetable oils (e.g. olive, canola, sunflower oils) and nuts.

Moreover, dietary cholesterol intake should be less than 300 mg/day. Indeed, reduction of dietary cholesterol intake decreases plasma LDL cholesterol. Furthermore, persons with diabetes appear to be more sensitive to dietary cholesterol than the general population. The intake of *trans* fatty acids should be minimized as the effect of *trans* fatty acids is similar to that of saturated fats in raising plasma LDL cholesterol. *Trans* fatty acids also lower plasma HDL cholesterol. The main sources of *trans* fatty acids in the diet include products made from partially hydrogenated oils such as baked products, cookies, and pies.

The "Carbohydrate–Monounsaturated Fat Balance"

Carbohydrate and monounsaturated fat together should provide 60–70% of energy intake. The metabolic profile of the patient and the need for weight loss should be considered when determining the proportion of carbohydrate and monounsaturated fat intake. Indeed, high-carbohydrate diets increase postprandial levels of glucose and triglycerides and, in some studies, decrease plasma HDL cholesterol level when compared to isocaloric high-monounsaturated fat diets. On the other hand, high-monounsaturated fat diets may

result in increased energy intake and weight gain. Therefore, when weight reduction is the major goal in a diabetic patient reducing monounsaturated fat intake is preferred, thus increasing the relative carbohydrate intake. When the metabolic profile of the diabetic patient is the major concern, reducing carbohydrate intake is recommended, increasing the relative monounsaturated fat intake.

Proteins

The recommended protein intake in patients with diabetes is 15–20% of energy intake, if renal function is normal. This proportion is similar to the usual protein intake in the general population.

Minerals and Vitamins

A daily intake of 1000 to 1500 mg of calcium is recommended. This recommendation appears to be safe and likely to reduce osteoporosis in older persons. There is no clear evidence of benefit of vitamin or mineral supplementation in people with diabetes who do not have underlying deficiencies.

Alcohol and Diabetes

The same precautions apply regarding the use of alcohol as in the general population. Abstaining from alcohol should be advised for people with other medical problems such as pancreatitis, advanced neuropathy, severe hypertriglyceridemia, or alcohol abuse. If individuals choose to drink alcohol, daily intake should be limited to one drink per day for adult women and two drinks per day for adult men.

Special Considerations for Type 1 Diabetes

Nutrition recommendations for a healthy lifestyle for the general public[14] are also appropriate for persons with type 1 diabetes. Since the body weight of patients with type 1 diabetes is usually normal, energy intake does not have to be modified. Many type 1 diabetic patients are now treated with intensive insulin therapy (insulin pumps or basal-bolus insulin regimen). For these patients, the total carbohydrate content of meals (and snacks) is the major determinant of the premeal insulin dose and the postprandial glucose response. Thus, patients treated with intensive insulin therapy are advised to adapt the premeal insulin dose to the carbohydrate content of the meal.

For planned exercise, reduction in insulin dosage may be the preferred choice to prevent hypoglycemia. Additional carbohydrate may be needed for unplanned exercise. For instance, a 70 kg person would need between 10 and 15 g carbohydrate per hour of moderate physical activity.

Practical Recommendations

For practical purposes, the ADA Diabetes Food Pyramid is recommended (Figure 24-1).

This pyramid divides food into five groups. The largest group (breads, grains, and other starches) is on the bottom. This means that one should eat more servings of grains, beans, and starchy vegetables than of any of the other groups. The smallest group (fats, oils, sweeteners, and alcohol) is at the top of the pyramid, which means that only a few servings from this group are recommended.

Bread, Grains, and Other Starches

At the base of the pyramid are bread, cereal, rice, and pasta. These foods contain mostly carbohydrates. The foods in this group are made mostly of grains, such as wheat, rye, and oats. Starchy vegetables (like potatoes, peas, and corn) and dry beans also belong to this group because they have about as much carbohydrates in one serving as a slice of bread. Starchy vegetables and dry beans also provide vegetable proteins.

All grains and starches contain carbohydrates. However, their glycemic index (a measure of the glycemic effect of the type of carbohydrate) may be different according to the type of food and the cooking preparation. For instance, mashed potatoes have a higher glycemic index than unmashed potatoes and pasta "al dente" has a lower glycemic index than overboiled pasta.

Vegetables and Fruits

Five servings of fruits or vegetables are recommended each day in patients with diabetes.

Most vegetables are naturally low in fat and are good choices to include often in meals or to have as a low-calorie snack. Vegetables are full of vitamins, minerals, and fiber. This group includes spinach, chicory, lettuce, broccoli, cabbage, Brussels sprouts, cauliflower, carrots, tomatoes, cucumbers, French beans, etc.

Fruits have plenty of vitamins, minerals, and fiber. They also contain carbohydrates. This group includes blackberries, strawberries, oranges, apples, bananas, peaches, pears, apricots, grapes, etc. Some fruits such as grapes and cherries have a higher glycemic index than other fruits. However, the glycemic index of fruits is attenuated when fruits are consumed at the end of a complete meal.

Some vegetables such as olives or avocados and some fruits such as nuts also contain monounsaturated fats.

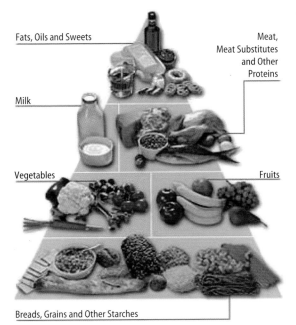

Fats, Oils and Sweets

Meat, Meat Substitutes and Other Proteins

Milk

Vegetables

Fruits

Breads, Grains and Other Starches

Figure 24-1. The ADA (American Diabetes Association) Diabetes Food Pyramid.

Milk and Dairy Products

Milk products contain a lot of protein and calcium as well as many other vitamins. Since a daily intake of 1000 to 1500 mg of calcium is recommended, the advice is to consume milk or dairy products three times a day. Non-fat or low-fat dairy products (milk, yoghurt, etc.) should be chosen to reduce saturated fat.

Meat, Meat Substitutes, and Other Proteins

This group includes beef, chicken, turkey, fish, eggs, tofu, cheese and cottage cheese. Meat and meat substitutes are good sources of protein and many vitamins and minerals. The fattest meat such as mutton and beef should be limited because they are rich in saturated fat; lean meat such as chicken or turkey would be preferred. Pork-butchery products are rich in protein. However, many of them (for instance, sausages, lard) contain large amounts of saturated fat. Ham and bacon that have less than 10% of saturated fat should be preferred.

Two or three servings of fish per week are recommended because fish provides proteins and n-3 polyunsaturated fatty acids. Indeed, n-3 polyunsaturated fatty acids lower plasma triglycerides in type 2 diabetic patients and have been shown, in the general population, to have cardioprotective effects.

Cheese provides protein and calcium but is rich in saturated fat. Thus, it is recommended to limit the amount and to choose low-fat cheese.

Fat, Oil, Sweets, and Alcohol

Fat

Many foods contain fat as we have previously discussed (for instance, cheese, meat). We also use fats for cooking such as butter and oil. Fat is calorie-dense: per gram, it has more than twice the calories of carbohydrate or protein. Since overweight is frequent in patients with type 2 diabetes, the amount of fat should be limited in order to lose weight or to maintain a healthy weight.

Foods that contain saturated fats, such as butter or some vegetable oils (palm oil), must be used in small amounts. Instead of butter, skimmed cream could be used.

Oil

Since foods containing mono- and polyunsaturated fats must be favored in patients with diabetes for their cardioprotective effects, a good choice for cooking should be olive or groundnut oils rich in monounsaturated fats and colza or nut oils rich in n-3 polyunsaturated fatty acids. Foods like potato chips, candy, cookies, cakes, crackers, pastries, and many ready-cooked dishes contain excessive amounts of fat or sugar, so they must be limited to small servings and saved for a special treat!

Sweets

Except in hypoglycemia, sweet products are not recommended in patients with diabetes due to their high glycemic index. Sodas and some concentrated fruit juices can be very rich in sugar. It is possible to substitute sodas with diet drinks, and concentrated fruit juices with pure fruit juices with no sugar added.

Alcohol

Intake of alcohol should be limited to one glass a day (100 mL) for women and two glasses a day for men except when contraindications are present, as we have seen previously. Beer, which contains sugar and alcohol, must be avoided in patients with diabetes. Moreover, it increases plasma triglyceride levels.

Useful Nutritional Tips for Diabetic Patients

Cooking Tips

Here are some ideas to help patients with diabetes to make healthy recipes. It is recommended:

- to reduce fat in baked products
- to use olive, groundnut, colza or nut oils or unsaturated fat margarines instead of butter
- to use skimmed milk instead of whole milk
- to skim the fat off meat and opt for broiling or roasting rather than frying
- to reduce the amount of sugar in baked foods and desserts. Non-nutritive sweeteners may be used to replace sugar. It is also possible

to add spices to increase the flavor in addition to reducing the amount of sugar in the recipes.

Take a Closer Look at the Label

To make wise food choices at the grocery store, diabetic patients must take an attentive look at the labels and the list of ingredients in the products. The information on the label provides total amounts of different nutrients per serving. Total amounts are shown in grams (g) or in milligrams (mg). Therefore, it is advised:

- to check the total amounts of calories, total fat, total carbohydrate and sugar alcohols
- concerning fat, to look precisely at the proportion of saturated and *trans* fats and of mono- and polyunsaturated fat
- concerning carbohydrates, to note the percentages of sugar, complex carbohydrates and fiber
- concerning "sugar-free" products, to look for the type of sweeteners used. Non-nutritive sweeteners (saccharin, aspartame, acesulfame potassium, and sucralose) are safe to consume. The sugar alcohols (xylitol, mannitol, and sorbitol) have some calories and do slightly increase plasma glucose. Eating too much of them can cause intestinal complaints. Patients should also be advised that some "sugar free" or low-carbohydrate products are richer in fat than usual products.

Guide to Eating Out

Eating out is a part of our lives (business meetings, meals with friends, fast-food with the children), often leading to the consumption of much more than at home, with more calories, sugar, and fat! Some tips are needed to order a healthy meal. It is advised to keep in mind the rules of good nutrition, to know the nutritional value of the foods you order, and to try to eat the same portion as you would at home. It is very important to watch calories, especially if it is necessary to lose weight. Many restaurants are trying to meet health needs. Some of them offer foods lower in fat, sugar, salt, and cholesterol, and diet drinks. A variety of choices will increase the chances of finding healthy foods.

When having a meal at a restaurant, it is recommended to avoid fried foods and choose broiled or roasted vegetables, meat or fish and with no extra butter. Ask for sauces and salad dressings to be served on the side. We advise the substitution of high-calorie foods with more favorable nutrients (e.g. vegetables instead of French fries) and limiting alcohol, which adds calories but no nutrition.

Larger portions mean more calories, fat, salt, sugar! Thus, when having a fast-food meal, it is recommended to watch out for words such as "giant, super-sized, double burger." It is suggested to fill salads with a lots of different vegetables full of good nutrients and to end the meal with sugar-free, fat-free yoghurt.

When having a meal out, diabetic patients should choose healthier foods like fruits and vegetables for the other meals of the day and increase their physical activity.

Nutrition counseling is important for patients with diabetes. It should not mean being restricted to a boring diet. Nutrition counseling in diabetic patients leads to a healthy and pleasant diet allowing a wide variety of food and a normal social life.

References

1. Garcia MJ, McNamara PM, Gordon T, Kannel WB. Morbidity and mortality in diabetics in the Framingham population: sixteen year follow-up study. Diabetes 1974;23:105–111.
2. Rytter L, Troelsen S, Beck-Nielsen H. Prevalence and mortality of acute myocardial infarction in patients with diabetes. Diabetes Care 1985;8:230–234.
3. Donahue RP, Orchard TJ. Diabetes mellitus and macrovascular complications. Diabetes Care 1992;15:1141–1155.
4. Takaishi H, Taniguchi T, Fujioka Y, Ishikawa Y, Yokoyama M. Impact of increasing diabetes on coronary artery disease in the past decade. J Atheroscler Thromb 2004;11:271–277.
5. Zeller M, Cottin Y, Brindisi MC, et al. The RICO survey working group. Impaired fasting glucose and cardiogenic shock in patients with acute myocardial infarction. Eur Heart J 2004;25:308–312.
6. Maki KC, Abraira C, Cooper RS. Arguments in favor of screening for diabetes in cardiac rehabilitation. J Cardiopulm Rehabil 1995;15:97–102.

7. World Health Organization (WHO) Screening for type 2 diabetes. 2003. www.who.int/diabetes.
8. American Diabetes Association (ADA). Screening for diabetes. Diabetes Care 2005;28(suppl 1):S5–S7.
9. International Diabetes Federation (IDF)/Europe. A desktop guide to Type 2 diabetes mellitus. European Diabetes Policy Group 1999. Diabet Med 1999;16: 716–730.
10. Drouin P, Blickle JF, Charbonnel B. Diagnostic et classification du diabète sucré les nouveaux critères. Diabetes Metab 1999;25:72–83.
11. American Diabetes Association (ADA). Standards of medical care in diabetes. Diabetes Care 2005;28(suppl 1):S11–S13.
12. American Diabetes Association (ADA). Nutrition principles and recommendations in diabetes. Diabetes Care 2004;27(suppl 1):S36–S46.
13. Monnier L, Slama G, Vialettes B, Ziegler O. Nutrition et diabète. Diabetes Metab 1995;21:371–377.
14. Dietary Guidelines for Americans. www.healthierus.gov/dietaryguidelines.

25
Nutritional Counseling for Overweight Patients and Patients with Metabolic Syndrome

André J. Scheen and Nicolas Paquot

Introduction

An alarming rise in overweight and obesity is occurring worldwide.[1,2] Obesity is more common than cardiovascular disease, diabetes, and cancer combined, and may be a leading cause of these three disorders and numerous other morbid states. Despite some advances in research into genetic, metabolic, behavioral, psychological, and environmental factors, children, adolescents, and adults are continuing to become overweight and obese in increasing numbers. In the United States, the Centers for Disease Control and Prevention report a doubling of the obese population in the period between 1976–1980 and 2001–2003. Currently, in this country, nearly two-thirds of adults are overweight, nearly one-third are obese, and almost 5% are extremely obese. Especially impressive is the progression of overweight and obesity in children and adolescents. Because of this high prevalence of overweight and obesity, approximately 1 in 5 adults has a metabolic syndrome (MetS), that is, a cluster of metabolic abnormalities leading to cardiovascular diseases, increased morbidity, and premature death, and MetS is now increasingly observed in young individuals.[3,4]

Even if genetics is important in body weight regulation, there is no doubt that the epidemic of obesity, MetS and type 2 diabetes is due to recent environmental changes, promoting a high-energy diet and reduced physical activity. The diets of the developing world are shifting rapidly, particularly with respect to fat, caloric sweeteners (from refined carbohydrates), and animal source foods.[5] This changing dietary composition promotes excess caloric intake. Diets high in fats and sugars are conducive to weight gain because they increase the energy density in foods, especially in individuals with limited physical activity.

In this chapter nutritional counseling for overweight/obese patients and individuals with MetS is described. Although MetS is intimately linked to overweight/obesity, especially abdominal adiposity,[2,3] and thus advice given for the treatment of both clinical entities is similar in most aspects, we will consider the specific status of overweight/obesity first, and thereafter we will focus on nutritional management of MetS.

Overweight/Obese Patients

Obesity is not a single disorder but a heterogeneous group of conditions with multiple causes, the outcome of an imbalance between energy intake and energy expenditure.[1,2] Although genetic components are very important, the principal causes of the accelerating obesity problem worldwide are best explained by changing behaviors and environment. Obesity research areas are numerous and include studies of genetics, basic mechanisms that regulate body composition, optimal nutrition from prenatal age to late adulthood, lifestyle strategies to maintain healthy weight, and effective nutritional care following weight loss.

Definition of Overweight/Obesity and Health Implications

Obesity specifically refers to an excess amount of body fat sufficient to harm health.[2] Obesity is most commonly assessed by a single measure, the body mass index (BMI). Individuals with a BMI of 25–29.9 kg/m^2 are considered overweight, while those with a BMI of 30 and above are considered obese (Table 25-1). Obesity is classified as moderate (class I), severe (class II), or extreme (class III) according to BMI (30–34.9, 35–39.9 and >40 kg/m^2, respectively). It is associated with a high risk of cardiovascular disease and type 2 diabetes which increases gradually as BMI increases.[1,2]

Waist circumference is increasingly recognized as a simple means of identifying abdominal obesity. A waist size greater than 102 cm for men and 88 cm for women, at least in Europid populations, markedly increases the risk of most weight-related illnesses. A moderately increased metabolic risk (including MetS) is already observed in individuals with waist circumference greater than 94 cm for men and 80 cm for women. Although the measurement of waist circumference gives little additional information in individuals with severe or extreme obesity, it is much more informative regarding the health risk in subjects with overweight (BMI: 25–29.9 kg/m^2) or mild obesity (BMI: 30–34.9 kg/m^2).[1,2]

Objectives in the Management of Overweight/Obese Subjects

The goals of obesity treatment have changed dramatically in the past two decades. Where once the goal was the reduction to "ideal" weight, the new goal is the attainment of a healthier weight.[2] Interestingly, modest weight loss as low as 5–10% of initial body weight can reduce or eliminate disorders associated with obesity, especially MetS components and type 2 diabetes.[6] The proposed explanation is that 5–10% weight loss is sufficient to induce a 30% reduction in visceral adipose tissue, an entity closely linked to various metabolic disturbances.

Thus, initially, the target of a weight loss program should be to reduce body weight by about 10%. Individuals will generally want to lose more weight than this but it should be remembered that even a 5% weight reduction in those who are overweight or obese lessens the risk of complications such as heart disease. Once this has been achieved, a new target can be set, either weight maintenance or further weight reduction. Indeed, numerous studies highlight the problem of weight regain that occurs following treatment by hypocaloric diets. Factors responsible for weight regain are poorly understood but are likely to include both metabolic and behavioral factors.

Nutritional Counseling for Overweight Patients

General Recommendations

The primary approach for achieving weight loss, in the vast majority of cases, is therapeutic lifestyle change, which includes a reduction in energy intake and an increase in physical activity.[1,2,4] There is no evidence to suggest that specific components of the diet (carbohydrate, fat, protein, vitamins, and micronutrients) influence the ways in which food energy is absorbed or used up. Therefore, the main dietary method for reducing weight is to reduce the total amount of calories consumed, and this is best achieved by a reduction in the amount of fat from the diet and calories from soft drinks. A moderate decrease in caloric balance (500–1000 kcal/day) will result in a slow but progressive weight loss. For most patients, weight loss diets should supply at least 1000–1200 kcal/day for women and 1200–1600 kcal/day for men.

Many different diets have been proposed for the treatment of overweight/obesity.[7] These dietary

TABLE 25-1. WHO classification of adult categories of body mass index (BMI)

Classification	BMI (kg/m^2)	Risk of co-morbidities
Underweight	<18.5	Low (*)
Normal range	18.5–24.9	Average
Overweight (**)	>25	
Pre-obese	25.0–29.9	Mildly increased
Obese:	>30.0	
Class I	30.0–34.9	Moderate
Class II	35.0–39.9	Severe
Class III	>40	Very severe

(*) But risk of other clinical problems increased.
(**) The term overweight refers to a BMI >25, but is frequently adapted to refer to the BMI 25–29.9, differentiating the pre-obese from the obese categories.

approaches vary in their total energy prescription, macronutrient (fat, carbohydrate, and protein) content, and other characteristics such as energy density, glycemic index, and portion control.

Reduction in Energy Content

The energy content of a diet is the primary determinant of weight loss. A decreased caloric intake is classically recommended as part of a weight loss and weight maintenance regimen. A balanced-deficit diet usually provides >1500 kcal/day, low-calorie diets (LCDs) generally contain 800 to 1500 kcal/day, and very-low-calorie diets (VLCDs) provide <800 kcal/day (Table 25-2).

Balanced Hypocaloric Diet

The Expert Panel on the Identification, Evaluation, and Treatment of Overweight and Obesity in Adults[1] recommended a 500 to 1000 kcal/day deficit for obese persons, which will initially result in a weekly weight loss of 0.5 to 1 kg. It is often difficult, however, to accurately determine a patient's daily energy requirements. Therefore, calorie intake guidelines for a weight loss diet have been suggested based between 1000 and 2000 kcal/day. Most recent pharmacological randomized trials comparing orlistat, sibutramine or rimonabant versus placebo used a diet with a 500–600 kcal deficit. The calorie content of any prescribed diet must be adjusted regularly, based on the patient's weight loss response and treatment goals.

Low- Versus Very-Low-Calorie Diets

The results from clinical trials may not reflect the experience in clinical practice because these trials involved subjects who volunteered for a weight loss study and often included formal behavior modification as part of the study protocol. An LCD usually causes an ≈8% loss of body weight at ≈6 months of treatment while the use of a VLCD usually produces a weight loss of ≈15% to 20% within 4 months. However, this initial greater weight reduction associated with VLCD results from water loss (especially during the first few days or weeks) and an undesirable reduction in fat-free mass, and not only from a greater diminution in fat mass. Therefore, VLCDs are associated with poorer weight loss maintenance and a greater weight regain than are LCDs, so weight

TABLE 25-2. Different types of diet used in overweight/obese subjects

Diet type	Characteristics	Comments
(A) Reduced calorie diets (quantitative approach):		
Starvation diet	<200 kcal/day	Serious medical complications
VLCD	<800 kcal/day	Rapid initial weight loss
		Supply all essential nutrients
		Require medical supervision
LCD	800–1500 kcal/day	Use fat-reduced foods
		Long-term use
Balanced hypocaloric diet	500–1000 kcal/day deficit	Slow progressive weight loss
		Long-term use
(B) Modified diet composition (qualitative):		
Low-fat diet	Reduce diet's energy density	Increase in triglycerides
		Reduction in HDL cholesterol
"Ad libitum" low-fat diet	No energy intake restriction	Reduced food intake because of satiating effect of fat
"Ad libitum" low-CHO diet	<25 g CHO/day	Short-term weight loss by reducing appetite
		Increase in LDL cholesterol
		Concerns about long-term safety

VLCD: very-low-calorie diet; LCD: low-calorie diet; CHO: carbohydrate.

loss at 1 year after treatment with a VLCD does not differ from treatment with an LCD. Indeed, even if VLCDs can induce very rapid weight loss over a 2- to 3-month period, these diets do not modify eating behavior and nutritional knowledge and skills, which seem to be required for long-term maintenance. In addition, VLCDs, which consist of 250 to 800 kcal/day, should only be administered to select patients under proper medical supervision. Individuals on VLCDs are more likely to suffer adverse effects than are those on LCDs (800–1500 kcal/day) because of the metabolic consequences of semi-starvation. They are also at increased risk for gallstones and nutritional deficiencies unless the VLCD is supplemented with vitamins and minerals.

Macronutrient Composition of the Diet

The macronutrient composition of a diet does not affect the rate of weight loss unless macronutrient manipulation influences total energy intake or expenditure. Nevertheless, changes in macronutrient composition of the diet have been tested in various clinical trials.[8]

Low-Fat Diet

A low-fat diet is considered the standard approach for the treatment of obesity. Based on several studies suggesting that there are benefits to restricting fat intake as well as calories, many programs also prescribe dietary fat goals to produce a 20–25% fat intake. High-fat diets are often highly palatable, but are energy dense and low in complex carbohydrates and water. Moreover, high-fat diets appear to be less satiating and the thermic effect of dietary fat is low, as compared to diets containing complex carbohydrates and/or proteins. Thus, low-fat diets reduce the diet's energy density while maintaining satiety as a result of their high content of complex carbohydrate and protein. These characteristics lead to a modest but predictable weight loss, which is further marked in the more obese individuals. However, although low-fat diets can enhance weight loss and may be particularly useful in selected persons, they are not necessarily more effective than LCDs. A negative influence of low-fat, high-carbohydrate diets on triglycerides

and HDL cholesterol concentrations has been reported, although this negative influence could be dampened by selecting carbohydrate with a low glycemic index. Whereas low glycemic index foods may be beneficial in established type 2 diabetes,[9] there is currently no agreement on whether they are beneficial in weight reduction.

Low-Carbohydrate Diet

The use of low-carbohydrate diets has become increasingly popular.[7,8] Several randomized controlled trials compared the effect of low-carbohydrate, high-protein, high-fat diets (e.g. the Atkins diet) with a conventional low-fat diet (≈30% energy from fats) in adults. In all studies, weight loss at 3 and 6 months in subjects randomized to the low-carbohydrate diet was almost two times as great (i.e. 4 to 5 kg greater weight loss) as in those randomized to the low-fat group. Low-carbohydrate diets usually produce initial rapid weight loss, but this is not real loss of body fat, but of body water. This induces an unbalanced metabolism of fat (ketosis), which suppresses hunger, and helps the maintenance of a restricted diet and further weight loss. However, in studies that observed patients for a longer period of time, weight loss at 1 year was not significantly different between groups. In general, these studies also found that a low-carbohydrate diet was more beneficial with respect to serum triglycerides and HDL cholesterol concentrations as compared with the low-fat diet, but the low-fat diet was more beneficial with respect to serum LDL cholesterol concentrations. Although these changes in triglycerides and HDL cholesterol after weight reduction on low-carbohydrate diets appear favorable (especially in subjects with MetS – see section below on the influence of qualitative modification of dietary fats), it is not known whether these alterations are associated with long-term beneficial effects on coronary heart disease. Furthermore, when weight loss fades out (resulting in an attenuation of the short-term favorable effects on insulin resistance, triglycerides, and HDL cholesterol), the high content of saturated fat may exert an adverse effect on blood lipids, especially total and LDL cholesterol levels. Therefore, the long-term impact of sustaining such a high-fat diet may be an increased risk of cardiovascular disease.

Supportive Approaches

Low-Energy Food, Portion Control, Prepackaged Prepared Meals

Although all popular hypocaloric diets have proven to reduce body weight and several cardiac risk factors at one year, overall dietary adherence rate is rather low.[8] More research is needed to identify practical techniques to increase dietary adherence.

The use of low energy-dense foods may be another effective approach for treating obesity. The energy density of a diet is defined as the calories present in a given weight of food. A food's energy density is directly correlated with its fat content and inversely correlated with its water content. Energy intake during a meal is partially regulated by the weight of ingested food and is inversely correlated with energy density.

Portion control is another important aspect of reducing energy intake. During ad libitum feeding, a direct relationship is found between portion size served and intake; therefore, increasing the size of the portion served increases the amount of food consumed and vice versa.

Providing prepackaged prepared meals, either as frozen entrees of mixed foods or liquid-formula meal replacements, improves portion control and can enhance weight loss. Data from clinical trials have shown that obese persons who were given such special foods lost several kilograms more weight than did those who were randomized to a standard diet.

Meal Plans to Improve Weight Loss/Maintenance

Using an LCD together with frequent meetings with health professionals, supplemented in some cases with group therapy and behavior modification, can usually lead to a 5–10% weight loss in the majority of individuals. Weight maintenance, however, is much more of a challenge.

Educating patients about food labels, recipe modification, restaurant ordering, social eating, and healthy cooking methods is also important to help patients understand portion size, energy intake, and macronutrient composition during meals and snacks.

Nutritional Intervention to Prevent Type 2 Diabetes in Overweight/Obese Subjects

Because much of the risk of developing type 2 diabetes is attributable to obesity,[10] maintenance of a healthy body weight is strongly recommended as a means of preventing this disease. The relationship between glycemic index and glycemic load and the development of type 2 diabetes remains unclear at this time.[9]

Studies have been initiated in the last decade to determine the feasibility and benefit of various strategies to prevent or delay the onset of type 2 diabetes. A majority of subjects included in these trials were overweight/obese and had impaired glucose tolerance. In well-controlled studies that included a lifestyle intervention arm, substantial efforts were necessary to achieve only modest changes in weight and exercise, but those changes were sufficient to achieve an important reduction in the incidence of diabetes (58% in both the Finnish Diabetes Prevention Study and the US Diabetes Prevention Program). In the Finnish Diabetes Prevention Study,[11] weight loss average 4.6 kg at 1 year, 3.8 kg after 2 years, and 2.3 kg after 5 years. In this study, there was a direct relationship between adherence to the lifestyle intervention and the reduced incidence of diabetes. In the Diabetes Prevention Program, the lifestyle group lost about 6 kg at 2 years and 4.5 kg at 3 years. A low-fat diet (<25% fat) was initially recommended.[12] If reducing fat did not produce weight loss to goal (reduction of 7% of initial body weight), calorie restriction was also recommended and the total calorie intake was reduced to 1200–2000 kcal/day according to initial body weight. The greater benefit of weight loss and physical activity with lifestyle change as compared to pharmacological intervention (relative risk reduction of 31% with metformin as compared to 58% with diet plus exercise in the Diabetes Prevention Program) strongly suggests that lifestyle modifications should be the first choice to prevent or delay diabetes. Modest weight loss (5–10% of body weight) and modest physical activity (30 min daily) are the recommended goals. Because this intervention not only has been shown to prevent or delay diabetes, but also has a variety of other benefits, healthcare providers should urge all overweight and sedentary individuals to adopt these changes, and such recommendations should be made at every opportunity.

Nutritional Prevention of Overweight/Obesity in Childhood

There are some indications that the likelihood of a particular individual of becoming obese may be reduced if the following modifiable nutritional risk factors are given attention:

- adequate maternal nutrition during pregnancy while avoiding excessive maternal weight gain and hyperglycemia and hypertriglyceridemia
- restricting the extent of "catch-up growth" in those infants born small (because of less than adequate maternal nutrition during pregnancy), an objective assisted greatly by breastfeeding and delayed weaning
- introduction to a variety of tastes during weaning and immediately afterwards
- development of a taste for fruit and vegetable consumption early in life and the lack of a taste for high-fat and high-sugar foods
- strict controls with regard to the availability of food and drinks for preschool, primary and middle school and preferably senior school children
- maintenance of a low energy-dense diet (fruits and vegetables), drinking water and doing an appropriate level of physical activity into adult life.

Major industrial concerns in food and drink production, manufacturing, retailing, and catering have targeted children. New policies to prevent overweight/obesity require children to be protected at the most vulnerable and important stages in their development.

Patients with Metabolic Syndrome

The increased cardiovascular risk associated with overweight/obesity is closely linked to the presence of insulin resistance and the related cluster of metabolic abnormalities. Therefore, nutritional counseling for overweight/obese patients should not only focus on weight reduction and weight maintenance, but also target the various disturbances included in MetS. Targeting abdominal

obesity has been proposed as a main goal in individuals with MetS.[2,3]

Definition of MetS and Health Implications

MetS (also called deadly quartet, syndrome X, insulin resistance syndrome, plurimetabolic syndrome, dysmetabolic syndrome, cardiometabolic syndrome) comprises a cluster of abnormalities that occur as a result of perturbations in multiple metabolic pathways, leading to insulin resistance and hyperinsulinemia, hyperglycemia, atherogenic dyslipidemia, hypertension, fibrinolytic abnormalities, etc.[3] Numerous other disturbances have been progressively added to the syndrome, including a prothrombotic state, endothelial dysfunction and inflammation, all conditions associated with cardiovascular diseases (CVD). In 1998, the World Health Organization (WHO) recommended a unifying definition and chose the term "metabolic syndrome" (MetS). However, an alternative definition has been proposed in 2001 by the National Cholesterol Education Program Adult Treatment Panel III (NCEP ATP III).[14] This definition is easier to use in clinical practice and now widely accepted.[3] According to this definition, patients are considered to have MetS if they exhibit three or more of the following criteria: (1) abdominal obesity; (2) hypertriglyceridemia; (3) low HDL; (4) high blood pressure; and (5) high fasting glucose (see cut-off values in Table 25-3). Individuals with MetS are at increased risk for type 2 diabetes mellitus and CVD, which justifies adequate management with lifestyle changes and when necessary with pharmacological approaches.[14,15]

TABLE 25-3. Definition of the metabolic syndrome according to the National Cholesterol Education Program – Adult Treatment Panel III (NCEP ATP III)[13]

Presence of at least three or more of the following criteria:
1. Abdominal obesity: waist circumference >102 cm in men and >88 cm in women
2. Hypertriglyceridemia: ≥150 mg/dL
3. Low HDL cholesterol: <40 mg/dL in men and <50 mg/dL in women
4. High blood pressure: ≥130/85 mm Hg
5. High fasting glucose: ≥110 mg/dL

According to the new definition of the International Diabetes Federation (IDF), central obesity (defined as waist circumference ≥94 cm for Europid men and ≥80 cm for Europid women, with ethnicity specific values for other groups) is considered as a prerequisite plus any two of the other four factors mentioned in Table 25-3 (with fasting glucose level threshold decreased from 110 to 100 mg/mg/dL).

Objectives in the Management of Individuals with MetS

Patients with MetS have a 1.5- to 3-fold increase in the risk of coronary heart disease and stroke.[3] The NCEP ATP III guidelines emphasize the importance of treating patients with MetS to prevent CVD.[14] The association between MetS and CVD raises important questions about the underlying pathological process(es), especially for designing targeted therapeutic interventions. Cardiovascular risk reduction in individuals with MetS should include at least three levels of intervention: (1) control of obesity and lack of physical activity; (2) control of insulin resistance; and (3) control of the individual components of MetS, especially hypertension and atherogenic dyslipidaemia.[14,15]

MetS can precede and is often associated with type 2 diabetes.[3] Because of this intimate relationship, appropriate management of MetS should be able to prevent the progression from impaired glucose tolerance to frank diabetes and thus to prevent type 2 diabetes. The importance of prevention of diabetes in high-risk individuals (such as people with MetS are) is highlighted by the substantial and worldwide increase in the prevalence of diabetes in recent years.[5,10]

Owing to the complex pathophysiology and phenotypic expression of MetS, lifestyle changes are crucial as they are able to positively and simultaneously influence almost all components of the syndrome. If such measures are not sufficient or not adequately followed, a pharmacological intervention should be considered.[15]

Nutritional Counseling for Patients with MetS

MetS has been identified as a target for dietary therapies to reduce CVD risk other than LDL cholesterol lowering by the NCEP ATP III.[13-15] Clear evidence from metabolic studies, epidemiological studies, and clinical trials supports the consumption of unsaturated fats from natural liquid vegetable oils and nuts at the expense of saturated and *trans* fats (rather than simply lowering total fat) in the treatment of various components of the MetS (e.g. dyslipidemia, insulin resistance, and

TABLE 25-4. Suggested dietary nutrient composition for overweight/obese patients, especially those with metabolic syndrome

Nutrient	Recommended intake
Saturated fat	<7% of total calories
Monounsaturated fat	≤20% of total calories
Polyunsaturated fat	≤10% of total calories
Total fat	25–35% or less of total calories
Carbohydrates	50–60% or more of total calories (complex carbohydrates from a variety of vegetables, fruits, wholes grains)
Fiber	20–30 g/day
Protein	≈15% of total calories
Cholesterol	<200 mg/day

glucose intolerance) and in the prevention of CVD.[16,17]

NCEP ATP III recommendations for diet composition for patients with MetS are consistent with general dietary recommendations (Table 25-4).[13] Guidelines for healthy anti-atherogenic diet call for: (1) low intake of saturated fats, *trans* fats, and cholesterol; (2) reduced consumption of simple sugars; (3) increased intakes of fruits, vegetables, and whole grains.[17] Such principles also concern diet recommendations for the treatment and prevention of diabetes mellitus and related disorders.[5,9] The so-called Mediterranean diet is in agreement with these basic recommendations and may be expected to improve some of the main metabolic abnormalities present in MetS and thus to reduce the incidence of CVD.

Effects of Weight Loss on MetS Components

Although obesity is thought to be the main predisposing factor for MetS, how it relates to insulin resistance is not precisely established. Abdominal obesity was identified as being particularly associated with several of the components of MetS,[2,3] and weight gain has been shown to be strongly correlated with MetS.[1,2] Although the precise answer to the question whether it is nature (genetic) or nurture (environment) is not known, it seems that it is probably both, to some extent. Nevertheless, it is clear that the current epidemic of obesity, and as a correlate of MetS, is related to modern lifestyles that emphasize overconsumption of high-caloric food and lack of physical activity.[1,2]

Effective for long-term weight loss are reduced-energy diets, consisting of a 500- to 1000-calorie/day reduction. A realistic goal for weight reduction is to reduce body weight by 7–10% over a period of 6 to 12 months. Numerous studies have shown that significant improvement of several abnormalities of MetS, including dyslipidemia, hyperglycemia, and hypertension, can be observed, even with a modest amount of weight loss.[6,10] For every kilogram of weight loss the following favorable changes occur: fasting serum cholesterol, −1.0%; LDL cholesterol, −0.7%; triglycerides, −1.9%; HDL cholesterol, +0.2%; systolic blood pressure, −0.5%; diastolic blood pressure, −0.4%; and fasting glucose, −0.2 mmol/L. The impact of weight reduction on diabetes mellitus is particularly impressive.[10]

Effects of Lifestyle Change on MetS Components

The underlying conditions that promote the development of MetS are overweight and obesity, physical inactivity, and an atherogenic diet.[16,17] Therefore, lifestyle modification is first-line therapy to prevent and treat MetS.[14,15] The most important therapeutic intervention effective in subjects with MetS should focus on modest weight reduction and regular leisure-time physical activities. The Finnish Diabetes Prevention Study[11] and the Diabetes Prevention Program (DPP) in the United States[12] performed in overweight subjects with impaired glucose tolerance (IGT) have both shown that as little as a 5% reduction in weight, obtained with a balanced moderately hypocaloric diet and regular physical activity, can reduce the risk of developing diabetes by over 50%. Further data from the DPP (only published as abstracts) showed that the subjects enrolled in the intensive lifestyle intervention group have lower levels of LDL cholesterol, lower triglyceride concentrations, and less hypertension than subjects in other groups. In addition, intensive lifestyle intervention lowered the level of C-reactive protein and improved fibrinolytic potency as expressed by the level of tissue plasminogen activator. Although the 3 years of follow-up seem insufficient to draw conclusions applicable at large, lifestyle modifications seem to substantially reduce the need for both lipid-lowering and antihypertensive therapies in subjects with impaired glucose tolerance.

Finally, the influence of intensive lifestyle intervention on the emergence of MetS was studied in the DPP. At baseline, about one-half of the participants showed at least three constituents of MetS. Lifestyle modification was superior to other treatments in reducing abdominal obesity and offered the best protection against the development of MetS. This highly successful lifestyle intervention applied in the DPP was based on empirical literature in nutrition, exercise, and behavioral weight control. The program has been described extensively[12] and was designed to achieve and maintain at least a 7% weight loss and 700 calories/week of physical activity (a minimum of 150 minutes of exercise equivalent to brisk walking) in all lifestyle participants.

Influence of Qualitative Modification of Dietary Fats

There has been clear understanding for decades that dietary fat subtypes have very different effects on many metabolic variables of importance in the etiology of MetS.[16,17] While the differing effects of saturated versus polyunsaturated fatty acids (PUFA) on cholesterol were identified decades ago, effects of dietary fats on plasma triglycerides have been recognized more recently. Plasma triglyceride levels are increased by some fats but decreased by n-3 PUFA. Furthermore, evidence for differential effects of fat subtypes on insulin action was published and consistent results were obtained in animal intervention and human cross-sectional and prospective studies. Animal studies have shown that increasing the percentage of calories from some, but not all, fats leads to impaired insulin action (insulin resistance) without the necessity of overconsumption of calories. Saturated fats are deleterious while n-3 PUFAs are protective. Monounsaturated fatty acids and n-6 PUFAs are also, somewhat surprisingly, deleterious. This means that increasing the proportion of PUFA in the diet is only beneficial if the n-6/n-3 ratio is low. In human studies, while fat intake, and in particular saturated fat intake, was still related to insulin resistance even after adjustment for adiposity, in many cases the evidence points to effects of fat intake on obesity as the linking variable. In contrast to the effects of saturated fats, PUFA intake is not associated with obesity and the pattern of changes in metabolic rate is opposite to that of saturated lipids.

An important question is whether individuals with MetS will benefit from a shift to relatively more unsaturated fats. Indeed, the risk that very high-carbohydrate diets may accentuate atherogenic dyslipidemia may be reduced by isocalorically substituting a higher intake of unsaturated fats. However, recent small clinical trials indicate that improvement of atherogenic dyslipidemia by increasing unsaturated fat consumption is relatively small when compared with standard dietary recommendations.[17]

Influence of Carbohydrate Type and Content

The optimal types and amounts of carbohydrates in the diet remain controversial.[18] It is now well established that low-fat, high-carbohydrate diets not only lower HDL and raise triglycerides but also generally produce higher postprandial glucose and insulin responses. However, metabolic consequences of carbohydrates depend not only on their quantity but also on their quality. The glycemic response of a given carbohydrate load depends on the food source, which has led to the development of the glycemic index, ranking foods by their ability to raise postprandial blood glucose levels.[19] In addition, effects on blood glucose and lipid metabolism by carbohydrate-rich foods depend on fiber content and type. Controlled feeding studies have found benefits of whole grains on insulin sensitivity and glucose and lipid metabolism compared with refined grains. In addition, several epidemiological studies found that diets rich in whole grains may protect against CVD, stroke, and type 2 diabetes. However, epidemiological studies are unlikely to yield detailed evaluations of the pathways, and basic and experimental research is clearly warranted.

The concept of glycemic index remains controversial.[19] The concept of glycemic load is appealing because it captures both the quality and the quantity of carbohydrates as well as potential interactions between them. In practice, glycemic load can be lowered by reducing the total amount of carbohydrates in the diet, the overall dietary glycemic index, or both. However, reducing the amount of carbohydrates (especially refined carbohydrates) is more effective in lowering glycemic load than is reducing the overall dietary glycemic index alone.

With the growing epidemic of obesity, MetS, and type 2 diabetes, reduction in the consumption of refined carbohydrates and sugar, replaced by either minimally processed whole grain products or healthy sources of fats and protein, should become a major public health priority, together with regular physical activity and weight maintenance.

Dietary Influence on Blood Pressure Regulation

Medical nutrition therapy for the management of hypertension has focused on weight reduction and reducing sodium intake.[20] In both normotensive and hypertensive individuals, a reduction in sodium intake lowers blood pressure. In hypertensive patients, the goal should be to reduce sodium intake to 2400 mg (100 mmol) or sodium chloride (salt) to 6000 mg/day. Other nutritional variables that have been considered include alcohol, potassium, calcium, and magnesium intake. An association between high alcohol intake (>3 drinks/day) and elevated blood pressure has been reported. However, there is no major difference in blood pressure between people who consume <3 drinks/day and non-drinkers. Clinical trials have reported a beneficial effect of potassium supplementation on lowering blood pressure. Such high potassium intake can be provided by high intake of fruits and vegetables (five to nine servings/day). In contrast, evidence for a beneficial effect from calcium and magnesium supplementation is lacking.

Conclusions

Reducing energy intake is the cornerstone of weight management therapy. Current recommendations suggest that overweight/obese patients who are trying to lose weight consume a diet that induces an energy deficit of 500 to 1000 kcal/day and has a macronutrient composition that is known to reduce the risk of CVD, especially in patients with MetS. This diet involves (1) consuming a variety of fruits, vegetables, grains, low-fat or nonfat dairy products, fish, legumes, poultry, and lean meals; (2) limiting intake of foods that are high in saturated fat, *trans* fatty acids, and cholesterol. These recommendations may require modification, based on the results of ongoing and future dietary therapy studies. The key to successful weight management is to provide patients with a dietary regimen that results in long-term compliance. Indeed, poor sustainability and adherence rates result in modest weight loss and cardiac risk factor reduction, whatever the type of diet. Adherence level rather than diet type appears to be the key determinant of clinical benefits. The available data suggest that it is unlikely that one approach is appropriate for all patients. Practical techniques to increase dietary adherence should be implemented, including techniques to match individuals with the diet best suited to their food preferences, lifestyle, and medical conditions.

Providing appropriate nutrition counseling and the behavior modification therapy needed to implement dietary changes is difficult if not impossible for most physicians because they do not have the time or expertise to provide this kind of care. Therefore, referral to a reputable weight loss program or experienced dietitian should be considered, if these resources are available.

Individuals with MetS have an increased risk of diabetes mellitus and CVD. The occurrence of multiple risk factors necessitates multifactorial therapy that includes glycemic control, lipid-lowering therapy, blood pressure control, and antiplatelet treatment. The most important therapeutic intervention effective in subjects with MetS is change in lifestyle, with the focus on modest weight reduction and regular leisure-time physical activities. However, some patients would require the aid of pharmacological therapy.

From a practical point of view, lifestyle modification, including regular physical exercise, healthy diet, and smoking cessation, should be recommended first in individuals with MetS. In addition, treatments specifically targeting dyslipidemia, hypertension, or hyperglycemia should be considered for patients with any of these conditions. In many cases, a combination of different drugs has to be proposed to reduce the risk of major adverse outcomes. However, the optimal manner in which the existing drugs should be used in patients with MetS has yet to be defined, including the optimal doses, regimens, and treatment combinations.

Public health trends and lifestyle patterns clearly suggest that nurture is the biggest contributor to the epidemic, and serious attention and public health measures are needed to curb the epidemic of obesity, MetS, diabetes, and CVD. Early identification, treatment, and prevention of MetS present a major challenge for healthcare professionals and public health policy makers facing an epidemic of overweight and sedentary lifestyle.

References

1. NHLBI Obesity Education Initiative Expert Panel. Clinical guidelines on the identification, evaluation, and treatment of overweight and obesity in adults – the evidence report. Obesity Res 1998;6: 51S–209S.
2. National Task Force on the Prevention and Treatment of Obesity. Overweight, obesity and health risk. Arch Intern Med 2000;160:898–904.
3. Grundy SM, Brewer HB Jr, Cleeman JI, Smith SC, Lenfant C, for Conference Participants. Definition of metabolic syndrome: report of the National Heart, Lung, and Blood Institute/American Heart Association conference on scientific issues related to definition. Circulation 2004;109:433–488.
4. Klein S, Burke LE, Bray GA, et al. Clinical implications of obesity with specific focus on cardiovascular disease. A statement for Professionals from the American Heart Association Council on Nutrition, Physical Activity, and Metabolism. Circulation 2004;110:2952–2967.
5. Franz MJ, Bantle JP, Beebe CA, Brunzell JD, Chiasson J-L, Garg A, et al. Evidence-based nutrition principles and recommendations for the treatment and prevention of diabetes and related complications (Technical Review). Diabetes Care 2002;25: 148–198.
6. Goldstein DJ. Beneficial health effects of modest weight loss. Int J Obes 1992;16:397–415.
7. Freedman MR, King J, Kennedy E. Popular diets: a scientific review. Obes Res 2001;9(suppl 1):1S–40S.
8. Dansinger ML, Gleason JA, Griffith JL, Selker HP, Schaefer EJ. Comparison of the Atkins, Ornish, weight watchers, and zone diets for weight loss and heart disease reduction. A randomized trial. JAMA 2005;293:43–53.
9. American Diabetes Association. Position Statement. Evidence-based nutrition principles and recommendations for the treatment and prevention of diabetes and related complications. Diabetes Care 2003;26 (suppl 1):S51–61.

10. Scheen AJ. Current management strategies for coexisting diabetes mellitus and obesity. Drugs 2003;63:1165–1184.

11. Tuomilehto J, Lindstrom J, Eriksson JG, et al. for the Finnish Diabetes Prevention Study Group. Prevention of type 2 diabetes mellitus by changes in lifestyle among subjects with impaired glucose tolerance. N Engl J Med 2001;344:1343–1350.

12. The Diabetes Prevention Program (DPP) Research Group. The Diabetes Prevention Program (DPP). Description of lifestyle intervention. Diabetes Care 2002;25:2165–2171.

13. Expert Panel on Detection, Evaluation, and Treatment of High Blood Cholesterol in Adults. Executive summary of the third report of the National Cholesterol Education Program (NCEP) Expert Panel on detection, evaluation, and treatment of high blood cholesterol in adults (Adult Treatment Panel III). JAMA 2001;285:2486–2497.

14. Grundy SM, Hansen B, Smith SC, Cleeman JI, Kahn RA, for Conference Participants. Clinical management of metabolic syndrome. Report of the American Heart Association/National Heart, Lung, and Blood Institute/American Diabetes Association Conference on scientific issues related to management. Circulation 2004;109:551–556.

15. Scheen AJ. Management of the metabolic syndrome. Minerva Endocrinol 2004;29:31–45.

16. Krauss RM, Eckel RH, Howard B, Appel LJ, Daniels SR, Deckelbaum RJ, et al. AHA Dietary Guidelines: revision 2000: a statement for healthcare professionals from the Nutrition Committee of the American Heart Association. Circulation 2000;102:2284–2299.

17. Hu FB, Willett WC. Optimal diets for prevention of coronary heart disease. JAMA 2002;288:2569–2578.

18. Sheard NF, Clark NG, Brand-Miller JC, et al. Dietary carbohydrate (amount and type) in the prevention and management of diabetes: a statement by the American Diabetes Association. Diabetes Care 2004;27:2266–2271.

19. Ludwig DS. The glycemic index: physiological mechanisms relating obesity, diabetes, and cardiovascular disease. JAMA 2002;287:2414–2423.

20. Guidelines Committee. 2003 European Society of Hypertension. European Society of Cardiology guidelines for the management of arterial hypertension. J Hypertens 2003;21:1011–1053.

26
Nutritional Counseling: Practical Models

Catherine Monpère

Introduction

Hippocrates' famous aphorism "we are what we eat" is more than ever pertinent at the present time. Indeed, strong scientific evidence has demonstrated that dietary patterns are important determinants of health status, especially concerning the cardiovascular system. However, nutrition must be considered not only as an energetic source, but must be integrated with its other components: culture, beliefs, tradition, and pleasure. This complexity explains why behavioral modifications in nutrition are so difficult to promote and sustain in subjects, often needing deep changes in the ways of being and thinking. Moreover, as cardiovascular prevention is multifactorial, healthy food choices must often be associated with other behavioral modifications, such as smoking cessation or physical exercise, so our main task will be to help patients to cope with all these recommendations.

Even if some aspects remain unclear, a wide range of epidemiological and randomized trials have clearly documented the association between dietary behaviors and cardiovascular prevention, beyond blood total cholesterol reduction. It is now recognized that a diet rich in fruits, vegetables, whole grains, fish, and calcium, and low in saturated and transunsaturated fats is effective in lowering cardiovascular morbidity and mortality. Most of the guidelines are concordant on those facts, and our challenge is to translate these recommendations into daily-life practice in our patients.

Although this chapter focuses on dyslipidemic patients, the concept and the practical models of nutritional counseling are applicable to all types of patients with metabolic diseases, such as diabetes, metabolic syndrome, or obesity.

Nutritional Counseling: From Evidence-Based Medicine to Recommendations

The Facts

Previous epidemiological studies showing the correlation between cholesterol levels, dietary patterns, and incidence of cardiovascular diseases have been subsequently confirmed by randomized interventional trials.

The Seven Countries Study,[1] one of the landmark observational studies, investigated associations between the intake of different food groups, blood cholesterol levels, and trends in coronary death (sudden coronary death and fatal myocardial infarction) in 12,763 men. They were aged from 40 to 59 years, located in five European countries, the US and Japan, and were followed up for 25 years. Relative risk of 25-year cardiovascular mortality was calculated for cholesterol quartiles and per 20 mg/dL cholesterol increase. Adjustment was made for age, smoking, and systolic blood pressure. The main results showed that across the different countries, cholesterol is linearly correlated to coronary heart disease mortality, and that a relative increase of 20 mg/dL in total cholesterol corresponded to an increase of 12% in cardiovascular mortality risk (except for Japan). Moreover, this study showed that mortality from coronary heart disease changed at different periods when comparing early phases of follow-up with later ones, and these variations were preceded by large changes in population mean levels of serum cholesterol. However, at a given cholesterol level, there are large differences in absolute coronary heart disease mortality rates among cultures: for a cholesterol level around 200 mg/dL cardiac death varies from 4% to 5% in Japan and Mediterranean countries to about 15% in northern Europe, suggesting that other factors than cholesterol may play a role, such as diet. For this purpose, 18 different food groups and combinations were considered for comparison among cohorts: large differences in food intake were seen in the different countries, with high consumption of dairy products and meat in northern Europe and the US, vegetables, fish and wine in southern Europe, and cereals, soy products and fish in Japan. Animal food groups (except fish) were directly correlated with cardiovascular mortality, whereas vegetables, as well as fish and alcohol, were negatively correlated.

The results of a more recent standardized case-control study, InterHeart,[2] performed in 52 countries all around the world, dealing with modifiable risk factors associated with myocardial infarction, are consistent with the above findings: 15,152 cases (patients with a first presentation of myocardial infarction) and 14,820 controls were enrolled. Odds ratios and their 99% confidence intervals for the association of risk factors to myocardial infarction, and the population attributable risk (PAR) were calculated. Current smoking and abnormal lipid profile (raised ApoB/ApoA1 ratio) were the two strongest risk factors accounting for about two-thirds of the PAR, followed by hypertension, diabetes, and psychological factors. In addition, nutritional factors such as daily consumption of fruits and vegetables and moderate alcohol intake two to three times a week were protective (respective odds ratio 0.70 and 0.91). It is noteworthy that lifestyle modifications such as smoking cessation, eating fruit and vegetables, and taking regular exercise could lead to nearly an 80% reduction in relative risk for myocardial infarction, worldwide, in both sexes and all ages in all regions! This new knowledge about risk factors for coronary disease in most regions of the globe makes it possible to base cardiovascular prevention on similar principles worldwide, and the role of cardiovascular prevention and rehabilitation is underlined by the fact that 90% of the PAR of myocardial infarction is linked to nine modifiable factors.

These results on dietary factors linked to cardiovascular prevention are reinforced by controlled intervention trials, aimed at evaluating the role of different categories of nutriment or dietary behaviors in cardiovascular morbidity and mortality. These trials focus mainly on the changes in intake of total, saturated, monounsaturated and polyunsaturated (PUFA) fats and cholesterol, and on the effects of omega-3 intake.

Lee Hooper et al. performed a systematic review[3] of the literature concerning the effects of dietary fat intake (except for omega-3 fatty acids) on the prevention of cardiovascular disease. Twenty-seven studies (39,902 person-years of observation) were included, showing that reduction or modification of intake of dietary fats reduced the incidence of combined cardiovascular events by 16% (rate ratio 0.84; 95% CI, 0.72 to 0.99), and cardiovascular death by 9% (0.91; 0.77 to 1.07) with no effect on total mortality. Beneficial effects on combined cardiovascular events are significant in trials of at least 2 years' duration; however, these trials support only limited and inconclusive evidence on total and cardiovascular mortality.

The following studies deal with the cardiovascular effects of a moderate-fat diet enriched with omega-3 (n-3) fatty acids. The Diet and Reinfarction Trial (DART)[4] in 1989 tested three simultaneous and independent interventions: reduction in fat intake with an increase in the ratio of polyunsaturated to saturated fat, an increase in cereal fiber intake, and an increase in the intake of fatty fish (200 to 400 mg/week, or "Maxepa" capsules). There were 2033 post myocardial infarction patients with a mean follow-up of 2 years: no differences versus control groups were attributable to fat or fiber advice, whereas the "fish group" had a significant 29% lower death rate, but surprisingly reinfarction plus cardiac death were not significantly affected by any of the dietary regimens. Later, Singh et al.[5] performed a randomized placebo-controlled trial evaluating the protective effects of n-3 fatty acids via fish oil or mustard oil in post myocardial infarctions patients: this trial revealed rapid protective effects of this diet in post myocardial patients, with a reduction in nonfatal myocardial reinfarction (respectively 13% and 15% vs. 25.4%, $P < 0.05$) and cardiac death (11.4% vs. 22.0%, $P < 0.05$) for fish oil.

The GISSI-Prevenzione Trial[6] is a randomized open label study, involving 113,244 patients surviving from recent myocardial infarction supplemented either with n-3 PUFA 1 g/daily (2836 patients), vitamin E 300 mg/day (2830 patients), both (2830 patients), or none (2828 patients). The mean follow-up was 3.5 years, and only the n-3 PUFA diet was effective, not vitamin E, with a 20% decrease in the risk of death, 30% for cardiac death (especially sudden death − 40%), but no difference for nonfatal cardiac events.

Finally, the Lyon Diet Heart Study[7] aimed at testing whether a Mediterranean type diet might reduce the rate of recurrence after myocardial infarction in 423 patients followed up for a mean of 46 months versus a prudent Western-type diet. The low-fat Lyon Diet Heart Study comprised a high intake of bread, fruit and vegetables, more fish, less meat and the replacement of butter and cream by a special margarine enriched in n-3 PUFA. These results were impressive in favor of the Mediterranean diet, with a 72% reduction in cardiovascular death and nonfatal myocardial infarction. Moreover, traditional risk factors (high blood cholesterol, hypertension, etc.) were independent and joint predictors of risk, indicating that this low-fat Mediterranean diet did not alter the relationship between risk factors and secondary prevention. Taken together, these results show that a diet focused only on reduction of fat intake with an increase in the ratio of PUFA to saturated fats has a poor compliance and no clear effect on mortality, whereas n-3

PUFA associated with fruit and vegetables confers early cardioprotection, especially for cardiovascular death and sudden death, whose mechanisms need further research.

Epidemiologic Studies and Intervention Trials on Diet and Cardiovascular Protection

- Total blood cholesterol levels are correlated positively with cardiovascular mortality.
- Mediterranean-type diet confers a rapid cardioprotective effect, independently of lipid levels, likely due to omega-3 fatty acids.
- Low-fat diets have moderate but beneficial effects on cardiovascular events, especially after 2 years of follow-up, but do not seem to alter total mortality.

Guidelines

The recommendations concerning dietary counseling in coronary patients, or patients at high risk of coronary heart disease are usually put together with the other facets of cardiovascular prevention such as smoking cessation or physical exercise. Dietary recommendations from the Third Joint Task Force of European and other Societies on Coronary Prevention,[8] and from the Third Report of the National Cholesterol Education Program (NCEP) Expert Panel on Detection, Evaluation and Treatment of High Blood Cholesterol in Adults (Adult Treatment Panel III[9] are summarized (Table 26-1). These two guidelines are the main references for cardiovascular prevention in Western countries.

From Recommendations to Practice

Despite the worldwide consensus on nutritional recommendations in cardiovascular prevention, their application in everyday life is far from optimal. Western countries are facing a significant increase in obesity, metabolic syndrome, and diabetes directly linked to unhealthy dietary and sedentary habits. However, studies are still needed to orient strategies dealing with this multifac-

TABLE 26-1. Comparison of dietary counseling between European and North American Guidelines

	ESC	Adult Treatment Panel III
Target population	Patients with CHD or other atherosclerotic disease Healthy high-risk individuals Absolute CHD risk ≥20% over 10 years, or will exceed 20% if projected to age 60	Patients with CHD Patients with CHD risk equivalents: – other clinical forms of atherosclerotic disease (peripheral arterial disease, abdominal aortic aneurysm and symptomatic carotid artery disease – diabetes – multiple risk factors that confer a 10-year risk for CHD >20%
Dietary recommendations		
Saturated fat	<7% total calories	<10% of total energy intake
Polyunsaturated fat	<10%	Replacement of saturated fats in part with
Monounsaturated fat	<20%	monounsaturated and polyunsaturated fats from both
Carbohydrate	50–60%	vegetable and margarine sources, as well as with complex
Fiber	20–30 g/day	carbohydrates
		To increase the intake of fresh fruits cereals and vegetables
Total fat	25–35% total calories	<30% total calories
Protein	≈15% of total calories	
Cholesterol	<200 mg/day	<300 mg/day
Total calories	Balance energy intake and expenditure to maintain desirable body weight/prevent weight gain	Reduce total calorie intake when weight reduction is needed
Salt/alcohol		Reduce salt and alcohol use when blood pressure is elevated

eted public health problem, both at population and individual levels.

Target Populations

Target populations are well defined by the European recommendations, represented by subjects "who have developed symptoms of coronary artery disease or other major atherosclerotic disease, and those who are at high risk of developing such diseases in the future" (Table 26-1). To increase the effectiveness of nutrition counseling this population should be extended not only to the family environment, but also the professional environment. Workplaces, via their occupational health service, may also deliver counseling on healthy food habits. Moreover, dietary surveys show that in the working population, nearly half of all meals are taken outside the home, most often in workplace cafeterias. To enable patients to follow their cardioprotective diet, and generally speaking for the good health of their employees, firms should train their "chefs" to prepare a well-balanced diet, and offer meals in line with the above recommendations. Studies evaluating the feasibility and the medico-economical consequences of this concept are to our knowledge not available.

Concerning the family, the partner must be involved in the process of nutritional education, especially if he or she is the usual family cook (it is most often the spouse even today). As for smoking cessation, mutual support in the couple strengthens motivation and adherence to new lifestyle behaviors, key factors for the long-term success of prevention. In this way, the STRIP project,[10] which is a child-targeted coronary artery disease intervention trial, performed in Finland, confirms the impact of nutrition counseling on the whole family. In this study of primary prevention, the families were instructed at 3–6-month intervals to reduce their child's intake of saturated fat and cholesterol from the ages of 7 months to 5 years while the control group ($n = 522$ families) received only brief counseling. During the follow-up, the mothers and fathers of the intervention children modified their diet, using less butter, more margarine and more skim milk than those of the control children, with a moderate but significant decrease in the intake of total and saturated fats in the parents, and a lower serum cholesterol concentration in mothers.

Which Health Professionals?

Although dietitians are specially trained to provide dietary advice, other health professionals such as registered nurses, general practitioners, or cardiologists may also provide it. Even if dietitians seem the best qualified, the effects of dietary advice given by a dietitian compared with another health professional, and occasionally through the use of self-help resources, are debated. In a Cochrane Review involving 12 studies,[11] participants receiving advice from dietitians experienced greater reduction in blood cholesterol than those receiving counsel only from doctors (0.25 vs. 0.12 mmol/L); however, there were no significant changes between dietitian and self-help resources. Compared to counselors the dietitians obtained greater weight reduction (5.8 vs. 2.69 kg). There was no evidence that dietitians provided better outcomes than nurses. However, due to the limited number of trials, these results should be interpreted with caution. Nevertheless, the presence of a dietitian in a cardiac rehabilitation setting leads to a greater variety of nutrition services offered, especially one-to-one nutrition counseling and cooking demonstrations, very helpful in the patient's daily practice.[12] The association of a doctor with a dietitian appears to be more cost-effective with less dropout from the nutritional program and better results on weight loss and decrease in blood pressure.[13]

Organizational Issues

The settings for nutritional counseling differ widely from one country or region to another, depending on the local health network. Nutrition services may be implemented in hospitals, in cardiology units, or cardiac rehabilitation centers, delivering inpatient or outpatient nutritional programs. Lifestyle counseling, especially concerning diet, in coronary patients is underused for many reasons. Lack of time is the first cause mentioned in cardiology wards, which are focused more and more on emergencies and interventional cardiology. Moreover, the patient's length of stay is decreasing and it is difficult to expect that physicians and staff nurses will be able to give substantial dietary advice.

Cardiac rehabilitation units are adequate structures, usually providing a wide range of nutrition services (individualized consultations, group nutrition classes, practical cooking lessons) on behalf of a multidisciplinary team. Unfortunately, these services are underused, as in several countries less than 20% of eligible patients are offered cardiac rehabilitation: younger age, male gender, and high socioeconomic status being associated with participation. The physician's attitude is a strong predictor of a patient's participation.

In general practice, despite the widespread diffusion of guidelines encouraging doctors to promote healthy eating and exercise among high-risk patients, less than half of such patients are given lifestyle advice. Beyond the lack of time due to the increasing patient volume, other factors may compromise dietary counseling, including available resources but also physician skills.

Nutrition science and generally speaking preventive aspects of cardiovascular diseases are poorly represented in medical school curricula, which explains mostly why physicians' readiness to provide lifestyle counseling is so low. This point has been highlighted by a study involving 290 medical students[14] in their first, second, and third year showing that they were generally knowledgeable about cardiovascular risk factors but not about body mass index and specific nutrition and physical activity recommendations. Upper-level students held less positive attitudes about providing lifestyle counseling. Moreover, few medical students apply healthy behaviors to themselves: only 23% were involved in 30 minutes of moderate activity at least five days per week, and half of them reported regularly unhealthy dietary choices.

Organizational Issues: Key Points

– Underuse of dietary counseling in general practice and cardiac hospitals due to medical lack of time and sometimes absence of expertise.
– Cardiac rehabilitation centers offer a large range of nutritional services, but less than 20% of patients undergo cardiac rehabilitation.
– Effective nutrition counseling should be ideally provided by a dietitian via a great variety of services with medical reinforcement.

Practical Modalities

Dietary counseling must be considered as a component of therapeutic education of coronary patients, and follow the same step-by-step process: educational diagnosis, setting of the goals, adherence to nutritional sessions, and evaluation of the dietary behavior modifications. For these purposes, a real partnership must be engaged between health professionals and the patient, with a transfer of knowledge and competencies. However, this type of partnership is rather new in clinical care, where the subject is often "obedient" and passive in front of a doctor's prescription. This type of behavior, adequate in case of emergency or acute illness (only 10% of these situations in general practice), is not adapted to the management of chronic diseases, which requires new skills for the professional team such as communication, pedagogy, or psychology.

Nutrition Educational Goals

A specific nutritional diagnosis is the basis of a tailored dietary counseling. Indeed, to be effective, dietary advice should take into account not only the metabolic disease, but also the patient (what he knows, his psychological status, his goals) and his environment (job, family support).

What Does the Patient Have: Medical and Nutritional Status

The question "What does the patient have?" includes medical diagnosis and risk stratification, type of metabolic abnormality (dyslipidemia, diabetes, overweight) and the associated risk factors which may have an influence on the dietary counseling (smoking, hypertension, sedentariness).

Dietary intake, as an index of atherogenicity and thrombogenicity, must be measured before counseling, as in most of western Europe more than 40% of energy derives from fat, far from the recommendations that only 20–30% of energy should be derived from lipid intakes. The major problem of dietary intake assessment is that no method is the universal "gold standard." Usually, three types of questionnaires are used:

• Recall methods based on the last 24 hours, or a 3-day period where subjects are asked to remember what they have eaten (this may be difficult because of problems of remembering or because certain days are not representative of usual daily intake).
• Prospective method based on exhaustive one week-record.
• Food frequency questionnaires, easy to use, inexpensive, valid and reliable, and less time-consuming than other methods, are increasingly being used.

What Does the Patient Do: Professional and Socioeconomic Context

This item deals with the characteristics of the job, in terms of energy expenditure, working hours, shift work, place where meals are taken, and salaries (in order to adapt food choices for the lowest incomes). Mean energetic requirements during leisure activities must also be assessed.

Moreover, socioeconomic context is associated with different attitudes and beliefs about diet and healthy lifestyles: subjects (especially male) with a low level of education have a higher intake of total and saturated fat, a lower consumption of vegetables and fruit, more frequently use butter and less frequently oil compared to those with a higher level of education.[15] Moreover, lower socioeconomic status seems associated with less health consciousness, stronger belief in the influence of chance on health, and lower life expectancies; these attitudes were in general linked to an unhealthy eating pattern.[16]

Who Is the Patient: Psychological Factors

Readiness to Change

Health professionals' knowledge of the different phases of a patient's acceptance of chronic disease is fundamental. It is often a long period of time from the initial phases of psychological shock, denial, opposition or anger, to coping strategies and progressive acceptance. It would be unrealistic to propose major nutritional behavior modifications for a patient in the denial phase, which may be felt as a partial loss of their identity or familial culture, or even aggression. Readiness to change is one of the first items to assess before embarking on nutritional education with a patient, for the content of the program may differ widely from one patient to another depending on the stage of change.

Several years ago Prochaska and DiClemente[17] identified six stages relating to the process of behavioral modification (Figure 26-1), conditioning our educational approach to a patient. An acute event, such as the occurrence of myocardial infarction, often shortens the three first stages, so patients in cardiac rehabilitation are most often in an action stage. At this phase, emphasis will be put on encouraging self efficacy for dealing with obstacles, counteracting the feeling of loss by reiterating health and quality of

life benefits, and help in managing nutritional aspects of prevention among all other aspects (i.e.: how to combine smoking cessation and weight loss).

The challenge is the maintenance stage with the long-term sustaining of the new behavior: planning for formal or "on request" follow-up support, evocation of relapse, and coping strategies will increase long-term adherence to healthy nutritional habits. Moreover, stages of change may differ within the different items of dietary recommendations: Frame et al.[18] showed in a cross-sectional, longitudinal evaluation or cardiac patients, with a 2-year follow-up after group nutritional education sessions, that results on fat reduction and increase in fruit and vegetable intake were not concordant: reduction in fat intake was effective in the population (from 83.1% at baseline to 87.3% at 2 years for action and maintenance stages) whereas precontemplation and contemplation stages increased from 37.6% to 58.5% for fruit and vegetable intake, indicating that cardiac rehabilitation patients were in different stages of change for food behaviors linked to the same disease.

Locus of Control

An other important psychological component to assess is the patient's locus of control, which means the tendency for the patient to attribute life events to "internal" factors depending on his willingness and behavior or to "external factors" such as a hazard or other people. In the latter, the process of nutritional change will be longer and more difficult, involving the need to improve the patient's health beliefs, self-efficacy and empowerment. A person's social life may also present barriers to implementing new ways of eating. In a study involving 362 male coronary heart disease patients, which evaluated the barriers in following nutritional advice, Koikkalainen et al.[19] showed that sensitivity to social influence was the most important factor explaining noncompliance with dietary advice among patients with high dietary fat intake, compared with other barriers (eating

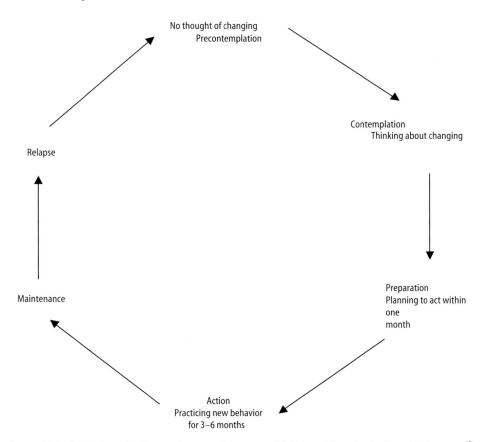

FIGURE 26-1. Prochaska and DiClemente's stages of change model. (Adapted from Prochaska and DiClemente.[17])

at work, food price, shopping, taste or level of knowledge).

What Does the Patient Know: Level of Knowledge

It is essential for health professionals to assess a patient's current knowledge and beliefs on diet, in order to give effective and adequate counseling. Classical evaluation tools, such as open or closed questionnaires or case problems, identify selective knowledge, but not the way this knowledge is organized nor the emotional factors that are implicated. A new tool, recently implemented in therapeutic education, includes this information: concept mapping[20] can be defined as the cartog-

raphy of an individual's knowledge and feelings about a given theme such as "diet," "fat," or "sugar." This graphic representation can be reassessed regularly to follow and guide the educational process (Figure 26-2). Despite its exhaustiveness and interest, this tool needs skilled physicians and is time-consuming in daily routine.

The educational diagnosis is concluded by discussing the patient's short- and long-term plans, and the setting of goals. These objectives must be realistic (in terms of weight reduction for example), easy to reach in daily life, with step-by-step aims. They engage the patient and the health professional in a long-term partnership.

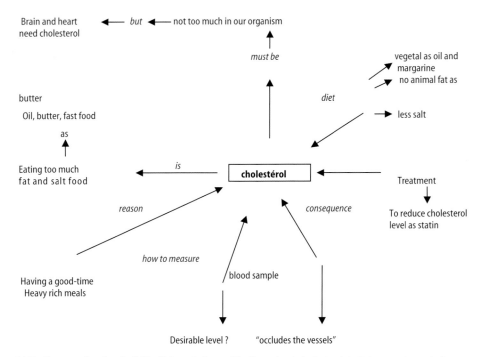

FIGURE 26-2. Cartography of an individual's knowledge and feelings about cholesterol: initial concept map before counseling.

Nutritional Counseling Sessions

For greater effectiveness, interventions should be varied and complementary, both at group and individual levels, including nutritional face-to-face consultations, interactive conferences, or cooking sessions on different themes (diabetes, weight loss, fat and cooking, how to choose fresh fruit or vegetables, or information on ready-to-eat meals) (Figure 26.3). To enhance a patient's adherence and skills, group nutritional counseling should be friendly, pragmatic, simple, with effective practice from the patient, and if possible, his or her partner.

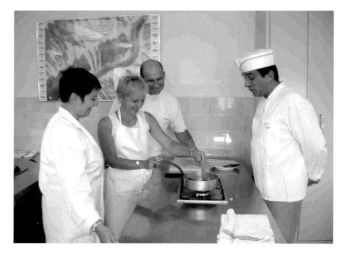

FIGURE 26-3. Cooking course.

Moreover, nutritional counseling sessions should involve the cultural context of attitudes to food in each country.[21] A study conductedin 1999 in four countries (US, Japan, Belgium, and France) dealt with beliefs about the diet–health link, worries about food, the tendency to associate foods with nutritional versus culinary contexts, the healthiness of one's own diet: the group associating food most with health and least with pleasure were US citizens. In contrast, the French were the most culinary oriented and the least health oriented, mainly among men. However, paradoxically, despite their knowledge about diet and health, the US group did not classify themselves as healthy eaters.

These sessions must be associated with periodic follow-up, in order to assess the progression to the goals, the difficulties met, and to reinforce the patient's motivation. In addition to this formal follow-up, individual help may be provided in the case of problems or relapse.

Practical Modalities: Key Points

- Coronary artery disease is a chronic disease, in which prognosis is highly dependent on the maintenance of a healthy diet.
- Dietary counseling is a part of the therapeutic education of coronary patients, and nutritional education diagnosis is the first step for tailored dietary advice.
- A patient's nutritional diagnosis includes not only medical status and assessment of dietary intake, but also socioeconomic factors, psychological context (readiness to change, locus of control) and level of knowledge.

Impact of Counseling on Dietary Behaviors

Because of the important differences across studies in outcome measures, study design, analysis strategy, and intervention techniques, it is difficult to reach definitive conclusions on the type of dietary counseling that is the most successful, even if some characteristics seem to improve the effectiveness of behavioral interventions in modifying dietary patterns.

Ammerman et al.[22] conducted an evidence-based review of existing literature on the efficacy of behavioral interventions in modifying dietary fat and fruit and vegetable intake. From 907 articles originally identified, the authors retained 92 independent studies meeting the research criteria (randomized controlled studies, not based on controlled diets, with at least a sample size of 40 subjects at follow-up). Intervention groups were similarly successful in reducing total fat (7.3% reduction in the percentage of total calories from fat) and saturated fat intakes, and in increasing fruit and vegetable intake (+0.6 servings per day). The interventions seemed to be more effective in high-risk populations rather than in primary prevention populations but results on long-term changes are unclear. High-intensity interventions were more likely to produce changes than low-intensity interventions, and counseling using a research clinic setting was more effective than counseling conducted by primary care doctors in the course of their usual activity. The researchers also noted that the variety of the types of counseling, such as individual dietary assessment, face-to-face consultations, group counseling, techniques aimed at improving the patient's skills and motivation produced more significant changes in diet behavior than brief counseling.

Only very limited data have evaluated the cost-effectiveness of different types of intervention: however, the combination of referral to a dietitian with brief medical counseling seems to have more positive medico-economic effects than referral alone.

Characteristics of Effective Nutritional Counseling in High-Risk Individuals

- Multidisciplinary approach (i.e. at least dietitian counseling and medical reinforcement).
- Hospital setting.
- High level of intervention with varied types of individual and group activities.
- Regular assessment and support.

Conclusion

Even though the "diet-heart hypothesis" has become a reality with proven facts, the translation of recommendations to daily eating practice is far from optimal. Today, further research is needed in human sciences to improve nutrition counseling at both an individual and population level: the different components of nutrition counseling, dietary assessment tools, intensity of dietary counseling, optimal organizational issues, and evaluation of cost-effectiveness are the key issues for an effective implementation of healthy food choices in the population.

References

1. Verschuren WMM, Jacobs DR, Bloenberg B, et al. Serum total cholesterol and long-term coronary heart disease mortality in different cultures. Twenty-five-year follow-up of the Seven Countries Study. JAMA 1995;274:131–136.
2. Yusuf FS, Hawken S, Ounpuu S, et al. Effect of potentially modifiable risk factors associated with myocardial infarction in 52 countries (the InterHeart Study): case control study. Lancet 2004; 364:937–952.
3. Hooper L, Summerbell CD, Higgins JP, et al. Dietary fat intake and prevention of cardiovascular disease: systematic review. BMJ 2001;322:757–763.
4. Buer ML, Fehily AM, Gilbert JF, et al. Effects of changes in fat, fish and fibre intakes on death, and reinfarction: Diet and Reinfarction Trial (DART). Lancet 1989;ii:757–761.
5. Singh RB, Niaz MA, Sharma JP, Kumar R, Rastogi V, Moshiri M. Randomized, double-blind, placebo controlled trial of fish oil and mustard oil in patients with suspected acute myocardial infarction: The Indian experiment of infarct survival. Cardiovasc Drugs Ther 1997;11:485–491.
6. GISSI Prevenzione Investigators. Dietary supplementation with n-3 polyunsaturated fatty acids and vitamins after myocardial infarction: results of the GISSI-Prevenzione trial. Lancet 1999;354:447–455.
7. De Lorgeril M, Salen P, Martin JL, Monjaud I, Delaye J, Mamelle N. Mediterranean diet, traditional risk factors and the rate of cardiovascular complications after myocardial infarction. Final report of the Lyon Diet Heart Study. Circulation 1999;99:779–785.
8. De Backer G, Ambrosioni E, Borch-Johnsen K, et al. Third Joint Task Force of European and Other Societies on Cardiovascular Disease Prevention in Clinical Practice. European guidelines on cardiovascular disease prevention in clinical practice. Eur Heart J 2003;24(17):1601–1610.
9. National Cholesterol Education Program (NCEP) Expert Panel on Detection, Evaluation and Treatment of High Blood Cholesterol in Adults (Adult Treatment Panel III). Third Report of the National Cholesterol Education Program (NCEP). Expert Panel on Detection, Evaluation and Treatment of High Blood Cholesterol in Adults (ATP III) final report. Circulation 2002;106:3143–3421.
10. Lagstrom H, Seppanen R, Jokinen E, et al. Nutrient intakes and cholesterol values of the parents in a prospective randomised child-targeted coronary heart disease risk factor intervention trial. The STRIP Project. Eur J Clin Nutr 1999;53:654–661.
11. Thompson RL, Summerbell CD, Hooper L, et al. Dietary advice given by a dietician versus other health professional or self-help resources to reduce blood cholesterol (Cochrane Review). In: The Cochrane Library Issue 3, 2003. Oxford: Update Software.
12. Cavallaro V, Dwyer J, Houser RF, et al. Influence of dietician presence on outpatient cardiac rehabilitation nutrition services. J Am Diet Assoc 2004;104: 611–14.
13. Pritchard DA, Hyndman J, Taba F. Nutritional counselling in general practice: a cost effective analysis. J Epidemiol Community Health 1999;53: 311–316.
14. Foster KY, Diehl NS, Shaw D, et al. Medical students' readiness to provide lifestyle counselling for overweight patients. Eat Behav 2002;3:1–13.
15. Erkkila AT, Sarkkinen EJ, Lehtos S, Pyomala K, Uustitupa MI. Diet in relation to socio-economic status in patients with coronary heart disease. Eur J Clin Nutr 1999;53:662–668.
16. Wardle J, Steptoe A. Socio-economic differences in attitudes and beliefs about healthy lifestyles. J Epidemiol Community Health 2003;57:440–443.
17. Prochaska JO, DiClemente CC. Stages of change in the modification of problem behaviors. Prog Behav Modif 1992;28:183–218.
18. Frame CJ, Green CG, Herr DG, Taylor ML. A 2-year stage of change evaluation of dietary fat and fruit and vegetables intake behaviours of cardiac rehabilitation patients. Am J Health Promot 2003;17: 361–368.
19. Koikkalainen M, Mykkanen H, Erkilla A, Julkunen J, Saarinen T, Pyorala K. Difficulties in changing the diet in relation to dietary fat intake among patients with coronary heart disease. Eur J Clin Nutr 1999;53:120–125.

20. Marchand C, Divernois JF, Assal JP, Slama G, Hivon R. An analysis using concept mapping of diabetic patients' knowledge, before and after patient education. Medical Teacher 2002;24:90–99.

21. Rozin P, Fischler C, Imada S, Sarubin A, Wrzesniewski A. Attitudes to food and the role of food in life in the USA, Japan, Flemish Belgium and France: possible implications for the diet health debate. Appetite 1999;33:163–180.

22. Ammerman AS, Lindquist CH, Lohr KN, Hersey J. The efficacy of behavioural interventions to modify dietary fat and fruit and vegetable intake: a review of the evidence. Prev Med 2002;35(1):25–41.

Section V
Tobacco Addiction

The burden of cardiovascular disease due to cigarette smoking is enormous, both in the Western world and in developing countries. To stop smoking is healthy at all ages. This section not only focuses on the burden of disease, but also gives information on the latest guidelines to help patients quit smoking, based on the fact that dependency is the main factor that has to be overcome. Therefore, assisting the coronary patient to give up smoking remains one of the main tasks of comprehensive cardiac rehabilitation and all team members should have a basic knowledge in this field.

Main Messages

Chapter 27: The Burden of Smoking on Cardiovascular Disease

Among the risk factors for cardiovascular disease, smoking still ranks as main cause of premature coronary disease. In this chapter the present epidemiology of smoking is described. The relation between both active and passive smoking and coronary heart disease (CHD) and the causal mechanisms are discussed. Severe consequences for public health are demonstrated.

Physicians and other health workers in the field of CHD prevention and rehabilitation should play an active role in smoking cessation.

Chapter 28: The Role of Tobacco Dependence and Addiction

In successful counseling of coronary patients on quitting smoking, physicians as well as other cardiac rehabilitation team members need to understand the role of dependence on and addiction to nicotine. This complex mechanism and the highly individual combination of contributing factors implies a diagnostic and therapeutic challenge. The aim of this chapter is to give insight into the theoretical background of nicotine addiction and thus provide a basis for smoking cessation as part of a cardiac rehabilitation program.

Chapter 29: Treatment of Tobacco Dependency

In most patients the traumatic experience of an acute cardiac event will be the starting point of serious efforts to give up smoking. Here, the engagement, knowledge, and support from all health professionals and the cardiac rehabilitation team is required. After information on the willingness and the stage of change of the patient to stop smoking, the method used to support the patients is described in this chapter, including indications for and use of pharmacotherapy. Insight into smoking addiction, information, support, and understanding are important success factors for the cardiologist in helping the patient to stop smoking and prevent relapse.

27
The Burden of Smoking on Cardiovascular Disease

Ulrich Keil

Introduction

According to the World Health Organization (WHO) the number of smokers in the world was estimated to be 1.1 billion in the year 2000. Of those, 300 million lived in the developed world, while 800 million lived in developing countries.

According to Ezzati and Lopez[1] the number of premature deaths caused by smoking in the year 2000 on a worldwide basis was estimated to be 4.83 million. Of these, 2.41 million were confined to developing countries and 2.43 to the developed world; 3.84 million occurred in men and about 1 million in women. Major causes of death were cardiovascular disease (CVD) with 1.69 million, chronic obstructive pulmonary disease (COPD) with 0.97 million, and lung cancer with 0.85 million.

For the year 2030, the estimates for premature deaths from smoking on a worldwide basis are 10 million, of which 3 million will happen in the developed countries and 7 million in the developing world. Half of all premature deaths from tobacco happen in people aged 35–69 years. If we do not succeed in persuading a large part of those who smoke today to quit their habit, the number of premature deaths from smoking will rise dramatically within the next 50 years. On epidemiological and demographic grounds it does not suffice to prevent "only" children and adolescents from taking up smoking because the large cohort of today's smokers will be exposed to the hazards of smoking over decades.

Among the ten most important risk factors for the burden of disease in Western societies, tobacco consumption ranks first before high blood pressure, alcohol consumption, high cholesterol, high body mass index (BMI), low fruit and vegetable intake, physical inactivity, etc. (Figure 27-1).[2]

Frequency of Smoking in Men and Women in 2002

According to data from the World Health Organization for the year 2002,[3] the frequency of smoking in men and women depicts a large variability internationally. Table 27-1 shows for men a range from 67% in China to 19% in Sweden and for women a range from 31% in Germany to 1% in Saudi Arabia. Germany belongs to the countries with the highest percentage of smokers in the world. In the age group 30–39 years about 50% of men and more than 40% of women are smokers.

In developed countries we see strong associations between indicators of social status (class) and the frequency of smoking.[4] Data from the MONICA Augsburg survey in 1994/95 in men and women, aged 25–74 years, also show strong associations between years of education and cigarette consumption. The higher the number of years of education the lower the percentage of smokers. This finding was true for men of all age groups (25–74 years) and for women of younger age groups (25–44 years).[5]

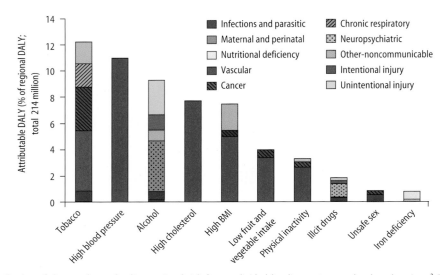

FIGURE 27-1. Burden of disease due to leading regional risk factors divided by disease type – developed regions.[2] DALY: disability-adjusted life year.

Smoking and Cardiovascular Diseases

In the first half of the last century German clinicians were among the first who contributed to our knowledge on the relationship between smoking and lung cancer.[6] The classical epidemiological studies on this relationship were started at the end of the 1940s and the beginning of the 1950s in England and in the US.

A cohort study of 34,000 British male physicians was started by Doll et al. in 1951 with follow-up periods of 20, 40, and 50 years.[7–9] For the 20-year follow-up, the relative risk for smokers

compared to non-smokers of developing lung cancer was 14. On the other hand, the relative risk for the relationship between smoking and coronary heart disease (CHD) mortality turned out to be only 1.6.

Because of the greater number of deaths from CHD compared to those from lung cancer the attributable risk for smoking and CHD was nearly twice as big as the respective figure for smoking and lung cancer (Table 27-2). With these data, Doll and Peto could show that a reduction in smoking would save more people from heart disease than from lung cancer.[7]

TABLE 27-1. Frequency (%) of smoking in men and women in selected countries 2002[3]

Country	Men	Women
China	66.9	4.2
Russia	63.2	9.7
Poland	44.0	25.0
Germany	**39.0**	**31.0**
France	38.6	30.3
Italy	32.4	17.3
Denmark	32.0	29.0
UK	27.0	26.0
USA	25.7	21.5
Saudi Arabia	22.0	1.0
Sweden	19.0	19.0

TABLE 27-2. Relative and attributable risks of mortality from lung cancer and CHD among cigarette smokers in a prospective cohort study of 34,000 male British doctors, 1951–1971

	Annual mortality rates per 100,000	
	Lung cancer	Coronary heart disease
Cigarette smokers	**140**	**669**
Nonsmokers	**10**	**413**
Relative risk	$\dfrac{140/10^5}{10/10^5} = \mathbf{14.0}$	$\dfrac{669/10^5}{413/10^5} = \mathbf{1.6}$
Attributable risk	**130/10⁵/year**	**256/10⁵/year**

Source: Doll and Peto.[7] © 1976 BMJ Publishing Group Ltd. Reprinted with permission.

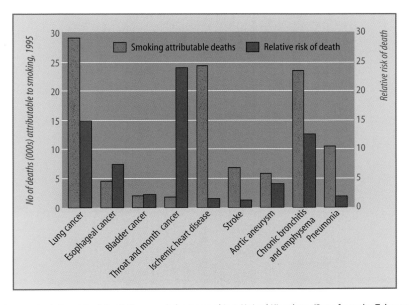

FIGURE 27-2. Numbers and relative risk of death (by cause) due to smoking, United Kingdom. (Data from the Tobacco Advisory Group of the Royal College of Physicians and Doll et al.[8,9])

Figure 27-2 depicts relative risks of causes of death due to smoking and attributable deaths for a number of cancer sites and for CHD, stroke, aortic aneurysm, and COPD based on data from the Tobacco Advisory Group of the Royal College of Physicians.[4] The relative risk of death is small for CHD and big for throat and mouth cancer, while the number of deaths attributable to smoking is big for CHD and small for throat and mouth cancer.

The 50-year follow-up of the British physicians study was published in 2004.[9] It revealed that smokers compared to non-smokers lost about 10 years of their life. Furthermore, this study clearly showed that it is practically never too late to stop smoking. Those physicians who stopped at age 25–34 had about the same survival as the non-smoking physicians. Those physicians who stopped smoking at age 55–64, did not lose 10 years of their life but "only" 7 years.[9]

Calculations of relative risks for smoking and CHD turn out to be around 2.0 in many cohort studies.[10] Relative risks are higher in younger compared to older people and in those who consume larger numbers of cigarettes.[7–9] There is a dose–response relationship between CHD and the number of cigarettes smoked per day.[8] Relative risks for CHD morbidity are higher than for CHD mortality.[11]

Of special interest for countries with high serum total cholesterol values is the synergism between smoking and hypercholesterolemia. Figure 27-3 is derived from the Augsburg cohort study of 1984/85 with an 8-year follow-up. It shows that men with high cholesterol values who are also smokers have a relative risk of 8.3 (1.5 + 2.8 ≠ 4.3 but 8.3!) to develop CHD (fatal and nonfatal) compared to men without any of the three classic risk factors.[12]

According to Figure 27-3, more than 65% of all CHD events in men could be avoided if the three classic risk factors were eliminated or controlled for; this is the message conveyed by the population attributable fraction of >65%. The risk factor combination smoking and hypercholesterolemia alone produced 23.1% of all CHD events in this cohort from southern Germany.[12] The data in Figure 27-3 have been calculated without adjusting for the "regression-dilution bias." Studies which have applied this adjustment came up with attributable risks of 80% and more[13] for the three classic CHD risk factors.

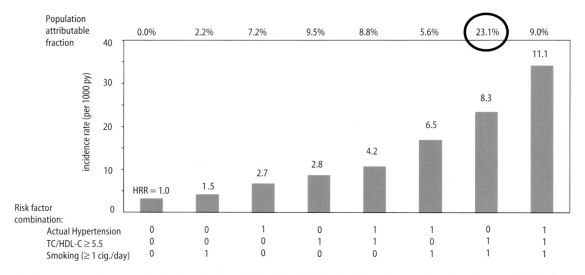

FIGURE 27-3. Relative risks and attributable risks (population attributable fraction) of CHD (fatal and nonfatal) in men of the Augsburg region caused by smoking, hypertension, and hypercholesterolemia and their various combinations.[12] PY, person years.

For northern European countries with a high consumption of animal fat and high mean total cholesterol values this interaction or synergism between smoking and hypercholesterolemia is of great importance. Ancel Keys and the Seven Countries Study have already taught us that a diet high in animal fat intake (saturated fatty acids) and cigarette smoking are the most important factors for high CHD rates in different countries.[14] The interaction between smoking and hypercholesterolemia shown in the Augsburg cohort data has already been seen much earlier in the Seven Countries Study. Figure 27-4 shows that the 10-year CHD incidence rate regression line has a much steeper slope with increasing cigarette consumption in northern Europe compared to southern Europe.[15] This steeper slope of the regression line in the northern

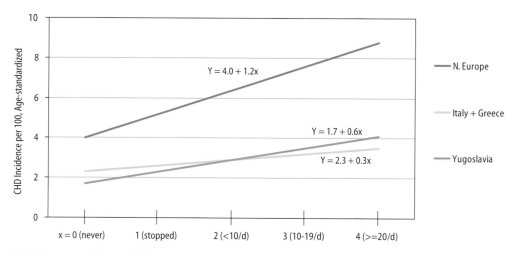

FIGURE 27-4. Regression of 10-year CHD incidence rate on smoking class of 8717 men free of cardiovascular disease at entry in northern Europe, Italy and Greece, and Yugoslavia.[15]

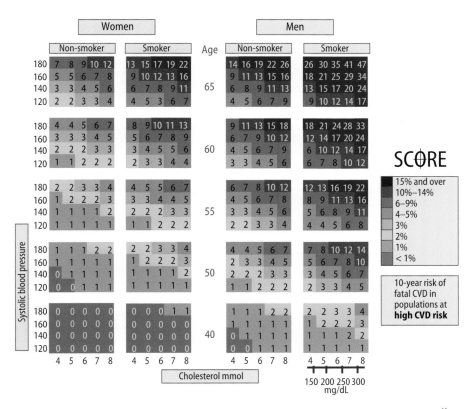

FIGURE 27-5. Prediction of 10-year risk for fatal cardiovascular disease in Europe: the SCORE project.[10]

European countries compared to southern Europe can be explained by the synergism between smoking and the high cholesterol values in northern Europe.[15]

The European SCORE (Systematic Coronary Risk Evaluation) project[10] provides 10-year risk estimates for fatal cardiovascular events including stroke in Europe by age, cholesterol level, systolic blood pressure, and smoking status. Figure 27-5 clearly shows that smoking doubles the (relative) risk for fatal cardiovascular events in any of the systolic blood pressure and total cholesterol constellations (boxes). This statement applies to men and women and to the age group 50–65 years.

Figure 27-5 provides for each risk factor profile the 10-year risk (= absolute risk) for a fatal CVD event according to age separately for men and women. Obviously smoking nearly doubles the (relative) risk for a fatal cardiovascular event. This finding applies to populations at high CVD risk (shown here) and to those at intermediate and low CVD risk.[10]

Passive Smoking and Cardiovascular Diseases

More than 19 epidemiological studies have focused on passive smoking or second hand smoke and CHD. A meta-analysis by Law et al.[16] demonstrated that never-smokers have a 30% higher risk for CHD, if they live with a smoker.

Active smoking of one cigarette per day increases the risk for CHD by 39%, which is similar to the risk of a non-smoker who lives with a smoker. Law et al. did not find any bias for this association. The impact of better food habits in non-smokers was estimated to amount to only 6%. If this is taken into account, a risk increase of about 24% for CHD in non-smokers exposed to second hand smoke remains (30%–6% = 24%).[16] This finding was substantiated by two more recent meta-analyses.[17,18]

The burden of cardiovascular disease from second hand smoke in the US is estimated to amount to about 35,000–62,000 deaths from CHD per year.[19] Conservative estimates for Germany come up with 3700 cases of CHD (fatal and non-fatal) and 1800 cases of stroke (fatal and nonfatal) due to second hand smoke.[20]

Smoking and Acute Myocardial Infarction: Mechanisms

Tobacco smoke is a complex mixture of aerosols and particulate matter containing about 4000 different chemical compounds of which many are highly toxic and more than 40 are carcinogenic.

Tobacco smoke interferes with the cardiovascular system in the following ways: Smoking increases the risk of thrombosis by increasing platelet aggregation, blood viscosity, and fibrinogen levels. C-reactive protein, a marker of inflammation, is also increased by cigarette smoking. The inhaled carbon monoxide produces carboxyhemoglobin, which leads to an imbalance between oxygen demand of and supply to the myocardium. Polycyclic aromatic hydrocarbons (PAH) and other toxic compounds damage the endothelium. LDL cholesterol is oxidized by cigarette smoke and it is the oxidized LDL cholesterol which exerts its atherogenic effect. VLDL cholesterol and triglycerides are also increased by inhaled cigarette smoke. In addition, cigarette smoke decreases the protective HDL cholesterol.

The Effects of Tobacco on Public Health

According to recent data from McNeill[21] for the 25 countries of the EU, there were 656,000 deaths caused by smoking in the year 2000. This amounts to more than one in seven of all deaths across the EU. In the ten new member states smoking alone caused nearly one in five of all deaths.

Table 27-3 shows the number of deaths due to smoking as a proportion of all deaths in the EU, stratified by cause of death. From Table 27-3 we learn that 10% of all deaths from cardiovascular disease in the EU are caused by smoking; in men this figure is 16% while in women it is only 5%.

Whether smoking-attributable deaths from cancer exceed those from cardiovascular disease varies across the different EU countries, depending on the background risk of cardiovascular disease in specific countries or regions and the age of the population studied. Death rates from stroke are higher in central and eastern Europe than in the other regions, and death rates from CHD are generally higher in northern, central, and eastern Europe than in southern and western Europe.[21] This relates to other risk factors for CHD and also to their synergistic effects with smoking. This refers to the interaction between smoking and cholesterol levels, smoking being more dangerous for those who also have high blood cholesterol levels.[21]

Cancers, cardiovascular diseases, and respiratory diseases together account for the great majority of deaths caused by smoking, representing 43%, 28%, and 18% of all deaths due to smoking, respectively (Figure 27-6).

TABLE 27-3. Number of deaths (in 1,000) caused by smoking in the (25 countries) EU, year 2000 [21]

Cause of death	Men	Women	Total
lung cancer	156/171 (91%)	34/53 (65%)	190/224 (85%)
all cancers	**239/626 (38%)**	**46/493 (9%)**	**285/1119 (25%)**
cardiovascular disease	**136/846 (16%)**	**48/1028 (5%)**	**184/1873 (10%)**
diseases of the respiratory system	78/194 (40%)	34/178 (19%)	113/371 (30%)
total	**508/2214 (23%)**	**148/2238 (7%)**	**656/4452 (15%)**

Source: Peto et al. Mortality from smoking in developed countries 1950 to 2010, 2nd ed. © 1995 Oxford University Press. Data updated in: Tobacco or Health in the European Union. Data from Peto R et al. Luxembourg: European Communities 2004, p 40.

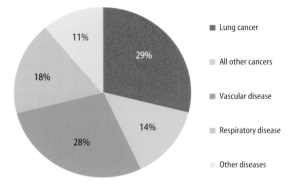

11%

29%

18%

14%

28%

- Lung cancer
- All other cancers
- Vascular disease
- Respiratory disease
- Other diseases

FIGURE 27-6. Proportion of deaths from smoking by disease group, European Union, 2000.[21]

Smoking Cessation in Patients with Coronary Heart Disease

Patients with CHD who smoke can halve their risk for a recurrent CHD event[22] if they quit smoking. Although physicians and patients may both be aware of this fact, smoking cessation is not easily achieved. Surveys within the framework of the EUROASPIRE project revealed that in the year 2000 on average 21% of CHD patients in Europe smoked (had continued their smoking or had taken it up again after their CHD event).[23]

EUROASPIRE data from Münster have shown that evidence-based smoking cessation procedures such as nicotine replacement therapy and behavioral therapy are seldom practiced by cardiologists. Of the 64 CHD patients who smoked in the EUROASPIRE Münster study of the year 2000 only 6% (= 4) reported that their physician had prescribed a nicotine replacement therapy. An independent survey of 681 ambulatory care physicians of the Münster region[24] revealed that only 16% of them were in favor of smoking cessation courses and only 5% had prescribed nicotine replacement therapy to their smoking CHD patients. Obviously, there is a lot of room for improvement in physician and patient education concerning the treatment of tobacco addiction. Smoking cessation measures should be conveyed to physicians as one of the most efficient prevention programs in medicine.

References

1. Ezzati M, Lopez AD. Estimates of global mortality attributable to smoking in 2000. Lancet 2003;362: 847–852.
2. Ezzati M, Lopez AD, Rodgers A, Vander Hoorn S, Murray CJL, and the Comparative Risk Assessment Collaborating Group. Selected major risk factors and global and regional burden of disease. Lancet 2002;360:1347–1360.
3. http://www.who.int/tobacco/en/atlas40.pdf (2002).
4. Edwards R. The problem of tobacco smoking. BMJ 2004;328:217–219.
5. Maziak W, Hense HW, Döring A, Keil U. Ten-year trends in smoking behaviour among adults in southern Germany. Int J Tuberc Lung Dis 2002;6: 824–830.
6. Schönherr E. Beitrag zur Statistik und Klinik der Lungentumoren. Z Krebsforsch 1928;27:436–450.
7. Doll R, Peto R. Mortality in relation to smoking: 20 years' observations on male British doctors. BMJ 1976;2:1525–1536.
8. Doll R, Peto R, Wheatley K, Gray R, Sutherland I. Mortality in relation to smoking: 40 years' observations on male British doctors. BMJ 1994;309:901–911.
9. Doll R, Peto R, Boreham J, Sutherland I. Mortality in relation to smoking: 50 years' observation on male British doctors. BMJ 2004;328:1529–1537.
10. Conroy RM, Pyörälä K, Fitzgerald AP, et al., on behalf of the SCORE project group. Estimation of ten-year risk of fatal cardiovascular disease in Europe: the SCORE project. Eur Heart J 2003;24:987–1003.
11. Yusuf S, Hawken S, Õunpuu S, et al., on behalf of the INTERHEART Study Investigators. Effect of potentially modifiable risk factors associated with myocardial infarction in 52 countries (the INTERHEART study): case-control study. Lancet 2004;364: 937–952.
12. Keil U, Liese AD, Hense HW, et al. Classical risk factors and their impact on incident non-fatal and fatal myocardial infarction and all-cause mortality in southern Germany. Results from the MONICA Augsburg cohort study 1984–1992. Eur Heart J 1998;19:1197–1207.
13. Magnus P, Beaglehole R. The real contribution of the major risk factors to the coronary epidemics: time to end the "only-50%" myth. Arch Intern Med 2001;161:2657–2660.
14. Kromhout D, Menotti A, Blackburn H (eds). Prevention of Coronary Heart Disease. Diet, Lifestyle and Risk Factors in the Seven Countries

Study. Dordrecht: Kluwer Academic Publishers; 2002.

15. Keys A. Seven Countries. A multivariate analysis of death and coronary heart disease. Cambridge, MA: Harvard University Press; 1980:151.

16. Law MR, Morris JK, Wald NJ. Environmental tobacco smoke exposure and ischaemic heart disease: an evaluation of the evidence. BMJ. 1997; 315:973–980.

17. He J, Vupputuri S, Allen K, Prerost MR, Hughes J, Whelton PK. Passive smoking and the risk of coronary heart disease – a meta-analysis of epidemiologic studies. N Engl J Med 1999;340:920–926.

18. Thun M, Henley J, Apicella LF. Epidemiologic studies of fatal and nonfatal cardiovascular disease and ETS exposure from spousal smoking. Environ Health Perspect 1999;107(suppl):841–846.

19. Davis RM. Passive smoking: history repeats itself. BMJ 1997;315:961–962.

20. Keil U, Becher H, Heidrich J, et al. Passivrauchbedingte Morbidität und Mortalität in Deutschland. In: Rote Reihe DKFZ. Die Gefahren der Passivrauchexposition in Deutschland, Heidelberg: Deutsches Krebsforschungszentrum; 2005.

21. McNeill A. Tobacco use and effects on health. In: Tobacco or Health in the European Union. Luxembourg: European Communities; 2004:40.

22. Wilson K, Gibson N, Willan A, Cook D. Effect of smoking cessation on mortality after myocardial infarction. Meta-analysis of cohort studies. Arch Intern Med 2000;160:939–944.

23. EUROASPIRE II Study Group. Lifestyle and risk factor management and use of drug therapies in coronary patients from 15 countries. Eur Heart J 2001;22:554–572.

24. Heidrich J, Behrens T, Raspe F, Keil U. Knowledge and perception of guidelines and secondary prevention of coronary heart disease among general practitioners and internists. Results from a physician survey in Germany. Eur J Cardiovasc Prev Rehabil 2005;12(6):521–529.

28
The Role of Tobacco Dependence and Addiction

Trudi P.G. Tromp-Beelen

Most smokers do want to quit smoking. That this is not always an easy task can be attributed to the fact that dependence plays an important role. Nicotine dependence meets all criteria of addiction. The use is compulsive, it is hard to quit even when there is clear damage, withdrawal symptoms appear when stopping, and there is always a risk of falling back when trying to quit a chronic behavior. Smoking dependence fits the criteria given in the *Diagnostic and Statistical Manual of Mental Disorders* system, version IV (DSM IV),[1] grading dependence and addiction to a substance (Table 28-1).

The estimated percentage of smokers who are addicted varies from 50% to 92%.[2,3] Yearly, about half of all smokers are planning to quit and about 25% are taking action to quit smoking. Only 7% of these attempts to quit are successful.[4]

Tobacco smoke consists of more than 2000 different substances, among which are gases and a very fine mixture of tar (solid and liquid substances). Nicotine is the main component in tobacco smoke that causes and maintains addiction. Nicotine addiction is a complex of pharmacological, behavioral and conditioned factors, predisposition, and social circumstances.

Pharmacological Mechanism of Addiction and Craving

All known addicting substances influence the mesolimbic reward system in the brain. This system initiates and maintains behavior that is essential to survive (for instance eating, sex, and taking care of the offspring) and is present in all mammals.

Dopamine plays the most important role in this system. Nicotine interferes with this dopamine rewarding system by influencing the concentration of dopamine directly at the receptor or indirectly influencing the neurotransmission via GABA, opioid, serotonin, acetylcholine or norepinephrine, thus being an inhibitor or stimulator of this dopamine rewarding system.[5] Nicotine, alcohol, heroin, and cocaine influence this system at various levels. Direct activation of the rewarding system leads to euphoric feelings. This is essential in the development of dependency and addiction. Neuroadaptation develops when nicotine is used regularly. The change in the brain is permanent at molecular, cellular, structural, as well as functional levels. This is the cause of craving. Craving can remain, even when the nicotine has been stopped for a very long time. Craving is closely related to the phenomenon of relapse, the essence of addiction. As a result of this neuroadaptation, tolerance and withdrawal symptoms may occur.

Nicotine Pharmacokinetics

The risk of addiction is greater when nicotine comes more quickly into the brain, as it increases the level of concentration in the blood faster and has a short-term effect, so it has to be taken more often. When nicotine is inhaled, it will reach the brain after approximately 7 seconds. Nicotine not only works quickly, is also works

TABLE 28-1. Dependency according to the criteria of DSM IV[1]

Three or more of the following characteristics occurring in a 12-month period:
- tolerance
- withdrawal
- smoking larger amounts or over a longer period of time than intended
- persistent desire or unsuccessful efforts to reduce smoking
- spending a great deal of time obtaining or using cigarettes or recovering from its effects
- reducing important activities (social, occupational, or recreational) because of smoking
- continuing smoking despite knowledge of smoking-related physical or psychological problems

briefly so it has to be dosed frequently, making it very addictive. Smoking *light* or *mild* cigarettes does not result in a lower intake of nicotine, because these cigarettes are inhaled more deeply and more frequently to meet the smoker's needs.[6]

Chewing and sniffing tobacco, as well as nicotine chewing gum, are made alkaline in order to promote resorption via the oropharyngeal mucous membrane. This way of administration is much slower, making it less addictive. Highest blood nicotine levels are reached after only 30 minutes, but remain at this level for a couple of hours (Figure 28-1).[7]

Nicotine Pharmacodynamics

It is not only due to the pharmacokinetic properties of nicotine administered by smoking, mentioned earlier, that nicotine is as addicting as it is, its pharmacodynamics play an important role as well. Nicotine interacts with the nicotinic cholinergic receptors in both the central and peripheral nervous system. The effect of nicotine can be stimulating but in a high dose it can be dampening too, due to complex electrochemical processes.

Stimulation of the nicotinic cholinergic receptor causes the release of many different neurotransmitters including acetylcholine, norepinephrine, dopamine, serotonin, beta-endorphin, gamma-aminobutyric acid, and glutamate. It also causes the release of hormones such as growth hormone, prolactin, vasopressin, and adrenocorticotropic hormone (ACTH).[8]

Smokers report many different pleasant, rewarding effects of their habit, such as arousal, relaxation (especially in stressful situations), improved attention, and an increased performance on certain tasks. Furthermore, nicotine can improve one's mood, reduce anxiety, relieve hunger, and prevent weight gain. Benowitz has linked these positive effects in a (hypothetical) model shown in Figure 28-2.[8]

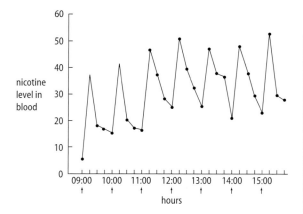

FIGURE 28-1. The nicotine level in blood after smoking one cigarette an hour. Blood samples every 15 minutes. The vertical axis shows the nicotine level in the blood (ng/mL blood). On the horizontal axis, the time is indicated on a scale of 1–24. (From Goldstein.[7] With permission from Oxford University Press.)

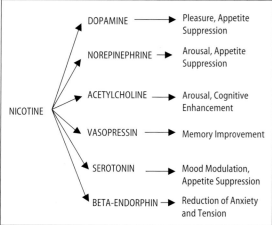

FIGURE 28-2. Neurochemical effects of nicotine. (From Benowitz.[8])

Dependence

From the DSM-IV standard definition of dependence[1] (Table 28-1) follows nicotine's addictiveness. In the long term, tobacco users experience tolerance, withdrawal symptoms, and continue the use of tobacco despite the desire to quit and knowledge of the harmful effects. This can be explained by nicotine's pharmacokinetic and pharmacodynamic properties. In the initial phase of tobacco use, the positive effects of tobacco are especially important. During this phase the smoker starts to associate the context in which he or she smokes with the rewarding effects of smoking by conditioning. These contexts can be specific moods or situations, such as after dinner, with a cup of coffee or alcoholic beverage, or among a group of friends. This conditioning is one of the causes leading to the next phase, the maintenance phase, which is characterized by tolerance and withdrawal symptoms, both mental and physical, when quitting smoking.

As with alcohol and heroin use, prolonged use of nicotine leads to neuroadaptation in the brain, caused by pharmacological, contextual, and behavioral factors. This neuroadaptation is responsible for the tolerance and physical withdrawal symptoms. Physical withdrawal symptoms of nicotine include a decrease in the heart rate, increased appetite, constipation, and hyperreactivity of the bronchial tubes. Some of the mental withdrawal symptoms are bad mood or depression, insomnia, irritability, anxiety, restlessness, and aggravation of psychiatric co-morbidity.

Craving

Apart from the physical dependence, long-term use results in mental dependence too, causing addiction behavior, the desire or craving for a cigarette. This can be triggered by the exposure to nicotine, stressful situations, or certain cues associated with smoking.

Craving can be explained by Schoffelmeer's sensitization theory.[9] This theory describes the phenomenon of increased sensitivity of the brain's mesolimbic dopamine system to psychoactive substances in people susceptible for this. During the use of nicotine, this increased sensitivity results in an increased dopamine release in the nucleus accumbens and the cerebral cortex and in euphoria, a powerful reinforcement, causing the desire to smoke.[8,10] With chronic use this desire can develop into obsessive craving. Individual differences in the limbic system and genetic predisposition play an important role in the development of sensitization, which happens as a result of neurochemical changes in the limbic dopamine system.

Many factors causing craving and possibly relapse on their own, like stress, mood disorders, the use of other drugs and cigarette-related cues, interact with the sensitization mechanism. It still remains unknown if the hypersensitivity to the effects of nicotine is permanent, but certainly it lasts for a long time, promoting relapse.

Factors Influencing the Development of Dependence

Genetic Factors

Having parents or siblings who smoke is associated with an increased risk of becoming a smoker.[11] It is hard to distinguish between the environmental factors and genetic factors. Some genetic factors influencing the development of nicotine dependence are known. These include individual differences concerning neuroreceptors as well as differences in nicotine metabolism.[12]

Other Addictions

There appear to be clear relations between nicotine addiction and other addictions. Those who started smoking at an early age often develop other addictions such as alcoholism later in their lives. Over 80% of alcoholics smoke and 30% of heavy smokers have alcohol problems.[13] The combined use of both drugs is highly conditioned. Heroin and methadone boost the desire for nicotine and vice versa. Of all heroin addicts and methadone users, 98% smoke.[14] Cocaine is highly addictive, just like nicotine. Nicotine can lead to increased cocaine use.

Psychiatric Co-morbidity

Smokers more often suffer from psychiatric diseases, namely depression, anxiety disorder and schizophrenia, than do non-smokers. At least 70–90% of all schizophrenia patients smoke.[15] There is a clear connection between smoking and depression and anxiety disorders. On the one hand, depression makes smoking lead to nicotine addiction more easily and, on the other hand, smoking promotes the development of depression. The same holds for anxiety and panic disorders. Smoking cessation can cause a temporary aggravation of the depression or anxiety.[15]

Other Factors

The younger one starts smoking the greater is the chance of becoming addicted.[9,16] Tobacco is widely available and relatively affordable, which promotes the development of an addiction. Social class also plays a role. In lower social classes there is a relatively higher influx of new smokers in the age group of 15- to 18-year-olds. People in these classes in general also quit smoking at an older age when confronted with severe health problems.[4] In the last decade there has been a rise in the number of smokers among girls and women. Of all women who quit smoking during pregnancy one-third recommence within a month after giving birth.[4] Women find it harder to quit smoking then men.[17]

References

1. American Psychiatric Association. Diagnostic and Statistical Manual of Mental Disorders, 4th edn (DSM-IV). Washington DC; 1994.
2. Prochazka AV. New developments in smoking cessation. Chest 2000;117:169S–175S.
3. Glantz LH, Annas GJ. Tobacco, the Food and Drug Administration, and Congress. N Engl J Med 2000; 343:1802–1806.
4. Willemsen M. Welke groepen hebben speciale aandacht nodig? CaraVisie 2001;14:44–46.
5. Tomkins DM, Sellers EM. Addiction and the brain: the role of neurotransmitters in the cause and treatment of drug dependence. Can Med Assoc J 2001; 164:817–821.
6. Janssen-Heijnen MLG, Coebergh JW, Klinkhamer PJJM, et al. Is there a common etiology for the rising incidence of and decreasing survival with adenocarcinoma of the lung. Epidemiology 2001;12: 256–258.
7. Goldstein A. Addiction; from Biology to Drug Policy. New York: Freeman & Co; 1995:105.
8. Benowitz NL. Nicotine addiction. Primary Care 1999;26:611–631.
9. Schoffelmeer ANM, Vanderschuren LJMJ, Mulder AH, et al. Terugval in drug- en alcoholgebruik: een kwestie van overgevoeligheid. Acta Neuropsychiatr 2000;12:5–8.
10. Koob GF, Le Moal L. Drug abuse: hedonic homeostatic dysregulation. Science 1997;278:52–58.
11. Mathias R. Study shows how genes can help protect from addiction. NIDA NOTES 2000;vol.13(6).
12. Vink JM, Willemsen G, Engels RCME, et al. Smoking status of parents, siblings and friends: Predictors of regular smoking? Findings from a longitudinal twin-family study. Twin Research 3(3):209–217.
13. Tromp-Beelen PG, Boonstra MH. Verslaving aan alcohol en nicotine. Bijblijven 2001;17(4):44–54.
14. Rook L, Buster M. Luchtwegaandoeningen en druggebruik. Rapport GG & GD. Amsterdam; 2000:1–40.
15. Bakker JB, Hovens JE, Loonen AJM. Soms is roken beter. Med Contact 2001;56(44):1607–1609.
16. Hanna EZ, Grant BF. Parallels to early onset alcohol use in the relationship of early onset smoking with drug use and DSM-IV drug and depressive disorders. Alcohol Clin Exp Res 1999;23(3):513–522.
17. Perkins KA. Smoking cessation in women: Special consideration. CNS Drugs 2001;15(5):391–411.

29
Treatment of Tobacco Dependency

Trudi P.G. Tromp-Beelen and Irene Hellemans

Stopping Smoking

When stopping smoking, the patient deals on the one hand with physical and on the other hand with psychosocial withdrawal, in other words getting out of smoking behavior. The patient has to learn how to deal with smoking needs and has to change habit patterns and to replace the function of smoking by, for example, learning to relax and deal with stress without cigarettes.

Stages of Change

As in all types of addiction, there is also a process of change in behavior with respect to the recognition of dependency. In order to counsel the patient in becoming aware of his problem, it is important to recognize the stages of change as they are outlined by Prochaska and DiClemente (Figure 29-1).[1] (See also Figure 26-1.)

Stage 1: Precontemplation

In the precontemplation phase, one does not realize there is a problem – the "happy smoker."

It is extremely important in this stage to inform the patient in a respectful, non-sermonizing way about the harmful effects of smoking and the possible connection with current complaints, both physical and psychological. One can ask if he or she has ever considered quitting and if so, is this in the near future. If the patient refuses to contemplate, then it is important to leave it for the moment and talk about this again at a later time.

Stage 2: Contemplation

Only in the second stage, the contemplation phase, will the patient be open to information about the short-term and long-term effects of quitting smoking. Short-term advantages are: being in better shape and feeling more energetic, having a better skin, better taste and smell, a better voice, and whiter teeth. Long-term effects are: a better prognosis, adding years to life, less chance of, or improvement of, lung diseases and heart and vascular diseases, less chance of lung cancer and other forms of cancer. In this stage possible misconceptions must be dispelled. These topics must be discussed to help the patient make a conscious decision.

Stage 3: Decision

In this stage the patient is prepared for stopping with smoking. It is important to prepare him or her for the possible withdrawal symptoms (see Table 29-1) and give advice on the problems that may occur. A date to quit should be set and help with medication must then be discussed.

Stage 4: Action

After the decision, a concrete quitting appointment can be made. From the Prochaska and DiClemente model it can be concluded that the client has a long way to go after his decision. After a successful attempt to quit, the smoker must maintain.

Stage 5: Maintenance

Stopping might be difficult but not starting again is much more difficult. In this stage a series of supporting contacts, for example starting one week after the set quitting date, is extremely important and medication must be considered again to prevent a relapse.

Stage 6: Relapse

In cardiac patients relapse may be present in 30–40% after discharge from the hospital. Relapse

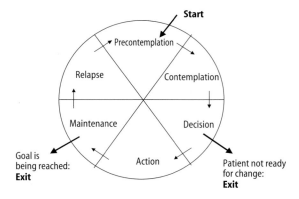

FIGURE 29-1. The wheel of change, based on the stages of change by Prochaska and DiClemente.[1]

TABLE 29-1. Nicotine withdrawal symptoms according to the criteria of DSM-IV

• depression	• concentration problems
• insomnia	• restlessness
• anger	• reduced heart frequency
• anxiety	• weight gain

is an essential part of the pathological process and although everything has to be done to avoid this, it is important to use a possible relapse as an educational tool. This means a positive attitude instead of disappointment when patients admit that they have started again. Both physician or nurse and patient should not give up right away! The smoker must be motivated to stop again as soon as possible. Many smokers have only stopped after various attempts. Relapse does not imply the patient has to start all over again, but has proven he can stop. The relapse can especially be explained on the basis of craving, as discussed in Chapter 28. This must slowly die; it needs time.

Effects of Type of Intervention

Advice given by physicians is effective for smoking cessation.[2] Interventions involving professionals from different disciplines have more effect than interventions carried out by professionals from a single discipline.[2] In their Cochrane review of interventions by nurses in the area of smoking cessation, Rice and Stead indicate that intensive telephone support after discharge from hospital is an essential component of an effective intervention for heart patients.[3] Brief advice given by nurses to patients with a coronary bypass is also effective. Patients with a myocardial infarct are twice as likely to be successful in stopping than are patients after a bypass operation.[4]

Patients with heart failure who during their stay in hospital had a twice-weekly group session and in addition to this received telephone follow-up on several occasions until 6 months after discharge

had (after 12 months) a biochemically confirmed chance of stopping of 57% compared to 37% in the group of patients who only received advice to stop (numbers needed to treat = 5 (95% CI: 3–6)).[5] Medicinal support for patients increases the chance of successfully stopping and is safe.[6,7] More intensive behavioral counseling increases the chances of successfully stopping by a factor two to three.[3,7]

One-off and Brief Supportive Interventions

One-off brief interventions during normal care contacts are the most relevant for physicians. One-off advice or a brief supportive intervention has an odds ratio of 1.69 (95% CI: 1.45–1.98) equivalent to an absolute difference of 2.5%.[2,7] Therefore the advice is that every doctor should always address the topic of smoking and focus on the issue of quitting.

Intensive Interventions

A meta-analysis revealed that the effectiveness of interventions increases if the intervention is more intensive, lasts longer. or contains more points of contact. Adding follow-up consultations was more effective than no follow-up.[7] This applies to all interventions which in total last for at least 40 minutes and take place in at least four sessions or contacts, including all psychological or psychosocial forms of influencing behavior.

Addressing the Patient

Patients who are not motivated to stop smoking should first of all be motivated. Cardiologists and nurses involved should record the smoking behavior and motivational level (Figure 29-1)[1] of their patients with a smoking-related disorder and then support motivated smokers in their attempt to stop. This should also include attention and support for the period following discharge from hospital, especially in cardiac rehabilitation programs.

Many smokers succeed without aid. Just as various factors may contribute to a some patients getting addicted more quickly to nicotine than others, so some people can stop easily than others. Some smokers can quit smoking after one single advice to stop; others will need the help of quit-smoking-groups. The best results are gained by the more intensive forms of support, for example a group course.[7] For those who cannot succeed in quitting this way, medication might increase their chance of success. The treatment with medication is preferably combined with psychosocial support. The five As ("ask," "assess," "advise," "assist," "arrange") shown in Table 29-2 are a simple guideline in this aspect. In cardiac patients relapse is an important issue to address during cardiac rehabilitation. A lot of patients quit smoking during their hospital stay, but find it very hard once they are in their own environment again (Table 29-3).

Pharmacotherapy

Nicotine Replacement Therapy

Before starting the nicotine replacement therapy the user has to quit smoking. Nicotine replacement therapy provides an alternative form of nicotine to relieve symptoms of withdrawal in a smoker who is abstaining from tobacco use.[8] The pharmacokinetic properties of available products differ, but none deliver nicotine as fast as does inhaling nicotine. The patch provides a relatively stable, fixed dose of nicotine over a period of 16 or 24 hours. The other products have a more rapid onset and a shorter duration of action, allowing the user to adjust the dose of nicotine. Blood nicotine levels peak 5 to 10 minutes after the adminis-

TABLE 29-2. The five As: intended for every smoker who wants to stop

Action	Implementation strategy
"Ask": systematically ask (preferably every year) whether he/she is a smoker	
Design a department-wide/organization-wide manner in which, for every patient, it is established (preferably yearly) whether he/she smokes and record this. Exception: adults who have not smoked for a considerable period of time, and for whom the status is clearly established.	Implement prompts for health professionals to systematically inquire about smoking behavior, for example stickers on the status or by placing a reminder in the patient's electronic record. Smoking status: smoker, has stopped, never smoked.
"Advise": emphatically advise him or her to stop smoking	
Advise the smoker to stop smoking, in a clear, strong, and person-specific manner.	Clear: I think that it is important that you stop and I think that I can help you. Emphatic: You should know that giving up smoking is the best way of keeping your health in the future. Specific to the person: Look at personal motives for the smoker: relationship with disease, cost-savings, in the children's interest, etc.
"Assess": establish the willingness to stop smoking	
Establish whether the smoker is willing to undertake an attempt to stop at this moment (e.g. within the next 30 days)	Prepared to stop now; proceed to assistance. Needs intensive support; offer this or refer. Not prepared to stop now; intervene at the motivation level. Special circumstances (child, pregnant, etc.) consider giving additional information.
"Assist": help him/her in undertaking the attempt to stop	
Make a 'stop plan' together with the smoker.	Agree on a stop date. Arrange social support from others (tell everybody). Anticipate difficult moments (withdrawal symptoms). Remove tobacco products from places (home and work) where the smoker might be.
Give practical support	Stop completely; do not even smoke half a cigarette. Evaluate previous failed attempts. Establish how the person can recognize a difficult moment. Suggest avoiding difficult moments (e.g. whilst having an alcoholic drink). Try to get partners, relatives, and friends to stop at the same time.

TABLE 29-2. *Continued*

Action	Implementation strategy
Offer support	Where can the smoker always go to in the event of questions and problems?
Try to arrange support from others	Ask partners, parents, and colleagues to support the smoker in the attempt to stop.
Advise pharmacotherapy, except in special situations	Consider advising pharmacotherapy if a smoker smokes more than 10 cigarettes per day. Explain why this increases the chances of stopping.
Obtain additional information	
"Arrange": care for follow-up as a form of preventing relapse	
Determine dates for follow-up contact, in person or over the telephone.	Timing: follow-up contact must take place soon after the planned stop date, preferably within one week, and a within second one month. Actions in follow-up: celebrate the success; if the person has still smoked, evaluate why and try to once more obtain a commitment for a complete stop; remind the smoker that failure can be seen as a learning step; discuss difficult moments and anticipate future ones; evaluate pharmacotherapy and consider more intensive treatment.

TABLE 29-3. Guidelines for relapse prevention

Problem: lack of support
Solution:
- make agreements for follow-up (if need be by telephone)
- try to find sources of support in the neighborhood of the stopped smoker
- refer to a relevant organization which can provide support

Problem: negative mood/depression
Solution:
- provide support, see if medication can help and refer to a relevant health professional

Problem: strong withdrawal symptoms
Solution:
- see if medication or an adjustment to the medication is needed

Problem: weight increase
Solution:
- emphasize the importance of a good diet, discourage strict dieting and try to encourage extra physical activity. State that an increase in weight is normal, but that after a while the weight no longer increases
- consider continuing to use medication which postpones the weight increase, for example bupropion
- refer to a relevant organization which can provide support

Problem: decreased motivation and slackness
Solution:
- emphasize that this is a normal reaction
- recommend rewarding activities
- discourage temporary tobacco use and emphasize that smoking (even one cigarette) only makes it more difficult to stop

tration of the nasal spray, 20 minutes after the user begins the chewing gum, sublingual tablet, sucking tablet or uses a inhaler, and 2 to 4 hours after the application of a nicotine patch. The dose depends on the number of cigarettes smoked a day. If more than two packets of cigarettes are smoked each day, two patches are recommended (twice a day) or one patch combined with some other form of nicotine replacement. Different nicotine forms of replacement therapy can be combined safely. The side-effect of these products varies according to the manner in which nicotine is administrated.[9]

Although nicotine increases the myocardial workload, nicotine replacement therapy is safe in patients with cardiovascular disease, including stable angina. The risk of cardiac complications should be lower than with smoking. Unlike smoking, nicotine replacement therapy does not increase the coagulability of blood or expose a patient to carbon monoxide or oxidizing gases that damage endothelium. In women who are pregnant or breastfeeding, the risk of smoking can be more severe than nicotine replacement therapy.

In a meta-analysis of placebo-controlled trials, nicotine replacement therapy was found to result in higher rates of smoking cessation, especially when combined with counseling.[9]

TABLE 29-4. Drugs used for smoking cessation

Product	Daily Dose	Maintenance	Duration of Treatment	Common Side Effects	Contraindications
Nicothine – replacement therapy (1) (3)					(2) instable angina, serious cardiac arythmics, recent myocardial infarction or cerebrovasculair accidents
Trandermal patch 7-, 14-, 21- or 15 mg (1) (3)	7-, 14- or 21 mg for 24 hours or 15 mg for 16 hours	idem, after 4–6 weeks halve the dosage	6–12 weeks	skin irritation, insomnia (remove during the night)	(2) serious eczema, allergic to patches
Chewing gum 2-, 4 mg (1) (3)	2–4 mg each 2 hour (maximum 48 mg/day)	idem, after 4–6 weeks halve the dosage	maximum 1 year	mouthe irritation, sorc jaw, dyspepsia, hiccups	(2) jaw problems, esophagitis
Sublingual tablets 2-, 4 mg (1) (3)	2–4 mg each 1–2 hour (maximum 60 mg/day)	idem, after 2–3 months phase out	6 months	mouthe irritation, dyspepsia, hiccups	(2)
Sucking tablets 1-, 2-, 4 mg (1) (3)	1–4 mg each 1–2 hour (maximum 25 mg/day)	idem, after 2–3 months phase out	6 months	mouthe irritation, dyspepsia, hiccups	(2)
Vapor inhalor 4-, 10 mg (1) (3)	6–12 cartridges/day	idem, after 2–3 months phase out	6 months	mouthe irritation, dyspepsia, hiccups	(2) asthma, rhinitis, nose polyps, allergic to menthol
Nasal spray 0.5 mg (1) (3)	1–2 doses each hour in each nostril (maximum 40 mg/day)	idem, after 2–3 month phase out	6 month	nasal irritation, sneezing, cough ,teary eyes	(2)
Bupropion sustained-release (3) (6)	150 mg/day (6 days)	after 6 days 150 mg twice a day 4) when predisposed to seizures: maintain 150 mg/day	7–9 weeks	insomnia, dray mouth, agitation	allergic to bupropion, epilepsy or seizures in the past, tumor of the central nerve system, abrupt cessation of benzodiazepines or alcohol, anorexia nervosa, boulimia, serious livercirrose
Nortiptyline (3) (5) (6)	25 mg/day (3 days) 50 mg/day (4 days)	after 7 days 75 mg/day 4)	7–12 weeks	dry mouth, sedation, dizziness	see bupropion except the seizures

(1) Different nicotine-replacement products can be combined safely.
(2) Contraindication for all nicotine-replacement therapy is instable angina, serious cardiac arytmics, recent myocard infarction or cerebrovascular accidents.
(3) Bupropion and nortriptyline can be combined with nicotine-replacement therapy.
(4) Smoking cessation 10 days after start medication.
(5) Nortriptyline has not been approved by the Food and drug Amministration as a smoking-cessation aid. The Public Health Service clinical guidelines recommend it as a second-line drug for smoking cessation.
(6) Bupropion and nortriptyline should not be combined with MOA-inhibitors.

Antidepressants and Other Pharmacotherapy

The withdrawal symptoms of smoking cessation can be stress, depression, anxiety, anger, insomnia, and weight gain. For that reason antidepressants can be helpful.[10]

Bupropion is an antidepressant with dopaminergic and norepinephrenic activity. It relieves the withdrawal symptoms and the craving for a cigarette. Because bupropion lowers the threshold for seizures it is contraindicated in patients who are at risk for seizures. The daily dose is 150 mg/day for 6 days, then 150 mg twice a day. In those predisposed to seizures, in elderly people, or those with decreased kidney or liver function, the maintenance dose should be taken once a day only. Smoking cessation starts about 10 days after the start of medication.[9] An overview of drugs used for smoking cessation, contraindications and side-effects is given in Table 29-4.

Nortriptyline is an antidepressant with serotonergic and norepinephrenic activity. This antidepressant is not approved as a smoking cessation aid but is recommended in many public health services guidelines for smoking cessation. The daily dose is 25 mg/day for 3 days, then 50 mg/day 4 days, then 75–100 mg/day. Smoking cessation starts from the tenth day after the start of medication. Duration of treatment is 7–12 weeks.

Both bupropion and nortriptyline can be combined with all kinds of nicotine replacement therapy. In randomized, controlled trials they double smoking cessation rates as compared with placebo treatment especially when combined with counseling.[9]

No other antidepressant has had demonstrated efficacy for use in smoking cessation.

There is research on the efficacy of other medications, for example rimoabant and varenicline,[11] as well as a vaccination against nicotine.

Acupuncture, Hypnosis, Laser Therapy

There are no good randomized, controlled trials to support the efficacy of these options.

Relapse Control

When one wants to check if the patient has quit smoking one can measure the CO level in expired air. About 6 hours after the last cigarette this level should be <10 ppm.

In urine, blood, or saliva one can measure the cotinine level. These determinations should be normalized within 24 hours. The topic should be addressed in all patients during the first years of follow-up.

Summary and Conclusion

Smoking is not just a bad habit. Because of nicotine, smoking is quickly and strongly addictive. This will result in a chronic change in the brain, causing a strong craving and a high chance of relapse after quitting. Greater understanding of the neurophysiological background of addiction, that is, the disruption of the neuroreceptors, has increased the possibilities of treatment with medication.

Cardiac rehabilitation plays an important role in supporting the patient to quit smoking. Furthermore, all health professionals should address the topic of quitting smoking from the moment the patient is admitted to the hospital. If there is a combined strategy, the success rate for cardiac patients may be very high, up to 50%. For patients who still smoke, the cardiac rehabilitation program offers a perfect setting for more intensive counseling or addition of medication in those patients that need this support.

References

1. Prochaska JO, DiClemente CC. Toward a comprehensive model of change. In: Miller WR, Heather N, eds. Treating Addictive Behaviors: Processes of Change. New York: Plenum Press; 1992:3–27.
2. Fiore MC, Bailey WC, Cohen SJ, et al. Treating tobacco use and dependence. Clinical Practice Guideline. Rockville, MD: US Department of Health and Human Services. Public Health Service; 2000.
3. Rice VH, Stead LF. Nursing interventions for smoking cessation [Cochrane review]. The Cochrane Library. Issue 3. Oxford: Update Software, 2002.
4. Hajek P, Taylor TZ, Mills P. Brief intervention during hospital admission to help patients to give up smoking after myocardial infarction and bypass surgery: randomised controlled trial. BMJ 2002; 324:641–645.
5. Quist-Paulsen P, Gallefoss F. Randomised controlled trial of smoking cessation intervention after admission for coronary heart disease. BMJ 2003;327: 1254–1257.
6. Tonstad S, Farsang C, Klaene G, et al. Bupropion SR for smoking cessation in smokers with cardiovascular disease: a multicentre, randomised study. Eur Heart J 2003;24:946–955.
7. Silagy C, Stead LF. Physician advice for smoking cessation [Cochrane review]. The Cochrane Library. Issue 3. Oxford. Cochrane Database Syst Rev. 2004;(3):CD000146.
8. Silagy C, Lancaster T, Stead L, Mant D, Fowler G. Nicotine replacement therapy for smoking cessation. Cochrane Database Syst Rev 2004;(3): CD000146.
9. Rigotti NA. Treatment of tobacco use and dependence. N Engl J Med 2002;346(7):506–512.
10. Jørenby DE, Leischow SJ, Nides MA, et al. A controlled trial of sustained-release bupropion, a nicotine patch or both for smoking cessation. N Engl J Med 1999;340:685–691.
11. Gonzales D, Rennard SI, Nides M, et al. Varenicline, an α4β2 nicotinic acetylcholine receptor partial agonist, vs sustained-relaese bupropion and placebo for smoking cessation. JAMA 2006;296:47–55.

Section VI
Psychological and Behavioral Support

This section addresses important psychosocial issues and their implications for cardiac patients. The section starts with a broad overview of psychosocial research in cardiac populations. This provides some historical perspective and covers issues such as the influence of the workplace and economics on well-being and cardiovascular function. Many notable associations have been documented but the causal mechanisms, and thus methods of intervention, are much less clear.

The overall goals of cardiac rehabilitation have been described as promoting secondary prevention and improving quality of life. The second contribution in the section describes the concept of health-related quality of life and shows how this patient-focused marker of success in the clinical setting is becoming much more important in medicine in general, including in cardiac populations. Clearly, since much of the prevention and management of cardiac conditions is in the hands of the patient, activities and interventions that have a serious cost to quality of life will not be easily undertaken by patients. One of the challenges facing professionals is to understand the quality of life impact of health recommendations on patients. In parallel, cardiology needs an agreed set of instruments to assess these issues if it is to become as focused as other specialties in arguing for resources for patient care. This challenge is discussed and the most widely used instruments described.

Managing mental health challenges such as stress and depression is the focus of two chapters

in this section. These are important in their own right but also as important barriers to adherence. The epidemiology and impact of depression in cardiac settings is described, as is the challenge of assessing and treating this depression. What is clear is both the damaging nature of depression for cardiac patients and the fact that it is not a short-term response to an acute cardiac event.

The concept of stress and of stress management procedures suited to a cardiac setting is described. This is coupled with a general chapter on the educational role intrinsic in good care for cardiac patients. It is a reminder of the need to see the busy cardiac setting from the perspective of the patient and family members and to be ever mindful that what is a daily job for professionals is a unique, almost always anxiety-provoking and even possibly a very frightening experience for the patient and family.

Promoting secondary prevention is essentially about promoting adherence to professional guidelines. It is notable how little attention this essential component in the management of patients has been given. The chapter on adherence shows just how big a challenge this is and highlights aspects of patients, professionals and systems that promote or militate against adherence.

Overall, the section aims to demonstrate the important psychosocial issues in cardiac patient care, to show that there is already a wealth of knowledge and informed practice in the area, and to provide a flavor of the research and clinical challenges in this area in the coming decades.

Main Messages

Chapter 30: Psychosocial Aspects in Prevention and Rehabilitation

Evidence that psychosocial factors are important in the development and prognosis of cardiovascular disease is outlined. Psychosocial problems are common among patients with psychosocial risk factors fitting broadly into two categories; external factors (such as financial and socioeconomic circumstances, life events, and work stress); and internal factors (such as anxiety, depression, hostility anger, and perception of external circumstances). The most extensive evidence that psychosocial factors are involved in prognosis in coronary heart disease (CHD) derives from work related to depression. In established CHD, depression is associated with a significantly increased risk for recurrent major cardiac events, particularly if there is also a lack of social support. The exact pathophysiological nature of the influence of psychosocial factors remains to be determined, as does the temporal sequence of events. Several interventions have been investigated, both to reduce psychosocial risk factors and to improve outcomes in cardiac patients. These include exercise training, psychosocial interventions, and pharmacotherapy. There is as yet little evidence that pharmacological treatment for depression can improve cardiac outcomes. Evidence suggests that exercise may modify psychosocial risk factors, including depression, while psychosocial interventions in post-MI patients have found some but not uniformly positive results. Even though there is now substantial evidence of the importance of psychosocial factors in CHD, there is still a lack of systematic knowledge about intervention approaches. An ever-increasing literature on psychosocial factors, with significant investment in psychosocial intervention studies including randomized trials, means that evidence in the coming decade is likely to dramatically increase our understanding of psychosocial contributors to both prevention and rehabilitation in cardiac disease.

Chapter 31: Health-Related Quality of Life in Cardiac Patients

This chapter deals with the concept of health-related quality of life (HRQoL) in the cardiac context. It overviews definitions of HRQoL and the main uses for the concept in research, clinical, and policy settings. The various categories of measures are then described – generic, health-related, disease-specific, individualized, and utility measures. Illustrations for the cardiac setting are provided. Examples of the HRQoL research endeavor are provided by condition (e.g. myocardial infarction and heart failure) and by procedure or intervention (e.g. cardiac surgery and cardiac rehabilitation). There is increasing evidence of incorporation of HRQoL measures in cardiovascular clinical trials. The current challenges in the cardiac research area are described. A major challenge is lack of consensus on instrument choice. This limits comparability across studies and conditions and slows the development of a cumulative evidence base on HRQoL in cardiac conditions. Projects that advise on instrument selection and use for the future are described.

Chapter 32: Depression Following Myocardial Infarction: Prevalence, Clinical Consequences, and Patient Management

Depressive symptoms and major depression have been consistently reported as common psychological reactions to myocardial infarction (MI). It has also been argued, on the basis of prospective observational evidence, that depression following MI constitutes an independent, that is, causal, risk for subsequent mortality and morbidity. Two recent meta-analyses have examined this evidence. Unadjusted pooled analyses of both meta-analyses indicate that depression following MI is associated with a 2-fold increased risk of death and recurrent cardiac events. However, with adjustment for potential confounders the associations between depression and these outcomes were attenuated. In addition, two recent randomized trials addressing depression in MI patients (SADHART and ENRICHD) observed a relative reduction in depression with treatment, but found no effects of treatment on mortality, nonfatal reinfarction, or indices of disease severity such as left ventricular ejection fraction. On balance, the evidence at this stage suggests that claims of causality should be treated with caution. Further randomized controlled trials are needed, as are observational studies that adjust for potential confounders, most importantly for measures of disease severity. Irrespective of the implications of depression following MI for mortality and morbidity, the high incidence of depression in this population and the link between depression and impaired quality of life should, however, be sufficient to suggest changes to patient management practices.

Chapter 33: Educating Cardiac Patients and Relatives

Spouses and family have a very important place in the rehabilitation of patients with coronary heart disease (CHD). Their involvement has the potential of facilitating the process and improving the outcome. The most important source of social support for a cardiac patient is family, particularly his or her spouse. Positive social support is important for the prognosis of CHD patients. This entails emotional (understanding and acceptance of feelings), appraisal (good advice and opportunity to discuss how to manage the new life situation), informational (knowledge about CHD, risk factors, and lifestyle), and instrumental (help with practical problems) support. These aspects should be included in comprehensive cardiac rehabilitation and secondary prevention. In terms of support, it is also the case that "too much" support from family to the patient can create over-protectiveness and decrease the patient's self-efficacy and own initiatives in rehabilitation.

A cardiovascular event is of course also a major negative event for family members. In order for spouses and family members to be able to provide adequate social support, they themselves need support. Spouse and family support can be offered in a group format in cardiac rehabilitation programs. There is evidence that socially isolated CHD patients are at significantly increased risk of further events. These patients need more active support interventions. In sum, the family can be an important asset in the care of the cardiac patient but this must be done in a way that addresses the family's own needs and concerns and enables them to be informed, confident supporters of the patient in their midst.

Chapter 34: Stress Management

Stress management training aims to change environmental triggers to the stress response and/or change inappropriate behavioral, physiological, or cognitive responses that occur in response to this event. High levels of muscular tension can be reduced through relaxation techniques; triggers can be identified and modified using problem-solving strategies; cognitive distortions can be identified and changed through cognitive techniques such as cognitive restructuring; and "stressed" behaviors can be changed through consideration and rehearsal of alternative behavioral responses.

Many stress management programs teach simple relaxation techniques to minimize high levels of arousal. More complex interventions try to change cognitive (and therefore emotional) reactions to environmental triggers. A few address factors that initiate the stress response. Given the idiosyncratic nature of both the stressors that individuals experience and the complexity of changing their cognitive response, such interventions are often led by stress management specialists, and are best targeted at individuals experiencing significant stress. Relaxation skills are learned through three phases: learning basic relaxation skills; monitoring tension in daily life; and using relaxation at times of stress. Two strategies for changing cognitions are used. Self-instruction training interrupts the flow of stress-provoking thoughts by replacing them with pre-rehearsed stress-reducing or "coping" thoughts. Cognitive restructuring involves identifying and challenging the accuracy of stress-engendering thoughts. Basic interventions, particularly relaxation, can be taught by most healthcare professionals in a group context. The problem-focused or cognitive interventions can be taught by professionals familiar with the issues. However, where an individual reports high levels of stress, these may best be implemented by more specialist mental health professionals.

Chapter 35: Adherence to Health Recommendations

Adherence is the single most important modifiable factor that compromises therapeutic outcome across a wide spectrum of diseases. The most efficacious treatment is made ineffective if the patient fails to adhere to it. Non-adherence produces unnecessary medical and psychosocial consequences of CHD, reduces quality of life, and wastes valuable healthcare resources. Adherence to health-related recommendations is thus a major challenge for prevention and rehabilitation in cardiovascular disorders. As many as half of all patients advised about long-term management of their condition do not adhere to recommendations. Cardiac rehabilitation (CR) provides a method of promoting patient adherence in secondary prevention for cardiovascular patients. Adherence can be considered to have illness-related aspects, patient aspects, and health professional/health system aspects. Side-effects of medications and complex regimens discourage adherence. However, sociodemographic factors such as age, gender, ethnicity, socioeconomic status, and education have not been consistently related to adherence. Patient beliefs about treatments and health conditions appear to make a difference while negative psychological states such as depression and anxiety increase non-adherence. Non-adherence has also been associated with poorly developed health services, lack of training in chronic disease management for health, and short consultation times. Interventions to improve adherence have had weak to moderate effects. However, even modest improvements in adherence may result in substantial mortality and economic savings. Adherence has been identified as a core outcome goal for cardiac rehabilitation services. Future research thus needs to identify those patients at highest risk for non-adherence and strategies that facilitate long-term adherence to recommendations since long-term behavior change is intrinsic to much of the potential to benefit.

30
Psychosocial Aspects in Prevention and Rehabilitation

Annika Rosengren

Introduction

According to popular opinion, stress is one of the most important risk factors for coronary heart disease (CHD). This view has not, however, so far been altogether accepted by the medical profession. However, accumulating evidence does demonstrate that it is likely that stress and other psychosocial factors are causally related to CHD, and possibly to stroke. Other than stress, some of the psychosocial factors that have been investigated in relation to CHD include socioeconomic factors, social support, adverse life events, personality factors, perceived control, anxiety, and depression.

Prognosis after acute myocardial infarction (AMI) has improved considerably over the last decades, both through treatment and interventions in the acute stage and through secondary prevention in the post-AMI stage. Similarly, there is increasing knowledge about the causes of cardiovascular disease, such as dyslipidemia, obesity, smoking, and inactivity. To a large extent, this is due to systematic research into pathophysiological mechanisms and scientific evaluation of medical treatment. Although there is, by now, evidence that psychosocial factors are important in the development and prognosis of cardiovascular disease, there is far less knowledge about prevention and management in this area.

Many patients are, in fact, themselves convinced that the external circumstances in which they live probably contributed to their event, whether it was an AMI or stroke. One patient might describe a situation at work, with multiple and often conflicting demands, time constraints, and very little appreciation. Another might describe a problematic family situation, elderly and demanding parents, difficult teenagers, or financial trouble. Depressed or anxious patients may also want to know if their state of mind contributed to their event. Even though much of this does not fall into the traditional domain of the medical profession, there is an increasing need to impart knowledge and to respond to the patient's concerns. Similarly, in secondary prevention, providing advice and sometimes treatment with respect to psychosocial factors should form part of an integrated treatment plan. However, whereas there are many proven therapies with respect to pharmacological interventions and lifestyle interventions, such as non-smoking advice, physical activity, and diet modification, much less is known about modifying psychosocial risks. In particular, there is a lack of knowledge about whether psychosocial interventions are effective in prolonging event-free survival.

Psychosocial problems are common among patients. In the recent INTERHEART study of 12,461 post-AMI patients and 14,637 matched controls from 52 countries, 27% of cases had had either several periods of stress at home or at work or permanent stress in the year before their AMI, 15% admitted to severe financial stress, 16% had had two or more adverse life events, and 24% had felt depressed for 2 weeks or more. These factors were all less common among the healthy controls of the study.[1] Taken together, the odds ratio for a composite of all psychosocial factors and population-attributable risk for AMI by this subjective measure of psychosocial stress were substantial, and comparable to those noted for other major coronary risk factors.[2] Similarly, in a large annual survey of the US non-institutionalized civilian population, psychological distress was assessed with a standardized questionnaire and heart disease diagnoses were based on self-report. Among healthy individuals, the estimated prevalence of psychological distress was 2.8%, whereas the estimates were 6.4%, and 4.1% among those with self-reported AMI and CHD, respectively, implying that psychological distress is a significant co-morbid factor with cardiovascular disease.[3]

There are, however, several methodological problems in the study of psychosocial factors and health outcomes. First, compared to other biological and lifestyle risk factors, psychosocial factors represent a more problematic construct in that there is little uniformity with respect to either definition or measurement of these factors. Second, most of the dimensions involved are subjective, and hence potentially open to biases and confounding. Third, even though some persons may be more vulnerable than others with respect to adverse circumstances, exposure probably varies considerably over a lifetime. Hence, prospective follow-up studies with extended follow-up may not adequately capture short-term influences.

Evidence That Psychosocial Factors Predict CHD Events

During the last two decades, considerable evidence has accumulated with respect to the association of markers of stress and other psychosocial factors with coronary disease.[4,5] However, compared to other major risk factors, psychosocial variables are more difficult to define objectively, because several different dimensions are involved. Despite this, several separate constructs within the broad conceptual framework of psychosocial factors are increasingly considered as being causally related to CHD. Stress at work[6] and in family life,[7] life events,[8] low perceived control,[1] lack of social support,[9] socioeconomic status,[10,11] and depression[12,13] are some of the dimensions that have been shown to either

influence the risk of CHD or affect prognosis in CHD patients.

Psychosocial risk factors fall broadly into two different categories; first those that represent external factors, such as financial and socioeconomic circumstances, life events, work stress, and second, those that have to do with factors within the individual, such as anxiety or depression, as well as hostility and anger, and perception of external circumstances. To some extent, perceived control and social support may modify other psychosocial factors, whether external or internal.

Of the external stressors, work stress has received a great deal of attention with respect to a potential adverse effect on the cardiovascular system. One model is the "job strain" model developed by Karasek et al.,[14] where jobs are evaluated according to two factors: "job demand" and "job latitude." The combination of high job demand and low job latitude is defined as "job strain." Other work parameters, such as low job control, have been demonstrated to account for a major part of the inverse gradient between socioeconomic status and cardiovascular disease.[15] Studies have also linked work stress to measures of subclinical atherosclerosis.[16–18] One recent study found triggering effects of sudden, short-term situations of increased workload or work competition.[19] Shift work has been described to increase future risk of CHD, in both women and men.[20,21] In the Helsinki Heart Study, the relative risk of CHD associated with shift work was 1.5 (95% CI 1.1–2.1) when only age was adjusted for and 1.4 (1.0–1.9) when adjustments were made for lifestyle factors, blood pressure, and serum lipids.[20] Also, shift work seemed to trigger the effect of other lifestyle-related risk factors of CHD, such that the joint effects of shift work and risk factors were at least multiplicative.[21]

In addition to perceived stress at work, stressful conditions in family life have been shown to increase CHD risk. In Stockholm, marital discord was found to worsen prognosis in women with an acute coronary syndrome and to reduce event-free survival over and above the effects of standard clinical prognostic factors.[7] Although a majority of the women were employed outside the home, the hazards of marital stress were stronger than those of stress at work in these women. Among working women ($n = 200$), work stress did not significantly predict recurrent coronary events. Other measures of stress have also been used. In a prospective survey of middle-aged Swedish men, self-reported permanent stress, using a stress question similar to the one used in the INTERHEART study, was associated with an increased risk of incident CHD (OR 1.5; 95% CI 1.2–1.9) after adjustment for conventional coronary risk factors during a 12-year follow-up.[22] There was also an association with stroke. Similar results were observed in a large prospective study involving 281 cases in 73,424 Japanese men and women, which reported an association between perceived mental stress and CHD mortality.[23]

Some studies have investigated the effect of other external influences like financial stress or life events on risk of coronary disease. In a previous case-control study, having experienced one life event or more during the year preceding an AMI and dissatisfaction with one's financial situation were twice as common among cases than controls among men, but no significant relation was found among women.[8] In 5021 middle-aged, white-collar men in the UK's Whitehall II study, associations between economic difficulties and incident coronary events were determined over an average follow-up of 7 years, with steep gradients in the incidence of coronary events with economic difficulties, independently of other markers of socioeconomic position.[24] The increase in risk was only partially mediated by conventional risk factors in mid-life. An extreme external stressor such as the death of a child was demonstrated to be associated with increased risk of future AMI in a Danish registry-based study,[25] particularly if it was a death from sudden infant death syndrome.

Men and women with low socioeconomic status (SES) have an increased risk of coronary disease. Several population-based studies have examined this relationship.[26–29] Controlling for standard risk factors reduced the size of the gradient, but a relevant proportion of the variance according to SES was explained by distinct psychosocial factors which either mediate or modify the effect of SES on CHD.[15]

People with poor social networks have also been demonstrated to have higher mortality from several causes.[30–31] However, data are less consistent with respect to the effect of social ties and activities on cardiovascular disease, but some studies have reported an association with coronary disease.[9,32,33] In a recent follow-up study of 6861 Swedish women and men, persons with low social participation had a 2-fold risk of CHD. After adjustment for education, housing tenure, and smoking habits, the hazard ratio was 1.69 (95% CI 1.21–2.37).[32] Similarly, lack of social support has been found to lead to decreased survival and poorer prognosis among people with clinical manifestations of CHD. When emotional support was assessed before AMI, in a group of post-MI patients, it was independently related to risk for death in the subsequent 6 months.[34]

Depression is one of the most common chronic conditions encountered in clinical practice and is a also significant problem in cardiac patients, although frequently unrecognized and untreated. Depressive disorders vary from mild depressive symptoms to classic major depression and are characterized by severely depressed mood and often also somatic complaints. Clinical depression, depressive symptoms, and other negative emotions have been associated with an increased risk of AMI in both men and women.[12,13,35,36] Similarly, in the NHANES I survey, depression was associated with an independently increased risk of CHD incidence in both men and women, as well as CHD mortality in men.[13] However, depression had no effect on CHD mortality in women. In the INTERHEART study,[1] 24% of patients with recent AMI could be identified as having had at least mild depression during the year before the event, compared to 17.6% among controls, with no gender difference in effect size.

Prognosis and Psychosocial Factors

The most extensive evidence that psychosocial factors are involved in prognosis in CHD derives from work related to depression. In established CHD, depression is associated with a significantly increased risk for recurrent major cardiac events,[35–37] particularly if there was also a lack of social support.[38] Not all studies, however, have found depression to predict survival post-MI.[39–40] Lack of a close confidant was associated with adverse outcome after MI in a British study, possibly mediated by unhealthy behaviors and lack of compliance with medical recommendations, but tentatively also compatible with difficulties in early life leading to heart disease.[40] Further discussion of depression and its management is provided in Chapter 32.

Mechanisms of Psychosocial Impact

The mechanisms by which psychosocial factors increase the risk of cardiovascular disease are complex. In experimental studies, worsened coronary atherosclerosis[41] and endothelial dysfunction[42] occur in response to social disruption. Decreased heart rate variability, a marker of autonomic imbalance, has been related to shift work exposure.[43] Several studies have demonstrated links between psychosocial variables and vascular function,[44–45] inflammation,[46] increased blood clotting and decreased fibrinolysis.[47,48] In women without known coronary disease, recurrent major depression was associated with subclinical atherosclerosis.[49] The exact pathophysiological nature of the influence of psychosocial factors remains to be determined, as does the temporal sequence of events.

Management of Psychosocial Risk Factors

Several behavioral and psychosocial interventions have been investigated in cardiac patients, both to reduce psychosocial risk factors and to improve outcomes.[50] These interventions include exercise training, psychosocial interventions and psychopharmacotherapy.

There is little evidence that pharmacological treatment for depression can improve outcome. In addition, there has been concern with respect to safety. However, the SADHART (Sertraline Antidepressant Heart Attack Randomized Trial),[51] which randomized patients with recent hospitalization for AMI or unstable angina and depression to treatment with sertraline or placebo, found no difference in cardiovascular events or any other safety measure, indicating that this agent is safe to use. Nonetheless, there is no evidence, as yet, that antidepressant treatment increases survival in cardiac patients.

In the ENRICHD trial,[52] 2481 post-MI patients with major or minor depression and/or low perceived social support were randomly assigned either to usual medical therapy or to an intervention consisting of up to 6 months of cognitive behavior therapy at a median of 17 days after the index MI, with sertraline added for patients with persistent depressive symptoms. The intervention improved depression and social isolation but not event-free survival. The failure to demonstrate any survival benefit was thought, in part, to have been due to the fact that a large proportion of patients with mild, transient, depression were involved. An ensuing subgroup analysis of those patients enrolled in the ENRICHD with the most severe symptomatology, however, also failed to demonstrate any survival benefit.[53] In addition, it was shown that intervention patients whose depression did not improve were at substantial risk for late mortality.

Exercise training is of particular interest because of the general beneficial effect of exercise and physical activity on several cardiovascular parameters. Evidence suggests that exercise may also modify psychosocial risk factors, including depression. Cross-sectional studies of patients as well as healthy men and women have demonstrated lower depression scores among those who are most active. The ability of exercise to reduce depression also has been demonstrated in randomized controlled trials, although many of these studies have had methodological limitations.[54] In a randomized controlled trial of 134 US patients (92 male and 42 female; aged 40–84 years) with stable ischemic heart disease (IHD) and exercise-induced myocardial ischemia, exercise and stress management training reduced emotional distress and improved markers of cardiovascular risk, such as left ventricular ejection fraction and wall motion abnormalities, flow-mediated dilation, and cardiac autonomic control more than usual medical care alone.[55] In a post-hoc analysis of the ENRICHD (Enhancing Recovery in Coronary Heart Disease) clinical trial, the association between self-reported physical exercise and all-cause mortality and cardiovascular morbidity among 2078 men and 903 women was studied 6 months after an AMI.[56] During an average 2-year follow-up, 187 fatal events occurred. Patients reporting regular exercise had less than half the events (5.7%) of those patients who did not exercise regularly (12.0%). The adjusted hazard ratio for fatal events was 0.62 (95% CI 0.44–0.86). The rate of nonfatal AMI among the exercisers was 6.5% compared with 10.5% among those who reported no regular exercise. After adjustment for covariates, the hazard ratio for nonfatal AMI was 0.72 (95% CI 0.52–0.99), demonstrating the potential value of exercise in reducing mortality and nonfatal reinfarction in AMI patients who were either depressed or who had low social support.

Studies on psychosocial interventions in post-MI patients have not yielded uniformly positive results. For instance, one study assessing the impact of a program of monthly screening for psychological distress in patients with AMI, combined with supportive and educational home nursing interventions, found no overall benefit for distressed patients.[57] Furthermore, cardiac and all-cause mortality was greater for women in the intervention group. While definitive conclusions cannot be drawn from the results of one study, it suggests that safety issues are a concern even in non-pharmacological trials.

Even though there is now substantial evidence that psychosocial factors are important in the development and prognosis in CHD, there is still a lack of systematic knowledge about how this dimension should be handled. With respect to primary prevention, this aspect is virtually unexplored. In cardiac and stroke patients, there is sketchy evidence, as outlined above. The contrast to the multitude of clinical trials demonstrating the effectiveness of various pharmacological interventions in these patients is striking. At the same time, patients with external stress factors are often themselves firmly convinced that these factors played a significant role in why they became ill in the first place. From the patient's point of view, the physician in charge needs to listen and acknowledge that there is, by now, scientific evidence that psychosocial factors are important as causal agents in CHD and probably also in stroke. What support can be offered will depend on what is available in a particular healthcare system. In some situations brief counseling may be offered. (Further discussion on related issues is included in other chapters in this section. Depression and its management in cardiac patients is discussed further in Chapter 32, while stress management is the focus of Chapter 34). In other situations, the patient's employer should be contacted to ensure a change in employment conditions, or work hours. This issue is discussed in further detail in the chapter on vocational rehabilitation. An ever-increasing literature on psychosocial factors, with significant investment in psychosocial intervention studies including randomized trials, means that evidence in the coming decade is likely to dramatically increase our understanding of psychosocial contributors to both prevention and rehabilitation in cardiac disease.

References

1. Rosengren A, Hawken S, Ounpuu S, et al. Association of psychosocial risk factors with risk of acute myocardial infarction in 11119 cases and 13648 controls from 52 countries (the INTERHEART study): case-control study. Lancet 2004;364:953–962.
2. Yusuf S, Hawken S, Ounpuu S, et al. Effect of potentially modifiable risk factors associated with myocardial infarction in 52 countries (the INTERHEART study): case-control study. Lancet 2004;364: 937–952.
3. Ferketich AK, Binkley PF. Psychological distress and cardiovascular disease: results from the 2002 National Health Interview Survey. Eur Heart J 2005;26(18):1923–1928.
4. Hemingway H, Marmot M. Evidence based cardiology: psychosocial factors in the aetiology and prognosis of coronary heart disease. Systematic review of prospective cohort studies. BMJ 1999;318:1460–1467.
5. Rozanski A, Blumenthal JA, Kaplan J. Impact of psychological factors on the pathogenesis of cardiovascular disease and implications for therapy. Circulation 1999;99:2192–2217.
6. Kivimaki M, Leino-Arjas P, Luukkonen R, Riihimaki H, Vahtera J, Kirjonen J. Work stress and risk of cardiovascular mortality: prospective cohort study of industrial employees. BMJ 2002;325:857–861.
7. Orth-Gomer K, Wamala SP, Horsten M, et al. Marital stress worsens prognosis in women with coronary heart disease: The Stockholm Female Coronary Risk Study. JAMA 2000;284:3008–3014.
8. Welin C, Rosengren A, Wedel H, Wilhelmsen L. Myocardial infarction in relation to work, family and life events. Cardiovasc Risk Factors 1995;5:30–38.

9. Rosengren A, Wilhelmsen L, Orth-Gomer K. Coronary disease in relation to social support and social class in Swedish men. A 15 year follow-up in the study of men born in 1933. Eur Heart J 2004;25:56–63.

10. Kaplan GA, Keil JE. Socioeconomic factors and cardiovascular disease: a review of the literature. Circulation 1993;88:1973–1998.

11. Marmot MG. Socio-economic factors in cardiovascular disease. J Hypertens 1996;14:S201–S205.

12. Rugulies R. Depression as a predictor for coronary heart disease. A review and meta-analysis. Am J Prev Med 2002;23:51–61.

13. Ferketich AK, Schwartzbaum JA, Frid DJ, Moeschberger ML. Depression as an antecedent to heart disease among women and men in the NHANES I study. National Health and Nutrition Examination Survey. Arch Intern Med 2000;160:1261–1268.

14. Karasek R, Baker D, Marxer F, Ahlbom A, Theorell T. Job decision latitude, job demands, and cardiovascular disease: a prospective study of Swedish men. Am J Public Health 1981;71:694–705.

15. Marmot MG, Bosma H, Hemingway H, Brunner E, Stansfeld S. Contribution of job control and other risk factors to social variations in coronary heart disease incidence. Lancet 1997;350:235–239.

16. Lynch J, Krause N, Kaplan GA, Salonen R, Salonen JT. Workplace demands, economic reward, and progression of carotid atherosclerosis. Circulation 1997;96:302–307.

17. Muntaner C, Nieto FJ, Cooper L, Meyer J, Szklo M, Tyroler HA. Work organization and atherosclerosis: findings from the ARIC study. Atherosclerosis Risk in Communities. Am J Prev Med 1998;14:9–18.

18. Nordstrom CK, Dwyer KM, Merz CN, Shircore A, Dwyer JH. Work-related stress and early atherosclerosis. Epidemiology 2001;12:180–185.

19. Moller J, Theorell T, de Faire U, Ahlbom A, Hallqvist J. Work related stressful life events and the risk of myocardial infarction. Case-control and case-crossover analyses within the Stockholm heart epidemiology programme (SHEEP). J Epidemiol Community Health 2005;59:23–30.

20. Tenkanen L, Sjoblom T, Kalimo R, Alikoski T, Harma M. Shift work, occupation and coronary heart disease over 6 years of follow-up in the Helsinki Heart Study. Scand J Work Environ Health 1997;23:257–265.

21. Karlsson B, Alfredsson L, Knutsson A, Andersson E, Toren K. Total mortality and cause-specific mortality of Swedish shift- and day-workers in the pulp and paper industry in 1952–2001. Scand J Work Environ Health 2005;31:30–35.

22. Rosengren A, Tibblin G, Wilhelmsen L. Self-perceived psychological stress and incidence of coronary artery disease in middle-aged men. Am J Cardiol 1991;68:1171–1175.

23. Iso H, Date C, Yamamoto A, et al. Perceived mental stress and mortality from cardiovascular disease among Japanese men and women: the Japan Collaborative Cohort Study for Evaluation of Cancer Risk Sponsored by Monbusho (JACC Study). Circulation 2002;106:1229–1236.

24. Ferrie J, Martikainen P, Shipley M, Marmot M. Self-reported economic difficulties and coronary events in men: evidence from the Whitehall II study. Int J Epidemiol 2005;34:640–648.

25. Li J, Hansen D, Mortensen PB, Olsen J. Myocardial infarction in parents who lost a child: a nationwide prospective cohort study in Denmark. Circulation 2002;106:1634–1639.

26. Salomaa V, Niemela M, Miettinen H, et al. Relationship of socioeconomic status to the incidence and prehospital, 28-day, and 1-year mortality rates of acute coronary events in the FINMONICA myocardial infarction register study. Circulation 2000;101:1913–1918.

27. Engstrom G, Tyden P, Berglund G, et al. Incidence of myocardial infarction in women. A cohort study of risk factors and modifiers of effect. J Epidemiol Community Health 2000;54:104–107.

28. Wamala SP, Mittleman MA, Horsten M, et al. Job stress and the occupational gradient in coronary heart disease risk in women. The Stockholm Female Coronary Risk Study. Soc Sci Med 2000;51:481–489.

29. Lawlor DA, Davey Smith G, Patel R, Ebrahim S. Life-course socioeconomic position, area deprivation, and coronary heart disease: findings from the British Women's Heart and Health Study. Am J Public Health 2005;95:91–97.

30. House JS, Landis KR, Umberson D. Social relationships and health. Science 1988;241:540–545.

31. Berkman LF, Melchior M, Chastang JF, et al. Social integration and mortality: a prospective study of French employees of Electricity of France-Gas of France: the GAZEL Cohort. Am J Epidemiol 2004;159:167–174.

32. Sundquist K, Lindstrom M, Malmstrom M, Johansson SE, Sundquist J. Social participation and coronary heart disease: a follow-up study of 6900 women and men in Sweden. Soc Sci Med 2004;58:615–622.

33. Barefoot JC, Gronbaek M, Jensen G, Schnohr P, Prescott E. Social network diversity and risks of ischemic heart disease and total mortality: findings from the Copenhagen City Heart Study. Am J Epidemiol 2005;161:960–967.

34. Berkman LF, Leo-Summers L, Horwitz RI. Emotional support and survival after myocardial infarction. A prospective, population-based study of the elderly. Ann Intern Med 1992;117:1003–1009.

35. Welin C, Lappas G, Wilhelmsen L. Independent importance of psychosocial factors for prognosis after myocardial infarction. J Intern Med 2000;247:629–639.

36. Barefoot JC, Brummett BH, Helms MJ, Mark DB, Siegler IC, Williams RB. Depressive symptoms and survival of patients with coronary artery disease. Psychosom Med 2000;62:790–795.

37. Frasure-Smith N, Lesperance F. Depression and other psychological risks following myocardial infarction. Arch Gen Psychiatry 2003;60:627–636.

38. Horsten M, Mittleman MA, Wamala SP, et al. Depressive symptoms and lack of social integration in relation to prognosis of CHD in middle-aged women. The Stockholm Female Coronary Risk Study. Eur Heart J 2000;21:1072–1080.

39. Lane D, Carroll D, Ring C, Beevers DG, Lip GY. In-hospital symptoms of depression do not predict mortality 3 years after myocardial infarction. Int J Epidemiol 2002;31:1179–1182.

40. Dickens CM, McGowan L, Percival C, et al. Lack of a close confidant, but not depression, predicts further cardiac events after myocardial infarction. Heart 2004;90:518–522.

41. Kaplan JR, Pettersson K, Manuck SB, Olsson G. Role of sympathoadrenal medullary activation in the initiation and progression of atherosclerosis. Circulation 1991;84:VI23–V132.

42. Strawn WB, Bondjers G, Kaplan JR, et al. Endothelial dysfunction in response to psychosocial stress in monkeys. Circ Res 1991;68:1270–1279.

43. van Amelsvoort LG, Schouten EG, Maan AC, Swenne CA, Kok FJ. Occupational determinants of heart rate variability. Int Arch Occup Environ Health 2000;73:255–262.

44. Ghiadoni L, Donald AE, Cropley M, et al. Mental stress induces transient endothelial dysfunction in humans. Circulation 2000;102:2473–2478.

45. Kop WJ, Krantz DS, Howell RH, et al. Effects of mental stress on coronary epicardial vasomotion and flow velocity in coronary artery disease: relationship with hemodynamic stress responses. J Am Coll Cardiol 2001;37:1359–1366.

46. Lewthwaite J, Owen N, Coates A, et al. Circulating human heat shock protein 60 in the plasma of British civil servants: relationship to physiological and psychosocial stress. Circulation 2002;106:196–201.

47. Brunner E, Davey Smith G, Marmot M, et al. Childhood social circumstances and psychosocial and behavioural factors as determinants of plasma fibrinogen. Lancet 1996;347:1008–1013.

48. von Kanel R, Mills PJ, Fainman C, Dimsdale JE. Effects of psychological stress and psychiatric disorders on blood coagulation and fibrinolysis: a biobehavioral pathway to coronary artery disease? Psychosom Med 2001;63:531–544.

49. Agatisa PK, Matthews KA, Bromberger JT, Edmundowicz D, Chang YF, Sutton-Tyrrell K. Coronary and aortic calcification in women with a history of major depression. Arch Intern Med 2005;165:1229–1236.

50. Rozanski A, Blumenthal JA, Davidson KW, Saab PG, Kubzansky L. The epidemiology, pathophysiology, and management of psychosocial risk factors in cardiac practice: the emerging field of behavioral cardiology. J Am Coll Cardiol 2005;45:637–651.

51. Glassman AH, O'Connor CM, Califf RM, et al. Sertraline treatment of major depression in patients with acute MI or unstable angina. JAMA 2002;288:701–709.

52. Berkman LF, Blumenthal J, Burg M, et al. Effects of treating depression and low perceived social support on clinical events after myocardial infarction: the Enhancing Recovery in Coronary Heart Disease Patients (ENRICHD) Randomized Trial. JAMA 2003;289:3106–3116.

53. Carney RM, Blumenthal JA, Freedland KE, et al. Depression and late mortality after myocardial infarction in the Enhancing Recovery in Coronary Heart Disease (ENRICHD) study. Psychosom Med 2004;66:466–474.

54. Lawlor DA, Hopker SW. The effectiveness of exercise as an intervention in the management of depression: systematic review and meta-regression analysis of randomised controlled trials. BMJ 2001;322:763–767.

55. Blumenthal JA, Sherwood A, Babyak MA, et al. Effects of exercise and stress management training on markers of cardiovascular risk in patients with ischemic heart disease: a randomized controlled trial. JAMA 2005;293:1626–1634.

56. Blumenthal JA, Babyak MA, Carney RM, et al. Exercise, depression, and mortality after myocardial infarction in the ENRICHD trial. Med Sci Sports Exerc 2004;36:746–755.

57. Frasure-Smith N, Lesperance F, Prince RH, et al. Randomised trial of home-based psychosocial nursing intervention for patients recovering from myocardial infarction. Lancet 1997:350;473–479.

31
Health-Related Quality of Life in Cardiac Patients

Hannah McGee

Introduction

Increased longevity and the development of sophisticated healthcare technologies and treatments mean that many people now live with chronic health conditions such as cardiovascular disease over extended periods of their lives. In this context, health-related quality of life (HRQoL) has become an important endpoint in evaluations of health interventions. Its use reflects an increasingly biopsychosocial perspective in modern healthcare. HRQoL research first developed in cancer settings where the balance of quality and duration of life became a key concern in decisions to use novel treatments with very serious side-effects and only partial efficacy. However, over the past 20 years there has been a burgeoning of research activity in every major chronic illness category. In cancer, the European Organisation for Research on the Treatment of Cancer (EORTC) has been established by interested professionals.[1] They have developed a core HRQoL measure and disease-specific modules for various types of cancer. In rheumatology, there is an international, professionally endorsed cooperative called OMERACT (Outcome Measures in Rheumatoid Arthritis Clinical Trials).[2] They seek to improve HRQoL outcome measurement through consensus. The cardiology area is less well integrated. There is general support for HRQoL assessment. For instance, the US research funding agency, the National Heart Lung and Blood Institute, requires almost all clinical trials and many epidemiological studies that it funds to have an HRQoL component. The mission statement of the European Society of Cardiology, sets HRQoL as its primary goal:

To improve the quality of life of the European population by reducing the impact of cardiovascular disease.

However, there has been less attention to developing consensus on assessment with the result that many differing instruments are used across studies and it is not easy to identify and summarize findings in the area. These issues are discussed later after an introduction to the concept of HRQoL and to the range of instruments suitable for use in cardiac settings.

Defining Health-Related Quality of Life

There are many definitions of generic quality of life (QoL). Some mention specific aspects of life while others identify the relative nature of QoL – the fact that QoL requires a comparison between a present and an aspirational or ideal state. A widely adopted approach has been to acknowledge that it is not practical (or perhaps possible) to assess all that is meant by QoL in health research and to use a more limited and focused definition. The argument is that since health interventions have been developed to address health-related aspects of an individual's life, they should be judged against the yardstick of HRQoL. The widely accepted definition of HRQoL is:

The value assigned to the duration of life as modified by the impairments, functional states, perceptions and social opportunities that are influenced by disease, injury, treatment or policy.[3]

Roles of Health-Related Quality of Life Assessment in Cardiac Populations

There are four main uses of HRQoL assessments in cardiac settings:

- To enable treatment comparisons in clinical trials.
- To guide the treatment focus in individual patient care.
- To assess the gap between the HRQoL of patients and age- and gender-matched samples of the general population.
- To enable clinical and economic evaluations to determine the best use of healthcare resources involving cardiac and other patient populations.

HRQoL work has to date focused mainly on the group and research context rather than on informing individual patient care decisions. Only

in the area of cancer care has there been much development in individual care use of HRQoL information. Examples of the other types of uses are presented through the rest of this chapter in reference to specific presentations of coronary disease. First, the types of measures available are described.

Health-Related and General Quality of Life Measurement Instruments

QoL instruments can be divided into five main categories: generic, disease specific, dimension specific, individualized, and utility.[4] These types of measures are outlined in Table 31-1 with illustrations focusing on cardiac-related QoL research. This illustrates the wide variety of instrument types and instruments that can be used in a specific setting such as the cardiac patient population.

The types of measures outlined above are now discussed in relation to their particular uses and constraints.

TABLE 31-1. Typology of quality of life instruments illustrated with examples that can be used in research with cardiac patients

Type of instrument	Examples of instruments used in cardiac research
Generic: can be used across patient and general population groups	Short-Form 36 (SF-36)[5] Nottingham Health Profile (NHP)[6]
Disease specific: focus on aspects of QoL relevant to particular health problems	Seattle Angina Questionnaire (SAQ)[7] MacNew Heart Disease HRQoL Questionnaire (MacNew)[8,9] Minnesota Living with Heart Failure (MLHF)[10]
Dimension specific: focus on a particular component of QoL	Cardiac Depression Scale[11] Global Mood Scale[12] Heart Patients Psychological Questionnaire[13] Hospital Anxiety and Depression Scale[14,15]
Individualized: focus on aspects of life selected by the individual being assessed	Schedule for the Evaluation of Individual Quality of Life (SEIQoL)[16,17] Quality of Life Index (QLI-cardiac)[18]
Utility: focus on hierarchy of preferences assigned by general population or patients for particular health states	EuroQoL (EQ-5D)[19] Quality of Well-being Scale (QWB)[20]

Generic Measures

Generic measures of HRQoL can be used in both general or disease-focused population studies. They are typically profile measures, i.e. they assess a number of dimensions of HRQoL but do not usually sum them into one single scale. The general assumption is that scores on separate dimensions, for example sleep and social function, cannot readily be added together in a meaningful way. The three most commonly used generic instruments, as found in a recent review,[4] are outlined in Table 31-2. The Functional Limitations Profile (an English adaptation of an American instrument – the Sickness Impact Profile)[21] is an early and lengthy instrument that, despite its name (SIP), can be completed by any member of

the adult population. Another long-established measure is the Nottingham Health Profile (NHP).[6] More recently the Short-Form 36 item scale has been developed from a large American series of studies. The SF-36 has become the most widely used measure internationally and has been translated and validated in many languages.[5] The measures have differing strengths and weaknesses. The FLP is clearly very broad in its coverage but is also very long. It does not have a pain subscale, which may be important in some cardiac conditions. The NHP focuses on more severe levels of disability and thus is likely to be less sensitive to change in conditions where effects are in the milder range. Conversely, the SF-36 is more sensitive to lower levels of disability. An illustrative study in relation to heart disease used the SF-36

TABLE 31-2. Scale profiles of three commonly used generic health-related quality of life questionnaires

	Functional Limitations Profile (FLP)[21]	Nottingham Health Profile (NHP)[6]	Medical Outcomes Study Short-Form 36 (SF-36)[5]
Number of items	136	38 (part 1)	36
Number of subscales	12	7 (part 2)	8
Subscale summary scores?	Physical Psychosocial	No	Physical component Mental health component
Total score?	Yes	No	No
Subscales	Ambulation	Energy	Physical functioning
	Body care and movement	Pain	Role limitations due to physical problems
	Mobility	Emotional reactions	Role limitations due to emotional problems
	Household management	Sleep	Social functioning
	Recreation and pastimes	Social isolation	Mental health
	Social interaction	Physical mobility	Energy/vitality
	Emotion		Pain
	Alertness		General health perception
	Sleep and rest		
	Eating		
	Communication		
	Work		

to provide a profile of nine common chronic medical conditions.[22] This showed that cardiac conditions such as myocardial infarction and congestive heart failure had a greater overall negative impact on HRQoL than did other chronic conditions such as diabetes.

The next types of instrument discussed are heart disease specific.

Heart-Disease-Specific Measures

There now exists a large body of research on instruments developed to measure aspects of HRQoL for specific diseases. Here the focus is on those aspects of HRQoL seen as most relevant to the particular health problem. There are excellent summaries of many of the available instruments.[23,24] Examples in the cardiac area are given in Table 31-3.

Disease-specific instruments are developed to be sensitive to change (i.e. have high responsiveness) in aspects of life believed to be most affected by the condition concerned and its treatments. The research challenge when using specific instruments is that it is never possible to determine how different a group is in function from the general population. This makes such assessment problematic from a health comparison perspective – for instance if the aim is to show how disabled particular groups of heart failure patients are in terms of seeking resources for their care in a broader healthcare environment, this cannot easily be done in a comparative way with disease-specific measures. On the other hand, if the research is to detect small but important differences in two pharmacological regimens for heart failure patients, disease-specific instruments are more likely to give meaningful information. Many studies combine specific and generic measures in order to be able to make reference to patient function in relation to the general population while also having useful disease-specific information.

The challenge when doing this of course is to have questionnaires that do not place excessive burden on participants because of their length. This is one issue to consider when deciding if and how to assess QoL in a given health setting. Where HRQoL is an important variable, it is worth considering that many of the other assessments in clinical settings are complex (e.g. requiring laboratory assessment and specific equipment and training to assess and interpret) and that many of these will be repeated at regular intervals to monitor progress in the patient's condition. QoL may be the only assessment that offers the patient an opportunity to provide his or her perspective on the success or otherwise of the treatment being provided.

Dimension-Specific Measures

Many dimensions that contribute to HRQoL have been identified as important in patient

TABLE 31-3. Scale profiles of three disease-specific quality of life questionnaires

	MacNew Quality of Life after Myocardial Infarction (MacNew QLMI)[9]	Seattle Angina Questionnaire (SAQ)[7]	Minnesota Living with Heart Failure Questionnaire (MLHF)[10]
Number of items	27	19	21
Number of subscales	3	5	3
Subscale summary scores?	Yes	Yes	No
Total score?	Yes	No	Yes
Subscales	Physical	Physical limitations	Physical
	Social	Anginal stability	Psychological
	Emotional	Anginal frequency	
		Treatment satisfaction	
		Disease perception	

populations. Some of these have been widely studied before the concept of HRQoL was popularized. In the cardiac situation, the dimensions focus on social and emotional aspects of well-being. Some examples were highlighted in Table 31-1. This gives some idea of the variety of instruments – for instance in the area of emotional well-being there is a generic measure of depression available since 1983 (the Hospital Anxiety and Depression Scale,[14,15] a cardiac-specific measure of depression developed in the mid-1990s (Cardiac Depression Scale[11]), a measure of positive and negative affect developed with cardiac patients but not exclusive to them (the Global Mood Scale),[12] and the Heart Patients' Psychological Questionnaire – a disease-specific measure including subscales on well-being, feelings of disability, despondency, and social inhibition.[13] Use of these scales will depend on the focus of the research – for instance a cardiac rehabilitation intervention might aim to increase HRQoL for the overall sample while seeking to also reduce depression in the subgroup with clinically serious symptoms at the start of the program. Hence a broad assessment such as the SF-36 might be used in conjunction with the Depression subscale of the Hospital Anxiety and Depression Scales or the Cardiac Depression Scale. Debate on use of these instruments in part revolves on the perceived nature of HRQoL – for some HRQoL is seen as an amalgamation of many of these concepts while for others HRQoL is seen as an independent variable which is influenced by these concepts. This theoretical debate is ongoing. Use of these measures is considered further in the cardiac rehabilitation section.

Individualized Measures

Acknowledging the relative and variable nature of QoL across individuals and circumstances, a number of research teams have attempted to develop instruments to assess QoL which have a standardized framework but which allow individualization in various aspects of the assessment.[25] Possibly the most individualized QoL assessment system is the Schedule for the Evaluation of Individual Quality of Life (SEIQoL)[16] and its briefer direct weighting procedure.[17] The SEIQoL philosophy on QoL proposes that the definition of QoL is individual in nature, that the individual assesses his or her QoL on the basis of evaluation of current status on salient aspects of life and compared with his or her own set of standards concerning optimal function. The SEIQoL assessment asks individuals to nominate the five aspects of their life which most contribute to their overall QoL (these do not have to be health-related). They then rate current function from "best possible" to "worst possible" on each and provide relative values of weights to the separate areas. A summary QoL score is derived from this process. Studies have shown that SEIQoL is more sensitive to change than generic or illness-related measures, that health is not always listed as one of the salient aspects of QoL, even for groups with chronic health conditions assessed in medical settings, and that QoL rated in this way can remain high even in very ill patients.[25] The measure has been used with cardiac patients.[26–28]

Some instruments include some rather than total individualization. For instance, the Quality of Life Index has a cardiac-specific version (QLI-III)[18] – 32 preselected items in four domains of life to rate – health and functioning, social and economic, psychological/spiritual, and family. Each is rated twice – once to indicate level of satisfaction with the specific aspect of life and once to rate the importance of the aspect for the individual. Scoring is a sum of each item function by its weighting or importance. QLI-III has been used in various cardiac populations.[29–31]

Utility Measures

Utility measures have been developed from a health economics perspective (see also Chapter 60). They focus on a hierarchy of preferences assigned usually by general population samples for particular health or illness states. Their aim is to assess the value of health or other interventions in terms of a combination of increased QoL and length of life. The challenge here is how to combine changes in length and quality of life, for instance how to compare two treatments for advanced cardiovascular disease – a surgical one which extends life by 5 years but with some early surgical risk and then a risk of cognitive impairment as a side-effect with a pharmacological intervention which will extend life by 3 years with minimal side-effects. The main way in which this has been done is to calculate quality-adjusted life years (QALYs). QALYs are an estimation of the number of life years gained (or lost) because of illness or health intervention multiplied by the change in the HRQoL of those treated. QALYs are calculated from population rather than individual data. HRQoL is rated from 1.0 (best possible life) to 0.0 (dead). Thus a treatment which lengthened life by 5 years and restored or maintained a person in perfect health ($5 \times 1.0 = 5.0$) would provide a health system gain of 5.0 QALYs. The cost per QALY can be calculated from the cost of the treatment in a traditional health economic calculation. Different treatments can thus be compared for the cost per QALY of the treatment. Comparisons can be done concerning the same patients, for example the cost of treating cardiac patients by medication, angioplasty or coronary artery bypass surgery.

QALYs have been criticized because the weights used in calculations are derived from general population rather than patient samples. Ratings might be quite different if the raters had some personal experience of the health condition. Furthermore, QALYs are inherently ageist since any improvement in HRQoL from a treatment, when multiplied by the number of subsequent years of life the individual can expect to benefit, will automatically indicate that the treatment is better value when provided to younger individuals. Such criticisms notwithstanding, the need for methods to inform explicit and objective criteria for societal spending on interventions to improve health is obvious. The most widely used utility measure is the EuroQoL Five Dimensions (EQ-5D). It comprises five questions and a visual analogue scale.[19] The person rates the severity of their problems for five dimensions of health – mobility, self-care, usual activities, pain/discomfort, and anxiety/depression. These can then be classified into 243 (3^5) health states which have pre-assigned population-based ratings. All five are summed to give an overall score. The visual analogue scale is a 100-point health rating from full health to worst imaginable health state. EQ-5D has been used in many cardiac studies.[32,33]

HRQoL Studies in Cardiac Conditions and Interventions

Having outlined the types of measures available to assess HRQoL in cardiac settings, an outline of studies and findings in this area follows. A thorough review of the areas is not possible because of the now extensive literature in many specific aspects. For instance, a recently completed literature review of HRQoL intervention studies in heart failure identified 151 studies.[34] The studies selected are thus illustrative of relatively recent research in the various presentations of cardiac conditions and the interventions provided for these conditions. Reviews are signaled where available.

Angina Pectoris

A variety of approaches including generic and utility HRQoL instruments have been used to evaluate HRQoL in patients with angina, as recently reviewed.[35] Two disease-specific HRQoL instruments have been developed for patients with angina[7,36] with one – the Seattle Angina Questionnaire (SAQ)[7] – being used increasingly in clinical studies. The SAQ is a symptom-specific HRQoL measure comprising 19 items in five domains: physical limitations, anginal stability, anginal frequency, treatment satisfaction, and disease perception.[7] There is evidence of the validity, reliability, and responsiveness of the scale from clinical trials and comparative studies.[7,37,38] In one intervention study, for instance, the SAQ demonstrated clinically meaningful improvement in levels over a one-year period for patients with refractory angina attending a coordinated program of activities.[39] Findings on the generic SF-12 also showed benefit for the intervention. Assessment of HRQoL (via the SF-36) has also been seen to add important clinical information to clinical evaluation of angina patients.[40]

Myocardial Infarction

Research in this area has been recently summarised.[41] Some studies of HRQoL following a myocardial infarction (MI) have used generic or utility instruments.[42–44] Others have opted for heart-disease-specific instruments.[8,9,12,13] A widely used MI-specific HRQoL instrument is the Quality of Life after Myocardial Infarction (QLMI) questionnaire.[8] Since development, it has been further modified to a version called the MacNew QLMI.[9] This consists of 26 items in three dimensions – Limitations, Emotions, and Social – with an overall HRQoL score as the sum of the MacNew QLMI dimensions (see Hoefer et al.[45] for a review). A number of studies with the MacNew QLMI have shown it predicts later adverse health events.[46,47] Predictors of quality of life have also been examined for MI patients. In a large British study, 288 MI patients were followed over the subsequent year. Levels of depression and anxiety during hospitalization did not predict mortality but did predict HRQoL, measured with a generic instrument, at one year.[48]

Heart Failure

A 1999 review summarized instruments used in clinical studies up to then.[49] A review to 2005 identified over 150 intervention studies in heart failure using HRQoL assessments.[34] This reflects in part the increased attention to pharmacological management of this population. Heart failure groups have been examined using a number of generic HRQoL instruments.[50,51] A number of disease-specific HRQoL measures have been published for use with patients with heart failure, for instance the Chronic Heart Failure Questionnaire,[52] the Minnesota Living With Heart Failure Questionnaire (MLHF),[10] and the Kansas City Cardiomyopathy Questionnaire (KCCQ).[53] The MLHF is the most widely used but there are promising psychometric profiles emerging in work with the more recently developed KCCQ. The MLHF questionnaire is a 21-item instrument which includes physical and psychological impairments that patients often relate to their heart failure. The KCCQ contains 23 items and measures physical limitations, symptoms, self-efficacy, social interference, and quality of life. Both have good psychometric properties and have been used in longitudinal evaluations of patient status and in clinical intervention trials (MLHF[54–56]; KCCQ[57–59]). For instance MLHF scores showed significant increases in heart failure patients randomized to an exercise training[55] or

cardiac rehabilitation program.[56] The KCCQ demonstrated the HRQoL advantage of reminder-based interventions to improve self-care management in a randomized study of heart failure patients.[58] It was also used to demonstrate the absence of a detrimental effect of moderate alcohol use on heart failure patients.[59]

An example of the use of a utility-based HRQoL instrument to "anchor" the severity of heart failure against other serious medical conditions is the use of the EQ-5D in the CArdiac REsynchronisation in Heart Failure (CARE-HF) clinical trial.[32] This study included patients with advanced heart failure (NYHA class III or IV) on optimal medical therapy. Baseline scores on the EQ-5D showed the major negative impact on HRQoL of this condition – patients were found to be equivalent to patients with moderate motor neuron disease, Parkinson's disease, those with non-small cell lung cancer, or patients 3 months after ischemic stroke. This type of information is important in educating both professionals and policy makers about the adverse impact of heart failure.

Other Cardiac Conditions

Research has shown the HRQoL improvements for a variety of other conditions and procedures such as cardiomyopathy, congenital heart disease, heart transplantation, and ICD implantation.[60–65] For instance, a major study of over 500 adults with congenital heart disease was conducted recently using individualized QoL assessment.[61] Since this type of research allowed key issues for these patients to emerge, this work is particularly valuable with a group about which less is known than the more common presentations of cardiovascular disease. A parallel study assessed factors determining generic QoL in adults with the condition.[62] Depressive disposition and experienced social support were more related to QoL than was the level of organic dysfunction.

Percutaneous Coronary Interventions

Percutaneous coronary interventions (PCI) are now very widely used with cardiac patients. In an early study demonstrating the value of HRQoL, the physical function scale of the SF-36 was found to be more responsive to change after angioplasty than was the Canadian Cardiovascular Society anginal classification.[66] A number of studies have compared stent-assisted PCI with coronary artery bypass grafting (CABG) surgery for multivessel disease, for example the "Stent or Surgery" trial.[67] Using the SAQ, CABG patients showed greater improvements and better HRQoL at 6 months and a year later (although differences decreased somewhat between 6 and 12 months). The advantage in HRQoL outcomes for CABG patients mirrored that found on clinical variables. A recent randomized trial reflects current developments in relation to PCI. It compared PCI with conservative strategies for management of acute coronary syndromes. It showed greater benefits for PCI at 4 months and one year.[33] These were evident on both disease-specific (SAQ) and generic (EQ-5D) measures.

Cardiac Surgery

A series of clinical studies has compared PCI with CABG with most finding an HRQoL benefit for CABG.[68,69] The benefits of cardiac surgery appear to extend even into very old age. A Swedish study of octogenarians undergoing CABG or aortic valve replacement found that their HRQoL was equivalent to age-matched controls almost a decade later.[70] HRQoL has been shown to predict mortality following CABG. In a follow-up of 2480 patients completing the SF-36, preoperative scores on the Physical Component Summary score (but not the Mental Component Summary score) were an independent predictor of 6-month mortality following CABG surgery.[71] The authors noted the potential value of having a patient self-report measure that can assist in risk classification in cardiac settings.

Cardiac Rehabilitation

The explicit goals of cardiac rehabilitation are to promote secondary prevention and to improve quality of life.[72] Hence HRQoL is a key outcome in this area. Many, but not all, cardiac rehabilitation intervention studies have found HRQoL to be improved in the intervention group compared with controls.[73–76] For instance, a recent 8-week program for MI or PCI patients resulted in HRQoL

increases still evident after 2 years when compared with randomized controls in Hong Kong.[76] The HRQoL improvements complemented lower costs per QALY gained. Some did not report benefits.[77,78] Somewhat in between, a study using the QLMI found early benefits for the intervention group in a cardiac rehabilitation trial but found no differences between groups at one year.[8] This issue also arose in a number of studies as outlined earlier – where differences between intervention and reference group reduced over time. Some of this effect may be a consequence of cross-contamination of groups, for example. a patient randomised to PCI who later has CABG surgery. More may be due to questionnaire items selected as sensitive to differing aspects or stages in time of the rehabilitation and recovery process. This needs further investigation. One dimension that is important to consider in HRQoL assessment is whether socio-demographic factors influence outcomes. Gender and age are briefly considered here as illustrations. While changes in the more physical components of HRQoL with cardiac interventions appear to occur across age groups, changes in more mental health components in HRQoL appear more common in older patients.[79,80] For instance, Lavie and Milani[79] found a smaller level of improvement in physical components (exercise capacity and peak oxygen consumption) in those over age 70 attending cardiac rehabilitation but conversely a larger improvement in HRQoL (SF-36) than in younger groups. In parallel, there is observational evidence that HRQoL is more negatively affected by the onset of cardiac conditions, such as MI, in younger groups.[81] A large 2-year follow-up study of angina or acute coronary syndrome patients undergoing coronary interventions found that, controlling for baseline scores, HRQoL scores improved most for men, younger patients, and those of higher socioeconomic status.[82] These population distribution issues are important to consider when comparing across studies.

Despite the many studies available, HRQoL has not been routinely measured in most clinical or research settings. The Cochrane review of trials of exercise rehabilitation found HRQoL measures used in only 11 studies.[83] Eighteen instruments were used so there was little opportunity to build an overall profile of HRQoL effects. In parallel work, a systematic review of HRQoL assessment in cardiac rehabilitation from 1986 to 1995 reported a wide variety of instruments in use with few instruments used in more than two or three studies.[84] The review also identified the low responsiveness of instruments in many studies. HRQoL instruments that are not responsive to change are unsuitable as outcome tools in cardiac rehabilitation as they underestimate the HRQoL benefits of program attendance. A follow-on study to address this issue selected the best performing instruments in terms of responsiveness from the systematic review and compared their performance within a single cardiac rehabilitation program format in over 700 patients.[85] Nine published instruments (including 27 subscales) were assessed and a high degree of variability in responsiveness was observed. This in effect means that choice of instrument could underestimate the HRQoL benefits of a program – a serious problem in an era of accountability and provision of only those services demonstrated to show benefit. The most responsive scale was the Global Mood Scale (the positive affect subscale). The Global Mood Scale (GMS) comprises 10 negative and 10 positive mood terms.[12] Thus the biggest difference in those attending cardiac rehabilitation versus usual care was in a positive sense of well-being. This encourages useful reflection on what exactly is measured in HRQoL instruments. While the phrase "quality of life" has positive connotations, many of the issues measured focus on negative experience or its absence. Since the majority of cardiac patients do not present with clinical levels of negative affect, instruments that focus only on this dimension may not adequately capture the benefits of interventions on HRQoL. The importance of resolving measurement challenges in HRQoL are considered next.

Measuring Health-Related Quality of Life in Cardiac Populations: The Importance of Getting Consensus

As highlighted in a recent editorial,[86] cardiology is behind other specialties such as rheumatology and oncology in having a coherent approach to HRQoL assessment. Lack of consensus on instru-

ment use limits comparability across studies, conditions, and interventions. This slows the development of a cumulative evidence base on HRQoL in cardiac conditions. This is problematic both within cardiology but also in resource-related discussions with policy makers and health planners, and in projects that advise on instrument selection and use for the future. Among a range of international activities, a project called EuroCardioQoL has been developed to address this challenge.[87] Its aim is to develop a single core coronary heart-disease-specific HRQoL questionnaire, to be called the HeartQoL, and ultimately to be available in 13 European languages. This will allow comparison of outcomes with the same, or different, treatments among pure or mixed populations of patients such as myocardial infarction, angina pectoris, and heart failure. The major advantage of having a single core heart disease HRQoL instrument is to optimize efficiency of inter- and intra-study comparisons by being able to make both across-diagnosis, within-treatment comparisons, and also across-treatment, within-diagnosis comparisons with the same instrument. It thus will create a common HRQoL "language" across cardiac conditions which will enable information to be combined and expertise pooled much more efficiently and effectively in the future.

Conclusion

There is now a burgeoning literature on HRQoL in cardiac conditions and it is increasingly accepted as an important outcome in health settings. The challenge for the cardiology community is to synthesize and build on the research to date in order to be able to use HRQoL information in a more routine and informed manner to guide policy and practice in the future.

References

1. Sprangers MA, Cull A, Groenvold M, Bjordal K, Blazeby J, Aaronson NK. The European Organization for Research and Treatment of Cancer approach to developing questionnaire modules: an update and overview. EORTC Quality of Life Study Group. Qual Life Res 1998;7:291–300.
2. Brooks P, Hochberg M. Outcome measures and classification criteria for the rheumatic diseases. A

compilation of data from OMERACT (Outcome Measures for Arthritis Clinical Trials), ILAR (International League of Associations for Rheumatology), regional leagues and other groups. Rheumatology 2001;40:896–906.

3. Patrick DL, Erickson P. Health Status and Health Policy. Quality of Life in Health Care Evaluation and Resource Allocation. New York: Oxford University Press; 1993.

4. Garratt A, Schmidt L, Mackintosh A, Fitzpatrick R. Quality of life measurement: bibliographic study of patient assessed health outcome measures. British Medical Journal 2002;324:1417–1421.

5. Ware JE Jr, Sherbourne CD. The MOS 36-item short-form health survey (SF-36). I. Conceptual framework and item selection. Med Care 1992;30:473–483.

6. Hunt S, McEwan J, McKenna S. Measuring health status: a new tool for clinicians and epidemiologists. J R Coll Gen Pract 1985;35:185–188.

7. Spertus JA, Winder JA, Dewhurst TA, et al. Development and evaluation of the Seattle Angina Questionnaire: A new functional status measure for coronary artery disease. J Am Coll Cardiol 1995;25:333–341.

8. Oldridge N, Guyatt G, Jones N, et al. Effects on quality of life with comprehensive rehabilitation after acute myocardial infarction. Am J Cardiol 1991;67:1084–1089.

9. Valenti L, Lim L, Heller RF, Knapp J. An improved questionnaire for assessing quality of life after myocardial infarction. Qual Life Res 1996;5:151–161.

10. Rector TS, Kubo SH, Cohn JN. Patients' self-assessment of their congestive heart failure: Content, reliability, and validity of a new measure, the Minnesota Living with Heart Failure questionnaire. Heart Failure 1987;3:198–209.

11. Hare D, Davis C. Cardiac Depression Scale: validation of a new depression scale for cardiac patients. J Psychosom Res 1996;40:379–386.

12. Denollet J. Emotional distress and fatigue in coronary heart disease: the Global Mood Scale (GMS). Psychol Med 1993;23:111–121.

13. Erdman R, Duivenvoorden H, Verhage F, Krazemier M, Hugenholtz P. Predictability of beneficial effects in cardiac rehabilitation: a randomised clinical trial of psychosocial variables. J Cardiopulm Rehabil 1996;6:206–213.

14. Zigmond A, Snaith R. The Hospital Anxiety and Depression Scale. Acta Psychiatr Scand 1983;67:361–370.

15. Hermann C. International experiences with the Hospital Anxiety and Depression scale – a review of validation data and clinical results. J Psychosom Res 1997;42:17–41.

16. McGee HM, O'Boyle CA, Hickey AM, Joyce CRB, O'Malley K. Assessing the quality of life of the individual: the SEIQoL with a healthy and a gastroenterology unit population. Psychol Med 1991;21:749–759.

17. Hickey AM, Bury G, O'Boyle CA, Bradley F, O'Kelly FD, Shannon W. A new short-form individual quality of life measure (SEIQoL-DW): application in a cohort of individuals with HIV/AIDS. BMJ 1996;313:29–33.

18. Ferrans CE, Powers MJ. Quality of life index: development and psychometric properties. Adv Nurs Sci 1985;8:15–24.

19. Brooks R and the EuroQoL Group. EuroQoL: the current state of play. Health Policy 1996;37:53–72.

20. Kaplan RM, Anderson JP, Ganaits TG. The Quality of Well-being Scale: rationale for a single quality of life index. In: Walker SR, Rosser RM, eds. Quality of Life Assessment: Key Issues in the 1990s. Dordrecht: Kluwer Academic; 1993.

21. Charlton JR, Patrick DL, Peach H. Use of multivariate measures of disability in health surveys. J Epidemiol Community Health 1993;37:296–304.

22. Stewart AL, Greenfield S, Hays RD, et al. Functional status and well-being of patients with chronic conditions: results from the Medical Outcomes Study. JAMA 1989;262:907–913.

23. Bowling A. Measuring Disease. Buckingham: Open University Press; 2001.

24. The Patient-Reported Outcomes and Quality of Life Outcomes Instruments (PROQOLID) database (www.proqolid.org).

25. Joyce CRB, O'Boyle CA, McGee HM. Individual Quality of Life: Approaches to Conceptualisation and Assessment. Amsterdam: Harwood; 1999.

26. Smith HJ, Taylor R, Mitchell A. A comparison of four quality of life instruments in cardiac patients: SF-36, QLI, QLMI, and SEIQoL. Heart 2000;84:390–394.

27. Dempster M, Donnelly M. Measuring the health related quality of life of people with ischaemic heart disease. Heart 2000;83:641–644.

28. Moons P, Van Deyk K, Marquet K, et al. Individual quality of life in adults with congenital heart disease: a paradigm shift. Eur Heart J 2005;26:298–307.

29. Papadantonaki A, Stotts NA, Paul SM. Comparison of quality of life before and after coronary artery bypass surgery and percutaneous transluminal angioplasty. Heart Lung 1994;23:45–52.

30. Deshotels A, Planchock N, Dech Z, Prevost S. Gender differences in perceptions of quality of life

in cardiac rehabilitation patients. J Cardiopulm Rehabil 1995;15:143–148.

31. Carroll DL, Hamilton GA, McGovern BA. Changes in health status and quality of life and the impact of uncertainty in patients who survive life-threatening arrhythmias. Heart Lung 1999;28:251–260.

32. Calvert MJ, Freemantle N, Cleland J. The impact of chronic heart failure on helath-0realted quality of life data acquired in the baseline phase of the CARE-HF study. Eur J Heart Failure 2005;7:243–251.

33. Kim J, Henderson RA, Pocock SJ, et al. Health-related quality of life after interventional or conservative strategy in patients with unstable angina or non-ST-segment elevation myocardial infarction. J Am Coll Cardiol 2005;45:221–228.

34. Morgan K, McGee H, Shelley E. Quality of life assessment in heart failure interventions: a systematic review. (submitted for publication).

35. Gandjour A, Lauterbach KW. Review of quality-of-life evaluations in patients with angina pectoris. Pharmacoeconomics 1999;16:141–152.

36. Wilson A, Wiklund I, Lahti T, Wahl M. A summary index for the assessment of quality of life in angina pectoris. J Clin Epidemiol 1991;44:981–988.

37. Dougherty CM, Dewhurst T, Nichol WP, Spertus J. Comparison of three quality of life instruments in stable angina pectoris: Seattle Angina Questionnaire, Short Form Health Survey (SF-36), and Quality of Life Index-Cardiac Version III. J Clin Epidemiol 1998;51:569–575.

38. Spertus JA, Dewhurst T, Dougherty CM, Nichol P. Testing the effectiveness of converting patients to long-acting antianginal medications: The Quality of Life in Angina Research Trial (QUART). Am Heart J 2001;141:550–558.

39. Moore RK, Groves D, Bateson S, et al. Health-related quality of life of patients with refractory angina before and one year after enrolment onto a refractory angina program. Eur J Pain 2005;9:305–310.

40. Chen AY, Daley J, Thibault GE. Angina patients' ratings of current health and health without angina. Med Decis Making 1996;16:169–177.

41. Simpson E, Pilote L. Quality of life after acute myocardial infarction: a systematic review. Can J Cardiol 2003;19:507–511.

42. Taylor R, Kirby B, Burdon D, et al. The assessment of recovery in patients after myocardial infarction using three generic quality of life measures. J Cardiopulm Rehabil 1998;18:139–144.

43. Brown N, Melville M, Gray D, Young T, Skene AM, Hampton JR. Comparison of the SF-36 health survey questionnaire with the Nottingham Health Profile in long-term survivors of a myocardial infarction. J Public Health Med 2000;22:167–175.

44. O'Brien BJ, Buxton MJ, Patterson DL. Relationship between functional status and health-related quality-of-life after myocardial infarction. Med Care 1993;31:950–955.

45. Hoefer S, Lim L, Guyatt G, Oldridge N. The MacNew Heart Disease health-related quality of life instrument: a summary. Health and Quality of Life Outcomes 2004;2:3.

46. Lim LL-Y, Johnson NA, O'Connell RL, Heller RF. Quality of life and later adverse health outcomes in patients with suspected heart attack. Aust N Z J Public Health 1998;22:540–546.

47. Dixon T, Lim LL, Heller RF. Quality of life: an index for identifying high-risk cardiac patients. J Clin Epidemiol 2001;54:952–960.

48. Lane D, Carroll D, Ring C, et al. Mortality and quality of life 12 months after myocardial infarction: effects of depression and anxiety. Psychosom Med 2001;63:221–230.

49. Berry C, McMurray J. A review of quality-of-life evaluations in patients with congestive heart failure. Pharmacoeconomics 1999;16:247–271.

50. Gorkin L, Norvell NK, Rosen RC, et al. Assessment of quality of life as observed from the baseline data of the studies of left ventricular dysfunction (SOLVD) trial quality-of-life substudy. Am J Cardiol 1993;71:1069–1073.

51. Martensson J, Stromberg A, Dahlstrom U, Karlsson JE, Fridlund B. Patients with heart failure in primary health care: effects of a nurse-led intervention on health-related quality of life and depression. Eur J Heart Failure 2005;7:393–403.

52. Wolinsky FD, Wyrwich KW, Nienaber NA, Tierney WM. Generic versus disease-specific health status measures. An example using coronary artery disease and congestive heart failure patients. Evaluation & the Health Professions 1998;21:216–243.

53. Green CP, Porter CB, Bresnahan DR, Spertus JA. Development and evaluation of the Kansas City Cardiomyopathy Questionnaire: a new health status measure for heart failure. J Am Coll Cardiol 2000;35:1245–1255.

54. Bouvy ML, Heerdink ER, Leufkens HG, Hoes AW. Predicting mortality in patients with heart failure: a pragmatic approach. Heart 2003;89:605–609.

55. Belardinelli R, Georgiou D, Cianci G, Purcaro A. Randomized, controlled trial of long-term moderate exercise training in chronic heart failure: effects on functional capacity, quality of life, and clinical outcome. Circulation 1999;99:1173–1182.

56. Benatar D, Bondmass M, Ghitelman J, Avitall B. Outcomes of chronic heart failure. Arch Intern Med 2003;163:347–352.

57. Soto GE, Jones P, Weintraub WS, Krumholz HM, Spertus JA. Prognostic value of health status in

patients with heart failure after acute myocardial infarction. Circulation 2004;110:546–551.

58. Feldman PH, Murtaugh CM, Pezzin LE, McDonald MV, Peng TR. Just-in-time evidence-based e-mail "reminders" in home health care: impact on patient outcomes. Health Serv Res 2005;40:865–885.

59. Salisbury AC, House JA, Conard MW, Krumholz HM, Spertus JA. Low-to-moderate alcohol intake and health status in heart failure patients. J Card Failure 2005;11:323–328.

60. Cotrufo M, Romano GP, De Santo L, et al. Treatment of extensive ischaemic cardiomyopathy: quality of life following two different surgical strategies. Eur J Cardiothorac Surg 2005;27:481–487.

61. Moons P, Van Deyk K, Marquet K, et al. Individual quality of life in adults with congenital heart disease: a paradigm shift. Eur Heart J 2005;26:298–307.

62. Rose M, Koehler F, Sawitzky B, Fliege H, Klapp BF. Determinants of the quality of life of patients with congenital heart disease. Qual of Life Res 2005;14:35–43.

63. Rector TS, Ormaza SM, Kubo SH. Health status of heart transplant recipients versus patients awaiting heart transplantation: a preliminary evaluation of the SF-36 questionnaire. J Heart Lung Transplant 1993;12:983–986.

64. Bainger EM, Fernsler JI. Perceived quality of life before and after implantation of an internal cardioverter defibrillator. Am J Crit Care 1995;4:36–43.

65. Carroll DL, Hamilton GA, McGovern BA. Changes in health status and quality of life and the impact of uncertainty in patients who survive life-threatening arrhythmias. Heart Lung 1999;28:251–260.

66. Krumholz HM, McHorney CA, Clark L, et al. Changes in health after elective percutaneous coronary revascularisation. Med Care 1996;34:754–759.

67. Zhang Z, Mahoney EM, Stables RH, et al. Disease-specific health status after stent-assisted percutaneous coronary Intervention and coronary artery bypass surgery. Circulation 2003;108:1694–1700.

68. Pocock SJ, Henderson RA, Seed P, et al. Quality of life, employment status and anginal symptoms after coronary angioplasty or bypass surgery: 3-year follow-up in the Randomised Intervention Treatment of Angina (RITA) Trial. Circulation 1996;94:135–142.

69. Wahrborg P. Quality of life after coronary angioplasty or bypass surgery: 1-year follow-up in the Coronary Angioplasty versus Bypass Revascularisation Investigation (CABRI) trial. Eur Heart J 1999;20:653–658.

70. Sjogren J, Thulin LI. Quality of life in the very elderly after cardiac surgery: a comparison of SF-36 between long-term survivors and an age-matched population. Gerontology 2004;50:407–410.

71. Rumsfeld JS, MaWhinney S, McCarthy M, et al. Health-related quality of life as a predictor of mortality following coronary artery bypass graft surgery. JAMA 1999;281:1298–1303.

72. World Health Organization. Needs and action priorities in cardiac rehabilitation and secondary prevention in patients with coronary heart disease. Geneva: WHO Regional Office for Europe; 1993.

73. Dugmore LD, Tipson RJ, Phillips MH, et al. Changes in cardiovascular fitness, psychological well-being, quality of life and vocational status following a 12-month cardiac exercise rehabilitation programme. Heart 1999;81:359–366.

74. Pasquali S, Alexander K, Coombs L, Lytle B, Peterson E. Effects of cardiac rehabilitation on functional outcomes after coronary revascularisation. Am Heart J 2003;145:445–451.

75. Koertge J, Weidner G, Elliott-Eller M, et al. Improvement in medical risk factors and quality of life in women and men with coronary artery disease in the Multicenter Lifestyle Demonstration Project. Am J Cardiol 2003;91:1316–1322.

76. Yu C-M, Lau C-P, Chau J, et al. A short course cardiac rehabilitation program is highly cost-effective in improving long-term quality of life in patients with recent myocardial infarction or percutaneous coronary intervention. Arch Phys Med Rehabil 2004;85:1915–1922.

77. Hawkes A, Nowak M, Speare R. Short form-36 survey as an evaluation tool for cardiac rehabilitation programmes: is it appropriate? J Cardiopulm Rehabil 2003;23:22–25.

78. Chan DSK, Chau JPC, Chang AM. Acute coronary syndromes: cardiac rehabilitation programmes and quality of life. J Adv Nurs 2005;49:591–599.

79. Lavie CJ. Milani RV. Benefits of cardiac rehabilitation and exercise training programs in elderly coronary patients. Am J Geriatr Cardiol 2001;10:323–327.

80. Pasquali SK, Alexander KP, Peterson ED. Cardiac rehabilitation in the elderly. Am Heart J 2001;142:748–55.

81. Brown N, Melville M, Gray D, et al. Quality of life four years after acute myocardial infarction: short form 36 scores compared with a normal population. Heart 1999;81:352–358.

82. Veenstra M, Pettersen KI, Rollag A, Stavern K. Association of changes in health-related quality of life in coronary heart disease with coronary procedures and sociodemographic characteristics. Health and Quality of Life Outcomes 2004;2:56.

83. Jolliffe JA, Rees K, Taylor RS, Thompson D, Oldridge N, Ebrahim S. Exercise-based rehabilitation for

coronary heart disease. The Cochrane Database of Systematic Reviews, 2001.

84. McGee HM, Hevey D, Horgan JH. Psychosocial outcome assessments for use in cardiac rehabilitation service evaluation: a 10-year systematic review. Soc Sci Med 1999:48;1373–1393.

85. Hevey D, McGee HM, Horgan JH. Responsiveness of Health-Related Quality of Life Outcome Measures in Cardiac Rehabilitation: Comparison of cardiac rehabilitation outcome measures. J Consult Clin Psychol 2004;72:1175–1180.

86. McGee H, Oldridge N, Hellemans I. Quality of life evaluation in cardiovascular disease: a role for the European Society of Cardiology? Eur J Cardiovasc Prev Rehabil 2005;12:191–192.

87. Oldridge N, Saner H, McGee HM for the EuroCardioQoL Study Investigators. The Euro Cardio-QoL Project. An international study to develop a core heart disease health-related quality of life questionnaire, the HeartQoL. Eur J Cardiovasc Prev Rehabil 2005;12:87–94.

32
Depression Following Myocardial Infarction: Prevalence, Clinical Consequences, and Patient Management

Deirdre A. Lane and Douglas Carroll

Introduction

The search for psychological factors involved in the development and/or progression of coronary heart disease (CHD) has been a fairly persistent, although not always fruitful, activity over the last few decades. Both the clinical observation that CHD patients seem to exhibit certain psychological profiles and the apparent failure of traditional risk factors, such as smoking, high blood pressure and cholesterol, and low levels of physical exertion, to predict anywhere near all new instances of CHD have helped fuel an expectation that there may be other, psychological, predisposing factors at work.

The earliest psychological research was concerned with what came to be called type A behavior. Briefly, individuals displaying the type A behavior complex were considered to be engaged in "chronic and excessive struggle to achieve more and more from their own environment in too short a period of time, and against the opposing efforts of other persons or things in the same environment."[1] The subcomponents of the behavioral complex were regarded as excessive competitive striving, time urgency, and hostility. The strength of the evidence linking type A behavior to CHD reached its zenith in 1981 with the publication in the US of the Consensus Report[2]; type A behavior was agreed to be a risk factor of similar importance to high blood pressure and high cholesterol. Since that date, though, there has been increasing doubt expressed about such claims,[3] and a number of large-scale and well-conducted prospective studies, such as the Multiple Risk Factor Intervention Trial,[4] reported null findings. However, from extensive sub-factor analysis of type A behavior emerged another potentially cardio-toxic psychological factor: hostility.

Whether or not type A behavior was indicated as a risk factor for CHD in prospective studies, one of its subcomponents, hostility, almost invariably was. In addition, studies specifically focusing on hostility, particularly cynical hostility, reported an association with subsequent incident CHD.[5,6] Evidence on hostility as a psychological risk factor has stood the test of time, unlike that of type A behavior. However, a substantial number of unanswered questions remain. Hostility is strongly associated with the likelihood of engaging in unhealthy behaviors, such as smoking and physical inactivity, that increase CHD risk.[7] Hence it remains possible that variations in hostility are merely a proxy for variations in such behaviors, and it is the latter which have consequences for CHD. Further, hostility is steeply stratified by socioeconomic position, such that high hostility is more likely to characterize those in poorer social circumstances. Accordingly, it may be other exposures contingent on low socioeconomic position, and not hostility per se, that increase CHD risk.[8] Thus, the question of causality remains problematic. It is important to appreciate that the issue of statistical confounding (i.e. when an association between an independent variable and a health outcome results from their mutual association with another variable) has not always been well understood. Even when prospective associations remain following statistical adjustment for potential confounders, caution should still be exercised in inferring a causal link. Residual confounding by a poorly measured or an unmeasured variable is still possible (see Christenfeld et al.[9] for a recent discussion). This is an issue to which we shall return.

More recently, attention on psychological factors has again shifted: this time to affective disposition, and especially depression. There is now a fair body of evidence linking depression prospectively with the onset of CHD (see Wulsin and Singal[10] for a review), although there are exceptions to the generally positive relationship.[11] There has also been substantial recent interest in the impact of depression following myocardial infarction (MI) on subsequent prognosis, and, in particular, whether patients who are depressed following their MI are at increased risk of subsequent morbidity and mortality and whether the link between depression and prognosis is causal or not. This constitutes the focus of the rest of the chapter. Given the prevalence of depression in MI patients, this is an important public health matter. It is also an issue that impacts substantially on how MI patients should be managed, that is, assessed and treated.

Prevalence and Persistence of Depression Following Myocardial Infarction

Depressive symptoms and major depression have been consistently reported as common psychological reactions to MI. Major depression, a syndrome characterized by persistently depressed mood, and/or loss of interest and pleasure, with symptoms lasting for a minimum of 2 weeks, occurs with an annual prevalence of between 1% and 6% in the general population, with rates typically higher among patients following MI, at approximately 16–18%.[12] Apart from major depression, depressive symptoms are quite prevalent among the general population, with rates ranging from 10% to 29%. Earlier studies of MI patients reported levels of depressive symptoms varying markedly, from 18% to 60%, although the majority of more recent studies report relatively consistent prevalence rates ranging from 17% to 37%.[12]

Little is known about the persistence of depression after an acute MI since few studies have repeatedly measured depression in the months following the event. However, it would appear that depressive symptoms first emerge between 48 and 72 hours following MI.[12,13] In the majority of post-MI patients, symptoms of depression are reported to abate after 5 or 6 days.[14] However, in some patients distress persists for several months after discharge, with some patients only becoming depressed after discharge from hospital, in the first few months following the infarction.

The majority of the more recent studies of MI patients have limited the formal assessment of symptoms of depression to the period prior to discharge from hospital. However, there are at least two compelling reasons why the assessment of depression should be continued beyond discharge. First, there is the proposed prognostic significance of post-MI depression. Some, although by no means all studies, have found that depressive symptomatology following MI increases the risk of death and/or recurrent cardiac events (see Table 32-1). Second, depression also significantly impairs quality of life and reduces the likelihood of participation in cardiac rehabilitation. Third, it is necessary to establish whether symptoms of depression experienced in hospital are associated with cardiac disease severity or are largely a reaction to hospitalization per se.

Review of the Evidence Linking Depression Following MI and Subsequent Mortality and Morbidity

Observational Studies

Many observational studies have now examined the association between depression following MI and subsequent cardiac events (fatal and nonfatal) and/or cardiac and all-cause mortality (Table 32-1). Of these, nine studies have reported a positive relationship between depression and one or more of these outcomes: cardiac events,[15–17,20,23] cardiac mortality,[16,17,19,21,23,24,29] and all-cause mortality.[19,29,36] Further, after adjustment for potential confounders, such as age, sex, and markers of disease severity, eight studies concluded that depression was an independent (i.e. causal) risk factor for at least one outcome: cardiac events[35] (Table 32-1), cardiac mortality,[17,21,24,29,33] and all-cause mortality.[29,36] In contrast, 11 reports found no significant association between depression and prognosis[18,22,27,28,31,32,39] or describe equivocal findings.[25,26,30,38]

In the absence of compelling evidence from randomized controlled trials, the case for depression as an independent risk factor for prognosis following MI necessarily rests with the evidence from these observational epidemiological studies. Accordingly, it is important to determine the strength of that evidence. Two recent meta-analyses[40,41] have sought to determine whether the evidence strongly implicates depression as an *independent* risk factor for mortality (cardiac and all-cause) and recurrent cardiac events, and to provide a quantitative estimate of the magnitude of the independent association between depression and prognosis following MI.

The unadjusted pooled analyses of both meta-analyses indicate that depression following MI is associated with a 2-fold increased risk of death and recurrent cardiac events. This was true irrespective of whether depression was assessed by clinical diagnosis or questionnaire, and the strength of the association was not influenced by length of follow-up. However, the year of data collection (prior to and after 1992) influenced the magnitude of the link between depression and subsequent mortality; earlier studies reported a stronger association between depression following MI and clinical prognosis (OR, 3.22; 95% CI, 2.14–4.86) than later studies (OR, 2.01; 95% CI, 1.45–2.78).[40]

However, only the latter meta-analysis[41] undertook formal analyses using adjusted odds ratios, to assess the association between depression and outcome after controlling for possible confounders. In such analyses, depression was no longer a statistically significant predictor of cardiac mortality (OR, 1.95; 95% CI, 0.81–4.73). The associations between all-cause mortality and recurrent cardiac events were also attenuated, but remained statistically significant (OR, 1.66; 95% CI, 1.20–2.29 and OR, 1.41; 95% CI, 1.11–1.79, respectively), indicating that depression following MI conferred a 41% and 66% increased risk of death from any cause and of recurrent cardiac

events, respectively. van Melle et al.[40] also conceded that in those studies reporting multivariate analyses, the adjusted odds ratios were generally smaller than the corresponding unadjusted odds ratios.

Why are there differences in study outcomes exploring the link(s) between depression following MI and prognosis? The inconsistency in previous findings may be due, in part, to the dissimilar MI populations studied and other methodological differences. The sample populations varied markedly, with highly selected MI populations (e.g. patients with arrhythmias or significant left ventricular dysfunction), which may have heightened their mortality risk. Studies also vary markedly in the time delay between the occurrence of MI and measurement of depression. The variety of diagnostic instruments and standardized questionnaires used may also have contributed to the variations in the outcomes of studies. Further, small sample sizes and the failure to report multivariate analyses controlling for other risk factors suggests that caution should be exercised in interpreting the results. With such variations in population measurement, design, and statistical control, it might be expected that results would vary considerably.

However, as we have highlighted previously,[42] there is one other fairly consistent difference between prospective observational studies reporting a relationship between depression and cardiac events and mortality following MI and those that do not find such an association. This has to do with the issue of disease severity and its relationship with depression. Depression would appear to predict clinical prognosis following MI mainly in studies that have either not controlled for cardiac disease severity or in which disease severity is significantly correlated with depression. Others researchers have also noted that one of the main problems with attributing a causal role to depression in clinical prognosis following MI is the potential confounding of depression with disease severity in such patients.[9,11,42,43] In the prospective observational studies that have adjusted for measures of disease severity,[17,20,21,24–29,31–33,35–36,38] the association between depression and outcome was either no longer statistically significant[20,25,26] or was attenuated.[17,21,29,33,35,36,38]

TABLE 32-1. Observational studies assessing the relationship between depression following myocardial infarction and mortality and recurrent cardiac events

Author, year, place	Sample size, n (% women)	Depression measure	Baseline prevalence of depression (%)	Outcomes	Length of follow-up	Association between depression and outcome(s)
Silverstone (1987), UK[15]	108 (25.0)	MADRS	44.4	Cardiac events ACM	1 week	Depression measured within 24 hours of MI was predictive of increased risk of ACM or cardiac events
Ladwig (1991), Germany[16]	553 (0)	KSb-S	High: 14.5 Med: 22.2 Low: 63.3	Cardiac events CM	6 months	Depression predicted CM (P = 0.035) and cardiac events (P = 0.001) in bivariate analyses only
Frasure-Smith (1993), Canada[17]	222 (22.1)	Modified DIS	15.8	CM	6 months	Major depression predicted CM in both bivariate (HR, 5.74; 95% CI 4.61–6.87) and multivariate analyses (HR, 4.29; 95% CI, 3.14–5.44)
Jenkinson (1993)*, UK[18]	1376 (22.0)	Investigator tailored scale	5.7	ACM	6, 12, and 36 months	Depression did not predict ACM (P = 0.48)
Denollet (1995) Belgium[19]	105 (0)	MBHI	46.7	ACM CM	2–5 years	Depression predicted ACM (P < 0.005) and CM (P = 0.01) in bivariate analyses only
Frasure-Smith (1995), Canada[20]	222 (22.1)	Modified DIS BDI	MDD: 15.8 BDI ≥10: 31.2	Cardiac events	12 months	Both major depression (OR, 2.67; 95% CI, 1.22–5.85) and depressive symptoms (OR, 3.32; 95% CI, 1.69–6.53) were predictive of cardiac events in bivariate analyses only. After adjustment, depression did not predict cardiac events
Frasure-Smith (1995), Canada[21]	222 (22.1)	Modified DIS BDI	MDD: 15.8 BDI ≥10: 31.2	CM	18 months	Depressive symptoms predicted CM in bivariate (OR, 7.82; 95% CI, 2.42–25.26) and multivariate (OR, 6.64; 95% CI, 1.76–25.09) analyses. However, major depression only predicted CM in bivariate analyses (OR, 3.64; 95% CI, 1.32–10.05)
Carinci (1997), Italy[22]	2449 (12.4)	CBAF depression scale	1.3	ACM	6 months	Depression did not predict ACM (HR, 1.7; 95% CI, 0.9–3.1)
Denollet (1998), Belgium[23]	87 (6.9)	MBHI	50.6	Cardiac events CM	6–10 years	Depression predicted CM (OR, 7.5; 95% CI, 1.5–36.4) and cardiac events (OR, 4.3; 95% CI, 1.4–13.3) in bivariate analyses. Multivariate analyses not reported
Frasure-Smith (1999), Canada[24]	896 (31.6)	BDI	32.4	CM	12 months	Depressive symptoms predicted CM in both bivariate (OR, 3.23; 95% CI, 1.65–6.33) and multivariate (OR, 3.66; 95% CI, 1.68–7.99) analyses
Irvine (1999), Canada[25]	634 (17.2)	BDI	†	Cardiac events	2 years	Depression predicted cardiac events in those receiving placebo medication after controlling for previous MI and congestive heart failure (OR 2.45; 95% 1.14 = 5.35. However, after additional adjustment for dyspnea, depression did not predict cardiac events (RR, 1.73; 95% CI, 0.75–3.98).
Kaufmann (1999), US[26]	331 (34.4)	DIS	27.2	ACM	6 and 12 months	Major depression only predicted ACM at the 12 month follow-up in bivariate analyses (p = 0.04)
Lane (2000), UK[27]	288 (25.3)	BDI	29.8	Cardiac events	12 months	Depression did not predict cardiac events in either bivariate (OR, 0.97; 95% CI, 0.55–1.70) or multivariate (OR, 0.79; 95% CI, 0.43–1.43) analyses
Mayou (2000)*, UK[28]	347 (27.0)	HADS-D	7.6	ACM CM	6 and 18 months and 6 years	Depression did not predict ACM or CM in either bivariate (OR, 1.95; 95% CI, 0.83–4.56 and OR, 1.34, 0.44–4.10, respectively) or multivariate (OR, 2.69; 95% CI, 0.97–7.48 and OR, 2.07; 95% CI, 0.53–8.09, respectively) analyses

Study	N (%)	Instrument	Depression (%)	Outcome	Follow-up	Results
Welin (2000), Sweden[29]	275 (16.4)	Zung SRDS	36.7	ACM, CM	10 years	Depression predicted ACM and CM in both bivariate (OR, 2.45; 95% CI 1.49–4.02 and OR, 3.54; 95% CI, 1.85–6.79, respectively) and multivariate (OR, 1.75; 95% CI, 1.02–2.99 and OR, 3.16; 95% CI, 1.38–7.25, respectively) analyses
Bush (2001), US[30]	267 (58.0)	SCID, BDI	Mood disorder: 17.2; BDI ≥10: 19.0; Mood disorder ± BDI ≥10: 27.3	ACM	4 months	Only mood disorder ± depressive symptoms were predictive of ACM in bivariate analyses (RR, 3.8; 95% CI, †; $P = 0.008$). Multivariate analyses were not reported
Lane (2001; 2002)*, UK[31,32]	288 (25.3)	BDI	30.9	ACM, CM	4, 12, and 36 months	Depression did not predict ACM or CM in either bivariate (OR, 1.04; 95% CI, 0.50–2.16 and OR, 0.84; 95% CI, 0.37–1.90) or multivariate (OR, 0.77; 95% CI, 0.33–1.76 and OR, 0.56; 95% CI, 0.22–1.43) analyses
Lespérance (2002), Canada[33]	896 (31.6)	BDI	≥10: 32.4	ACM, CM, Cardiac events	5 years	BDI scores ≥10 predicted a 2- to 4-fold increased risk of ACM and CM in bivariate and multivariate analyses. Depression was associated with a 1.6- to 2.4-fold greater risk of cardiac events in bivariate analyses only. BDI scores <10 only predicted CM in bivariate analyses
Luutonen (2002), Finland[34]	85 (23.5)	BDI	21.2	ACM	18 months	†
Shiotani (2002), Japan[35]	1042 (19.6)	Zung SRDS	42.0	CM, Cardiac events	12 months	Depression predicted cardiac events in both bivariate (OR, 1.46; 95% CI, 1.11–1.92) and multivariate (OR, 1.41; 95% CI, 1.03–1.92) analyses. However, depression did not predict CM
Carney (2003), US[36]	766 (39.6)	DSM-IV, DISH, BDI	Any: 46.7; MDD: 45.5; Minor: 54.5	ACM	30 months	Depression (MDD/minor/combination) was associated with a 2- to 3-fold increased of ACM in bivariate and multivariate analyses
Lauzon (2003), Canada[37]	587 (19.8)	BDI	34.7	ACM	12 months	Depression did not predict ACM (HR, 1.3; 95% CI, 0.59–3.05) in bivariate analyses
Strik (2003), The Netherlands[38]	318 (0)	SCL-90 depression subscale	47.1	Cardiac events	1–70 months	Depression did not predict cardiac events in bivariate analyses. After adjustment for age, LVEF, and antidepressant use, depression was predictive of cardiac events (HR, 2.32; 95% CI, 1.04–5.18). However, after additional adjustment for anxiety and hostility, depression did not predict cardiac events ($P = 0.45$)
Steeds (2004), UK[39]	131 (32.8)	BDI (version II)	47.3	ACM	25–37 months	Depression did not predict ACM (OR, 1.8; 95% CI, 0.56–6.0) in bivariate analyses

ACM = all-cause mortality; BDI = Beck Depression Inventory; Cardiac events = fatal and nonfatal cardiac events combined; CI = confidence intervals; CM = cardiac mortality; CBAF = Cognitive-Behavioural Assessment Form; DIS = Diagnostic Interview Schedule; DISH = Depression Interview and Structured Hamilton; DSM-IV = Diagnostic and Statistical Manual of Mental Disorders (Fourth Edition); HADS-D = Hospital Anxiety and Depression Scale-Depression subscale; HDRS = Hamilton Depression Rating Scale; HR = hazard ratio; KSb-S = Kleinische Selbstburteilungsskalen; LVEF = left ventricular ejection fraction; MADRS = Montgomery-Asberg Depression Rating Scale; MBHI = Millon Behavioural Health Inventory; MDD = major depressive disorder; MI = myocardial infarction; NS = not significant; OR = odds ratio; PVCs = premature ventricular contractions; RR = relative risk; SADS = Schedule for Affective Disorders and Schizophrenia; SCID = Structured Clinical Interview for DSM-III-R; SCL-90 = Symptom Checklist-90; SD = standard deviation; SRDS = Self-Rating Depression Scale; < = less than; ≥ = greater than or equal to; † = not reported; * = the results from the longest follow-up period available are presented.

Further, the inference that some exposure or characteristic constitutes an independent, causal, risk factor for some health outcome is usually based on multivariate analyses in which a statistically significant bivariate association between the exposure or characteristic and the health outcome remains after adjustment for potential confounding variables. However, declarations of independence on this basis may be premature.[44] The ability of multivariate statistical models to determine independence depends on the accuracy of measurement of the potentially confounding variables; any inaccuracy will inevitably lead to underestimation of their true impact.[44] Therefore, "it can appear that a risk factor is related to disease after the adjustment for confounding factors, but this residual relationship only exists because of under-adjustment for these confounding factors" (Davey Smith and Phillips,[44] p. 257).

The indices of disease severity employed in observational studies in this area have been various and all are imperfect. Accordingly, characteristics such as depression can appear to have an independent association with mortality or recurrent cardiac events but this could arise as a consequence of the residual confounding of depression with disease severity, where disease severity is measured imprecisely. Since no single precise measure of cardiac disease severity exists, composite indices assessing the severity of the MI, degree of heart failure, left ventricular dysfunction, medication, presence of arrhythmias, and length of index hospital admission, among others, may be a better method of capturing exactly how ill patients are.[45]

Experimental Studies

The issue of whether depression is a cause of mortality, through some as yet identified pathway, or is a marker for some other cause, is an important one. If depression is a cause, its appropriate treatment should reduce subsequent mortality. However, if depression is only a marker of some other underlying cause, for example disease severity, the treatment of depression per se should not affect prognosis.

The reported association between depression and mortality and recurrent cardiac events has helped to initiate interventions aimed at reducing depression and thus mortality and morbidity. To date, two randomized controlled trials, one large-scale cognitive-behavioral trial, supplemented where necessary with antidepressant medication (Enhancing Recovery In Coronary Heart Disease: ENRICHD),[48] and one pharmacological trial (Myocardial INfarction and Depression-Intervention Trial: MIND-IT),[46] have examined the impact of reducing depression post-MI on subsequent morbidity and mortality (Table 32-2). Another pharmacological trial, SADHART (Sertraline Antidepressant Heart Attack Randomised Trial: SADHART),[47] assessed the safety and efficacy of SSRI antidepressants in unstable cardiac patients (Table 32-2). Both SADHART[47] and ENRICHD[48] observed a relative reduction in depression with treatment.

However, the interventions had no significant effect on nonfatal reinfarction or mortality[48] or on indices of disease severity, such as left ventricular ejection fraction, ventricular arrhythmias, or electrocardiogram profile.[47] We await the results of the MIND-IT trial.[46]

Summary of the Evidence Concerning Depression and Prognosis

The balance of evidence and argument suggests that it is right to be skeptical about a causal link between depression following MI and subsequent cardiac events and mortality. The recent meta-analyses suggest that depression following MI is associated with a slightly elevated risk of all-cause mortality and recurrent cardiac events after adjustment for potential confounders, including disease severity. However, few studies included in these meta-analyses reported statistical outcomes following adjustment. In addition, the possibility of residual confounding remains even in those studies which have undertaken multivariate analyses, given the difficulties surrounding the accurate assessment of disease severity in this context. Further, the one experimental study, to date, to have its findings published, found that an intervention effective in ameliorating depression did not influence mortality or recurrent nonfatal cardiac events.[48]

TABLE 32-2. Experimental studies examining the impact of interventions to reduce depression on outcomes in MI/unstable angina patients

Trial, year, country	Sample size, n (% women); study period	Intervention	Outcome(s)	Length of follow-up	Summary
MIND-IT (2002), The Netherlands[46]	320 (†) MI patients enrolled September 1999 to March 2002	Mirtazapine (or open-label citalopram**) ($n = 190$) vs. usual care ($n = 130$) for 24 weeks	Cardiac events (cardiac death or hospital admission for nonfatal MI, unstable angina, heart failure, or ventricular tachyarrhythmia)	12–27 months	Ongoing trial – results available late 2005/early 2006
SADHART† (2002), US, Europe, Canada, Australia[47]	369 (36.6) MI and unstable angina patients enrolled April 1997 to April 2001	Sertraline ($n = 186$) vs. placebo ($n = 183$) for 24 weeks	Change in baseline LVEF ECG parameters (e.g. PVCs) Reduction in depression	6 months	No significant differences between two groups in LVEF, ECG parameters, death, or recurrent cardiac events Sertraline significantly reduced depression compared to placebo
ENRICHD (2003), US[48]	2481 (43.7) MI patients enrolled October 1996 to October 1999	Cognitive-behavioral therapy* ($n = 1238$) vs. usual care ($n = 1243$) for maximum of 6 months	Death or nonfatal MI ACM CVM Recurrent nonfatal MI Reduction in depression	30 months	All events: HR (95% CI) = 1.01 (0.86–1.18) ACM: 0.98 (0.79–1.21) CVM: 0.83 (0.64–1.10) Recurrent nonfatal MI: 0.90 (0.71–1.14) Cognitive-behavioral therapy significantly reduced depression

ACM = all-cause mortality; CI = confidence interval; CVM = cardiovascular mortality; ECG = electrocardiogram; ENRICHD = Enhancing Recovery In Coronary Heart Disease; HR = hazard ratio; LVEF = left ventricular ejection fraction; MI = myocardial infarction; MIND-IT = Myocardial INfarction and Depression Intervention Trial; PVC = premature ventricular complexes; SADHART = Sertraline Antidepressant Heart Attack Randomised Trial; * = given if mirtazapine was refused or not tolerated; ** = 249 patients received adjunctive antidepressant medication; † = SADHART was designed to assess the safety and efficacy of sertraline use in unstable cardiac patients.

Depression Following MI and Quality of Life

Whatever the case regarding depression following MI and clinical prognosis, it is clear that depression has substantial lifestyle consequences for MI patients. Several studies have now demonstrated a link between depression and subsequent quality of life.[28,31] In this context, it is worth noting that cardiology has started to embrace outcomes other than morbidity and mortality, such as quality of life. As an influential editorial argued, "We should not lose sight of the fact that an intervention that improves well-being, but fails to change survival, is still a very valuable treatment" (Lespérance and Frasure-Smith,[49] p. 20). Quality of life is discussed in more detail in Chapter 31. Aside from overall quality of life and subjective well-being, depression has been linked to a range of behavioral outcomes in MI patients: non-attendance at cardiac rehabilitation,[50] delayed return to work,[51] and poor adherence to medication.[52]

Implications for Patient Management

The research on depression following MI has clear implications for patient management. As soon as MI patients are medically stable, as determined by a cardiologist, they should undergo routine screening to identify those that are severely distressed. There are many self-report questionnaires available[53] to assess depression, with the Beck Depression Inventory,[54] and the Hospital Anxiety and Depression Scale[55] being among those most commonly employed. Symptoms of depression should be assessed using a self-report instrument during hospitalization (3 to 7 days post-MI), and 6 weeks or so after discharge (usually when formal cardiac rehabilitation classes begin), to identify those patients who are experiencing significant emotional distress. Appropriate referral to a mental health professional should be considered for those patients demonstrating persistent elevated symptoms of depression, to allow for assessment of clinical depression and appropriate treatment. For those patients who are depressed or have a history of depression, therapy, in addition to health education and exercise rehabilita-

tion, should be made available. For most, intervention with cognitive behavior therapy, supplemented where appropriate with selective serotonin reuptake inhibitors, is advised. Cognitive behavior therapy has proved to be an effective treatment for depression in the general population, and in the ENRICHD trial,[48] relative to usual care, it significantly improved levels of depression following MI. In addition, treatment with selective serotonin reuptake inhibitors, regardless of treatment arm, was associated with decreased mortality.[48]

Conclusions

The issue of whether depression following MI is a causal factor in subsequent mortality and cardiovascular morbidity remains to be resolved. Only further randomized control trials will truly advance our understanding. In addition, future observational studies should report multivariate analyses in which adjustment is made for potential confounders, most importantly measures of disease severity. Better composite measures of disease severity need to be employed.[45] Irrespective of the implications of depression following MI for mortality and morbidity, the high incidence of depression in this population and the link between depression and quality of life should be sufficient to suggest changes to patient management practices.

References

1. Rosenman RH. The role of Type A behaviour pattern in ischaemic heart disease: modification of its effects by beta-blocking agents. Br J Clin Pract 1978;32: Suppl 1.
2. Review Panel. Coronary-prone behaviour and coronary heart disease: A critical review. Circulation 1981;63:1199–1215.
3. Bennett P, Carroll D. Type A behaviours and heart disease: Epidemiological and experimental foundations. Behav Neurol 1990;3:261–277.
4. Shekelle RB, Gale M, Ostfeld AM, et al. Hostility, risk of coronary disease and mortality. Psychosom Med 1983;45:219–228.
5. Barefoot JC, Dahlstrom WG, Williams RB Jr. Hostility, CHD incidence, and total mortality: A 25-year follow-up study of 255 physicians. Psychosom Med 1983;45:59–63.

6. Barefoot JC, Williams RB, Dahlstrom WG, et al. Predicting mortality from scores on the Cook-Medley Scale: A follow-up of 118 lawyers. Psychosom Med 1987;49:210.

7. Smith TW. Hostility and health: Current status of a psychosomatic hypothesis. Health Psychol 1992; 11:139–150.

8. Carroll D, Davey Smith G, Sheffield D, et al. The relationship between socio-economic status, hostility, and blood pressure reactions to mental stress in men: Data from the Whitehall II study. Health Psychol 1997;16:131–136.

9. Christenfeld NJS, Sloan RP, Carroll D, et al. Risk factors, confounding, and the illusion of statistical control. Psychosom Med 2004;66:868–875.

10. Wulsin LR, Singal BM. Do depressive symptoms increase the risk for the onset of coronary disease? A systematic quantitative review. Psychosom Med 2003;65:201–210.

11. Everson-Rose SA, House JS, Mero RP. Depressive symptoms and mortality risk in a national sample: Confounding effects of health status. Psychosom Med 2004;66:823–830.

12. Lane D, Carroll D, Ring C, et al. The prevalence and persistence of depression and anxiety following myocardial infarction. Br J Health Psychol 2002;7: 11–21.

13. Havik OE, Mæland JG. Patterns of emotional reactions after a myocardial infarction. J Psychosom Res 1990;34:271–285.

14. Thompson DR, Webster RA, Cordle CJ, et al. Specific sources and patterns of anxiety in male patients with first myocardial infarction. Br J Med Psychol 1987;60:343–348.

15. Silverstone PH. Depression and outcome in acute myocardial infarction. BMJ 1987;294:219–220.

16. Ladwig KH, Kieser M, Konig J, et al. Affective disorders and survival after acute myocardial infarction: results from the Post-Infarction Late Potential Study. Eur Heart J 1991;12:959–964.

17. Frasure-Smith N, Lespérance F, Talajic M. Depression following myocardial infarction: Impact on 6-month survival. JAMA 1993;270:1819–1825.

18. Jenkinson CM, Madeley RJ, Mitchell JRA, et al. The influence of psychosocial factors on survival after myocardial infarction. Public Health 1993;107:305–317.

19. Denollet J, Stanislas US, Brutsaert DL. Personality and mortality after myocardial infarction. Psychosom Med 1995;57:582–591.

20. Frasure-Smith N, Lespérance F, Talajic M. The impact of negative emotions on prognosis following myocardial infarction: is it more than depression? Health Psychol 1995;14:388–398.

21. Frasure-Smith N, Lespérance F, Talajic M. Depression and 18-month prognosis after myocardial infarction. Circulation 1995;91:999–1005.

22. Carinci F, Nicolucci A, Ciampi A, et al., on behalf of the Gruppo Italiano per lo Studio della Sopravvivenza nell' Infarto Miocardioco. Role of interactions between psychological and clinical factors in determining 6-month mortality among patients with acute myocardial infarction. Application of recursive partitioning techniques to the GISSI-2 database. Eur Heart J 1997;18:835–845.

23. Denollet J, Brutsaert DL. Personality, disease severity, and the risk of long-term cardiac events in patients with a decreased ejection fraction after myocardial infarction. Circulation 1998;97: 167–173.

24. Frasure-Smith N, Lespérance F, Juneau M, et al. Gender, depression, and one-year prognosis after myocardial infarction. Psychosom Med 1999;61: 26–37.

25. Irvine J, Basinski A, Baker B, et al. Depression and risk of sudden cardiac death after acute myocardial infarction: testing for the confounding effects of fatigue. Psychosom Med 1999;61:729–737.

26. Kaufmann MW, Fitzgibbons JP, Suusman EJ, et al. Relation between myocardial infarction, depression, hostility, and death. Am Heart J 1999;138: 549–554.

27. Lane D, Carroll D, Ring C, et al. Do depression and anxiety predict recurrent coronary events 12 months after myocardial infarction? Q J Med 2000;93:739–744.

28. Mayou RA, Gill D, Thompson DR, et al. Depression and anxiety as predictors of outcomes after myocardial infarction. Psychosom Med 2000;62: 212–219.

29. Welin C, Lappas G, Wilhelmsen L. Independent importance of psychosocial factors for prognosis after myocardial infarction. J Intern Med 2000;247: 629–639.

30. Bush DE, Ziegelstein RC, Tayback M, et al. Even minimal symptoms of depression increase mortality risk after acute myocardial infarction. Am J Cardiol 2001;88:337–341.

31. Lane D, Carroll D, Ring C, et al. Mortality and quality of life 12 months after myocardial infarction: effects of depression and anxiety. Psychosom Med 2001;63:221–230.

32. Lane D, Carroll D, Ring C, et al. In-hospital symptoms of depression do not predict mortality 3 years after myocardial infarction. Int J Epidemiol 2002;31: 1179–1182.

33. Lespérance F, Frasure-Smith N, Talajic M, et al. Five-year risk of cardiac mortality in relation to initial severity and one-year changes in depression

symptoms after myocardial infarction. Circulation 2002;105:1049–1053.

34. Luutonen S, Holm H, Salminen JK, et al. Inadequate treatment of depression after myocardial infarction. Acta Psychiatr Scand 2002;106:434–439.

35. Shiotani I, Sato H, Kinjo K, et al., for The Osaka Acute Coronary Insufficiency Study (OACIS) Group. Depressive symptoms predict 12-month prognosis in elderly patients with acute myocardial infarction. J Cardiovasc Risk 2002;9:153–160.

36. Carney RM, Blumenthal JA, Cateillier D, et al. Depression as a risk factor for mortality after acute myocardial infarction. Am J Cardiol 2003;92:1277–1281.

37. Lauzon C, Beck CA, Huynh T, et al. Depression and prognosis following hospital admission because of acute myocardial infarction. Can Med Assoc J 2003;168:547–552.

38. Strik JJMH, Denollet J, Lousberg R, et al. Comparing symptoms of depression and anxiety as predictors of cardiac events and increased health care consumption following myocardial infarction. J Am Coll Cardiol 2003;42:1801–1807.

39. Steeds RP, Bickerton D, Smith MJ, et al. Assessment of depression following acute myocardial infarction using the Beck Depression Inventory. Heart 2004;90:217–218.

40. van Melle JP, de Jonge P, Spijkerman TA, et al. Prognostic association of depression following myocardial infarction with mortality and cardiovascular events. A meta-analysis. Psychosom Med 2004;66:814–822.

41. Lane D, Taylor RS, Lip GYH, et al. Is depression following myocardial infarction an independent risk factor for recurrent cardiac events and mortality? A systematic review and meta-analysis of the observational evidence. (submitted for publication)

42. Lane D, Carroll D, Lip GYH. Anxiety, depression, and prognosis after myocardial infarction. J Am Coll Cardiol 2003;42:1808–1810.

43. Mendes de Leon CF. Depression and social support in recovery from myocardial infarction: Confounding and confusion. Psychosom Med 1999;61:738–739.

44. Davey Smith G, Phillips AN. Declaring independence: Why we should be cautious. J Epidemiol Community Health 1990;44:257–258.

45. Lane D, Ring C, Lip GYH, et al. Indirect markers of cardiac disease severity and mortality following myocardial infarction. Heart 2005;91:531–532.

46. van den Brink RHS, van Melle JP, Honig A, et al., on behalf of the MIND-IT investigators. Treatment of depression after myocardial infarction and the effects on cardiac prognosis and quality of life: Rationale and outline of the Myocardial Infarction and Depression-Intervention Trial (MIND-IT). Am Heart J 2002;144:219–225.

47. Glassman AH, O'Connor CM, Califf RM, et al. Sertraline treatment of major depression in patients with acute MI or unstable angina. JAMA 2002;288:701–709.

48. Berkman LF, Blumenthal J, Burg M, et al., for the Enhancing Recovery in Coronary Heart Disease Patients Investigators (ENRICHD). Effects of treating depression and low perceived social support on clinical events after myocardial infarction: the Enhancing Recovery in Coronary Heart Disease Patients (ENRICHD) Randomised Trial. JAMA 2003:289:3106–3116.

49. Lespérance F, Frasure-Smith N. The seduction of death. Psychosom Med 1999;61:18–20.

50. Lane D, Carroll D, Ring C, et al. Predictors of attendance at cardiac rehabilitation after myocardial infarction. J Psychosom Res 2001;51:497–501.

51. Mayou R, Foster A, Williamson B. Psychosocial adjustment in patients one year after myocardial infarction. J Psychosom Res 1978;22:447–453.

52. Ziegelstein RC, Bush DE, Fauerbach JA. Depression, adherence behaviour, and coronary disease outcomes. Arch Intern Med 1998;158:808–809.

53. Albus C, Jordan J, Herrmann-Lingen C. Screening for psychosocial risk factors in patients with coronary heart disease: Recommendations for clinical practice. Eur J Cardiovasc Prev Rehabil 2004;11:75–79.

54. Beck AT, Ward CH, Mendelson M, et al. An inventory for measuring depression. Arch Gen Psychiatr 1961;4:561–571.

55. Zigmond AS, Snaith RP. The Hospital Anxiety and Depression Scale. Acta Psychiatr Scand 1983;67:361–370.

33
Educating Cardiac Patients and Relatives

Gunilla Burell

Please, Doctor, tell that to my wife!

Introduction

> PATIENT A: A post-MI male patient in his forties, as part of a cardiac rehabilitation program, participated in a stress management group for men. During a discussion of sexual issues the group leader presented a recently published report described in the newspaper under the heading "Sex is good for post-MI men." The patient's comment was immediate and intense: "Please, tell that to my wife! She is so damned scared."
>
> PATIENT B: A man in his fifties had attended a stress management group program after his MI. A few months after the program had ended, the participants of the group were invited for a follow-up session. By that time, this patient had to a large extent resumed his stressful lifestyle. Half-jokingly he told the group what his son kept saying: "Dad, you ought to go back to that stress doctor!"
>
> PATIENT C: A 60-year old woman still experienced angina after CABG surgery. This made it difficult for her to perform household work to the extent that she had been capable of previously. In a cardiac rehabilitation group setting she was offered advice concerning alternative ways of, in this case, cleaning the windows of her house. For instance, she was advised how she could best ask for help. She became very upset and offended by the idea, saying with tears in her eyes: "But I love window cleaning!"

> PATIENT D: The wife of a young post-MI patient was terrified by the wish of her husband to go sailing alone in his small boat. The patient was well recovered, and sailing had always been his great interest in vacation times. He was puzzled by his wife's reaction because she could not state a reason for her anxiety. However, the wife confided to a psychologist in the cardiac care unit that her fear came from a comment from a cardiologist. When the patient, her husband, was released from the ward after his acute event, the cardiologist told the wife: "One more MI like that, and he's dead." In her mind, sailing would kill him. She simply could not tell her husband this terrible verdict.

Which conclusions can be drawn from these clinical observations? One key message is that educating patients and spouses with the purpose of optimizing rehabilitation and secondary prevention is not just a matter of informing about facts. It is a process where professional caregivers must be sensitive to the social and emotional reality of the patient and spouse. Caregivers must also be very aware of the communicative interplay and the fact that both patient and spouse cognitions and interpretations may be very different from those of the professional. To health professionals, cardiological and surgical procedures are relatively routine aspects of their daily work. However, these procedures are not routine to the patient and his or her family – to them, it is a profoundly life-changing experience, and emotionally and spiritually a brush with death.

The first patient described above expressed a very common problem in the readjustment of cardiac patients. The research on sexual activities and satisfaction in CHD patients is scarce,[1] especially for female patients. Sexual activity is more common than previously estimated, even in relatively older patients. and can be an important contribution to a patient's quality of life. For instance, Addis et al.[2] report that in a sample of post-menopausal women with CHD (mean age 67 years), almost half of them were sexually active, although a majority experienced one of several sexual problems. Fear in the spouse can prevent resumption of joyful sexual activity. However, this issue is rarely discussed with patients and their spouses, despite the fact that erectile dysfunction is very common in male CHD patients.[1] The obstacle to discussion of sexual issues is usually not that of the patient.[3]

The situation of the stressed patient post-MI – the second case – entails at least two important observations. The first is related to the meaning of social support for successful rehabilitation. Spouses and family members of patients typically monitor carefully the patient's symptoms and behaviors. This can be of great value if the family member is actively included in the rehabilitation process.[4] The second observation from this case is that long-term maintenance of the new lifestyle is often difficult. Life is ever-changing, thus presenting threats and challenges to the patient's new healthy lifestyle. Therefore, cardiac rehabilitation and secondary prevention programs must contain strategies for long-term maintenance in the face of changing circumstances in life.

The woman who "loves window cleaning" is an illustration of the very different meaning that activities can have for patients and caregivers. An activity may seem trivial to the professional caregiver and the concerns may be responded to with simplistic advice for solutions. However, to the patient in this case, being able to clean her windows had the symbolic meaning of autonomy and self-esteem. Her reaction expressed her grief for the loss of so much that had been important and valuable to her. Professionals involved in cardiac rehabilitation need to refrain from giving premature advice in complex situations. Instead they need to listen carefully so that patients can reflect on the meaning and emotional significance of the problem they are addressing.

The wife who was terrified of her husband's sailing is an example of poor communication. The views of health professionals, particularly physicians, are extremely important for patients, especially in the vulnerable situation of cardiac care. Hence communication needs to be clear and realistic while also being supportive, and ongoing.

Overview of the Chapter

This chapter will focus on the role of spouses and family support in the rehabilitation of patients with coronary heart disease (CHD). It will describe some of the effects of CHD and its relationship to the rehabilitation process and review the importance of social support in the recovery, particularly how the interaction between patient and spouse may have an impact on rehabilitation outcomes. The chapter will be summarized in a set of brief recommendations.

Cardiac rehabilitation can be defined as the restoration of physical, psychological, and social functions after a cardiac event. The level of function may not be the same as before the event; however, optimal capacity and quality of life should be the goal. Secondary prevention can be defined as the development and practice of long-term strategies aiming at minimizing symptoms, preventing recurrence, and hopefully compressing morbidity and prolonging life. Such strategies entail healthy lifestyle, behavioral and emotional coping skills, stress management, problem solving, and adherence to medication. The involvement of spouse and family members in the rehabilitation has the potential of facilitating the process and improving the outcome.

Psychological Reactions to Coronary Heart Disease

A coronary event for most patients and their families is a traumatic experience with major consequences for daily life. Typically, to be diagnosed with CHD causes fears, anxiety, and depression,[5] and has implications for the dynamics within the family.[6] Research shows that prognosis may be more related to emotional factors than to the seriousness of the event. Outcome of rehabilitation is better predicted by emotional factors than by anatomical features and size of infarction. Thus, anxiety and depression may present major obstacles to successful rehabilitation and secondary prevention. A comprehensive cardiac rehabilitation program should allow a forum for patients to share experiences with other patients in similar situations. The opportunity to reflect on emotional reactions usually has a normalizing effect, reducing the uncertainties related to feelings that seem alien and strange. Patients learn that such previously unknown strong emotional reactions are normal in this stage, and that such negative emotions will not last forever. A sound "crisis intervention" can prevent many of these emotional obstacles to further rehabilitation from occurring. Often, the spouse experiences emotional reactions that are at least as strong as those of the patient.[5,6] However, he or she may be hesitant to express fears and concerns, in order not to "disturb" the patient. Thus, spouse reactions need to be directly addressed.

The Meaning of Social Support

Social support may have a direct effect on the course of cardiovascular disease.[7,8] There is evidence that socially isolated CHD patients are at significantly increased risk of recurrence.[9] The most important source of social support for a cardiac patient is the family, particularly his or her spouse. "Social network" refers to the number of people available to an individual for personal interaction, while "social support" refers to the quality and effects of interactions. Generally, research shows that for male patients, both social network and support is health-enhancing. For female CHD patients, on the other hand, a vast social network that entails many demands and duties may be a psychological burden, and lead to health hazards.[10] The reasonable interpretation of these data is that it is the non-directional ("just being there") positive quality of the support that contributes to health, and that this characteristic is sometimes lacking for women in traditional gender roles.[11]

Different forms of social support have been described, such as emotional, appraisal, informational, and instrumental support.[12] Research

shows that different forms of social support may have differential effects in terms of benefit for a CHD patient. For instance, "too much" instrumental support given by the spouse to the patient could create over-protectiveness and decrease the patient's self-efficacy and own initiatives in rehabilitation. A randomized intervention study by Berkhuysen et al.[13] showed that over-protectiveness by a spouse, as assessed by the patient, counteracted self-efficacy and thus decreased patients' confidence in their ability to make positive changes. Itkowitz et al.[14] showed that too much attention by the spouse to cardiac symptoms may contribute to negative outcomes of rehabilitation. Selective focus on the expression of CHD symptoms may unwittingly serve to reinforce emotional distress.

Two conclusions can be drawn from the above. First, positive social support is important for the prognosis of CHD patients. This entails emotional (understanding and acceptance of feelings), appraisal (good advice and opportunity to discuss how to manage the new life situation), informational (knowledge about CHD, risk factors, and lifestyle), and instrumental (help with practical problems). All of these aspects should be included in comprehensive cardiac rehabilitation and secondary prevention. Second, in order for spouses and family members to be able to provide adequate social support, they themselves need social support. There is evidence that when spouses exhibit higher levels of anxiety and depression and lower sense of control than the patient, the patient's psychosocial adjustment to illness is adversely affected.[6] It is a good investment to offer some structured support to spouses and family members of CHD patients. There are at least three reasons for this. First, family members are deeply affected by the cardiac event or intervention, and family dynamics and roles may change considerably. Those reactions need to be dealt with because of the risk that they would otherwise impact negatively with treatment and rehabilitation efforts. Second, spouses and family members need information and knowledge about the management of the disease, so as to understand what will happen to the patient. Third, CHD families may need instrumental support and help to deal with social and financial consequences of illness. A support program for spouses and family members has the potential to aid recovery and rehabilitation considerably.[14]

Clinical experience indicates that interventions with spouses do not need to be very extensive in most cases. Adequate information, opportunities to ask questions and reflect on emotional reactions, and sharing experiences with other spouses and family members on a few occasions in group counseling can be a very cost-effective use of time. Trained and experienced cardiac nurses are well suited to conduct such support groups. In our experience, both groups for spouses only and groups for patients and spouses together are very much appreciated by the participants.

Information Is Not the Whole Solution

In order to obtain effects on prognosis and manifestations of the disease, cardiac rehabilitation (CR) and lifestyle programs must achieve real and concrete behavior change (diet, exercise, coping with stress, and adherence to medication). Traditionally, in health promotion programs, too much emphasis has been put on information – it is assumed that if patients *know* what is right to do, they will do it. Behavioral science evidence, in combination with conclusions from many lifestyle interventions, shows that this is rarely the case. Those who are very well informed, nonetheless, could behave in self-destructive ways. Thus, CR and lifestyle interventions should not rely on information transmission only. Rather, one could argue that information works best when the individual has already been supported to change behavior. Gradually adopting a new behavior leads to change of attitudes, and to the awareness that relevant information and knowledge is needed to assist and support the change process. The patient will then seek and integrate information that he or she sees as personally relevant – thus teaching becomes true learning. The effects of information will be much more potent when it is linked to a behavioral intervention, where information and behavior change mutually reinforce each other. Thus, effective CR and lifestyle programs must be built on knowledge in the CR team about behavioral science and the dynamics of behavior change.

Who Should Be Referred?

Resources for cardiac rehabilitation and patient education may be limited, depending on local circumstances. It may also be the case that not all CHD patients are equally in need of intensive professional support. It is therefore of clinical importance to screen patients with respect to risk factors for prognosis. Screening for physiological and medical risk factors is covered elsewhere in this book. In the context of patient education, screening for psychological and psychosocial risk factors are very relevant.

Numerous studies consistently show that psychological and psychosocial factors contribute to increased risk for CHD. A cluster of negative emotions are related to increased risk, such as depression, anxiety, hostility, type D personality. Among psychosocial risk factors are low socioeconomic status (SES) and social isolation. These have been described in detail in Chapter 30. When CHD has manifested itself, the risk factor pattern is more complex, and findings are less consistent. However, the overall conclusions from studies point to hostility, depression, low SES, and social isolation contributing to increased risk for recurrence. Depression in particular has received considerable attention in recent studies.[15] These issues are discussed in other chapters, particularly depression (Chapter 32) and stress management (Chapter 34). Research has shown that such psychological risks are more prevalent among women. Since they are also generally older, the presence of social isolation and concomitant illness is more likely. For instance, more older women will be widowed or for other reasons without an intimate other to support them in their rehabilitation.

Ades et al.[16] showed that older women were less likely to enter cardiac rehabilitation than were older men. This was explained primarily by a greater likelihood of primary physicians to strongly recommend cardiac rehabilitation to men, but older women were also more likely to report having dependents than were older men. Thus these women in need of healthcare to maximize their own health and recovery were also more likely than men to also have the "burden" of caring for someone else with healthcare needs. These US findings have also been found in a

Swedish study – caring for a dependent husband often made it difficult for female patients to attend rehabilitation programs.[11] Once in CR programs, both groups improved aerobic capacity similarly. Thus, older female coronary patients are less likely to be referred for cardiac rehabilitation, despite a similar clinical profile and improvement in functional capacity from the training component. Similar results have been obtained in other studies; for instance Grace et al.,[17] reported that in a prospective study of CR referral and participation patterns, only 30% of participants were referred, with significantly fewer women being referred. Thus, female gender is a marker of increased risk for psychological ill-being and worse prognosis. Studies show that referral to CR by the cardiologist is one of the strongest predictors of actual participation in a CR program. The clinic may very well have adopted procedures where different professionals can refer to CR, such as cardiac nurses or physiotherapists. However, it is very important to make it clear to the patient that the physician is actively promoting his or her participation in the program.

To conclude, patients should be screened for negative emotions and psychosocial profiles known to be associated with poorer outcomes, since such factors could create obstacles to participation and benefit from cardiac rehabilitation and education. Social isolation means a lack of social support in difficult times for a cardiac patient. Patients with a psychosocially vulnerable profile need more active support interventions. The presence of a spouse or other close family member can be a particularly important asset. In order for them to contribute positively to the rehabilitation of the cardiac patient, they in turn need information and emotional support. Thus, some "diagnosis" of the spouse interaction is a valuable source of information for involving spouses.

Recommendations

Family Support

Spouse and family support can be offered in a group format in cardiac rehabilitation programs. One option is to offer educational courses for patients and spouses together, with different professionals participating in sessions as appropriate (e.g. cardiologist, nurse, physiotherapist, psychologist). These courses consist of 6–8 sessions and give opportunities for questions and discussions on topics like diet, exercise, stress, emotional reactions, etc. Another option is group meetings for spouses only; typically with 6–7 participants over 6–10 sessions. These groups focus more on the spouses' own reactions and adjustment. Such groups are *not* psychotherapy but more like self-help groups. In some countries, non-governmental organizations (NGOs) for patients exist which are very active and often have a high profile. Typically, such organizations offer educational and social activities which are available to members. Thus, they give opportunities for long-term social support and maintenance of lifestyle changes in a way that clinics cannot do. Active cooperation between cardiac rehabilitation personnel and such organizations is strongly recommended as a way to provide for the wider needs of patients and their families.

Communication

Traditionally, healthcare professionals have adopted a fairly authoritarian style of "providing" information *and* giving structured advice. However, adherence to lifestyle prescription is discouragingly low (see Chapter 35 on levels of non-adherence to professional advice).

Patients who need to change lifestyle go through a series of motivational stages,[18] and may be in the ambivalent stage and not yet ready to make the decision to change. Premature advice given in this situation may create opposition. To conclude: first, *ask questions*, do not give advice unless the patient asks for it; second, assess the patient's *motivational readiness* for change. Development of motivation may very well be the first change target, including the readiness to open up communication with spouse and family and allowing them to be involved.

Teamwork

Education, behavior change, and recovery from a serious medical condition takes time. Comprehensive CR programs need to offer frequent sessions over an extended period of time. In most clinical situations, it is not feasible that the physician is the one who conducts such group interventions. However, teamwork is well established in work with cardiac patients. Cardiac nurses, physiotherapists, dieticians, psychologists, social workers, etc. are very suitable to conduct this type of extended program. From our own and others' clinical experience with education and training of personnel, I would like to emphasize three criteria for the selection of staff for this work. The first requirement is considerable experience with cardiac patients, in order to have insight into and empathy with the realities of cardiac disease. The second is a reasonable degree of personal maturity, in order to maintain professional integrity and stability when dealing with profoundly emotional and spiritual issues. The third is special education, training, and supervision in the work. It is not something "anyone can just do." It is not lecturing. Helping people change is a specialist undertaking. It takes expertise to recognize, understand, and work with behavioral and emotional dynamics in other people. Doing it the wrong way can prove fatal.[19]

Back to Our Patients' Needs

PATIENT A: There are several fairly simple remedies for the first man. It helps for him to share experiences and concerns with the other men in his stress management group. Further, to reduce some anxiety in his wife, she can be offered an opportunity to express her thoughts, either in a group of spouses or in consultation with a cardiac nurse. The cardiologist or nurse may also meet with the two of them together. Some reassuring facts can be provided, but advice giving is not necessary. The therapeutic effect comes from the opportunity to express emotions and concerns.

PATIENT B: For stress management interventions, and other rehabilitation programs, follow-up "booster sessions" are a very good and cost-effective investment. With the basic program accomplished, the patient has a very good basis for maintenance even with only a few follow-up reminders. It is also highly recommended to offer family members a couple of occasions during the program to be informed about the contents of processes in the patient's

rehabilitation. This gives a much better understanding of how the family can support progress.

PATIENT C: The women who was grieving her window-cleaning needed to be listened to by a professional person who understands how to look and listen under and beyond the surface. Again, no psychotherapy sessions are needed for this, just an awareness that often listening with patience and refraining from advice is the best therapy for troubled emotions.

PATIENT D: The wife of the sailing husband needed more adequate information. A study by Moser et al.[6] found that patients and spouses after an acute MI identified information as the most important need; however, information requests were not well met by physicians and nurses. A number of studies have identified information needs such as symptom management, risk factors, pathophysiology, diet, medication, etc.[20] Since information needs vary with the course of recovery, the professional person providing the information must be sensitive to what is most relevant to the particular patient and spouse on that particular occasion. The best and easiest strategy is to just ask "what is it that you need to know?".

To conclude, for professional caregivers, too, education certainly has its place. It should be noted, though, that in most cases what is needed is not psychotherapy expertise in any traditional sense. The key issue is to understand behavioral dynamics and motivational processes, and to apply one's own communication skills. This will provide the best possible atmosphere for cardiac patients and their spouses to develop empowerment and optimism about the future.

References

1. Kloner RA, Mullin SH, Shook T, et al. Erectile dysfunction in the cardiac patient: how common and should we treat? J Urol 2003;170:2.
2. Addis IB, Ireland CC, Vittinghof E, Lin F, Stuenkel CA, Hulley S. Sexual activity and function in postmenopausal women with heart disease. Obstet Gynecol 2005;106(1):121–122.
3. Bedell SE, Duperval M, Goldberg R. Cardiologists' discussions about sexuality with patients with chronic artery disease. Am Heart J 2002;144:2.

4. Kärner A, Abrandt Dahlgren M, Bergdahl B. Rehabilitation after coronary heart disease: spouses' views of support. J Adv Nurs 2004;46(2):204–211.

5. Lukkarinen H, Kyngäs H. Experiences of the onset of coronary artery disease in a spouse. Eur J Cardiovasc Nurs 2003;2:189–194.

6. Moser DK, Dracup K. Role of spousal anxiety and depression in patients' psychosocial recovery after a cardiac event. Psychosom Med 2004;66:527–532.

7. Baker B, Szalai JP, Paquette M, Tobe S. Marital support, spousal contact and the course of mild hypertension. J Psychosom Res 2003;55:229–233.

8. Tsouna-Hadjis E, Vemmos KN, Zakapoulos N, Stamatelopoulos S. First-stroke recovery process: the role of family support. Arch Phys Med Rehabil 2000;81:881–887.

9. Berkman LF, Leo-Summers L, Horwitz RI. Emotional support and survival after myocardial infarction. A prospective, population-based study of the elderly. Ann Intern Med 1992;117:1003–1009.

10. Burell G, Granlund B. Women's hearts need special treatment. J Behav Med 2002;9:228–242.

11. Orth-Gomer K, Wamala SP, Horsten M, Schenck-Gustafsson K, Schneiderman N, Mittleman MA. Marital stress worsens prognosis in women with coronary heart disease. The Stockholm Female Coronary Risk Study. JAMA 2000;284:3008–3014.

12. Kristofferzon ML, Löfmark R, Carlsson M. Myocardial infarction: gender differences in coping and social support. J Adv Nurs 2003;44:360–374.

13. Berkhuysen MA, Nieuwland W, Buunk BP, Sanderman R, Rispens P. Change in self-efficacy during cardiac rehabilitation and the role of perceived overprotectiveness. Patient Educ Couns 1999;38:21–32.

14. Itkowitz NI, Kerns RD, Otis JD. Support and coronary heart disease: the importance of significant other responses. J Behav Med 2003;26:19–30.

15. Frasure-Smith N, Lespérance F, Talajic M. Depression following myocardial infarction: impact on 6-month survival. JAMA 1993;270:1819–1825.

16. Ades PA, Waldmann ML, Polk DM, Coflesky JT. Referral patterns and exercise response in the rehabilitation of female coronary patients aged greater than or equal to 62 years. Am J Cardiol 1992:69:1422–1425.

17. Grace SL, Abbey SE, Shnek ZM, Irvine J, France RL, Stewart DE. Cardiac rehabilitation II: referral and participation. Gen Hosp Psychiatr 2002;24:127–134.

18. Miller WR, Rollnick S. Motivational Interviewing. New York: Guilford Press; 1991.

19. Cossette S, Frasure-Smith N, Lesperance F. Clinical implications of a reduction in psychological distress on cardiac prognosis in patients participating in a psychosocial intervention program. Psychosom Med 2001;63:257–266.

20. Stewart DE, Abbey SE, Shnek ZM, Irvine J, Grace SL. Gender differences in health information needs and decisional preferences in patients recovering from an acute ischemic coronary event. Psychosom Med 2004;66:42–48.

34
Stress Management

Paul Bennett

What Is Stress?

Early models of stress considered it to arise from our environment, and to impact on us all equally. Holmes and Rahe[1] established a hierarchy of severity for various stressors. They also attempted to provide a link between stress and health, suggesting that the more stressful life events an individual experiences, the more their risk of ill-health. Unfortunately, this hypothesis was rarely substantiated. What has emerged from subsequent research is that the impact of potentially stressful events is mediated by our psychological responses to those events. The meaning attributed to events, and the coping responses we use, profoundly influence our emotional and behavioral responses to them. Accordingly, more recent models of stress consider stress to have a number of components: a cognitive response ("I am worried I won't cope with this problem"), a physiological component usually involving increased autonomic arousal, a behavioral element involving more or less useful coping responses, and an emotional experience involving a variety of negative emotional states such as anger or anxiety (Figure 34-1).

Clinicians such as Beck[2] argued that feelings of stress or distress are a consequence of "faulty" or "irrational" thinking. That is, they considered stress to be the result of negative misinterpretations of environmental events. Such thoughts have been referred to as automatic negative assumptions. These form the individual's first response to a particular situation and are without logic or grounding in reality. Beck

identified a number of categories of such thoughts, including:

- Catastrophic thinking: considering an event as completely negative, and potentially disastrous: "That's it – I've had a heart attack . . . I'm bound to lose my job, and I won't be able to pay the mortgage."
- Over-generalization: drawing a general (negative) conclusion on the basis of a single incident: "That's it – my angina stopped me going to the cinema – that's something else I can't do . . ."
- Arbitrary inference: drawing a conclusion without sufficient evidence to support it: "The pain must mean my condition is getting worse . . . I just know it."
- Selective abstraction: focusing on a detail taken out of context: "OK, I know I was able to cope with going out, but I was worried about my angina, and I know that will stop me going out in future . . ."

Of course, some events may be inherently "stressful" and a negative cognitive response may be accurate – something which may have significant implications for any intervention aimed at reducing stress.

The Impact of Stress Management

In terms of summarizing a large body of evidence, a recent Cochrane review[3] reported that stress management procedures are effective in reducing distress. Other goals may be to improve the rehabilitation process, improve health, and/or prevent

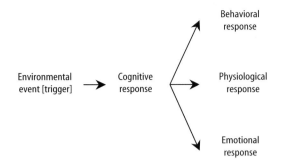

FIGURE 34-1. A simplified representation of the event–stress process.

disease progression. Unfortunately, from a scientific perspective, many stress management interventions are combined with other interventions such as exercise programs, making it difficult to isolate a specific therapeutic effect of the stress management. Nevertheless, the relatively small number of studies that have used stress management in isolation suggest a beneficial impact on these other goals. For instance, a meta-analysis of 27 trials of relaxation therapy in the rehabilitation of cardiac patients found that intensive supervised relaxation practice contributed to many secondary prevention outcomes – psychological, vocational, physiological, and clinical.[4]

Reducing Symptoms

Angina may be triggered by emotional as well as physical stresses. Accordingly, several studies have explored the potential benefits of stress management procedures in people with angina. One of the first studies[5] found that patients who participated in a stress management program reported reductions in the frequency of angina symptoms, were less reliant on medication, and tolerated higher levels of exercise on a treadmill than those in a usual treatment control group. A larger study, involving a very large sample,[6] compared a less intensive intervention involving a stress management program delivered in booklet form combined with three group meetings. At 6-month follow-up, compared to a no treatment control group, participants reported a significant reduction in stress-, but not exercise-related, angina.

Preventing Reinfarction

The largest study involving the use of stress management in post-MI patients[7] targeted type A men (i.e. those who scored highly on measures such as time urgency, competitiveness, hostility, and easily aroused anger: a form of "self-stress") who had experienced a recent MI. Over a 4-year intervention, participants in the type A management program were at half the risk for further infarction than those in a similarly long, but traditionally focused, rehabilitation program, with total infarction rates over the 4.5-year study of 6% and 12% in the groups, respectively.

Other studies have shown positive gains following shorter and more general stress management interventions. Blumenthal and colleagues,[8] for example, assigned patients to a 4-month program of exercise or stress management training or usual treatment control. Participants in the stress management group were significantly less likely to have a cardiac event over the follow-up period than participants in either other condition. Appels and colleagues[9] used a simpler intervention program involving a relaxation and controlled breathing program following angioplasty. This resulted in a 50% lower risk of further intervention or a new coronary event than that of participants in a no treatment group in the following 18 months.

Although the evidence is not always strong, there is a general consensus that depression may increase risk for infarction or reinfarction.[10] Such a relationship suggests that interventions that reduce depression should reduce risk of reinfarction. Evidence in support of this hypothesis, however, is still lacking. In one of the first studies to examine this issue, Black et al.[11] found lower use of hospital services in the year following MI among patients offered cognitive behavior therapy to help reduce their distress than among those in a usual care control group. Whether this difference was a consequence of physiological or psychological changes such as less anxiety over cardiac symptoms is not clear. Evidence from the largest study conducted in this area[12] proved more disappointing. The ENRICHD study included 2481 patients and provided an intervention for up to one year for people identified as depressed immediately following an MI. All participants in the active intervention arm received two or three treatment components: group cognitive behavior therapy, provision of social support, and, if necessary, antidepressant medication. A comparison group received usual care. Although the intervention appeared to lower levels of depression more than reductions achieved in the usual care condition, there were no differences in survival between the two groups in the 2 years following infarction. More detailed discussion of depression and cardiovascular events is considered in Chapter 32.

Stress Management Training

Strategies to help people cope with stress are many and varied. Some may be as simple as the provision of reassuring information. Others require a more complex technology. This chapter will focus specifically on strategies that fall within the rubric of "stress management training." The approach is based on the model of stress described above and aims to:

- Change environmental triggers to the stress response.
- Change inappropriate behavioral, physiological, or cognitive responses that occur in response to this event.
- These goals may be achieved through a variety of strategies:
- High levels of muscular tension can be reduced through relaxation techniques.
- Triggers can be identified and modified using problem-solving strategies.
- Cognitive distortions can be identified and changed through a number of cognitive techniques such as cognitive restructuring:
- "Stressed" behaviors can be changed through consideration and rehearsal of alternative behavioral responses.

Many stress management programs simply teach relaxation techniques to minimize the high levels of arousal associated with stress. More complex interventions try to change cognitive (and therefore emotional) reactions to environmental triggers. Few address the factors that initiate the stress response. Given the idiosyncratic nature of both the stressors individuals may

experience and the complexity of changing their cognitive response to them, interventions that address these factors are often led by specialists in stress management, and may best be targeted at individuals who are experiencing significant levels of stress. By contrast, relaxation techniques are relatively easy to teach and incorporate into "real life," and may benefit most cardiac patients. As a consequence, they can be taught by non-specialists, and may usefully be integrated into the core syllabus of any group rehabilitation program.

Teaching Relaxation Skills

The goal of teaching relaxation skills is to enable patients to relax as much as is possible and appropriate both throughout the day and at times of particular stress. This contrasts with procedures such as meditation, which provide a period of deep relaxation and "time out" as sufficient in themselves. Relaxation skills are best learned through three phases:

- learning basic relaxation skills
- monitoring tension in daily life
- using relaxation at times of stress.

The first stage involves practice under optimal conditions such as a quiet room in a comfortable chair – where there are no distractions and it is relatively easy to relax. Initially, a trained practitioner should lead the individual through the process of deep relaxation. This is augmented by continued practice at home, typically using taped instructions. The relaxation process most commonly taught involves alternately tensing and relaxing muscle groups throughout the body in an ordered sequence. As the individual becomes more skilled, the emphasis of practice shifts towards relaxation without prior tension, or relaxing specific muscle groups whilst using others, in order to mimic the circumstances in which relaxation will be used in "real life." The order in which the muscles are relaxed varies, but a typical exercise may involve the following stages (the tensing procedure is described in brackets):

- hands and forearms (making a fist)
- upper arms (touching fingers to shoulder)

- shoulders and lower neck (pulling up shoulders)
- back of neck (touching chin to chest)
- lips (pushing them together)
- forehead (frowning)
- abdomen/chest (holding deep breath)
- abdomen (tensing stomach muscles)
- legs and feet (push heel away, pull toes to point at head: not lifting leg).

At the same time as practicing relaxation skills, individuals can monitor their levels of physical tension throughout the day using a diary to record their level of tension on some form of numerical scale (0 = no tension, 100 = the highest tension possible) at regular intervals through the day or at times of particular stress. This helps teach people how and when they become tense, and acts as a baseline against which to assess their progress when learning relaxation. As a prelude to the cognitive or behavioral interventions considered below, diaries may also focus on the thoughts, emotions, or behaviors experienced at times of stress (Table 34-1).

After learning relaxation techniques and monitoring tension, individuals can begin to integrate relaxation into their daily lives. At this time, relaxation involves monitoring and reducing tension to appropriate levels while engaging in everyday activities. Initially this may involve trying to keep as relaxed as possible at times of relatively low stress and then, as the individual becomes more skilled, implementing relaxation at times of increasing stress. An alternative strategy involves relaxing at regular intervals (such as coffee breaks) throughout the day.

Changing Triggers

The triggers to each person's stress necessarily differ, as will any strategies used to cope with them. Nevertheless, clinicians such as Egan[13] have developed a relatively simple set of procedures for both identifying and changing stress triggers. It involves a three-phase process as outlined in the following sections:

- Problem exploration and clarification: what are the triggers to stress?
- Goal setting: which triggers does the individual want to change?
- Facilitating action: how do they set about changing the triggers to stress?

Problem Exploration and Clarification

The goal of this stage is to help an individual identify the problems he or she is facing that are contributing to the stress. Some of these may be immediately obvious; some require a more detailed exploration. However, detailed and careful work here prevents errors and failed attempts to resolve inappropriate issues subsequently. A number of techniques were identified to elicit relevant information at this stage. The most obvious method is to ask direct questions, which should be open-ended to discourage one-word answers. Requests for information may also take the form of prompts ("Tell me about . . ."). It is important to mix direct questioning with other strategies, including the use of silence or minimal prompts ("uh-huh") or empathic feedback, in

TABLE 34-1. Excerpt from a stress diary noting stress triggers, levels of tension, and related behaviors and thoughts

Time	Situation	Tension level	Behaviors	Thoughts
8.32	Driving to work – late!	62	Tense – gripping steering wheel Cursing at traffic lights	Late again!! . . . the boss is bound to notice . . . – Come on – hurry up – I haven't got all day! Why do these bloody traffic lights always take so long to change?!
10.00	Couldn't catch my breath while exercising	100	Got agitated Phoned home and said thought I was having a heart attack	Oh no . . . I'm havinganother heart attack . . . is this the time I die? My chest hurts just like last time . . .

which the health professional reflects back their understanding of the situation reported by the patient: "So, you find it scary when you are away from people who know about your heart condition, in case you experience problems . . .". Such feedback also shows that the health professional understands the situation and facilitates rapport with the patient.

Goal Setting

Once problems have been identified, some people may have the resources to deal with them and need no further help in making appropriate changes. Others, however, may need support in determining what they want to change and how to change it. The first stage in this process is to help them decide the goals they wish to achieve, and to frame their goals in specific rather than general terms ("I will walk for 20 minutes a day" versus "I will try to exercise more"). If any goal seems too difficult to achieve in one step, the elaboration of sub-goals should be encouraged. Some goals may be apparent following the problem exploration phase. However, should this not be the case, a series of strategies has been designed to help the patient identify and set them. Of critical importance is that the individual is invited to explore their own new perspectives – to think about new ways of doing things. Advice giving, however well phrased ("Well, why don't you take some time out each day to relax?"), is likely to result in resistance to change or feelings of defeat.

Facilitating Action

Having identified what they want to change, some people may remain unsure of how to achieve their goals. Accordingly, the final stage of this element of stress management is to plan ways of achieving the identified goals. Stress may have multiple sources, and some areas of stress may be easier to change than others. It can be helpful to work towards relatively easy goals at the beginning of any attempt at change, before working towards more serious or difficult to change goals as the individual gains skills or confidence in their ability to change.[13]

Cognitive Interventions

Two strategies for changing cognitions that contribute to stress are frequently employed. The simplest, known as self-instruction training, was developed by Meichenbaum[14] and is intended to interrupt the flow of stress-provoking thoughts by replacing them with pre-rehearsed stress reducing or "coping" thoughts. These can be considered as three categories:

- Reminders to use any stress coping techniques the person has learned ("You're winding yourself up here – take it easy, remember to relax . . . deep breathe, relax . . .").
- Reassurance, reminding the individual that they can cope effectively with their feelings of distress ("Come on you've dealt with this before – you should be able to again – keep calm – things will not get out of control.").
- Reducing the stress inherent in the situation ("OK . . . this feels bad, but you've had this feeling before . . . it doesn't mean you are having another heart attack . . . you've just been trying too hard. Relax and the feelings will go like last time.").

To ensure relevance to the individual, and to help them to evoke these thoughts at times of stress, Meichenbaum suggested that particular coping thoughts should be thought through and rehearsed, wherever possible, before the stressful events occur – whether in a therapy session or minutes before a known stressor is likely to occur.

A more complex intervention, known as cognitive restructuring, involves identifying and challenging the accuracy of stress-engendering thoughts.[14] It asks the individual to consider them as hypotheses, not facts, and to assess their validity without bias. The best way of challenging stressogenic thoughts may initially be taught within therapy sessions. In this, the health professional uses a process known as the Socratic method or "guided discovery"[2] to help patients identify distorted patterns of thinking that are contributing to their feelings of stress. Then, the health professional encourages the individual to consider and evaluate different sources of information that provide evidence of the reality or otherwise of the beliefs they hold. Patients may challenge their stressful assumptions by asking key questions such as:

- What evidence is there that supports or refutes my assumption?
- Are there any other ways I can think about this situation?
- Could I be making a mistake in the way I am thinking?

Once individuals can engage in this process within the therapy session, they are encouraged to use the Socratic process at times when they feel hooked into feelings of stress – to question the basis of those feelings. The following excerpt from a dialogue between a nurse and a patient who has had an MI shows the basics of the Socratic dialogue at work:

Tom: Well, that's it . . . I've had a heart attack . . . that's my health ruined now . . . and I know I'll lose my job now. Bound to . . . and what's going to happen about money. Wow, we are in a real mess now . . .

Nurse: Those are big worries to have . . . Tell me, why do you think you'll lose your job?

Tom: Well, most people do when they've had a heart attack I guess . . . Why should I be different?

Nurse: Some people do – but most don't lose their job. Having a heart attack does not necessarily disable you and stop you working . . . What sort of job do you have?

Tom: I'm a manager in a large manufacturing company.

Nurse: I imagine in a large company like that, many people must have serious illnesses at some time or other. How does the company treat them? Do you know?

Tom: Not bad actually. Most people do OK.

Nurse: Do they get made redundant?

Tom: In some ways that would be crazy, if they are a good worker and can still work, the company would keep them on.

Nurse: So as far as you know, the company tries to keep people on even if they are ill.

Tom: Well, yes, I suppose so . . . But I've had a heart attack . . . that has to be more serious than most things . . .

Nurse: Not necessarily at all . . . Most people go on to recover well from their heart attack. The heart can recover just like any other part of the body. And if you look after yourself you could be as fit if not fitter than you are now.

Tom: So there's no real need for the company to have a problem with me?

Nurse: Not really.

Tom: So, things might not be that bad after all . . . wow, I feel better after thinking that through.

Here Tom is encouraged to rethink some of the assumptions he has made and not simply to accept them as true. In addition, by giving some relevant information the health professional has aided his restructuring and encouraged him to reconsider his situation.

Behavioral Interventions

The goal of behavioral change is to help the individual respond to any stress triggers in ways that maximize their effectiveness in dealing with the trigger, and causes them minimal stress. Some behaviors can be relatively simple. Behaviors that reduce the stress of driving may involve, for example, driving within the speed limits, putting the handbrake on when stopped at traffic lights and taking time to relax, not cutting people up, and so on. Others may take practice – a person who becomes excessively angry, for example, may role play assertive responses within therapy sessions to prepare them for doing the same in "real life." Still others have to be thought through at the time of the stress. Here, the goal of stress management training may be to teach the individual to plan their response to any potential stressor to be one that minimizes their personal stress. A simple rule of thumb that can be useful here is to encourage individuals to stop and plan what they are going to do – even if this takes a few seconds – rather than to jump into action without thought, as this typically leads to more rather than less stress.

Putting It All Together

The various strands of cognitive therapy described above could be combined into a simple iterative learning process in one of two ways.[14]

Firstly, when an individual is facing a stressor, they need to keep three processes under review:

- check that their behavior is appropriate to the circumstances
- maintain relaxation
- give themselves appropriate self-talk.

In addition, where a particular stressor can be anticipated, the opportunity should be taken to rehearse these actions before the event itself. Once in the situation, the planned strategies should be enacted. Finally, after the situation has occurred, time should be given to review what occurred and successes or failures learned from – rather than treated as disasters that should be forgotten.

Conclusions

Strategies to cope with stress are many and varied. Some may be as simple as the provision of reassuring information. Others require a more complex technology. This chapter has considered strategies that fall within the rubric of "stress management" training. Basic interventions and, in particular, relaxation can be taught by most healthcare professionals – and are frequently taught in a group context. The core elements of the problem-focused approach or cognitive interventions can be taught to individuals or groups of cardiac patients by professionals familiar with the issues. Indeed, the basic strategies of the problem-focused approach may be key to successful rehabilitation, as patients may benefit from thinking through not just how they can manage their stress but how they implement some of the broad issues of risk behavior change or disease management in their own lives. However, where an individual is reporting high levels of stress of distress, these (and other) strategies may best be implemented by more specialist health professionals with a background in mental as well as physical health problems.

References

1. Holmes TH, Rahe RH. The Social Readjustment Rating Scale. J Psychosom Res 1967;11:213–218.
2. Beck A. Cognitive Therapy of Depression. New York: Guilford Press; 1977.
3. Rees K, Bennett P, Vedhara K, West R, Davey Smith G, Ibrahim S. Stress Management for Coronary Heart Disease. The Cochrane Library, Issue 2. Chichester: John Wiley & Sons; 2004.
4. Van Dixhoorn J, White A. Relaxation therapy for rehabilitation and prevention in ischaemic heart disease: a systematic review and meta-analysis. Eur J Cardiovasc Prev Rehabil 2005;12:193–202.
5. Bundy C, Carroll D, Wallace L, Nagle R. Psychological treatment of chronic stable angina pectoris. Psychol Health 1994;10:69–77.
6. Gallacher JEJ, Hopkinson CA, Bennett P, Burr ML, Elwood PC. Effect of stress management on angina. Psychol Health 1977;12:523–532.
7. Friedman M, Thoresen CE, Gill JJ, et al. Alteration of Type A behavior and its effect on cardiac recurrences in post myocardial infarction patients: summary results of the Recurrent Coronary Prevention Project. Am Heart J 1986;112:653–665.
8. Blumenthal JA, Jiang W, Babyak MA, Williams, DE, Rummans, TA, Gau GT. Stress management and exercise training in cardiac patients with myocardial ischemia. Arch Intern Med 1997;157:2213–2217.
9. Appels A, Bar F, Lasker J, Flamm U, Kop W. The effect of a psychological intervention program on the risk of a new coronary event after angioplasty: A feasibility study. J Psychosom Med 1997;43:209–217.
10. Sorensen C, Friis-Hasche E, Haghfelt T, Bech P. Post-myocardial infarction mortality in relation to depression: a systematic critical review. Psychother Psychosom 2005;74:69–80.
11. Black JL, Allison TG, Williams DE, Rummans TA, Gau GT. Effect of intervention for psychological distress on rehospitalization rates in cardiac rehabilitation patients. Psychosom 1998;39:134–143.
12. Berkman LF, Blumenthal J, Burg M, et al. Effects of treating depression and low perceived social support on clinical events after myocardial infarction: the Enhancing Recovery in Coronary Heart Disease Patients (ENRICHD) Randomized Trial. JAMA 2003;289:3106–3116.
13. Egan G. The Skilled Helper: A Problem-Management and Opportunity-Development Approach to Helping. Pacific Grove, CA: Brooks/Cole; 2002.
14. Meichenbaum D. Stress Inoculation Training. New York: Pergamon; 1985.

35
Adherence to Health Recommendations

David Hevey

Introduction and Definitions

The WHO[1] defines adherence as "the extent to which a person's behaviour – taking medication, following a diet, and/or executing lifestyle changes, corresponds with agreed recommendations from a health care provider" (p. 3). There are numerous ways in which behavior may not correspond with recommendations: non-adherence comprises behaviors such as not commencing performance of a recommended behavior (e.g. not exercising), cessation of a behavior too soon (e.g. stopping medication prematurely), not performing enough of the behavior (e.g. taking insufficient exercise to gain a benefit), and inconsistently performing the behavior (e.g. taking some medications some of the time). A distinction is made between intentional and unintentional non-adherent behaviors. Unintentional non-adherence arises from not knowing the treatment regimen, forgetting to perform the behavior, misunderstanding the treatment regimen, dementia or cognitive impairment, stress, or psychological disturbance. In contrast, intentional non-adherence arises from a deliberate decision, which may be based on perceptions of symptom reduction, fear of side-effects, fear of addiction, or perceived inefficiency of treatment.

Adherence in the Cardiac Context

Coronary heart disease (CHD) is a complex multifactorial disease and successful management places a variety of demands on the patient. The explicit goals of cardiac rehabilitation (CR) are to enhance secondary prevention and to improve health-related quality of life. In order to achieve these goals, patients are typically presented with a variety of recommendations, including:

1. Take medication.
2. Follow dietary recommendations.
3. Quit smoking.
4. Perform regular exercise.
5. Manage stress.
6. Change work practices.

Extent of the Problem of Non-Adherence

It has been estimated that 20–80% of patients do not adhere to the basic requirements of a medical regimen[2]; however, it is important to note that adherence rates vary across regimen, setting, and populations, with the highest levels of non-adherence reported for preventive regimens in asymptomatic patients. Adherence to long-term therapy for chronic illnesses in developed countries averages 50%,[1] and similar adherence rates have been reported in CHD patients.

Cardiac rehabilitation delivers secondary prevention for cardiovascular patients and promotes patient adherence. It is acknowledged that the major changes required of many patients are difficult to do on the basis of professional advice only. Cardiac rehabilitation is, effectively, a sophisticated adherence-promotion program using many techniques proven to promote and maintain behavior change in terms of promoting health and it has a beneficial effect on mortality, morbidity, and quality of life. However, despite these proven benefits, many eligible patients fail to attend: among those offered CR, the reported uptake rates range from 15% to 50%.[3] An evaluation of lifestyle changes among CHD patients in five European countries found that approximately 50% of patients changed lifestyles in accordance with recommendations.[4] Similarly, there is evidence that only 50% of patients adhere to cardiac medication (e.g. statins, ACE inhibitors) 1 year after commencing treatment, and of those taking the drug, approximately 50% follow the treatment sufficiently to gain a therapeutic benefit.[5] To date the majority of research on adherence among cardiac patients has focused on exercise adherence.[6] There is less evidence regarding adherence to other behavioral recommendations of CR.

Consequences of Non-Adherence

Across illnesses, adherence is the single most important modifiable factor that compromises therapeutic outcome. The most efficacious treatment is made ineffective if the patient fails to adhere to it. Irrespective of whether non-adherence is intentional or non-intentional, it has substantial health and societal costs in terms of increased morbidity, mortality, and economic costs. A recent meta-analysis reported a 50% increase in the risk of adverse outcomes in non-adherent CHD patients.[7] For example, in comparison to hypertensive patients who adhere, non-adherent hypertensive patients are four times more likely to be hospitalized or to die from CHD.[8] In addition, the economic costs of non-adherence in the United States are considerable; a decade ago, it was estimated that medication non-adherence required $25 billion to pay for additional treatment and hospital admissions, and lost productivity due to non-adherence was estimated at $100 billion.[9]

Non-adherence produces unnecessary medical and psychosocial consequences of CHD, reduces quality of life, and wastes valuable healthcare resources. These consequences impair the ability of healthcare interventions such as CR to achieve therapeutic goals. Non-adherence produces

increased need for expensive health services (e.g., hospitalization, outpatient clinic visits) due to disease progression or relapse. Furthermore, the patient's resumption and maintenance of normal social and vocational contributions is impaired. The development of strategies to promote adherence offers considerable potential to provide substantial medical, psychological, and economic gains. Before considering possible interventions, it is necessary to examine the main predictors of adherence identified in the literature.

Causes of Non-Adherence

Adherence has typically been regarded as an issue for the patient only; however, it is increasingly recognized that adherence is a multilevel issue[10] and consequently requires consideration of the illness and the treatment, the patient, the healthcare provider, and the healthcare system.

Illness and Treatment Factors

Adherence is related to the specifics of the illness and treatment recommendations. In general,[1] poor adherence is associated with treatments characterized by:

- long duration
- complex recommendations
- frequent changes in treatment
- side-effects
- treatment for asymptomatic conditions
- lack of immediate benefit
- high costs financially
- disruption to valued activities.

Behavior changes recommended for preventive purposes are at high risk for non-adherence. For example, in asymptomatic conditions such as raised cholesterol levels and hypertension, patients feel no obvious benefit after medicines are taken. Indeed, the patients may report negative side-effects to such medications. Furthermore, cardiac patients are often faced with a complex regimen involving a number of different components that may interfere with their daily routine. Non-adherence is associated with the presence of co-morbid conditions, and many cardiac patients have concurrent diagnoses of hypertension, hyperlipidemia, and type 2 diabetes that may compromise adherence.

Patient-Related Factors

Sociodemographic factors such as age, gender, ethnicity, socioeconomic status, and education have not been consistently related to adherence.[1,2] A number of psychological factors have been investigated, including traits, states, knowledge, and beliefs. There is little evidence of personality traits influencing adherence and the search for the "non-adherent" personality type has provided limited insight. Negative psychological states such as stress, depression, anxiety, and low levels of perceived social support increase the risk of non-adherence.[2]

Inadequate knowledge of illness and treatment, or misunderstanding of regimes could result in unintentional non-adherence. Nevertheless, knowledge alone is not sufficient for successful behavioral performance as there is substantial evidence that knowledge alone does not consistently predict behavior.[1] It has been suggested that the failure to adhere may reflect a failure to remember recommended behavior change, but even if the patient has adequate knowledge, accurate recollection of recommendations is not consistently associated with better adherence.[11]

The failure to find general patient-related factors as consistent predictors of adherence has resulted in a focus on specific beliefs that patients hold about their illness and treatment. A seminal series of investigations by Leventhal and colleagues in the 1970s revealed that patients make sense of illness in terms of five specific types of illness representations:

1. Identity: what is the illness and what are its symptoms?
2. Causal attributions: what caused the illness?
3. Time-line: how long will it last?
4. Consequences: what are the physical, social, and economic implications of the illness?
5. Control: what can be done to manage and control the illness?

The patient's beliefs about their illness and consequently how they think it should be managed may conflict with the healthcare provider's beliefs, and consequently the patient may not adhere. Of note, attendance at CR is related to illness representations. A recent randomized trial examined the efficacy of a brief three-session in-hospital intervention to change beliefs about a myocardial infarction in comparison to usual care.[12] Three months after discharge from the hospital, the intervention group returned to work at a significantly faster rate and had fewer angina symptoms. Having favorable attitudes towards the behavior and high levels of self-efficacy (confidence in one's ability to successfully perform the behavior) have been associated with successful performance of health behaviors.[13]

Healthcare Provider

Characteristics of the healthcare provider, such as communication style, can impact on rates of adherence. Communications associated with higher rates of adherence are characterized by providing information, being empathic, being clear, providing emotional support, allowing the patient to ask questions, and asking specific questions about adherence.[1,2,5] The patient's perceptions of being an active partner in the treatment process and being satisfied with the relationship with the healthcare provider also enhance adherence.

The multidisciplinary nature of CR offers a valuable forum for educating patients, motivating behavior change, monitoring behavior change, reinforcing messages, and providing feedback to patients. The multidisciplinary CR team's effectiveness at promoting adherence can be enhanced through the diverse skills base of the CR team. For example, the exercise specialist can encourage safe, effective, and regular practice of exercise strategies in a manner which promotes increased self-efficacy and habit formation: the dietician can illustrate how to "substitute" healthier behaviors or products rather than asking patients to undertake a loss-focused strategy of "removing" unhealthy aspects of their dietary lifestyle; the psychologist can help manage psychological distress that may inhibit adherence and, furthermore, may provide inputs to the other members of the CR team in relation to motivating and rewarding behavior change.

To date, research has typically examined the adherence behavior of cardiac patients; the adherence of healthcare professionals to evidence-based guidelines remains relatively understudied. Research evidence consistently reports non-adherence to recommended best practice. The EUROASPIRE I and II studies documented a substantial gap between standard clinical guidelines and actual clinical practice.[14] In general, secondary prevention of CHD is poorly integrated into clinical practice and this represents a substantial barrier to achievement of optimal health outcomes for patients. Furthermore, there is evidence that some health professionals lack confidence in changing patient behavior; for example, GPs and practice nurses reported a lack of confidence in their lifestyle counseling skills for cardiac patients.[15] Thus there is a critical need for healthcare professionals to receive appropriate training in the development and implementation of behavioral counseling skills in clinical practice. Such training requires the support of the healthcare system in which the service is embedded.

Healthcare System

Relatively little research has examined the effects of healthcare system-related factors on adherence. Non-adherence has been associated with poorly developed health services, poor medication distribution systems, lack of knowledge and training for health professionals on managing chronic illnesses, overworked professionals, underresourced services, lack of incentives and feedback on performance, short consultation times, poor provision of follow-up, and inability to establish community support.[1] Systems often fail to provide the continuity of care and ongoing contact (e.g. through telephone contact) that can help keep the patient engaged in the healthcare process. However, continuity of contact has cost and resource implications that may act as a barrier to implementation of such initiatives.

Summary

To fully understand adherence, we need to consider a particular patient experiencing a specific illness that requires a specific treatment in the context of a healthcare system. All of these factors contribute to the levels of adherence and to maximize adherence, interventions need to target the different levels. To date, research has typically only considered one of these levels – predominantly the patient – and consequently we have little evidence on the effectiveness of multilevel interventions.

Interventions

Numerous psycho-educational and behavioral strategies to enhance adherence have been examined (Table 35-1).

A meta-analysis which evaluated a range of interventions to improve adherence reported that they generally had a weak to moderate effect on adherence.[16] However, even modest improvements in adherence to behavioral recommendations could result in substantial mortality and economic costs. Combined-focus interventions were more successful than single-focus ones, and the most effective were a combination of educational, behavioral, and affective communications, which educated patients about their illness and treatment, taught behavioral strategies to enable people to cope better with symptoms and the behavior, and addressed emotions and moods. Thus multilevel interventions offer a more effective approach to enhancing adherence.

The CR team can use a number of the strategies presented in Table 35-1 in a coordinated manner. Education is a core component of CR and the team includes healthcare professionals who have the specific knowledge and skills to ensure patients understand their condition and their treatment. Healthcare providers should ask the patient about adherence at each visit. Acknowledgement that non-adherence occurs should be approached from an open, non-judgmental manner that avoids patient blaming. The use of open questions, showing empathy and following up on the patient's verbal clues makes it easier for the patient to discuss barriers to good adherence. A partnership approach to developing solutions emphasizes that adherence is an issue for both patient and healthcare provider. Improved communication between the professional and the patient should result in more informed decision-making by the patient and greater levels of patient satisfaction. The increased involvement of the patient in the clinical discussion of treatment

TABLE 35-1. Strategies for improving adherence to CHD secondary prevention behaviors

Strategy	Aim
Education	Communicate clearly the required information to the patient. Elicit what the patient understands about the illness and treatment. Clarify any misconceptions and provide written instructions if necessary.
Counseling	Treat patient depression and anxiety and provide coping strategies to help manage stress.
Self-efficacy enhancement	Increase patient confidence through provision of education, physiological feedback, vicarious experience, and mastery experiences.
Social support	Involve the patient's spouse/partner/significant others to reinforce behavior change.
Problem solving	Identify specific current or anticipated problems, generate potential solutions and determine a strategy, apply the strategy and evaluate in terms of successfully solving the problem.
Relapse prevention	Identify the high-risk situations, consider different approaches to manage the high-risk scenario, rehearse selected coping strategy during imaginary scenarios.
Patient-centered counseling	Assist patients in making plans for behavior change and to help patients adhere to such plans. Actively encourage patient involvement in the behavior change process.
Tailored behavioral change plan	Develop a feasible plan for behavior change that considers the patient's characteristics, values, and skills.
Behavioral skill learning and rehearsal	Provide instruction to help patient acquire and practice skills necessary to change behavior. Break behavior down into a series of manageable steps.
Stimulus control	Identify the potentially modifiable antecedents to the non-adherent behavior, change the environment to remove triggering stimuli.
Specific goal setting	Assist patients to make an explicit commitment outlining how specific behaviors are to be performed under specified circumstances.
Written agreement	Develop an agreed contract with patient outlining the behavior change process in an explicit time frame.
Reinforcement	Provide positive feedback to patient after successful achievement of a behavioral goal. Eventually the patient should be able to self-reward goal achievement.
Modeling	Provide the patient with an appropriate credible model successfully performing the behavior.
Self-monitoring	Review the patient's log/diary of the behavior over time and provide feedback on performance.
Cueing by patient	Establish a system of reminders for patient (e.g. notes in highly visible areas) to prompt the behavior.
Cueing by the healthcare providers	Remind the patient of appointment schedules, send letters after missed appointments, send reminders for medication refill, provide medication calendars and pill boxes.
Ongoing support	Contact the patient regularly to provide support to maintain behavior change. Support can be delivered through mail, phone, or e-mail.

Source: Adapted from Burke.[23] Copyright © 1999. Reproduced by permission of Routledge/Taylor & Francis Group, LLC.

recommendations can improve adherence, satisfaction, and outcome.

Cardiac patients require assistance in integrating new demands into their daily routine. A focus on the positive benefits of adherence, rather than the negative effects of non-adherence, will help to achieve a positive outcome. Emphasis should be placed on the fact that adherence provides patients with the means to control the disease rather than the disease controlling them. A focus on short-term behavioral goals while highlighting the long-term objectives can facilitate adherence. Short-term goals set around patient priorities, such as commencing regular exercise twice a week outside of the CR program, are achievable. Such successes should be reinforced and act as sources of confidence to achieve further goals. Strategies aimed at increasing self-management using individual assessment, problem solving, goal setting, and follow-up show significant potential for enhancing adherence.[17]

A number of prompts and reminders have been demonstrated to improve adherence and the CR team can provide such prompts through provision of individualized reminder charts or diaries, sending postcard reminders, and telephone calls. Furthermore, the family members and partners of the patients can be encouraged to provide such reminders. Indeed, partners are involved in the rehabilitation process in many CR services.

A recent systematic review[17] examined interventions to increase uptake of CR, patient adherence to CR, and healthcare provider adherence to CR. Provision of motivational communications using pamphlets, letters, or conversations with health professionals has been associated with improved uptake of outpatient CR. Improvements in CR referral have been reported in response to education of medical and nursing staff, electronic feedback and referral, and prompt card systems in the critical care pathway. A coordinated approach to transferring patients from hospital to general practice care, including cardiac liaison nursing support and patient self-management, can enhance uptake. The provision of support from trained lay volunteers offers another potentially useful strategy to increase adherence.

Few studies have examined ways to improve healthcare professionals' adherence with CR and such studies tend to be characterized by poor methodological reporting. The main interventions used to date include improvement of the referral process, coordination of the patient's post-discharge care, and formal recommendation of CR by the physician. Such approaches warrant further study as the conduct of the healthcare professionals is central to optimal CR utilization.

The CR program should be flexible in response to the patient's needs. The provision of opportunities for patients to make decisions about the treatment course should help establish a collaborative approach. The CR service may need to offer a variety of programs with varied time commitments. For example, CR non-attenders often cite inconvenient timing as one reason for not attending the program. Offering a variety of class times (including evening classes) should help attract those who may have other commitments (e.g. have returned to work). Innovative web-based technology combined with physician support may enhance adherence by healthcare staff in following up cardiac patients who leave the cardiac rehabilitation program. Services may need to respond to the needs of different client groups (e.g. women,[18] older people,[18] and those in lower socioeconomic status groups[19]) in imaginative and creative ways to increase uptake and reduce drop-out from the CR program.

Initial non-adherence predicts later non-adherence, and thus early intervention to promote adherence among patients is important in promoting more adherent behavior and enhancing long-term outcome. In essence, any approach to enhancing adherence has to be multidisciplinary

and multilevel and improving levels of adherence requires continued collaboration between healthcare providers involved in the CR.

The costs of such interventions tend to be minimal, and some data suggest a cost-to-savings ratio of 1:10 for self-management strategies, with savings in terms of health service use.[1] However, it should be noted that the cost-effectiveness of the interventions used in CHD patients remains unclear due to lack of detailed information on the resources used in the studies. Given the intensive nature of some of these strategies, there is an absence of efficacy data on strategies in clinical practice.

Recent scientific statements on cardiac rehabilitation and secondary prevention of CHD recommended that research should examine the effectiveness of interventions to promote adherence to secondary prevention recommendations.[20,21] In addition, adherence has been identified as a core expected outcome for cardiac rehabilitation services.[22] Future research needs to address the identification of those patients at highest risk for non-adherence, methods for assessing and improving compliance, and strategies that facilitate long-term adherence to recommendations.

Summary of Strategies

To date, no one single intervention strategy, or combination of strategies, has been found to be effective across different patient populations, conditions, and settings. Therefore, interventions that target adherence must be tailored to the specific illness and treatment-related demands experienced by the individual patient in light of the particular social and cultural setting of the patient.

Conclusion

Non-adherence is not simply a patient problem; aspects of health professional behavior and the healthcare system also contribute to non-adherence. Non-adherence needs to be routinely assessed as part of the therapeutic relationship between the patient and all professionals involved in disease management. Optimal secondary prevention is impeded by non-adherence to recommendations. Although non-adherence is associated with substantial costs, both medically and economically, it is potentially modifiable. Insights from behavioral science have highlighted the role of psychological factors in patient decision-making regarding adherence and a number of promising intervention strategies have been developed with documented evidence of efficacy. However, as yet, many of these strategies are not routinely incorporated into clinical practice. Further research is required to identify key factors that explain adherence, and an integrated theoretical framework is needed to account for the relationship among such predictors. Such information will facilitate the development, implementation, and evaluation of evidence-based interventions in clinical practice. The promotion of adherence strategies in a coherent, systematic manner offers great potential for decreasing health risks and unnecessary healthcare costs and improving patient outcomes. In the cardiac setting, since patient (and professional) adherence to long-term behavior change is intrinsic to much of the potential to benefit, activities to promote adherence must encompass individual patient, health professional, and system-related activities.

References

1. World Health Organization. Adherence to Long-term Therapies: Evidence for Action. Geneva: World Health Organization; 2003.
2. Dunbar-Jacob J, Schlenk E. Patient adherence to treatment outcomes. In: Baum A, Revenson T, Singer J, eds. Handbook of Health Psychology. Mahwah, NJ: Erlbaum; 2001:571–580.
3. Cooper AF, Jackson G, Weinman J, Horne, R. Factors associated with cardiac rehabilitation attendance: a systematic review of the literature. Clin Rehabil 2002;16:541–552.
4. Shepard J, Alcalde V, Befort P-A, et al. International comparison of awareness and attitudes towards coronary risk factor reduction: the HELP study. J Cardiovasc Risk 1997;4:373–384.
5. Ockene IS, Hayman LL, Pasternak RC, Schron E, Dunbar-Jacob J. Task Force #4 – Adherence issues and behavioral changes. J Am Coll Cardiol 2002;40: 579–651.
6. Emery CF. Adherence in cardiac and pulmonary rehabilitation. J Cardiopulmon Rehabil 1995;15: 420–423.
7. DiMatteo MR, Giordani PJ, Lepper HS, et al. Patient adherence and medical treatment outcomes: a meta-analysis. Med Care 2002;40:794–811.
8. Psaty BM, Koepsell TD, Wagner EH, LoGerfo JP, Inui TS. The relative risk of incident coronary heart disease associated with recently stopping the use of beta-blockers. JAMA 1990;263:1653–1657.
9. Berg JS, Dischler J, Wagner DJ, et al. Medication compliance: a healthcare problem. Ann Pharmacother 1993;27:S1–S24.
10. Miller NH, Hill M, Kottke T, Ockene IS. The multilevel compliance challenge: recommendations for a call to action. A statement for healthcare professionals. Circulation 1997;95:1085–1090.
11. Kravitz R, Hays RD, Sherbourne CD, et al. Recall of recommendations and adherence to advice among patients with chronic medical conditions: Results from the Medical Outcomes Study. Arch Intern Med 1993;153:1869–1878.
12. Petrie KJ, Cameron LD, Ellis CJ, Buick D, Weinman J. Changing illness perceptions after myocardial infarction: An early intervention randomised controlled trial. Psychosom Med 2002;64:580–586.
13. Burke LE, Dunbar-Jacob JM, Hill MN. Compliance with cardiovascular disease prevention strategies: a review of the research. Ann Behav Med 1997;19: 239–263.
14. Cohen JD. ABCs of secondary prevention of CHD: easier said than done. Lancet 2001;357:972–973.
15. Steptoe A, Doherty S, Kendrick T, Rink E, Hilton S. Attitudes to cardiovascular health promotion among GPs and practice nurses. Fam Pract 1999;16: 158–163.
16. Roter DL, Hall JA, Rolande M, et al. Effectiveness of interventions to improve patient adherence: a meta analysis. Med Care 1998;36:1138–1161.
17. Beswisk AD, Rees K, Griebsch I, et al. Provision, uptake and cost of cardiac rehabilitation programmes: improving services to under-represented groups. Health Technol Assess 2004;8(41). York: York Publishing Services.
18. McGee HM, Horgan JH. Cardiac rehabilitation programmes: are women less likely to attend? BMJ 1992;305:283–284.
19. Sykes DH, Hanley M, Boyle DM, Higginson JD, Wilson C. Socioeconomic status, social environment, depression and postdischarge adjustment of the cardiac patient. J Psychosom Res 1999;46:83–98.
20. Giannuzzi P, Saner H, Bjornstad H, et al. Secondary prevention through cardiac rehabilitation. Position paper of the Working Group on Cardiac Rehabili-

tation and Exercise Physiology of the European Society of Cardiology. Eur Heart J 2003;24:1273–1278.

21. Leon AS, Franklin BA, Costa F, et al. Cardiac rehabilitation and secondary prevention of coronary heart disease: an American Heart Association scientific statement from the Council on Clinical Cardiology (Subcommittee on Exercise, Cardiac Rehabilitation, and Prevention) and the Council on Nutrition, Physical Activity, and Metabolism (Subcommittee on Physical Activity), in collaboration with the American association of Cardiovascular and Pulmonary Rehabilitation. Circulation 2005; 111:369–376.

22. Balady GJ, Ades PA, Comoss P, et al. Core components of cardiac rehabilitation/secondary prevention programs: A statement for healthcare professionals from the American Heart Association and the American Association of Cardiovascular and Pulmonary Rehabilitation Writing Group. Circulation 2000;102:1069–1073.

23. Burke LE. Adherence to a heart-healthy lifestyle – what makes a difference? In: Wenger NK, Smith LK, Froelicher ES, McCall Comoss P, eds. Cardiac Rehabilitation. A Guide to Practice in the 21st Century. New York: Marcel Dekker, 1999:385–393.

Section VII
Social and Caring Support

A comprehensive cardiac rehabilitation program has to offer to the patient all the constitutive parts that have been defined by the World Health Organization and included in the different European or American specific guidelines. This section gives the "state of the art" in specific aspects of cardiac rehabilitation: the role of nurses, factors influencing return to work, counseling of the patient, long-term maintenance programs, national foundations or heart networks, and new perspectives in caring and support.

Cardiac rehabilitation includes prevention and heart failure rehabilitation programs. In Europe, these programs are usually led by medical doctors (most often cardiologists), as advised by the ESC working group's recently published guidelines on cardiac rehabilitation and exercise physiology. Nurses are thus part of the multidisciplinary team, which also includes physiotherapists, nutritionists, psychologists, social workers and others, as available given local circumstances, who deliver cardiac rehabilitation programs. Nurses are, in some settings, the main team who deliver these cardiologist-led programs. These aspects of nurse-led programs will be described by A. Cahill (Chapter 36) and A. Strömberg (Chapter 37).

The medical and socio-professional factors involved in work resumption after myocardial infarction or after coronary interventions (J. Perk) will be analyzed in Chapters 38 (J. Perk) and 39 (J. Perk). Return to work rate remains suboptimal and socioeconomic factors seem to play a major role, often more than medical factors.

Sexuality is a part of quality of life; so sexual counseling of the cardiac patient is an important goal, which may be offered to patients before resuming sexual activity (Chapter 40, T. Jaarsma and E. Steinke).

The last part of this section will deal with new perspectives in cardiac rehabilitation and prevention. There are in some patients some discrepancies between symptoms and objective evaluation of the patient. These symptoms may have a detrimental effect on quality of life and work resumption. The objective of cognitive behavioral rehabilitation in patients with angina (Chapter 41, R.J. Lewin) is to decrease the symptoms by educating patients to analyze their beliefs and by changing their symptom-related behavior.

S. Logstrup and colleagues (Chapter 42) will report on the role of national heart foundations (in Finland and Switzerland) and the European Heart Network in prevention of cardiovascular disease.

The importance of long-term maintenance programs in the field of cardiac rehabilitation maintaining the results obtained during the initial program is well known. M. Mendes (Chapter 43) will analyze the objectives, the methods, and the necessary means for such long-term maintenance programs.

Finally, new models of care and support, involving nurses, trained lay volunteers, or even internet will be proposed by J.F. Pattenden and R.J. Lewin (Chapter 44).

Main Messages

Chapter 36: Prevention Programs: The Role of the Nurse

International guidelines dictate multifactorial and multidisciplinary delivery of cardiac rehabilitation services. However, cardiac rehabilitation programs can often fail through a lack of appropriate coordination. Skilled coordination of programs is necessary to ensure an effective and efficient service. Nurses, who constitute the largest employee population of the health service workforce, are often recruited into these positions.

The coordination of the cardiac rehabilitation program requires the ability to work with patients and their families and also the ability to liaise with and coordinate other disciplines. The skills required of a program coordinator are varied and are dictated by the particular requirements of each phase of the program.

Chapter 37: Heart Failure Rehabilitation: The Role of the Nurse

Nurses' participation in heart failure rehabilitation has increased in Europe during the last decade. When evaluated in meta-analyses, heart failure programs, often nurse-led, have been shown to effectively reduce mortality and morbidity and improve self care in patients with chronic heart failure. In this chapter structural elements (setting, education, financing) and process of care (referrals, components, interventions) as well as the advantages and disadvantages with different models of nurse-based heart failure programs are discussed.

Chapter 38: Returning to Work after Myocardial Infarction

Assisting the patient to resume work after a myocardial infarction is one of the main aims of a comprehensive rehabilitation program after myocardial infarction. A majority of patients will be able to return to work but non-medical factors are more important predictors than medical factors of the likelihood of resuming work. Yet, through vocational counseling, adapted training models and adequate communication with work-place medical services cardiac rehabilitation can play an important supportive role.

Chapter 39: Return to Work after Coronary Interventions

Improving the work resumption rate after coronary interventions is an important goal of a cardiac rehabilitation program. The available data show us that the return to work rate is not optimal, that unless the presence of symptoms, the severity of heart disease has little impact, but that socioeconomic factors, including age, play a major role.

The specific role of cardiac rehabilitation after coronary interventions on work resumption remains to be clearly demonstrated.

Chapter 40: Sexual Counseling of the Cardiac Patient

Cardiovascular disease is a common cause of sexual dysfunction. Patients and their partners may experience sexual problems as a result of anxiety, symptoms or sexual dysfunction. They worry about the effect of the condition on sexual activity, the effect of sex on the heart, symptoms that may occur during sexual activity and possible effects of medication.

Healthcare providers may have difficulty addressing the issue but should take the initiative to bring up the topic of sexual functioning. There are several prerequisites to implementing successful sexual counseling. Environmental issues, communication issues, and confidentiality are important. Open-ended basic questions can be used to facilitate discussion and to assess patient concerns. In addition, specific questions are asked during this discussion, moving from general questions to more specific issues or problems as the counseling session continues. Health professionals are in key positions to provide this teaching and facilitate successful return to sexual activity after a cardiac event.

Chapter 41: Cognitive Behavioral Rehabilitation for Angina

Cognitive behavioral (CB) disease management programs are new techniques that can be applied in cardiac rehabilitation. Using the example of angina, this chapter will demonstrate the application of these techniques, and a brief practical description of the "Angina Management Programme" is presented.

Chapter 42: National Heart Foundations, European Heart Network

Heart Foundations in Europe fulfill many roles in their work to prevent cardiovascular diseases. An important role is to lend support to cardiovascular patients and their families.

This chapter presents two case studies, from Finland and Switzerland, illustrating patient education and rehabilitation programs offered by Heart Foundation in those countries. The chapter also describes recent EU developments on cross border patient mobility, on the High Level Group on Health Services and Medical Care and on the European Parliament report on patient mobility.

Chapter 43: Long-Term Maintenance Programs

After a phase II cardiac rehabilitation program the challenge is to keep the patients committed to risk factor control and regular exercise. Only long-term intervention can have positive consequences

for the patient's prognosis, since the benefits achieved in the earlier phases will quickly vanish if the program is not continued.

Although the maintenance phase program is the logical continuation of the previous program, it is very difficult to keep the patient committed to it, outside the protective atmosphere of the rehabilitation center, experiencing time conflicts due to job resumption and at risk of leaving the program for financial reasons. In this chapter, readers will find advice on how to design the exercise and risk factor control program, strategies to keep the patients motivated and coping with this comprehensive intervention in the long term, the only way to give patients a better and longer life.

Chapter 44: New Models of Care and Support

As the number of people living with cardiovascular disease continues to rise, new models of care and support need to be developed to integrate patient care between primary, secondary, and social care. This chapter describes some emerging methods: specialist nurse-led care; nurse facilitated self-management programs; lay-led programs of education, advice and support; and eHealth applications including web-based programs and use of internet resources.

36
Prevention Programs: The Role of the Nurse

Alison Cahill

Cardiac rehabilitation services have developed worldwide over the last few decades. The World Health Organization definitions of cardiac rehabilitation of 1969 and 1993 outlined what was required of a cardiac rehabilitation service for patients with coronary heart disease. However, as might be expected, different countries and health provision services developed different styles of programs in response to local funding, available staff, and patient profiles. As a result of this, many international bodies developed their own guidelines and policies for the provision of cardiac rehabilitation.[1-4] The CARINEX survey of current guidelines and practices within the European Union[5] identified 20 professional guidelines since 1990, in nine languages across Europe alone. Twelve separate countries had national guidelines.

A variety of program types have been developed. One strong common recommendation across the guidelines was that cardiac rehabilitation programs be multifactorial and multidisciplinary in nature. The provision of a program of this nature requires a wide range of expertise and skills, and access to a multidisciplinary team may be difficult with restricted healthcare budgets and smaller centers. Nurses, who constitute the largest employee population of the health service workforce, are often recruited into these positions.

Several recent reviews of cardiac rehabilitation service provision assessed staffing, and nurses appear to play a significant role. Lewin et al. assessed programs in the UK in 1998.[6] They reviewed 263 programs and identified nurse involvement in 89% of them. With the exception of physiotherapists, input from other disciplines was minimal. The British Association of Cardiac Rehabilitation indicated that in 1998 80% of cardiac rehabilitation services were coordinated by nurses.

The most recent review of cardiac rehabilitation services within the European Union, the CARINEX survey,[7] was carried out in 1995. Staffing was reviewed in centers which provided WHO-defined phase II and III cardiac rehabilitation. The staffing profile indicated that even though variation in the type of staff involvement was the norm across the European Union, nurses were involved in the majority of the programs.[8,9] The appointment of nurses to coordinator roles can be very strategic. Nurses are professionals with good communication skills, they have significant experience of working with patients and families, and they have the ability to interact easily with other disciplines. The cardiac rehabilitation service coordinator requires the skill to manage coronary heart disease which can result in a wide-range of residual symptoms depending on diagnosis.

Cardiac rehabilitation services are by definition "comprehensive, long-term programs involving medical evaluation, prescribed exercise, cardiac risk-factor modification, education and counseling. These programs are designed to limit the physiological and psychological effect of cardiac illness, reduce the risk of sudden death or re-infarction, control cardiac symptoms, stabilize or reverse the atherosclerotic process, and enhance the psychological and vocational status of selected patients."[10] Obviously, these rehabilitation activities do not take place all at once. They are carried out at different stages of recovery. To facilitate this, a nurse leading a cardiac rehabilitation program needs to develop many roles.

Jillings described nursing interventions in cardiac rehabilitation as falling into six categories: supportive, palliative, restorative, educative, protective, and preventative.[11] While all cardiac rehabilitation patients should be dealt with on the basis of individual needs, there are basic requirements that need to be met in each of the various phases of cardiac rehabilitation.

The Role of the Nurse in Phase I Rehabilitation

This initial phase of rehabilitation begins at admission. It may be administered at ward level by ward staff. Evidence-based practice has shown that early intervention of a cardiac rehabilitation nature has a positive effect on recovery.[12] The key areas to be addressed at this phase of rehabilitation are reassurance and information/education. If at all possible, partner or family involvement should be part of this phase.

Reassurance

Anxiety, depression, and reduced self-confidence are common reactions to a coronary event. Failure to address these issues means a prolonged negative response from a patient toward their illness and poor psychological adjustment is predictive of subsequent mortality.[13] The ideal means to reassure a patient is for the cardiac rehabilitation nurse to have an individual consultation with the patient and his or her family. It is important that the multidisciplinary approach is well coordinated with the involvement of all relevant staff as required.

Reassurance of patients and their families does elicit a positive attitude to recovery and can dispel the myths of "hearsay" often associated with cardiac illness. The best means to reassure patients is to inform and educate them about their illness and to provide a realistic approach to its management.

Information/Education

The education of the patient is the cornerstone of any cardiac rehabilitation program. Often the requirements of a patient are to change a lifestyle they have practiced since childhood. Educating patients requires more than knowledge acquisition. Patient profiles may differ but they will always require clear, concise information to assist them with their recovery.

When planning any information/education service there are some very important issues to be addressed regardless of who provides the service:

1. Identify any material, linguistic, and cultural barriers to learning.
2. All information and advice should be presented and delivered by both written and verbal means. If designing written information, the editing suggestions from Cox[14] and Pocinki[15] may prove useful. It is necessary to ensure that any written information provided is "user-friendly" to the overall patient population. Provisions (video- or audio-tapes) for patients with learning difficulties, for example visual/hearing difficulties, must be made.

Information Requirements

Information requirements may differ greatly between patients, hence the benefit of individual counseling, but nonetheless there are some integral components that must be included:

Risk Factor Profile

This activity is often described by patients as one of the most important pieces of information required.[16] The amount and type of data collected can vary and often might be dictated by the auditing policies in place. The identification of specific coronary risk factors must be performed for each patient. The information may be collected as per the British Cardiac Rehabilitation Association Guidelines.[3]

Diagnosis

Explanation of anatomy and physiology and definition of a clear diagnosis will help to clarify the rationale for treatment and future rehabilitation interventions. The cardiac rehabilitation nurse or medical team should liaise with each other so they are unified in their presentation to the patient.

Multidisciplinary Approach

The cardiac rehabilitation nurse, in their role as program coordinator, should use the consultation with the patient to identify those that need specific intervention from particular team disciplines; for example, patients are often concerned about vocational issues such as job suitability, job security, and financial aspects. By liaising with the vocational officer and medical team at an early stage, the patient may be reassured, providing a more positive approach to recovery and alleviating anxiety.

Advice Regarding Activities

Providing patients and their families with appropriate advice on activity levels, both the activities of daily living and social and leisure in nature, is necessary. Advising patients on activities after discharge can help identify patients who may need assistance in the early discharge period – the elderly, those living alone, or those with significant dependants. Social workers, occupational therapists, physiotherapists, and vocational counselors can be consulted on these issues. Providing patients with an exercise program for post discharge will ensure that recovery progresses at a suitable pace.

Symptom Management

Potential future symptoms and their management should be discussed prior to discharge to avoid panic and anxiety in the instance of their occurrence. Proper instruction on intervention techniques, for example the use of glyceryl trinitrate spray, and early medical attention should be addressed.

Further Rehabilitation

Outlining the rehabilitation process planned for the patient with the patient's family will provide structure for their recovery and help to maintain and promote motivation and compliance to advice given.

The Role of the Nurse in Phase II Rehabilitation

Phase II usually comprises a structured program of patient participation. Program formats can vary significantly. They can be residential, hospital based, or community based. Even though most are exercise based, coordination of all services into this program is essential. Most European countries follow the outpatient-based formula and even still display significant differences, i.e. program length, the use of ECG monitoring, supervising disciplines. The coordinator should be mindful that each patient should still be treated individually and progress monitored.

It is well established that the program should be multidisciplinary in nature and the nurse, as coordinator, should devise a program which encompasses all aspects of rehabilitation. Liaising with the other disciplines is required to develop a program that meets these needs, for example nutritional guidance, vocational guidance, psychological support, and education regarding medications.

Physical

Before commencing any physical program, an appropriate baseline assessment should be performed on every participant. This allows for individual prescription of exercise in a safe and efficient manner. The most basic of assessments should include the following: baseline physical assessment (risk factor profile, diagnosis, current symptoms, and previous or other associated medical history); inclusion and exclusion criteria for exercising as per the recognized guidelines (ACSM,[17] AACVPR[2]); risk stratification of patients should be performed according to recognized guidelines[1]; baseline exercise capacity assessment by an exercise stress test performed on a treadmill or bicycle, carried out according to National Cardiac Society recommendations.[18]

Once collected, these data provide the nurse with detailed information to devise a specific program. All programs should include the following features:

- Individual exercise prescription for the supervised exercise class.

- Baseline vital sign assessment at each session.
- Each exercise session should include a warm-up phase, aerobic exercise at a submaximal level, some resistance training and a cool-down period.
- All emergency responses should be in place.
- Staff to patient ratios will depend on the patient profile.
- Appropriately qualified staff should be in situ for class monitoring.
- Nutritional guidance should be included in the program.
- Psychological support should be included.
- Educational classes on coronary heart disease and its implications.
- Education regarding medications.

On completion of the formal program, a subsequent exercise stress test should be performed for comparison purposes.

Psychological Aspects

When coordinating the program, the cardiac rehabilitation nurse must ensure that psychological support is provided as part of the mainstream service. The psychological aspect should consist of group sessions or individual counseling, where appropriate. The most common evaluation is screening for levels of anxiety and depression and the most common assessment tools are the Hospital Anxiety and Depression Scale (HADS) and the Short Form 36 questionnaire (SF-36). Ideally a psychologist should provide this service and the nurse as coordinator will liaise with them to integrate the sessions into the program. In the absence of a psychologist, with appropriate training, the nurse would be able to provide the basic requirements of the service, but screening for patients who need further intervention must be carried out and patients referred on to specialists as required.

The Role of the Nurse in Phase III Rehabilitation

By its definition, the cardiac rehabilitation service promotes lifestyle amendments for patients but specifies that it must be by their own efforts. The goal of the cardiac rehabilitation nurse is to educate patients in the means to do this. Phase III rehabilitation mostly concerns maintenance of a heart-healthy lifestyle. The nurse can encourage this by completing the formal aspects to the rehabilitation program. This should include the following recommendations:

- Send a report of the patient's rehabilitation program containing all results and comments to the referring cardiologist and general practitioner.
- Arrange medical review for all patients on completion of the program.
- Ensure appropriate follow-up with the necessary disciplines as required, for example dietitian review, psychological follow-up.
- Ensure that the patient has formulated a plan for long-term maintenance and discuss this with them.
- Arrange return group sessions in some centers for patients at approximately 6 months and conduct some measurements – lipid profiles, psychological screening. This may depend on staffing issues or time constraints of existing staff.

There are some community-based exercise programs which offer long-term continued incentives for the patient but these are scarce. A "Heart-watch" program (Ireland) is a nurse-led program which was developed to assist in the continuous monitoring of coronary risk factors; patients should be encouraged to avail themselves of such services where they are available.

Training

As early as 1992, the British Cardiac Society Working Party Report on cardiac rehabilitation[19] identified the need for formal training for cardiac rehabilitation coordinators. At policy level, the Irish National Cardiovascular Health Strategy ("Building Healthier Hearts" 1999) is an example of a national directive which recommended trained coordinators be part of every cardiac rehabilitation program.[20] Appropriate training for the coordinator's role seems a logical step. In response to this need, a training program was published,[9] outlining the multidisciplinary approach to training. The authors identified that "formalized training contributes to acceptable standards of both clinical practice and service delivery and advances expertise in audit and service representation." This training program is now conducted to a Masters degree level. Training is provided worldwide by the British Association of Cardiac Rehabilitation and other national societies, European Society of Cardiology, the American Association of Cardiopulmonary Rehabilitation etc (see also Chapter 1).

Conclusions

Cardiac rehabilitation is a multidisciplinary service which needs to be delivered over a long period in the course of recovery from cardiac events and procedures. Such a program needs skilled coordination to ensure effective, efficient, and ongoing program delivery for all who can benefit. While many professional groups can coordinate such activities, nurses are well placed because of their broad-based training and likely availability in cardiac settings. Often cardiac rehabilitation programs do not commence or falter through poor coordination. Medical leadership is essential and frequently found in most European programs but less often is the coordination of the day-to-day services the sole commitment of a program director. In small centers where coordination requires only part-time staffing, the role of the cardiac rehabilitation coordinator can be easily facilitated as part of a senior cardiac nurse's role. Service provision can be enhanced by capitalizing on the broad-based training and holistic perspective of experienced cardiac nurses.

References

1. Irish Association of Cardiac Rehabilitation. Guidelines for Cardiac Rehabilitation. Dublin; 2002.
2. American Association of Cardiovascular and Pulmonary Rehabilitation. Guidelines for Cardiac Rehabilitation and Secondary Prevention Programs, 3rd edn. Champaign, IL: Human Kinetics; 1999.
3. British Association of Cardiac Rehabilitation. Guidelines for Cardiac Rehabilitation (Coats A, McGee H, Stokes H, Thompson D, eds). Oxford: Blackwell Science; 1995.
4. Giannuzzi P, Saner H, Bjornstad H, et al. Secondary Prevention through Cardiac Rehabilitation. Position Paper of the Working Group on Cardiac Rehabilitation and Exercise Physiology of the European Cardiac Society of Cardiology. Eur Heart J 2003;24:1273–1278.
5. Vanhees L, McGee HM, Dugmore LD, et al. The CARINEX Survey: Current Guidelines and Practices in Cardiac Rehabilitation within Europe. Leuven: Acco; 1999.
6. Lewin R, Ingleton R, Newens A, Thompson D. Adherence to Cardiac Rehabilitation Guidelines: a survey of rehabilitation programmes in the United Kingdom. BMJ 1998;316:1354–1355.
7. Vanhees L, McGee H, Dugmore L, et al. The CARINEX survey. A representative study of cardiac rehabilitation activities in European Union member states. J Cardiopulmon Rehabil 2002;22:264–272.
8. McGee H, Hevey D, Horgan J (On behalf of the Irish Association of Cardiac Rehabilitation). Cardiac Rehabilitation Service Provision in Ireland: The Irish Association of Cardiac Rehabilitation Survey. Ir J Med Sci 170;3:159–162.
9. Hevey D, McGee H, Cahill A, Newton H, Horgan J. Training cardiac rehabilitation coordinators. Coronary Health Care 2000;4:142–145.
10. Frigenbaum E, Carter E. Cardiac Rehabilitation Services. Health technology assessment report, 1987, No. 6. Rockville, MD: US Department of Health and Human Services, Public Health Service, National Center for Health Services Research and Health Care Technology Assessment. DHHS Publication No. PHS 88 – 3427, August 1988.
11. Jillings C. Cardiac Rehabilitation Nursing. Rockville, MD: Aspen Publishers; 1988.
12. Johnston M, Foulkes J, Johnston DW, Pollard B, Gudmundsdottir H. Impact on patients and partners of inpatients and extended cardiac counselling and rehabilitation: a controlled trial. Psychosom Med 1999;61:225–233.
13. Frasure-Smith N. In-hospital symptoms of psychological stress as predictors of long term outcome after acute myocardial infarction in men. Am J Cardiol 1991;167:121–127.
14. Cox B. The art of writing patient education materials. American Medical Writers Association Journal 1989;4:11–14.
15. Pocinki K. Writing for an older audience; ways to maximize understanding and acceptance. American Medical Writers Association Journal 1990;5:6–10.

16. Wingate S. Post MI patients perceptions of their learning needs. Dimensions of Critical Care in Nursing 1990;9:112–118.

17. American College of Sports Medicine. Guidelines for Exercise Testing and Prescription, 6th edn. Lippincott Williams & Wilkins; 2000.

18. Recommendations of the Medical Practice Committee and Council of the British Cardiac Society. Guidelines for exercise testing when there is not a doctor present. Br Heart J 1993;70:488.

19. Horgan J, Bethell H, Carson P, et al. British Cardiac Society Working Party Report on Cardiac Rehabilitation. Br Heart J 1992;67:412–418.

20. Department of Health and Children. Building Healthier Hearts. The Cardiovascular Health Strategy. Dublin; 1999.

37
Heart Failure Rehabilitation: The Role of the Nurse

Anna Strömberg

Why Is Heart Failure Rehabilitation Important?

Heart failure is a serious condition. More than two-thirds of individuals with moderate to severe systolic dysfunction are hospitalized yearly and one out of three die within one year after hospitalization. The heart failure group consumes >2% of the total healthcare costs and the main costs are due to hospitalizations.[1,2]

There are several issues in the management and rehabilitation of patients with heart failure that need to be taken into account in order to improve outcomes. Many patients are not adequately diagnosed[3] and do not have optimal treatment according to guidelines.[4] Patients hospitalized due to heart failure often have a short length of stay in the hospital and discharge planning and rehabilitation are often not provided, especially not to the majority of heart failure patients who are above the age of 65 years. Education for patients with heart failure in order to teach self-care is often insufficient.[5] Patients' satisfaction with care is sometimes low and patients ask for more support and education.[6] It has been shown that non-compliance with medication, diet or symptom monitoring caused up to 50% of hospital readmissions.[7]

The Contribution of Nurses in Heart Failure Rehabilitation

Nurses are increasingly involved in heart failure care, especially in patient education, follow-up, and drug titration. During the later part of the 1980s, the concept of heart failure clinics often run by nurses was initiated in the US. In 1995, the first randomized study evaluating a nurse-based, multidisciplinary intervention that combined telephone follow-up and home-based visits was published. The results of this study showed that a nurse-based intervention could decrease hospital admission and improve quality of life and these findings started a boom in nurse-led heart failure programs and randomized trials evaluating these initiatives.

Sweden was the first country in Europe to establish nurse-based heart failure clinics for patient education and follow-up and there are today heart failure clinics in 80% of the Swedish hospitals. There are now also heart failure clinics in more that one-third of the hospitals or more in Norway, Denmark, Iceland, the Netherlands, the United Kingdom, Greece, and Slovenia.[8] Several other European countries are rapidly developing heart failure programs. In the US, Australia, and New Zealand heart failure programs are also common, but there are few reports from Asia and Africa about nurse-based initiatives in heart failure care.

Some nurse-based heart failure programs are home-based, some are clinic-based or a combination of the two models. The majority also provide patient- or nurse-initiated telephone consultations. Specially educated heart failure nurses staff the programs and provide discharge planning, structured follow-up and patient education, both pre- and post-discharge. The nurses can be delegated the responsibility for making protocol-led changes in medications, such as uptitrating ACE inhibitors, beta-blockers, angiotensin- and aldosterone-receptor blockers as well as spirono-

TABLE 37-1. Advantages and disadvantages with different models of nurse-based heart failure programs

	Advantages	Disadvantages
Clinic visits	Convenient to be in a hospital setting with medical facilities and equipment available Physician easily reached if nurses need a second opinion or changes in medications or prescriptions	Fewer patients are suitable for this follow up. Transportation to the hospital can be tiring for the patient and needs organization of transport and support
Home care	The patients do not need to be mobile Easier to assess the patients' needs, capabilities and adherence to treatment in their own environment Convenient to do a follow-up visit shortly after hospitalization in the home	Time-consuming for nurses to travel to the patients Cars and mobile equipment are needed Nurses alone with the responsibility. Difficult to reach the medically responsible physician
Telemonitoring	Increasing need for this type of monitoring when more advanced care moving into the patients' homes New equipment is continually under development	Steep learning curve to use the equipment, for patient and/or caregiver and healthcare providers Unclear which variables are the most helpful to monitor

lactone, terminating treatment with interacting drugs, and decreasing or increasing the daily doses of diuretics. A cardiologist retains medical responsibility and initiates or confirms the medical changes.

The focus of the majority of these programs is to monitor symptoms, optimize treatment, and provide patient education and support in order to increase self-care behavior. Despite the many positive effects of exercise training in heart failure, this component is seldom included for all patients in the heart failure programs. In this area there is room for improvement.

Telemonitoring is a tool that allows the heart failure team to monitor daily the physiological variables and symptoms measured by patients or caregivers at home. Patients with heart failure can be kept under close supervision in their own homes. Telemonitoring uses the technology of special telecare devices and a telecommunication system standard telephone lines, cable network or broadband technology. The use of telemonitoring has increased in order to support chronically ill patients. Before telemonitoring can spread broadly in clinical practice, more widely available low-cost, user-friendly telemonitoring equipment as well as further evaluations of effects are needed.

In telemedicine blood pressure, pulse or ECG, saturation devices as well electronic scales, symptom response system and video consultation equipment can be installed in the patient's home. The collected data are sent to a server usually in a hospital setting. A nurse monitors the vital signs daily in order to detect changes suggesting deterioration of heart failure, and contacts the patient if signs of deterioration or no data occurs. The nurse reacts and takes action either on their own judgement or action algorithms or contacts the responsible physician when deterioration occurs. Compliance with monitoring has been good and technical failures quite low, so it seems to be a feasible and reliable model of care.[9] In Table 37-1, the advantages and disadvantages of follow-up through clinic visits, home visits, or telemonitoring are outlined.

Starting a Nurse-Based Heart Failure Rehabilitation Program

Goals and Key Components

Overall goals of the program should include both the patient and healthcare perspective. Examples of goals on the healthcare level are to improve follow-up after hospitalization, improve quality of life and survival in patients with heart failure, reduce the number of hospital readmissions, provide evidence-based medicine and care regarding diagnostics, treatment, education and support, and perform regular quality assurance and audits of the program. Goals on the patient level can be to provide individualized patient education and increase self-care management and adaptation of living with chronic heart failure.

The aim of nurse-based programs is to provide holistic, individualized, and evidence-based care. The key components are: a diagnosis verified by echocardiography, rehabilitation provided by a multidisciplinary team with the objectives to provide optimized drug therapy, patient education and counseling with special emphasis on self-care, as well as psychosocial support to patients and family. The rehabilitation is started with early follow-up after hospitalization with the focus on high-risk patients, and is either home or clinic based with increased access to healthcare through telephone consultation and long consultations (30–60 minutes).

It has been debated which of the components in the nurse-based heart failure follow-up is the most important and effective, but apart from education, which has shown isolated positive effects,[10,11] none of the present studies have been designed to answer this question. However, it might be more relevant to consider this type of follow-up as a concept of care composed of several components with synergism instead of believing that just one single component could be enough to improve outcomes such as survival, morbidity, and quality of life.

Economic and Organizational Frameworks

The most important aspect in terms of economic and organizational issues is to set up a heart failure program that is adapted to the means and organization of the local hospital or primary care setting. The economic resources influence how the service can be organized, for example the number of nurses, physicians, and other healthcare professionals that can be appointed, what facilities that can be afforded, and the type of follow-up. In some cases new recourses are provided from the start, in other cases the program is paid by relocating budgets. The goal is cost-effectiveness. Another important issue is whether it is most convenient for patients and the staff to provide hospital-based clinic visits or home visits. If the visits are be hospital-based, well-functioning premises are demanded. If it is home-based, transportation and mobile equipment are needed.

The timing of the first visit is still a matter of debate. Early follow-up after discharge is effective; it should be done within the first days or weeks after discharge. The number of visits and length of the program are also under debate. Recent data have shown that only the first 3 months of follow-up reduce readmissions, so a longer follow-up might not be needed in stable patients.[12] There is also evidence that the number of visits can be few and individualized according to the patient's needs and that stable, optimally treated and well-informed patients can be referred back to their family doctor, often a GP or cardiologist.[13]

Create Relations Throughout the Chain of Care

Establishing a well-functioning collaboration throughout the whole chain of care, especially between primary and secondary care, is important. Good relations ensure that the competence and potential of the nurse-based program is used in the best way. It is relevant to elucidate the referral of patients to the program and the type of service that can be provided. The responsibility for the total care and follow-up of stable heart failure patients must be defined in order to use human and material resources effectively; for example, the issue of discharge from the program or the need for readmission.

The patients need to be optimally diagnosed, treated, and educated according to guidelines irrespective of the caregiver. Therefore educational initiatives are needed for all caregivers in the chain of care, as are regular contact channels.

Choose the Patient Population

Before setting up a program it is important for planning purposes to have knowledge about patient needs. Patients with heart failure are a heterogeneous group covering a large age span, with differences in etiology, severity of heart failure, and social situation. The majority of the patients are over 70 years of age and have several other co-morbidities such as diabetes, arthritis, cancer, chronic obstructive lung disease, or kidney failure.

The number of patients hospitalized each year due to heart failure and the percentage that are suitable for follow-up need to be estimated as well as the number of patients that will be referred from other caregivers, for example primary healthcare. It is crucial to discuss which patients benefit the most from participating in the program.

Define the Content of the Program

The content of a follow-up visit or telephone call depends on how far a patient has reached in the course of the disease. It is important that optimal treatment according to guidelines and patient education are given directly after the diagnosis. A heart failure management program has a role in the uptitration of drugs such as ACE inhibitors, beta-blockers, angiotensin- and aldosterone-receptor blockers. Since most heart failure nurses do not prescribe drugs, titration protocols, delegations and treatment algorithms are needed as well as routines for prescriptions and consultations.

The first education session should include a definition of heart failure, rationale for and importance of following the prescribed pharmacological and non-pharmacological treatment, as well as what self-care behaviors need to be performed such as symptom monitoring, physical exercise, lifestyle changes, and immunization.[4]

The information about the diagnosis can trigger a crisis for both patients and families due to the feeling that their life might be threatened.[14] Support during the first session in order to adapt to the new situation of living with chronic illness might therefore be needed. One should emphasize that the goal of treatment and self-care is to live with as little limitation as possible in daily life. However, it is important to inform patients that they will not be cured, since many patients during periods of clinical stability feel that the do not suffer from heart failure anymore and might stop taking their medication or observe symptoms.

Patients with heart failure who have been hospitalized are considered as high-risk patients with a poor prognosis and at risk for readmission. The aim of an early outpatient visit is to assess the physiological status in order to detect signs of deterioration, optimize treatment, and discuss side-effects. Furthermore, educational needs should be assessed and additional education provided. Patients should learn to manage symptom monitoring and flexible intake of diuretics when signs and symptoms of fluid retention occur. After a period of deterioration, patients and families may experience insecurity and anxiety and need support. Consultations in nurse-based programs are often longer (30–60 minutes) than visits to the physician and enables a caring assessment, in-depth education and psychosocial support. In order to prevent readmission the cause of the previous admission should be determined and addressed in order to lower the risk for readmissions.

Easy access to care through daily telephone hours facilitates the opportunity to discuss, symptoms, treatment, and self-care behavior with a specialized nurse.

Each program needs documentation. Key parts are the physiological status, sign of heart failure, health and life situation, treatment changes, the education and psychosocial support provided, and the plan for further follow-up.

Recruit and Educate Staff

Defining the amount of staff, the roles and responsibilities for the team members, and what additional education and training they need is important. Is the program mainly run by nurses with medical back-up from a cardiologist or should a multidisciplinary team be involved that will be coordinated by nurses? Often, team members have long experience of cardiac care in combination with a personal interest in heart failure care and additional education within heart failure care and treatment. Since many nurses have extended responsibilities in regard to interpreting laboratory tests and echocardiography, assessing physiological status such as lung auscultation, symptom monitoring and titrating drugs for legal reasons, a written description of these tasks that goes beyond the nursing curriculum might be needed. In the US, many heart failure nurses are clinical nurse specialists or advanced nurse practitioners. Several nurses have master degrees. In Europe, nurses working in heart failure clinics often have quite long experience (>5 years) of cardiac care in combination with additional education in heart failure. In

Sweden and Scotland there are university courses at degree level in heart failure care. In several other European countries there are shorter courses on how to set up and run a heart failure program.[15]

The Role and Responsibilities of the Nurse

A central issue to explore is the role and responsibility of nurses in heart failure programs. Among all tasks, nurses have formal competence for some, delegated responsibility for others, while some extended tasks need additional training and education. There are huge differences both within and between countries regarding the education and competencies of registered nurses. There are legal differences as to what nurses are allowed to do within their license. The whole team needs to agree on the nurse's tasks, responsibilities, and competencies. The job description needs to be clear and in agreement with formal and real competence. Networks for heart failure nurses are important in the further development of the role of nurses as well as the improved possibilities to influence policy makers and stakeholders in healthcare systems. Such networks now exist both in Europe through the Heart Failure Association within the European Society of Cardiology and in the US through the American Association of Heart Failure Nurses and the Heart Failure of Society America.

Effects of Nurse-Based Rehabilitation

During the last few years, several meta-analyses have tried to evaluate the effects of heart failure management programs. One recent meta-analysis performed by McAlister et al.[2] was based on approximately 30 randomized trials of almost 5000 patients that were performed between 1993 and 2004, evaluating the effect of multidisciplinary, often nurse-led, interventions with follow-up and patient education sometimes also combined with optimization of treatment. They found that multidisciplinary, often nurse-led, follow-up in a clinic or home-based setting reduced mortality (RR 0.75, 95% CI 0.59–0.96). The numbers needed to treat in order to save one life was 17. The number of readmissions was decreased by follow-up in a heart failure clinic or home-based setting (RR 0.79, 95% CI 0.68–0.92). Since nurse-based rehabilitation at a quite limited cost reduces readmissions they are cost-effective.[2]

It was concluded that since nurse-based heart failure rehabilitation has positive effects, it should be considered for all patients hospitalized due to deterioration of heart failure.

References

1. McMurray JJ, Stewart S. Epidemiology, aetiology and prognosis of heart failure. Heart 2000;83:596–602.
2. McAlister F, Stewart S, Ferrua S, McMurray J. Multidisciplinary strategies for the management of heart failure patients at high risk for admission. A systematic review of randomized trials. J Am Coll Cardiol 2004;44:810–819.
3. Mejhert M, Holmgren J, Wändell P, Persson H, Edner M. Diagnostic tests, treatment and follow-up in heart failure patients – is there a gender bias in the coherence to guidelines? Eur J Heart Fail 1999;1:407–410.
4. Swedberg K, Cleland J, Dargie H, et al. Guidelines for the diagnosis and treatment of chronic heart failure: executive summary: The Task Force for the diagnosis and treatment of chronic heart failure of the European Society of Cardiology. Eur Heart J 2005;26:1115–1140.
5. Carlson B, Riegel B, Moser D. Self-care abilities of patients with heart failure. Heart Lung 2001;30:351–359.
6. Broström A, Strömberg A, Dahlström U, Fridlund B. Patients with congestive heart failure and their conceptions of their sleep situation. J Adv Nurs 2001;34:520–529.
7. Vinson JM, Rich MW, Sperry JC, Shah AS, McNamara T. Early readmission of elderly patients with congestive heart failure. J Am Geriatr Soc 1990;38:1290–1295.
8. Jaarsma T, Stromberg A, De Geest S, et al. Heart failure management programmes in Europe. Eur J Cardiol Nurs 2006;5:197–205.
9. Louis A, Turner T, Gretton M, Baksh A, Cleland J. A systematic review of telemonitoring for the management of heart failure. Eur J Heart Fail 2003;5:583–590.
10. Krumholz HM, Amatruda J, Smith GL, et al. Randomized trial of an education and support intervention to prevent readmission of patients with heart failure. J Am Coll Cardiol 2002;39:83–89.

11. Koelling T, Johnson M, Cody R, Aaronson K. Discharge education improves clinical outcomes in patients with chronic heart failure. Circulation 2005;111:179–185.

12. Ledwidge M, Ryan E, O'loughlin C, et al. Heart failure care in a hospital unit: a comparison of standard 3-month and extended 6-month programmes. Eur J Heart Fail 2005;7:385–391.

13. Strömberg A, Mårtensson J, Fridlund B, Levin L-Å, Karlsson J-E, Dahlström U. Nurse-based heart failure clinics improve survival and self-care behaviour in patients with heart failure. Results from a prospective, randomised study. Eur Heart J 2003;24:1014–1023.

14. Stull DE, Starling R, Haas G, Young JB. Becoming a patient with heart failure. Heart Lung 1999;28:284–292.

15. Blue L, McMurray J. How much responsibility should nurses take? Eur J Heart Fail 2005;7:351–361.

38
Returning to Work after Myocardial Infarction

Joep Perk

One of the main goals of a cardiac rehabilitation (CR) program is to support the patient in returning to work: strong economic and quality of life arguments exist. It has been stated that patients after an acute myocardial infarction (MI) without complications such as left ventricular dysfunction or exercise-induced myocardial ischemia may safely resume their previous work: for light office work 2 weeks of sickness absence are recommended, for average manual work 3 weeks, and for strenuous physical work 6 weeks. Thus, a majority of MI patients may well return to work (RTW) within the first month after discharge from hospital, as almost all industrial and other jobs require significantly less effort than the average maximum work capacity of a healthy population: only 25% is generally demanded for the modern workplace.

Yet few patients resume work early: the median time is 50 days in most countries but and there are considerable differences between individual countries. In Europe and the United States between 60% and 93% rates of RTW have been reported in surveys. This may well be an overestimate as less than 70% remain at work one year after MI, less than 50% after 4 years.

Is there an explanation for the discrepancy between the chance of an early RTW and the actual praxis? Can, or should, CR programs play a role? The answer is yes. Inability to work after MI is determined by medical, psychosocial, and economic or job-related factors. Among the medical and patient factors, the main determinants are age, sex, education, previous MI, severity of MI, residual angina pectoris, poor left ventricular function, and a low exercise capacity. The psychosocial factors include anxiety and depression post-MI, stress at the workplace, motivation to resume work, and the patient's own perception of the severity of the disease. Among the economic and job-related factors, health insurance benefits and other financial incentives, employment rates, physical and mental workload demands are important prognostic factors.

It has been shown that the medical factors only play a minor role, with the other factors dominating the prognosis of RTW. Here the role of a CR team to support a patient to return to work is a truly multidisciplinary task. Knowledge of the patient's expectations and physical limitations must be translated into individually adapted exercise training. Psychosocial needs must be addressed carefully and the economic benefits of an early RTW must be weighed against the possible risks for work-related recurrence of cardiac events. Therefore, at the onset of CR an individual strategy for a successful and lasting return to work should be created. This strategy builds upon elements from three phase: the period before, during, and after the MI.

Relevant Factors from the Period Before MI

The CR team has a variety of pre-MI factors to consider when planning the road back to work: elderly and female patients, persons with a low level of education, and those living far away from the workplace all tend to resume work to a lesser degree. Surveys have shown that these are the populations that have poor access to CR, low participation rates, and a considerable drop-out. They are clearly in need of special CR efforts, an adapted program design.

An analysis of the work environment and demands is mandatory including the degree of job satisfaction and economic reward, the physical burden and any perceived employment stress, and the presence of conflicts at the workplace. What is the role of the labor market, is there a threat of unemployment? Has the patient noted symptoms of angina pectoris during work or does he or she believe the disease is caused by the work environment? Have there been any thoughts of an early retirement or a change of job/profession? Any notable financial consequences or a loss of social status? The summary of this individual job analysis should be available for the CR team at the beginning of the program.

Relevant Factors from the Hospital Phase

In several programs cardiac rehabilitation does not start until the patient is referred to the CR center. This causes an unwanted delay in the recovery process. Over the years the average duration of the hospital admission has shortened; after an uncomplicated MI patients may remain 3–4 days before discharge, which gives the CR team ample time to inform and engage the patient in the aftercare. This unsatisfactory situation may even be aggravated if the acute care hospital lacks resources for cardiac rehabilitation and the patient may have to wait weeks before being enrolled in a comprehensive program. Acute care and the following rehabilitation should be a streamlined service in order to be effective.

The information from the acute phase is highly relevant for the tailoring of the post-MI care: Which acute interventions were performed? Were there any serious complications? Has the patient developed signs of heart failure or is there a risk of malignant arrhythmia? Is there any residual ischemia that can or will not be treated with further coronary intervention?

Is drug treatment considered to be optimal or is there a need for adaptation during the period after discharge and have there been any significant side-effects? Has smoking cessation been successful and were there signs of severe anxiety or depression that need attention? Which information has the patient and the family received during the hospital stay and at discharge?

As from the pre-MI period, a complete inventory of the acute phase should be available for the multidisciplinary CR team at the start of rehabilitation.

Relevant Factors from the Post-MI Period

Information from the patient's physical and mental recovery, from the social environment and from the workplace should be added to the information from the pre- and acute MI phase when preparing for an early return to work or for a decision to advise a change of job or even a permanent withdrawal from working life. For the CR team the following questions need answers: Has the patient regained the desired physical work capacity or is there a persisting disability? Is the patient motivated to resume work, or is he or she limited by poor self-confidence? Is there an exaggerated perception of disability with the onset of psychosomatic complaints, as tends to occur after 2–3 months of sickness absence?

Is the attitude of family and friends supportive and is there understanding and encouragement from the employer, supervisor, and colleagues? Is the employer willing to contribute to a change in the patient's work environment if needed?

Who decides formally about sick leave, the family doctor, factory health service, health insurance physicians, the cardiologist, others? Are generous sick leave benefits an obstacle for RTW? The answers to these questions may form the base of an action plan in which possible limiting factors are attended to. Thus, combining data from all three phases gives the information needed for the planning of an optimal RTW strategy. This may be expected to enhance an early and lasting RTW, but is this assumption evidence-based?

Survey of the Literature on RTW (Table 38-1)

The answer may be found in a recent review: fourteen studies from the past 25 years were assessed to be of sufficient quality according to the standard used by the Swedish Council on Technology Assessment in Health Care.[1] Two studies describe outcomes during the first year post-MI, six studies present predictors for RTW, and six studies describe the outcome of interventions aimed at limiting sickness absence.

RTW Post-MI

Herlitz et al.[2] in a prospective cohort study investigated all patients <65 years with MI and who were employed part-time or full-time prior to infarction: 37% had returned to full-time work and 12% to part-time work one year post-MI. Higher age and larger infarctions influenced the outcome negatively. Boudrez et al.,[3] in the city of Gent, Belgium, found that of all men <60 years who had experienced MI only a few were on long-term sick leave due to heart disease. During the course of the first year 85% had returned to work.

Predictors for RTW

Maeland et al.[4,5] followed 249 MI patients <67 years for half a year post-MI: 25% were still on sick leave. Social and psychological factors negatively influenced the possibility of return to work: high age, low education, residence (worse in rural areas), stress at the workplace and anxiety, depression, and poor self-confidence.

Wiklund et al.,[6] in a cohort study of 201 male MI patients <60 years at work prior to MI, showed that the motivation to return to work was the main predictive factor. Patients with physically demanding jobs returned to work to a lesser degree than patients with lighter jobs.

More recently, similar findings have been reported: a study of first-MI patients from New Zealand found that 58% of the patients were working after half a year.[7] The patients' perception that the disease was an obstacle for returning to work predicted longer sick leave. Soejima et al.[8] showed that 83% of male Japanese MI patients were back at work after 8 months. The prevalence of depression and worry concerning one's own health were predictive of lower RTW. Smith and O'Rourke[9] found in a study from the US that individuals with higher socioeconomic status had a greater chance of returning to work: 72% of all patients returned to work, a higher number in those with high socioeconomic status.

Interventions to Improve RTW

Dennis et al.[10] showed that advice from a cardiologist to the patient's family physician could shorten sickness absence. The intervention group reported a shorter sick leave duration (51 vs. 75 days). This could not be reproduced when advice was provided by a non-hospital-based cardiologist.[11]

Bengtsson[12] could not show a reduction in sickness absence in the study group. Hedbäck and Perk[13] did not find any effect after the first year in comparison with a study group and a control group (62% vs. 57%), even though regular contact was made with the workplace to reduce the duration of sick leave. However, increasingly more individuals in the control group were sick-listed, and at 5-year follow-up significantly more were still at work among the CR participants (52% vs. to 27%). Froelicher et al.[14] offered three alternatives for aftercare: participation in an exercise group, exercise including counseling, or only standard aftercare. In this study from the US only a few were sick-listed, and 94% were at work after 6 months regardless of the design of aftercare. Nursing-based psychosocial intervention as part of CR did not influence RTW, as shown by Burgess et al.[15]

In summary, the review has shown that at least half of the patients following MI return to work within the first year. Regarding the outcome of aftercare and CR programs several improvements in program design, access, and application are recommended below:

The Role of Cardiac Rehabilitation: Physical Training

The physical capacity of patients early post-MI is diminished due to physical deconditioning, a possible loss of cardiac reserve and the effect of drug treatment. Exercise training influences VO_{2max}, blood lipid levels, platelet aggregation, and fibrinolysis, and protects against malignant arrhythmia. Exercise-related dyspnea, fatigue, and angina may be alleviated.

TABLE 38-1. Return to work after myocardial infarction

Author, publication year, reference number and country	Aim	Focus of study	n	Mean age distribution	Type of sick leave data	Intervention	% return-to-work	Results
Herlitz, 1994,[2] Sweden	Outcome of morbidity and RTW 1 year post-MI	All patients admitted to a specific hospital for MI	921	72, 16–98	Percentage RTW of total groups and of groups <65 y	Standard medical treatment	49%	Under 65: 37% full-time, 12% part-time. Age and infarction size predicts RTW
Boudrez, 1994,[3] Belgium	RTW after MI	Males ≤60 years in a regional infarction register	295	57.5 years	Data via mailed survey 1991. Only RTW	60% participated in a rehabilitation program	85%	69% of all subjects RTW, 85% of those who worked before MI. Few cases of remaining sick leave
Maeland, 1986,[4] Norway	RTW 6 months post-MI in relation to job before, demographic factors, and disease severity	Consecutive group patients after MI <67 years	249	<67	RTW and sick leave 6 months post-MI	Standard medical treatment	72.7%	See below. Residence, age, education, stress at work and with complications predict RTW
Maeland, 1987,[5] Norway	RTW 6 months post-MI vs. psychological variables	Consecutive group patients after MI <67 years	249	<67	RTW and sick leave 6 months post-MI	Standard medical treatment	72.7%	73% RTW half a year post-MI, 25% remained sick listed. Perception, anxiety, depression at hospital predictors for RTW
Wiklund, 1985,[6] Sweden	Predictors of RTW 2 and 12 months post-MI	Male patients <60 years, working before MI	201	<60	Via mailed survey/telephone: return-to-work 2 and 12 months post-MI	Standard medical treatment	75%	Importance of psychological factors in RTW. Patients indicated association between work and MI
Petrie, 1996,[7] New Zealand	RTW 6 months post-MI in relation to patient's perception and participation in cardiac rehabilitation	Consecutive group patients after first MI <65 years	143	53.2 ± 8.4	RTW and sick leave 3 and 6 months post-MI	Participation a combined rehabilitation program	58%	40/105 RTW after 6 wk, 76 after 6 months. Initial perception of disease severity determines the prognosis
Soejima, 1999,[8] Japan	RTW 8 months post-MI in relation to psychological and clinical variables	First-time MI, men ≤65 years, in full-time job previously.	134	54.3	Via mailed survey/telephone: RTW on average 8 months post-MI	Standard medical treatment	82.9%	Age, depression, perception of health, difficulty in managing stress but not infarction size determine RTW
Smith, 1988,[9] US	RTW 1 year post-MI vs. work before, demographic factors and degree of severity of the disease	Consecutive group patients after first MI <70 years	151	51.2 ± 8	Via mailed survey/telephone: RTW 4 and 12 months post-MI	Standard medical treatment	72%	Educational level, physical demands of job, perception of disease, and economic motives mainly determine RTW

Study	Design/aim	Population	n	Age	Outcome measure	Intervention	Result	Findings
Dennis, 1988,[10] US	RCT of targeted advice based on cardiac stress test after uncomplicated MI	MI patients (male) ≤60, with uncomplicated MI, worked before	201: 102 vs. 90	49 and 50 ± 7	Detailed information on time, degree, and type of RTW 6 months post-MI.	Early stress test and targeted advice on sick-leave duration to primary care	91% vs. 88%	Shorter sick leave with targeted advice: 51 vs. 75 days post-MI. RTW: 32% reduction which gave $2102 as extra income in the study group
Pilote, 1992,[11] US	RCT of targeted advice based on stress-ECG in men after uncomplicated MI vs. standard care	Consecutive group patients after MI ≤60 years, working before MI	187: 95 vs. 92	50 vs. 51 ± 6 vs. 7	Via mailed survey/telephone: RTW 1,3 and 6 months post-MI	Early stress test and targeted advice on sick-leave duration to primary care	91% vs. 95%	No difference after 6 months. Patients without residual ischemia at work sooner 38 vs. 65 days.
Bengtsson, 1983,[12] Sweden	The outcome of a rehabilitation program after MI	Infarction patients <65 years	87: 44 vs. 43	39–65	Number of sick-leave days year 1, % RTW	Combined cardiac rehabilitation program	85%	No significant difference in RTW between CR and control. Av. 177 vs. 172 full-time sick-leave days, 58 vs. 98 part-time days
Hedbäck, 1987,[13] Sweden	The outcome of a rehabilitation program post-MI with standard treatment	All patients <65 years admitted for acute MI	305: 148 vs. 157	57.3 vs. 57.2	Return at 5 years post-MI	Combined cardiac rehabilitation program vs. standard treatment	51.8% vs. 27.4%	No difference after 1 year (61.5% vs. 56.5%, but after 2 years (64.9% vs. 43.1%) and after 5 years
Froelicher, 1994,[14] US	Two different interventions post-MI with standard treatment	All survivors ≤70 years with MI	258: 84 vs. 88 vs. 86	57.1 vs. 55.6 vs. 56.3	RTW 12 and 24 weeks after discharge	Physical exercise, vs. physical exercise + education vs. standard treatment	94%	83% returned to work at 12 weeks post-MI, 94% after 24 weeks. No difference between groups
Burgess, 1987,[15] US	RCT of psychosocial rehabilitation post-MI	MI patients who worked at least 20 hours/week before infarction	180: 89 vs. 91	50.9 ± 7.4	Numbers RTW 3–4 and 13 months after MI. Percent moved to another job and sick-listed	Nursing-based psychosocial intervention	88% vs. 88%	10% still sick-listed after 13 months, no effect from intervention

RCT: randomized controlled trial.

The benefits of physical training post-MI for RTW are a high degree of functional recovery, an improvement in psychological status, and enhanced self-confidence in the ability to perform physical work. In spite of this, conventional training programs appear to have a limited effect on RTW when compared to patients who have not participated in CR. Therefore CR training programs should adapt to the actual work conditions of the patient: even though the physiological effect of training may be equally beneficial for each patient, an office clerk will have different work capacity needs than a forestry worker. This applies even to exercise testing: the conventional treadmill or ergometer bicycle stress test has little resemblance to the average industrial job. Vocational exercise testing and training should simulate the patient's work environment. Based upon the medical information of the referring cardiologist and the background data from the workplace, the physiotherapist can choose the appropriate model of exercise training.

The Role of Cardiac Rehabilitation: Psychological Support and Stress Management

Psychosocial factors play an important role in the prevalence and in the progression of coronary artery disease. This has consequences for the provision of psychosocial support within the framework of a CR service. The psychological expertise within the CR team should advise the employer on means of limiting a stressful work environment in patients where mental stress or strain at the workplace has been reported. Patients may be helped by participating in stress management classes or in special cases through individual counseling by a psychologist. Overprotection by family and friends and the attitude of work colleagues and supervisors may extend sickness absence. Here clear and timely information from the CR team is invaluable! Anxiety and depression should be diagnosed early post-MI and treated if indicated with pharmacotherapy. Repeated mental reinforcement within the CR program may help the patient to regain self-confidence and trust in the ability to face work demands.

The Role of Cardiac Rehabilitation: Vocational Counseling

This area remains insufficiently developed in a majority of the programs around Europe. In general, physical training, dietary advice, smoking cessation, psychological support, and drug treatment are the core components. In some centers specialized occupational therapists have been engaged, in other centers cooperation with corporate health services in larger industries has been organized, but a structured program for RTW is often missing. A specific function within the multidisciplinary team is recommended (specialized nurse, occupational therapist, or physiotherapist) where relevant information from the patient, the social environment, and the workplace is gathered and an RTW plan is applied. The person performing this function will act as communicator between the CR service and the workplace. The main items for this service are shown as a checklist in Table 38-2. Early post-MI information to the employer is of special practical relevance. Is there a need for a short-term or permanent replacement for the patient? Is there a recommendation to change the present job or are adaptations at the workplace needed? Can a relation between the work environment and the MI be suspected and does this have consequences for other workers? Work task-adapted training programs and work-simulated exercise testing may be used. Interesting results have been reported from the use of Holter ECG monitoring during a test-run of 2 hours at the

TABLE 38-2. Checklist

- Are there any relevant limitations for RTW in the pre-MI job: heavy physical or mental demands, conflicts?
- Is the patient motivated?
- Early post-MI contact with employer, factory health services and/or family doctor
- Create an RTW plan, including expected length of sick leave
- Inform employer about length and degree of sickness absence
- Encourage regular and early contact between patient and workplace (at least weekly visits)
- Adapt the training program to physical demands at work
- Consider the appropriate exercise test before RTW when needed
- Use low-intensity work during sick leave as a bridge for RTW
- Use part-time work as a bridge for RTW
- Maintain contact between patient and CR team during the first months after RTW

patient's workplace. In patients with physically or mentally strenuous work demands, a gradual increase of work hours from part-time to full-time is often a valuable bridge between post-MI disability and a normal productive life. During this transition period continued support and encouragement from the CR team may be requested, even if the exercise training has been concluded.

Conclusion

Advances in emergency care, coronary intervention technique, and post-MI prevention have improved the medical prognosis, but the social prognosis, that is, the opportunity to return to work, appears to have remained unchanged over the past decades. It is time that the advances in medical care are translated into improvements in the socioeconomic sphere. Relevant medical, psychological, and socioeconomic information should be summarized in a concise definition of the needs and demands of the patient. A multidisciplinary CR team well connected to the acute care hospital but also to workplaces in the local community will then be able to provide a tailormade service contributing to a timely and lasting return to normal social life and work.

References

1. Perk J, Alexandersson K. Sick leave due to coronary artery disease or stroke. Scand J Public Health 2004; suppl 63:181–206.
2. Herlitz J, Karlson BW, Sjolin M, et al. Prognosis during one year of follow-up after acute myocardial infarction with emphasis on morbidity. Clin Cardiol 1994;17:15–20.
3. Boudrez H, De Backer G, Comhaire B. Return to work after myocardial infarction: results of a longitudinal population based study. Eur Heart J 1994;15:32–36.
4. Maeland JG, Havik OE. Psychological predictors for return to work after a myocardial infarction. J Psychosom Res 1987;4:471–481.
5. Maeland JG, Havik OE. Return to work after a myocardial infarction: the influence of background factors, work characteristics and illness severity. Scand J Soc Med 1986;14:183–195.
6. Wiklund I, Sanne H, Vendin A, Wilhelmsson C. Determinants of return to work after myocardial infarction. J Cardiac Rehabil 1985;5:62–72.
7. Petrie KJ, Weinman J, Sharpe N, Buckley J. Role of patients' view of their illness in predicting return to work and functioning after myocardial infarction: longitudinal study. BMJ 1996;312:1191–1194.
8. Soejima Y, Steptoe A, Nozoe S, Tei C. Psychosocial and clinical factors predicting resumption of work following acute myocardial infarction in Japanese men. Int J Cardiol 1999;72:39–47.
9. Smith R, O'Rourke DF. Return to work after a first myocardial infarction. JAMA 1988;259:1673–1677.
10. Dennis C, Houston-Miller N, Schwartz RG, et al. Early return to work after uncomplicated myocardial infarction. Results of a randomized trial. JAMA 1988;260:214–220.
11. Pilote L, Thomas RJ, Dennis C, et al. Return to work after uncomplicated myocardial infarction: a trial of practice guidelines in the community. Ann Intern Med 1992;117:383–389.
12. Bengtsson K. Rehabilitation after myocardial infarction. Scand J Rehabil Med 1983;15:1–9.
13. Hedbäck B, Perk J. 5-year results of a comprehensive rehabilitation programme after myocardial infarction. Eur Heart J 1987;8:234–242.
14. Froehlicher ES, Kee LL, Newton KM, et al. Return to work, sexual activity, and other activities after acute myocardial infarction. Heart Lung 1994;23:423–435.
15. Burgess AW, Lerner DJ, D'Agostino RB, Vokonas PS, Hartman CR, Gaccione P. A randomized control trial of cardiac rehabilitation. Soc Sci Med 1987; 24:359–370.

39
Return to Work after Coronary Interventions

Philippe Sellier

One of the objectives of coronary interventions is to enable patients to return to work. This is also one of the aims of the cardiac rehabilitation programs offered to these patients. The inability to resume professional activities after coronary interventions may constitute a stress (and therefore a risk factor) for the patient due to a loss of self-esteem and earnings.

The most frequent coronary interventions currently in use are aorto-coronary bypass graft surgery (CABG) and percutaneous coronary angioplasty or intervention (PCI). Both are expensive and contribute to the high cost of treating coronary disease. The economic consequences are even more severe if the patient does not return to work afterwards.

In this context, we need to improve our understanding of the factors increasing or decreasing the probability of a return to work, to make it possible to implement appropriate measures to facilitate the return to professional activity after coronary interventions.

Return to Work after Aorto-coronary Bypass Graft Surgery

Rate and Delay for Return to Work

Between 59%[1] and 100%[2] of patients who were working before surgery return to work after CABG (Tables 39-1, 39-3), with an average of about 75%. The mean delay to return to work is generally about 3 months, with a value of 3.2 ± 2.2 months reported in the prospective study

PERISCOP[3] and of 67 ± 58 days in the surgical arm of the study by Mark et al.[4]

Medical Factors

Many studies have attempted to analyze the factors that have a significant effect on return to work after CABG.

Medical History

Diabetes may be predictive of failure to return to work.[5] However, many authors have reported that diabetes has no effect on the likelihood of returning to work.[3,4,6,7] A history of myocardial infarction has no significant effect on the likelihood of returning to work.[3] In contrast, Mark et al. reported that diffuse peripheral vascular damage is a negative factor for return to work.[4]

Severity of Coronary Disease

Preserved left ventricular function is a positive factor for return to work.[8] In the study by Boudrez and De Backer,[8] mean left ventricular ejection fraction was 0.71 ± 0.12 in those who returned to work, and 0.62 ± 0.18 in those who did not ($P < 0.01$). Hlatky et al.[7] also reported that a good left ventricular function increased the probability of return to work at the end of a 4-year follow-up period. Conversely, other studies have reported that a depressed left ventricular function decreases the likelihood of returning to work.[5] According to Mark et al.,[4] congestive cardiac

TABLE 39-1. Studies on return to work after coronary artery bypass surgery

Authors	Period of study	Patients (n)	Average follow-up (months)	% RTW (active patients)
Perk[1]	1980–1985	49	12	59
Monpère[14]	1988	57	7	73
Speziale[10]	1995	213	38	78.7
Skinner[6]	1988–1989	353	12	84
Boudrez[8]	1995-1998	136	12	81
PERISCOP[3]	1998–1999	530	12	67.5

RTW: return to work.

failure also decreases the likelihood of returning to work, with an odds ratio of 0.20 (95% CI: 0.10–0.39; $P < 0.0001$).

The severity of coronary lesions also has a debatable effect. The number of coronary arteries affected has no significant effect on the likelihood of returning to work.[3,6,9] According to Boudrez and De Backer,[8] complete revascularization is a positive factor for return to work. In the PERISCOP study,[3] complete revascularization was observed in 78.2% of patients who returned to work and in 75% of those who did not; this difference is not significant.

Cardiac arrhythmias,[3] detected by Holter recording carried out after the end of bypass surgery, have no significant effect on the likelihood of returning to work, regardless of whether these problems result from numerous premature ventricular contractions or from residual ventricular tachycardia.

Cardiac Symptoms

Cardiac symptoms also play an important role in determining the likelihood of returning to work after CABG:

- *Persistent angina symptoms* decrease the likelihood of returning to work.[3,9,10] According to Skinner et al.,[6] the absence of angina increases the likelihood of returning to work. However, it should be noted that a positive effort test, showing an ST-segment depression at peak exercise >1 mm, has no significant effect[3] on the likelihood of returning to work. It therefore seems that only symptoms associated with myocardial ischemia are important.

- *Persistent dyspnea* has also been reported to decrease the likelihood of returning to work after CABG.[3]

Postoperative Physical Capacity

Good effort tolerance is a medical variable with a positive predictive value for return to work after CABG. In the PERISCOP study,[3] the duration of the exercise test was 543 ± 183 seconds in those who returned to work and 481 ± 168 seconds in those who did not ($P = 0.00024$). These results are consistent with those obtained by Engblom et al.[11]

Other Factors

Functional Class

Patients with a functional class I or II according to the New York Heart Association (NYHA) classification before surgery are more likely to return to work.[11]

Psychological Factors

The degree to which the patient is motivated to return to work plays a positive role according to Boudrez and De Backer,[8] Engblom et al.,[11] and Hlatky et al.[7]

The depression that may follow CABG decreases the likelihood of returning to work. In the study by Stanton et al.,[12] 56% of patients who were not depressed returned to work after surgery, versus only 16% of depressed patients.

Socio-Professional Factors

Many socio-professional factors have a significant effect on the likelihood of the patient returning to work after CABG.

Age

The older the patient, the less likely he or she is to return to work.[3,4,6,9,10,11,13] Speziale et al.[10] reported that age is a negative factor for return to work, with an odds ratio of 4.44 (95% CI: 1.3–15.0). In this study, 78.3% of patients below the age of 50 years returned to work compared to only 60.7% of patients over the age of 50.

In the PERISCOP study,[3] the mean age of the patients who had returned to work after CABG during the first year was 49.6 ± 5.7 years and the mean age of those who had not was 52.6 ± 5.4 years ($P < 0.001$).

The Patient's Educational Level

Generally, the more educated the patient, the more likely he or she is to return to work after bypass surgery.[4,7,10]

Socio-professional Category

Belonging to a high socio-professional category increases the chances of a patient returning to work after CABG.[4,8,10,14] Speziale et al.[10] reported that belonging to a low socio-professional category significantly decreased the likelihood of a patient returning to work, with an odds ratio of 0.65 (95% CI: 0.16–0.95). In contrast, Engblom et al.[11] found that socio-professional category had no significant effect on the likelihood of returning to work.

Physical Activity Associated with Work

The probability of returning to work is lower if the patient's former job involves intense physical activity. According to Boudrez and De Backer,[8] only 50% of patients with jobs involving heavy manual work returned to work, versus 80–88% of patients with moderately heavy or light jobs ($P < 0.02$). However, this difference did not remain significant in multivariate analysis.

Social Support

Boudrez and De Backer[8] found a relationship between the frequency of return to work and the presence of solid social support, particularly from the patient's colleagues. This relationship was significant only in univariate analysis, disappearing in logistic regression models.

Previous Employment Status

The employment status of the patient before surgery (in active employment, unemployed, or on sick leave) plays a key role in determining whether the patient will return to work. Patients who were not working before surgery rarely return to work.[6–11] According to Speziale et al.,[10] being in active employment before CABG is predictive of a return to work (odds ratio 4.20; 95% CI: 1.5–13.5). Similarly, the longer the patient is on sick leave before surgery, the less likely the patient is to return to work after surgery.[1,6,11]

Effect of Cardiac Rehabilitation after CABG on the Likelihood of Returning to Work

The effect of cardiac rehabilitation programs after CABG on the likelihood of returning to work is unclear. In a case-control study, Perk et al.[1] compared 49 patients following global rehabilitation programs after CABG with 98 patients who underwent surgery and then received the usual treatment. One year after bypass surgery, the rate of return to work was 59% for the group undergoing rehabilitation, and 64% for those on usual treatment (not significant). Other authors have also shown that cardiac rehabilitation programs have no significant effect.[11] In this last study, only the group of patients under the age of 55 years undergoing cardiac rehabilitation had a rate of return to work higher than the control group (60% vs. 35%, $P = 0.002$). Monpère et al.[14] compared the results of two non-synchronous studies and demonstrated that occupational health physicians played a positive role in the return to work, increasing the rate of return to work from 51% to 78%.

Return to Work after Coronary Angioplasty

Rate and Delay for Return to Work

The rate of return to work after PCI at one year is similar to that for CABG (Table 39-2). In a study by Danchin et al.,[15] the rate of return to work was 73%. In the subgroups of patients undergoing

TABLE 39-2. Return to work after coronary angioplasty

Authors	Period of study	Patients (n)	Average follow-up (months)	% RTW (active patients)
Danchin[15]	1980–1982	77	?	73
Ben-Ari[19]	1983–1984	175	18	74
Holmes[17]	1984	2250	18	81–86

RTW: return to work.

TABLE 39-3. Comparative studies on return to work rate after coronary artery bypass surgery or angioplasty

Authors	Publication (year)	CABG (n)	PCI (n)	Mean follow-up (months)	% RTW (CABG)	% RTW (PCI)	P value
Jang[20]	1982	151	163	19	69	79	NS
Laird-Meeter[9]	1989	125	94	12	63	76	NS
McGee[2]	1993	112	119	6–18	100	100	NS
Mark[4]	1994	449	312	12	79	84	NS
RITA[13]	1996	251	267	24	62	65	NS
BARI[16]	1997	217	192	48	82	82	NS

% RTW: rate of work resumption after revascularization, only in patients working before. CABG: coronary artery bypass graft surgery; PCI: percutaneous coronary intervention.

angioplasty in comparative studies (mostly comparing angioplasty with bypass surgery), the rates of return to work vary from 63% to 100% of the patients working before surgery (Table 39-3). The delay to return to work is also highly variable and has decreased over time. In 1984, Danchin et al.[15] reported that patients returned to work an average of 4 months after surgery. In the "PCI" arm of comparative studies, the median time to return to work was 27 days in the Mark et al. study,[4] 4.9 weeks (2.7 to 10.9) in the BARI study[16] and almost 20 days in the RITA study in 1990.[13]

Medical Factors

Several studies comparing the effects of PCI and CABG have investigated factors affecting the likelihood of returning to work, but none has identified the specific effect of each of these treatment strategies. However, certain factors making a return to work less likely have been identified. These factors are age,[11,15] the persistence of anginal pain,[13,15,17] and the result of angioplasty.[15]

Socio-professional Factors

According to Laird-Meeter et al.,[9] not working before angioplasty makes a return to work significantly less likely. However, the type of work done and job satisfaction have no significant effect on the likelihood of returning to work.

Role of Rehabilitation in the Return to Work

Hoffman-Bang et al.[18] randomized 150 patients undergoing coronary angioplasty into an intervention group (cardiac rehabilitation program) and a control group. The rate of return to work at 12 and 24 months was 74% and 78%, respectively, in the intervention group and 68% and 61%, respectively, in the control group (not significant). Ben-Ari et al.[19] found that the rate of return to work at 18 months was significantly higher for patients following cardiac rehabilitation programs than for other patients (84% vs. 64%; $P < 0.01$).

Comparison of Aorto-Coronary Bypass Surgery and Coronary Angioplasty

Many studies have shown that angioplasty only has a positive effect on delay to return to work, with the rates of return to work being similar at the end of follow-up for both therapeutic strategies.[2,4,7]

Conclusions

Only 60–80% of patients working before surgery return to work after myocardial revascularization. Patients return to work slightly sooner after PCI than after CABG, but the long-term results are similar for the two treatments.

The medical factors influencing return to work are essentially the presence of symptoms, which has a negative effect, and ability to tolerate effort, which has a positive effect. The severity of coronary disease, in patients without symptoms, has only a slight effect.

As after myocardial infarction, social factors such as age, educational level, socio-professional category, and level of physical activity involved in the patient's work play an important role in the likelihood of returning to work.

Cardiac rehabilitation, studied almost exclusively in patients undergoing CABG, has no significant demonstrated effect on the likelihood of returning to work. The promising results obtained in a study of cardiac rehabilitation after angioplasty require confirmation. However, specific interventions, particularly those of an occupational physician, facilitating the transfer of information to the company doctor and social reinsertion, are clearly of great value.

References

1. Perk J, Hedbäck B, Engwall J. Effects of cardiac rehabilitation after coronary artery bypass grafting on readmissions, return to work, and physical fitness. A case-control study. Scand J Soc Med 1990; 18:45–51.

2. Mc Gee HM, Graham T, Crowe B, et al. Return to work following coronary artery bypass surgery or percutaneous transluminal coronary angioplasty Eur Heart J 1993;14:623–628.

3. Sellier P, Varaillac P, Chatellier G, et al. on behalf of the investigators of the PERISCOP study. Factors influencing return to work at one year after coronary bypass graft surgery: results of the PERISCOP study. Eur J Cardiovasc Prev Rehabil 2003;10: 469–475.

4. Mark DB, Lam LC, Lee KL, et al. Effect of coronary angioplasty, coronary bypass surgery, and medical therapy on employment in patients with coronary artery disease. A prospective comparisons study. Ann Intern Med 1994;120:111–117.

5. Maor Y, Cohen Y, Olmer L, et al. Factors associated with health indicators in patients undergoing coronary artery bypass surgery. Chest 1999;116:1570–1574.

6. Skinner JS, Farrer M, Albers CJ, et al. Patient-related outcomes five years after coronary

7. Hlatky MA, Boothroyd D, Horine S, et al. Employment after coronary angioplasty or coronary bypass surgery in patients employed at the time of revascularization. Ann Intern Med 1998;129:543–547.

8. Boudrez H, De Backer G. Recent findings on return to work after an acute myocardial infarction or coronary artery bypass grafting. Acta Cardiol 2000;55(6):341–349.

9. Laird-Meeter K, Erdman RAM, van Domburg R, et al. Probability of a return to work after either coronary balloon dilatation or coronary bypass surgery. Eur Heart J 1989;10:917–922.

10. Speziale G, Bilotta F, Ruvolo G, et al. Return to work and quality of life measurement in coronary artery bypass grafting. Eur J Cardiothorac Surg 1996;10:852–858.

11. Engblom E, Hämäläinen H, Rönnemaa T, Vanttinen E, Kallio V, Knuts LR. Cardiac rehabilitation and return to work after coronary artery bypass surgery. Qual Life Res 1994;3:207–213.

12. Stanton SA, Jenkins CD, Denlinger P, et al. Prediction of employment status after cardiac surgery. JAMA 1983;249:907–911.

13. Pocock SJ, Henderson RA, Seed P, et al. Quality of life, employment status, and anginal symptoms after coronary angioplasty or bypass surgery. 3-year follow-up in the randomised intervention treatment of angina (RITA) trial. Circulation 1996;94:135–141.

14. Monpère C, François G, Rondeau du Noyer C, et al. Return to work after rehabilitation in coronary bypass patients. Role of the occupational medicine specialist during rehabilitation. Eur Heart J 1988; 9(suppl L):48–53.

15. Danchin N, Cuilliere M, Mathieu P, et al. Socio-professional rehabilitation after transluminal coronary angioplasty. Arch Mal Coeur Vaiss. 1984;9:993–997.

16. The writing group for the Bypass Angioplasty Revascularization Investigation (BARI) investigators. Five-year clinical and functional outcome comparing bypass surgery and angioplasty in patients with multivessel coronary disease. JAMA 1997;277:715–721.

17. Holmes DR Jr, Van Raden MJ, Reeder GS, et al. Return to work after coronary angioplasty: a report of the National Heart, Lung, and Blood Institute percutaneous transluminal coronary angioplasty Registry. Am J Cardiol 19984;53: 48C–51C.

18. Hoffman-Bang C, Lisspers J, Nordlander R, et al. Two-year results of a controlled study of residential rehabilitation for patients treated with percuta-

neous transluminal coronary angioplasty. Eur Heart J 1999;20:1465–1474.

19. Ben-Ari E, Rothbaum DA, Linnemeier TA, et al. Return to work after successful coronary angioplasty. J Cardiopulm Rehabil 1992;12:20–24.

20. Jang GC, Gruentzig AR, Black PC, et al. Work profile following coronary angioplasty or coronary bypass surgery: results from a national cooperative study. Circulation 1982;66(Suppl II):II, 123.

40
Sexual Counseling of the Cardiac Patient

Tiny Jaarsma and Elaine E. Steinke

Introduction

It is often expected that among seriously ill patients sexuality is not important. However, satisfaction with sexual functioning is recognized as a component that influences quality of life. Studies show that patients who are chronically or critically ill are concerned about sexual dysfunction. Sexual function has been studied in some chronic disease states, especially in diabetes, cancer, spinal cord injury, and some cardiac diseases. For example, sexual function in patients after myocardial infarction (MI) or after coronary artery bypass grafting (CABG) has been studied since the 1970s and 1980s. More recently sexual function in patients with heart transplantation or heart failure has been studied. It is known that there are many important links between sexual activity and heart disease:

- Heart disease can result in both reduced sexual activity and increase sexual dysfunction, for example due to fear or symptoms.
- Heart disease and erectile dysfunction share important risk factors such as diabetes and hypertension.
- Sexual activity, like all forms of exertion and/or stress, may trigger cardiac symptoms.
- Medications used to treat heart disease may impair sexual function.
- Drugs that are used to treat sexual dysfunction may have serious interactions with medications used to treat heart disease.

All these complicated relationships can keep healthcare providers from addressing the issue of sexuality in patients with heart disease. Healthcare providers may believe that discussing sexuality causes anxiety in the patient, that patients do not want to talk about it, or that another healthcare provider has discussed it. In this chapter we will discuss problems reported by cardiac patients related to resuming sexual activity, facts and myths related to sexual activity, and give some practical pointers in discussing sexuality with cardiac patients.

Problems

Cardiac patients often are worried about a safe return to sexual activity. They worry about the effect of the condition on sexual activity, the effect of sex on the heart, symptoms that may occur during sexual activity, and possible effects of medication.[1-3] Partners of cardiac patients also may be worried and may be overprotective. Some problems in returning to sexual activity are general to (cardiac) patients (Table 40-1), while others might be more disease specific.

Return to sexual activity might be stressful for both for patient and partner, including experiences of fear, anxiety, and overprotectiveness.

Cardiac patients also often report erectile difficulties. Vascular disease is a common cause of sexual dysfunction and can be assumed to be present in a proportion of the patients with heart disease. Steinke (2003) found that the areas of greatest concern reported by ICD patients were

TABLE 40-1. Problems of cardiac patients and partners related to sexual activity

Psychological problems
– General anxiety
– Fear of symptoms (chest pain, dyspnea)
– Fear of death
– Worries about the effect of medication on sexual function
– Change of self-esteem

Stress for couples
– Overprotectiveness
– Lack of communication

Symptoms (chest pain, fatigue, dyspnea)

Erectile difficulties

Reduced sexual desire

Effect of cardiovascular medications

Men:
– Decreased or absent libido
– Difficulty in maintaining and erection
– Priapism
– Premature retrograde ejaculation

Women:
– Decreased vaginal lubrication
– Decreased or absent libido
– Inability to achieve orgasm

overprotectiveness by the partner (56%) and erectile difficulties (57%).[4]

Myocardial Infarction

Myocardial infarction patients may have all the concerns described in Table 40-1. Specifically patients after an MI might fear a reinfarction and/or sudden death during intercourse.

Coronary Bypass Surgery

Patients recovering from bypass surgery or other cardiac surgery may have specific concerns about pain and support of incisions during sexual activity. In addition, changes in body image due to the operation may play a role in returning to sexual activity.

Heart Failure

From descriptive studies it is known that a considerable number of patients report a marked decrease in both sexual interest and the frequency of sexual relations caused by their heart failure. Symptoms of dyspnea and fatigue may hinder sexual activity. A relationship between higher levels of daily functioning and fewer sexual problems has been established, and a relationship between the number of co-morbidities and sexual problems.[1,5] Patients might fear deterioration as a result of sexual activity and death during intercourse.

Implantable Defibrillators

In addition to the general problems mentioned earlier, ICD patients and their partners often have concerns related to device discharge with sexual activity. Patients are concerned that sexual activity will trigger the device and may avoid sexual encounters. They also fear touching others when the device fires.[6]

Partners of ICD patients are also known to report a lack of interest in sex after the ICD was implanted. Spouses often describe fear and anxiety about cardiac arrest and ICD firing, often resulting in overprotectiveness towards their partner. Patients and partners may have been in a stressful period before the ICD implantation in which they also had reduced sexual activity.

Myths and Misconceptions

Myth 1: *Sex and sexuality are the same.*
Truth: The term "sex" is often used to refer to the sex act, whereas sexuality reflects both the psychosocial and physical aspects of intimacy. Engaging in sex can be fun, passionate, and has been called a "restorative force" that can be both healing and energizing.[7]

Myth 2: *Older adults with cardiac disease are less interested in information on resuming sex.*
Truth: Older adults have many of the same questions and sexual concerns as younger individuals. Studies with cardiac patients have shown that many older adults continue to be sexually active well into the 8th decade of life.[2,8]

Myth 3: *Sex after a heart attack often causes sudden death.*

Truth: A number of studies have been conducted in order to clarify whether sexual activity poses any significant risk to cardiac patients. Based on these findings, patients should be reassured that, in most cases, sexual activity carries little risk of causing a cardiac event. Although sexual activity increases the relative risk of MI, the absolute risk remains low for most patients. To communicate this important information to patients, the author of a study on cardiac events triggered by sexual activity suggests that simple analogies can be helpful.[9] For example, data from the Framingham Heart Study indicate that if a healthy, 50-year-old man exercises regularly, his absolute risk of MI is only 1 chance in a million per hour. If this same person engages in sexual intercourse, his absolute risk doubles to only 2 chances in a million per hour, and only for a 2-hour period. For a post-MI patient who has been in a rehabilitation program, the absolute risk of MI is 10 chances per million per hour. Although sexual activity transiently doubles this risk, the absolute risk is still only 20 per million per hour. A report from the Princeton Consensus Panel[10] provides guidelines that health professionals can use to evaluate the risk of sexual activity and recommended treatment (Table 40-2).

Myth 4: *Erectile dysfunction (ED) is always caused by psychological problems.*
Truth: Erectile dysfunction is a common problem in the healthy population, with around 10% of adult men being affected, and increasing with age. The most common cause of ED is so-called vasculogenic erectile dysfunction, which is associated with the development of atherosclerosis. Accordingly diabetes, hypertension, hyperlipidemia, and smoking are all risk factors for the development of ED. Erectile dysfunction is often seen in conjunction with other manifestations of atherosclerosis such as cardiovascular, cerebrovascular, and peripheral vascular disease.

Myth 5: *Impotence and lack of sex drive always occurs when one has heart disease.*
Truth: Both men and women can have a normal sex life after a cardiac event.

Myth 6: *If a cardiac patient can walk up two stairs, then they can resume sex.*

TABLE 40-2. Risks and management of sexual dysfunction[10]

Risk	Categories of CVD	Management recommendations
Low	− Asymptomatic <3 risk factors CVD − Controlled HT, − Mild stable angina − Post-successful revascularisation. − Uncomplicated post MI (>6–8 wk) − Mild valvular disease − LVD (NYHAI) − other cardiovascula conditions	− receive treatment for ED as needed − Reassess regularly (6–12 mo)
Intermediate	− Asymptomatic ≥ risk factors − modenater stable angina − recent MI (<2 <6 wk) − LVD/CHF class II − Noncardiac atherosclerotic disease	− Specialised CV testing − Restratification into high or low risk
high	− Unstable or refractory angina − Uncontrolled HT − LVD/CHF class III/IV − Recent MI (<2 wk) − High-risk arrhythmias − Obstructive hypeitrophic cardiomyopathy − Moderate/severe valvular disease	− Referral specialised CV management − Defer treatment for sexual problems

CVD = Cardiovascular disease; MI = Myocardial Infraction; CHF: heart failure; LVD = Left ventricular dysfunction; HT = hypertension; CV = Cardiovascular.

Truth: The energy cost to the cardiovascular system is often measured in metabolic equivalents (METs). The energy cost of sexual intercourse is 5 METs, while the energy expended during the pre- and post-orgasmic phase is estimated at 3.7 METs.[11] This is equivalent to walking a treadmill at 3 to 4 miles per hour, or 5 to 6 METs. This amount of energy expenditure has also been compared to climbing two *flights* of stairs at a brisk pace, 20 steps in 10 seconds.

Myth 7: *Alcohol is a great stimulant for sex.*
Truth: The role of alcohol and heart disease in general has been widely discussed. Studies have examined both the preventive or deleterious effect of alcohol for the cardiovascular system. We know that a small amount of alcohol may help reduce tension or fears; however, one also has to consider that alcohol may impair sexual performance.

Myth 8: *It is best for the cardiac patient to be on the bottom during sex.*
Truth: It was once believed that certain sexual positions increased cardiac workload; for example, the patient was advised to avoid the on-top position and to assume a passive position for sexual activity. It was believed that isometric exertion might lead to cardiac stress.[12] Studies have shown that blood pressure and heart rate do not change significantly when a variety of positions were used. In fact, elevations in these vital signs may occur when assuming an unfamiliar position. Patients can usually be advised to assume their usual position or one that is most comfortable for them.

Myth 9: *The heart needs to recover at least 6 months after an MI, before resuming sex.*
Truth: The rate of return to sexual activity is quite variable, with some patients returning as soon as a few weeks and others more than 6 months post-MI. Guidelines from the American College of Cardiology and American Heart Association suggest that patients with an uncomplicated MI can resume sexual activity in a week to 10 days,[13] and in the Second Princeton Consensus this is advised at 3 to 4 weeks.[10] Return to sexual activity is often gradual, sometimes at reduced frequency and some do not resume sexual activity at all. Most patients return to sexual activity in the first

month post-MI, although some may take more than 6 months to return to prior levels of activity.[2,8,14]

Myth 10: *If a doctor or nurse does not talk about it, then sex is prohibited.*
Truth: Health professionals have historically been reluctant to discuss sexual issues. However, studies have shown that cardiac patients want this information.[2] Sex is generally not prohibited unless cardiac function is seriously compromised. Health professionals must take the initiative in assessing sexual concerns of patients and partners and provide teaching that is individualized to the cardiac condition and the needs of the patient.

Sexual Counseling

Health professionals must take the initiative to bring up the topic of sex with the cardiac patient. Often, the patient may feel too embarrassed to ask questions about such a private area. By bringing up the topic, health professionals are acknowledging that sexual concerns are both normal and common for cardiac patients. Health professionals must be aware of their own biases in regard to sexuality, and be careful to approach sexual counseling in a non-judgmental way. Drench and Losee[15] provide a helpful guide for self-assessment of feelings and attitudes, particularly toward sexuality in older adults (Table 40-3).

TABLE 40-3. Self-assessment of sexual attitudes by health professionals

- When I think about people in their 60s and 70s, do I assume that intercourse ceases and they are no longer interested in sex?
- Do I think that sex among older adults is normal? Is it repulsive or immoral?
- When I think about sex, do I think it is limited to sexual intercourse? Does sex also include touching, stroking, and fondling?
- Do I think orgasm has to occur with sex?
- What do I think of my own parents engaging in sex? What about my grandparents?
- What would I think if my widowed parent engaged in sex without being married?
- How do I feel about masturbation, oral sex, and anal sex?
- How comfortable am I in discussing these issues with any of my patients, irregardless of age, young or old?
- Do I feel comfortable talking about sex to adults of both genders?

Source: Adapted from Froelicher et al.[14]

These can be used by health professionals to evaluate their own readiness to initiate sexual counseling.

There are several prerequisites to implementing successful sexual counseling. Environmental issues include providing a quiet environment in a private setting. Sexual counseling might be conducted in a conference room or other private area. Ask permission from the patient prior to beginning sexual counseling. Begin by asking more general questions about the patient's sexual concerns and then proceed to more sensitive topics.[16] Patients should be assured that confidentiality is maintained about sexual problems or issues that arise. Issues that require further intervention should be documented, however. The language used in sexual counseling is an important consideration. Using the language and terms used by the patient will enhance understanding of the content of sexual counseling. For example, some patients use slang terms to refer to body parts; if the health professional uses medical language, the message may not be understood by the patient.

Formulating Questions for Sexual Counseling

When beginning sexual counseling, start with a statement that stresses that concerns about sex and sexuality are normal after a cardiac illness. Often, open-ended questions are used to facilitate discussion and to assess patient concerns. For example, the health professional might use this statement: "Many people have concerns about sexual activity as part of living with heart failure. What concerns do you have?" This statement stresses that it is normal to have concerns, and it allows the individual to state any concerns to be addressed. This question can be used with any cardiac condition by inserting the appropriate health issue, for example heart attack or implantable defibrillator. In addition, specific questions are asked during this discussion, moving from general questions to more specific issues or problems as the counseling session continues (Table 40-4). This gives the health professional a better perspective of the issues and concerns. Evaluating usual sexual activities, current medications and supplements,

TABLE 40-4. Questions for sexual assessment[16]

- How would you describe your relationship with your partner?
- What concerns do you have about resuming sexual activity with your cardiac condition (insert appropriate term, e.g. heart attack, implantable defibrillator, heart failure, etc.)
- How important is sex and intimacy in your relationship? Are activities like hugging, kissing, and just being close an important part of your relationship?
- Were you sexually active before you were hospitalized? Is it important to you to be sexually active after you are discharged from the hospital?
- Did your previous sexual activity include sexual intercourse (vaginal or anal), masturbation, or oral sex? Note: this helps to gauge the amount of energy expenditure required and to plan sexual counseling strategies.
- Changes in sexual performance can occur as part of normal aging. Would you like me to review some of these changes?
- Have you noticed any changes in your sexual performance such as problems with erections or orgasm, vaginal dryness, or decreased desire for sex?
- What medications or supplements are you currently taking? (Note: evaluate for sexual side-effects.)
- What concerns has your partner expressed about resuming sex after you are discharged from the hospital? Would you like to include your partner in a discussion of resuming sexual activity after your cardiac condition?

sexual dysfunction, and specific sexual concerns assists in tailoring sexual counseling to each individual.

Specific Strategies for Sexual Counseling for Selected Cardiac Conditions

As there are some similarities in problems experienced by cardiac patients there are also some similarities in content in providing sexual counseling of cardiac conditions, although there are some distinct concerns described by patients. In all cases, sexual assessment questions should be used first, and followed with specific counseling strategies for the particular cardiac condition.

It is often helpful to briefly discuss myths about sexual activity and cardiac disease to help frame the discussion. Open communication about sexuality between patient and partner is particularly important. Health professionals can model appropriate communication by including partners in sexual counseling, framing the questions and discussion with sensitivity to the personal nature of the topic, and involving the partner in care activities that involve touch. Recommending that the couple take daily walks together is one way to encourage couple communication and to promote intimacy.

Myocardial Infarction

The importance of including information about return to sexual activity post-MI has been demonstrated in several studies and a few studies have specifically addressed sexual learning needs post-MI, although limited to one or two questionnaire items. In one study of the specific sexual counseling needs of MI patients, the importance and timing of 14 specific sexual teaching items were rated by patients as important to learn.[2]

Few studies have explored interventions for sexual counseling post-MI. Varvaro[17] found that patients who received a nursing instructional program had fewer concerns about sexual activity, and better adaptation to family role and work. The treatment group showed a trend for increased self-confidence ($P = 0.059$) in resuming sexual activity over time and the largest decrease in adjusting to sexual intercourse over time, reflecting the positive effect of the intervention. Froelicher and colleagues[14] used a teaching-counseling program on exercise to assess return to usual activities; participants completed eight sessions on risk factor modification and post-MI adjustment. The rate of return to physical activities was not significantly different between groups, and most patients returned to sexual activity, driving, and outdoor activities by 3 weeks post-MI. Steinke and Swan[8] tested a videotape for sexual counseling post-MI which demonstrated improved knowledge in the experimental group at 1 month. While these studies have added to the body of knowledge on sexual counseling post-MI, interventions and strategies for sexual counseling must be implemented in practice. Table 40-5 illustrates key points to be included in sexual counseling post-MI.

Coronary Bypass Surgery

For those patients having coronary artery bypass grafts (CABG), the topics discussed for MI should be followed. However, return to sexual activity occurs over a longer period of time, generally 3 to

TABLE 40-5. Sexual counseling topics post-MI[11,16]

- Ask the sexual assessment questions (Table 40-4).
- Effect of the MI on sexual function, such as energy requirements.
- Partner concerns such as anxiety, overprotectiveness, communication.
- Sexual activity can be resumed in an uncomplicated MI. Those with a complicated MI (e.g. cardiac arrest, arrhythmias) will need to resume sexual activity more slowly and will need to seek advice from their physician about this.
- The setting for sexual activity should be comfortable and the cardiac patient should be well rested.
- Avoid alcohol or a heavy meal for 2 to 3 hours before having sex.
- Avoid unfamiliar settings or partners.
- Use foreplay prior to sexual activity (decreases anxiety, less strain on heart, allows vital signs to rise gradually).
- Use a position for sex that is comfortable and relaxing.
- Report any warning signs that occur with sex such as unrelieved chest pain, shortness of breath, irregular heart rate, extreme fatigue the next day.
- Avoid anal sex unless approved by your physician; this puts added strain on the heart.
- Nitroglycerine, if prescribed, can be used for angina with sexual activity; stop and rest if chest pain is experienced.
- Discuss any medication with the physician that you think may be causing a sexual problem. Do not discontinue use of a medication without consulting the physician.
- Avoid drugs such as amphetamines, amyl nitrate (both are stimulants), marijuana (increases heart rate and oxygen consumption), and cocaine (chest pain, fatal MI).

6 weeks post-CABG or at the direction of the physician. Once the incisions have had time to heal, sexual activity can generally be successfully resumed.

Heart Failure

There are a few guidelines for heart failure patients and sexual activity in the literature (Table 40-6). Patients can be advised that a semi-reclining or on-bottom position may decrease the amount of physical effort needed for sexual activity. The suggestions for MI patients related to the setting and timing of sexual activity also apply to the heart failure patient. In addition, patients should be encouraged to stop and rest if shortness of breath occurs with sexual activity. Sexual foreplay can be beneficial in allowing the patient and the partner to determine tolerance to sexual activity. Patients should be encouraged to express their affection through hugging, kissing, and sexual foreplay. Activities such as mutual masturbation, oral sex, or intercourse may not be possible if exercise capacity is diminished. There is a correlation between the 6-minute walk test and improved patient levels of sexual function. The 6-minute walk test can be easily administered in the clinical setting and serve as a guide for overall physical function and sexual activity. Patients who are not able to manage the 6-minute walk or expend approximately 5 METs may not be able to handle the exertion required for sexual activity. Patients with symptoms at rest should be advised to be careful in engaging in coital activity. Although heart failure patients may experience sexual difficulties, they still may have a satisfying sexual relationship.[1]

Implantable Defibrillators

Specific guidelines for resuming sexual activity after ICD are largely unavailable. Some suggestions for teaching include normalizing fears and concerns about resuming sex; providing education on safe levels of activity, although not well defined; and the role of regular exercise in increasing confidence for sexual activity (see also Table 40-7). Patients frequently want to know when they can resume sexual activity. There are usually no restrictions as long as strain on the incision site is avoided in the immediate postoperative period.[6] The possibility of ICD discharge should be discussed with the patient and partner. The relative risk of arrhythmia with sexual activity is reported

TABLE 40-7. Sexual counseling topics for implantable cardioverter defibrillators

- Ask the sexual assessment questions (Table 40-4).
- Sexual activity can be normally resumed after hospital discharge; avoid strain on the incision.
- Report problems such as dyspnea, chest discomfort, or dizziness with sexual activity.
- Discuss the likelihood of ICD discharge with sexual activity. Discuss what to do if a shock occurs with sexual activity, and that the partner will not be injured.
- Discuss feelings of overprotectiveness by partner.
- Reinforce positive aspects of living with the ICD.
- Have a resource person, someone who has an ICD and is sexually active, discuss living with the ICD with the patient and partner.
- Advise patients regarding organic causes of sexual problems and also medications. Further sexual assessment may be needed if problems are detected, e.g. erectile dysfunction.

to be low, although it is possible for the ICD to sense increased heart rates with sexual activity and fire. The ICD settings may need to be adjusted. Other items to discuss include medications, vascular disease, and alternative causes of sexual difficulties or impotence.[4] The patient should be advised to report any dyspnea, chest discomfort, or dizziness with sexual activity. If patient anxieties persist, additional concerns of patients and partners must be identified and discussed.

Summary

Increased attention to the sexual counseling needs of cardiac patients is warranted. Health professionals are in key positions to provide this teaching and facilitate successful return to sexual activity after a cardiac event. Return to sexual activity is part of the recovery process and can lead to improved satisfaction and quality of life.

TABLE 40-6. Sexual counseling topics for heart failure

- Ask the sexual assessment questions (Table 40-4).
- Explore alternative means of sexual expression, e.g. hugging, kissing, fondling, sexual foreplay.
- Encourage the use of a semi-reclining or on-bottom position for the patient to minimize energy expenditure and strain on the heart.
- Sexual activity should be in a comfortable setting, including no extremes of room temperature, and when the patient is well rested and less short of breath.
- The patient should stop and rest if shortness of breath is experienced.
- Take nitroglycerine if needed for chest discomfort.
- Adjust diuretic use if needed.
- Some activities may not be possible with decreased exercise capacity.
- Use the 6-minute walk test as a guide to whether the patient can resume sexual activity.
- Patients with symptoms at rest should be careful in engaging in sexual activity.

References

1. Jaarsma T, Dracup K, Walden J, et al. Sexual function in patients with advanced heart failure. Heart Lung 1996;25:262–270.
2. Steinke E, Patterson-Midgley P. Importance and timing of sexual counseling after myocardial infarction. J Cardiopulmon Rehabil 1998;18:401–407.

3. Westlake C, Dracup K, Walden JA, et al. Sexuality of patients with advanced heart failure and their spouses or partners. J Heart Lung Transplant 1999; 18:1133–1138.

4. Steinke E. Sexual concerns of patients and partners after an implantable cardioverter defibrillator. Dimens Crit Care Nurs 2003;22:89–96.

5. Jaarsma T. Sexual problems in heart failure patients. Eur J Cardiovasc Nurs 2002;1:61–67.

6. Vitale MB, Funk M. Quality of life in younger persons with an implantable cardioverter defibrillator. Dimens Crit Care Nurs 1995;14:100–111.

7. Duffy LM. Lovers, loners, and lifers: Sexuality and the older adult. Geriatrics 1998;53(Suppl 1):S66–S69.

8. Steinke EE, Swan JH. Effectiveness of a videotape for sexual counseling after myocardial infarction. Res Nurs Health 2004;27:269–280.

9. Muller JE, Mittleman A, Maclure M, et al. Triggering myocardial infarction by sexual activity. Low absolute risk and prevention by regular physical exertion. Determinants of Myocardial Infarction Onset Study Investigators. JAMA 1996; 275:1405–1409.

10. Kostis JB, Jackson G, Rosen R, et al. Sexual dysfunction and cardiac risk: the Second Princeton Consensus Conference. Am J Cardiol 2005;96(12B): 85M–93M.

11. Seidl A, Bullough B, Haughey B, et al. Understanding the effects of a myocardial infarction on sexual functioning: A basis for sexual counseling. Rehabil Nurs 1991;16:255–264.

12. Franklin BA, Munnings F. Sex after a heart attack: Making a full recovery. Physician Sportsmed 1994;22:84–89.

13. American College of Cardiology American Heart Association. ACC/AHA Guidelines for the management of patients with ST-elevation myocardial infarction. 2004. Available at: http://circ.ahajournals. org/cgi/reprint/110/9/e82.

14. Froelicher ES, Kee LL, Newton KM, et al. Return to work, sexual activity, and other activities after acute myocardial infarction. Heart Lung 1994;23: 423–435.

15. Drench ME, Losee RH. Sexuality and sexual capacity in elderly people. Rehabil Nurs 1996;21: 118–123.

16. Steinke EE. Sexual counseling after myocardial infarction. Am J Nurs 2000;100:38–43.

17. Varvaro FF. Family role and work adaptation in MI women. Clin Nurs Res 2000;9:339–351.

41
Cognitive Behavioral Rehabilitation for Angina

Robert J. Lewin

Cognitive behavioral (CB) disease management programs were developed to help people with chronic back pain and have an extensive evidence base in that role. The same methods are now being adapted for use in other chronic illnesses.[1] Using the example of angina, this chapter will explain how these techniques can be applied in cardiac rehabilitation (CR) and concludes with a brief description of such a program.

The Cognitive Hypothesis

Our thoughts and beliefs about an illness lead us to choose how to behave. Therefore, to understand patients' behavior we have to examine their beliefs – to help them change their behavior we may have to encourage them to change some beliefs. For example, many people with angina believe that each "attack" leads to further damage to their heart. Quite reasonably they stop doing any activity likely to lead to angina and become inactive and physically deconditioned, an unhelpful reaction. Changing that specific belief is associated with patients becoming more active. Another common example is the belief that heart problems are caused by too much stress, worry, or overwork. Again the sensible action appears to be to avoid: any kind of exciting or "stressful" situations; sexual intercourse; promotion at work; playing with grandchildren, and so on. It is clear that this can lead to a failure to rehabilitate and, if too many pleasures are abandoned, a depressed and anxious patient and spouse. These beliefs have been called "cardiac misconceptions" and the effect they have

on recovery following a myocardial infarction (MI) was first shown more than 15 years ago[2] and more recently in angina.[3]

Cognitive *and* Behavioral – Both Are Required

It is important to *educate* people to understand that these beliefs are wrong and how they can be harmful. A simple method in a CR program is to ask patients to complete a questionnaire of common "cardiac misconceptions" as a group "quiz" and to then discuss each of the answers, pointing out how these beliefs have led people into trouble in the past. We have developed questionnaires for this purpose (available on request). The most essential things to discover are: what the patient thinks has caused the problem; what is likely to happen next with the illness; how much control they think they can exert on the illness and how they should best respond to protect their health. If conducted in the right manner, as a discussion rather than a lecture, most patients will find this a useful and rewarding exercise.

Important as it is, educating patients and their partners about wrong beliefs will not usually be sufficient to produce lasting behavior change. This is where the "behavioral" part of CB becomes important. CB programs use principles derived from "behavioral psychology" to help people develop new habits. The first law of behavioral psychology is that "behavior that is rewarded increases in frequency." A powerful behavioral strategy derived from this is to arrange for rewards to be given as soon as possible after a person has practiced a desired behavior. Self-recording of success in a task is a simple but effective way to do this. Patients set goals and work up through these in small steps, "ticking off the boxes" as they progress. A facilitator reviews the progress with the goals at regular times, also congratulating (rewarding) the patient. In a group program reporting these successes to the whole group is a powerful added reward for many people. The steps should always be set by the patient and be small to allow for many rewards. Each small step forward builds further confidence that the person can succeed (technically often called "self-efficacy") and makes it more likely that the they will attempt the next step. Deliberately building up "self-efficacy" in this way is a common element of CB treatments. A number of the other common techniques used in CB based programs have recently been summarized in a review by Michael Von Korff.[1]

The Relationship Between the Lesion and Disability

CB programs started because it was obvious that the amount of disability shown by a patient often had little or no relationship to the amount of damage to their back. There was little or no connection between the impairment (the lesion) and the disability (pain, functional capacity, anxiety, etc.). This is also true in cardiac illness.[4,5] For example, the degree to which angina interferes with a patient's daily life is not related to the extent of atheroma in their arteries. From a CB perspective this lack of association is to be expected because having a lot of mistaken beliefs, known as "cardiac misconceptions," is associated with increased disability but not with impairment. If the patient *does not* believe the angina misconception that every further attack of angina is damaging them, they are much more likely to stay active even if this sometimes causes angina. This repeated ischemic challenge can lead to an increase in the blood flow through capillaries to the ischemic area, lowering the threshold for angina. This has been shown experimentally by deliberately encouraging patients to exercise despite angina.[6] The opposite is also likely. If the patient thinks that every attack *is* a "mini-heart attack" and restricts their activity level, the threshold at which they experience angina will fall. In both cases the correlation between the extent of atheroma and exercise tolerance will become weaker. It is known that psychological and personality factors are related to the amount of disability and symptoms reported by a person with angina.[4]

Psychological Factors in the Production of Angina

Herberden named angina after the "*choking sensation of fear*" it produces and most patients will agree that it is a very frightening sensation. As many as 50% of ischemic episodes may be triggered by emotion rather than exertion.[7] This is most likely the result of raised autonomic drive leading to vasoconstriction; emotionally induced hyperventilation may also be involved. We teach patients a rapid relaxation technique to use if they feel angina starting.

Evidence for the CB Approach

A trial of a specially developed Angina Management Programme conducted by our group (described below) produced at 12 months: a 72% reduction in self-reported disability (Sickness Impact Profile); a 70% reduction in episodes of angina (30% reported no angina); a 65% reduction in the use of nitrates; a 57% improvement in exercise tolerance and a 30% increase in time to 1 mm ST depression.[8] We have translated aspects of this program into a patient-held workbook, home-based program that can be administered by a healthcare worker who has completed a brief distance learning intervention, the Angina Plan (www.anginaplan.org.uk). It is currently being used by CR programs in the UK in a number of ways: in a group format, in brief clinic visits, or though repeated phone contacts. In a randomized controlled trial we compared it to a "usual practice" 40-minute angina advice clinic for newly diagnosed patients. At 6 months the patients who had used the Angina Plan reported 43% fewer episodes of angina, fewer physical limitations

(Seattle Angina Questionnaire), and a lower level of anxiety and depression. They were also more likely to report having changed their diet and increased their daily walking.[9] This replicated the success of an earlier CB program for post-MI patients, the Heart Manual,[10] a rehabilitation method also now widely used in CR in the United Kingdom.

Protocol for a Group CB CR Program for Angina

Goal Setting and Pacing (40–60 Minutes for a Group of 8–10 People)

Patients select some activities that they have had to cut back on or give up but would like to get back to. These are their "*goals*." Walking is chosen by most patients, gardening, hobbies, sports and social activities are all popular choices. A "*baseline*" level for each activity, one that will not produce any symptoms and that they agree they can practice every day even if it is "a bad day," is set in individual discussion with each patient. It may be that initially they can only do a few minutes of an activity; this does not matter, in fact the lower the initial goal is set the better. The goals, that week's baselines, and the daily success with each is logged on charts by the patient, who "ticks off the box" as soon as they have done it. They may start with only one or two goals but as the weeks pass they usually add further goals; most patients choose to set between four and seven. At each subsequent session they report to the group their success with each goal and later and individually with a member of the rehabilitation team discuss the next week's baseline, either continuing at the same level for the next week, or increasing the duration by a small percentage, usually not more than 10%.

Exercise Program (10 Minutes per Patient)

Patients take part in a home-based, self-paced, exercise program of 5–8 different exercise sets. An individual baseline for each set is agreed in an initial session with a physiotherapist. A time limit of 10 minutes is set because one of the main reasons given by patients for stopping their exer-

cising program after CR is "no time": no one can claim not to have 10 minutes free once or twice during the day. The training effect comes from increasing the number of repetitions in that fixed time. Patients are asked to practice at least once per day. Initial levels are deliberately set low because of the behavioral laws that: (1) behaviors that are punished, (through pain, tiredness, soreness, etc.) die out; and (2) the easier it is, the more likely it is they will succeed, thus *rewarding* them and raising their self-efficacy for exercise at the same time. They rate each exercise on a 10 cm line on two qualities: (1) on a scale "very pleasant"/"very unpleasant" and (2) as "very high effort"/"very low effort." The center of both lines is marked as "just right." They record their program on charts and score each set on both 10 cm lines on each occasion. As they become fitter, the effort scores become easier, and after 3 successive days of scoring a set lower on effort than "just right" they can add one extra repetition to the number of repetitions for that exercise *but only* if the new level chosen would still be "about right" on the pleasant/unpleasant line: no pain, more gain!

Educational Sessions (45 Minutes per Week)

Discussion topics cover: cardiac misconceptions; mistaken ways of reacting to the diagnosis and symptoms; the psycho-physiology of stress; the physical symptoms of anxiety, panic attack, hyperventilation, and phobias; how thoughts interact with the autonomic system to produce vasoconstriction and hyperventilation; how psychological variables such as anxiety, depression, and hypochondriasis may all increase disability.

Relaxation and Stress Management

Techniques that may be used include relaxation training, breathing re-training, biofeedback, yoga, meditation, rapid relaxation and the identification (using questionnaires) of our own behavior and attitudes that lead to anger and stress. Each week one of the patients is asked to recall a recent event that had stressed them or made them very angry and the group is shown stress management techniques to avoid this. Patients are taught a rapid relaxation and distraction technique that they can perform, wherever they are, during an acute angina attack.

The Staff

Staff are aware of the rationale and methods of the CB techniques being used. They use "differential reinforcement," paying warm attention to success but ignoring or being emotionally neutral to self-defeating statements. Staff continually stress that the benefits the patient is experiencing are entirely a result of the patient's own efforts.

Patient-Held Materials

Each session is accompanied by written information reinforcing what has been taught. Over the weeks this builds up, in a clip file, into a substantial volume complete with the record sheets of the exercise and goal setting. Patients are encouraged to read this material regularly and if possible to use it to explain the program to their partner and family.

References

1. Von Korff M, Gruman J, Schaefer J, et al. Collaborative management of chronic illness. Ann Intern Med 1997;127:1097–1102.
2. Maeland JG, Havik OE. After the myocardial infarction. A medical and psychological study with special emphasis on perceived illness. Scand J Rehabil Med Suppl 1989;22:1–87.
3. Furze G, Bull P, Lewin RJ, Thompson DR. Development of the York Angina Beliefs Questionnaire. J Health Psychol 2003;8:307–315.
4. Lewin B. The psychological and behavioural management of angina. J Psychosom Res 1997;5:452–462.
5. Lewin RJ. Improving quality of life in patients with angina. Heart 1999;82:654–655.
6. Todd IC, Ballantyne D. Antianginal efficacy of exercise training: a comparison with beta blockade. Br Heart J 1990;64:14–19.
7. Deanfield JE, Maseri A, Selwyn AP, et al. Myocardial ischaemia during daily life in patients with stable angina: its relation to symptoms and heart rate changes. Lancet 1983;2(8353):753–758.
8. Lewin B, Cay EL, Todd I, et al. The Angina Management Programme: a rehabilitation treatment. Br J Cardiol 1995;1:221–226.
9. Lewin RJ, Furze G, Robinson J, et al. A randomised controlled trial of a self-management plan for patients with newly diagnosed angina. Br J Gen Pract 2002;52:194–196, 199–201 (see also www.anginaplan.org.uk).
10. Lewin B, Robertson IH, Cay EL, et al. Effects of self-help post myocardial infarction rehabilitation on psychological adjustment and use of health services. Lancet 1992;339:1036–1340.

42
National Heart Foundations, European Heart Network

Susanne Løgstrup, Ulla-Riitta Penttilä, Silvia Aepli, and Therese Junker

National Heart Foundations

Heart foundations in Europe fulfill many roles in their work to prevent cardiovascular diseases. They fund a great deal of research, they provide information to the general public on healthy lifestyles, and they undertake educational programs in specific settings targeting selected audiences. An important role for many heart foundations is to lend support to cardiovascular patients and their families.

The heart foundations provide services at various levels to the patients. They offer a wide range of patient activities including:

- providing written information to patients on their conditions, their options for treatment, healthy lifestyles etc.
- web pages dedicated specifically to heart patients and telephone services
- funding heart patients' centers
- establishing counseling groups for self-help and training patients to become supporters of other heart patients and their families
- running training courses in cardiac rehabilitation for professionals in order to give them the necessary skills and qualifications
- initiating new rehabilitation programs and services as well as rehabilitation guidelines
- providing guided physical training groups and keep fit groups in phase III of rehabilitation and events to introduce patient motivation programs.

The national heart foundations also work at a political level, advocating for more funds to be allocated to research, for bringing down waiting lists and for better access to rehabilitation and for continued improvement of the quality of rehabilitation services.

European Heart Network

Introduction

The European Heart Network (EHN) is a Brussels-based alliance of heart foundations and other like-minded non-governmental organizations throughout Europe. EHN has 31 member organizations in 26 countries.

The European Heart Network plays a leading role in the prevention and reduction of cardiovascular disease through advocacy, networking, and education so that it is no longer a major cause of premature death and disability throughout Europe.

To achieve this mission, the EHN's objectives are to:

- influence European policy-makers in favor of a heart-healthy lifestyle
- monitor EU policy
- create and nurture the ties between organizations concerned with heart health promotion and cardiovascular disease (CVD) prevention
- gather and disseminate information relevant to heart health promotion and CVD prevention
- encourage support for comprehensive CVD research.

EHN has a focus on population-based primary prevention through advocating for environments that are supportive of cardiovascular health and through establishing best practice for cardiovascular health promotion programs. Environments that are smoke-free and provide easy access to affordable healthy diets and to regular physical activity are a prerequisite for successful secondary prevention and cardiac rehabilitation.

European Union Developments on Patient Mobility

EHN also follows developments in the European Union that aim at setting standards for patient care and ensure quality services. Over the last 6 years, the European Court of Justice has on several occasions ruled on movements of patients across borders. These rulings led to the establishment of a high-level reflection group on patient mobility and healthcare developments in the European Union in June 2002, which submitted its report in December 2003.[1] The European Commission responded to it by adopting a Commission Communication in April 2004.[2] This Communication is concerned with four main areas, namely:

- European cooperation to enable better use of resources
- information requirements for patients, professionals, and policy-makers
- European contribution to health objectives
- responding to enlargement through investment in health and health infrastructure.

The Communication sets out responses to a wide range of issues, including rights and duties of patients, sharing spare capacity and transnational care, European centers of reference, health systems information strategy, and developing a shared European vision for health systems.

Case Studies

The Finnish Heart Association

In Finland, secondary prevention and cardiac rehabilitation are part of public healthcare by legislation. The Social Insurance Institution of Finland also offers rehabilitation to patients who are at work. During the last decade, however, the budget cuts and personnel shortages in the public

sector have reduced the availability of cardiac rehabilitation and secondary prevention. Finland participated in the EUROASPIRE study,[3] which proved that the present patient guidance system has been unsuccessful in addressing the risk factors of coronary artery disease according to the recommendations. The Finnish Heart Association and its local branches supplement the public services by offering patient education and rehabilitation courses, as well as by developing rehabilitation programs. Finland's Slot Machine Association, RAY, supports the rehabilitation programs of the Finnish Heart Association financially. Today, the Heart Association is quantitatively the biggest organizer of cardiac rehabilitation in Finland. Annually, some 3400 cardiac patients participate in rehabilitation offered by the Heart Association. This number represents 10% of cardiac patients discharged from hospitals. In addition, the Heart Association offers some rehabilitation courses for smaller patient groups, such as patients with cardiomyopathy, heart transplants, or implantable defibrillators.

The Finnish Heart Association has developed a new type of outpatient care program that can be implemented with reduced resources. The TULPPA program (the name is derived from the Finnish word for "thrombus") was designed to support the follow-up care of cardiac patients. The program has already been used in 30 municipalities in eastern and northern Finland. The program's primary goal is to strengthen the self-care skills and advocate lifestyle changes for patients, but also to alleviate any fears the disease may have brought on, intervene in good time if there are depressive symptoms, find the right level of exercise, and encourage patients to join peer and self-help groups. The rehabilitation is part of normal public healthcare work, with the Heart Association responsible for training the group leaders as well as producing the material.

The patients meet in groups of approximately 10 patients for 2 to 3 hours at a time for 10 weeks, and have follow-up meetings after 6 and 12 months. The program includes all the traditional cardiac rehabilitation topics: treatment and risks of coronary artery disease, medical treatment, exercise, moods, family and relationships, pain, recognizing the deterioration of the condition, and emergencies. Each meeting consists of theory, action, and exercise. The program framework includes selected themes, but the topics and focus can be modified to suit the group's needs.

The groups are led by a team consisting of a nurse and a physiotherapist, and the implementation of the program is largely up to them. Doctors evaluate the patients' fitness for rehabilitation and any eventual restrictions in areas such as exercising. The Finnish Heart Association trains the group leaders and they receive extensive educational material for the group. Group leaders from each region get together about once every 6 months to assess their activities and to receive further training.

The implementation method of the program differs from the traditional cardiac rehabilitation. Each participant chooses only one key risk factor and then commits to changing that factor. Since the risk factors of coronary artery disease are all interlinked, improving one risk factor also improves the others. This empowerment method,[4] based on the transtheoretical model of readiness for change,[5] facilitates the patient's motivation to make lifestyle changes. Special emphasis is placed on setting individual goals for patients and following up the results. The groups also combine professional knowledge with personal experience: each group includes a lay member from the local heart association, an experienced cardiac patient who acts as a peer guide. Their role is to set a positive survival example for new patients and their families.

Instead of lectures, the program consists of action, such as shopping expeditions to find out about the salt and fat contents of foods, cooking lessons, and various types of exercise. Patients also receive a lot of homework.

The changes in the patient's risk factors are monitored for a year. The monitored risk factors are blood pressure, lipids, body mass index, waist circumference, a 6-minute walking test, and smoking. Exercise and food diaries are also used.

An evaluation study was done of the program in 2002 (57 groups, $N = 547$). The average age of the patients was 64, and 54% were still working. Eighty-eight percent of the patients in the program had coronary artery disease, and the rest had metabolic syndrome. Over half of them had had cardiac infarction. Blood pressure, choles-terol, and waist circumference all decreased and the walked distance increased during the year by a statistically significant amount. For those patients whose initial blood pressure was over 140/85 mmHg, the systolic pressure decreased on average by 14.2 mmHg ($P < 0.001$), and for those patients who chose blood pressure as their key risk factor, the drop was 17 mmHg. For patients whose initial cholesterol level exceeded 5 mmol/L, cholesterol dropped by 0.67 mmol/L ($P < 0.001$) independent of medication. The distance walked lengthened on average by 83 meters ($P < 0.001$) and waist circumference decreased by 3 cm ($P < 0.001$). Only patients whose weight was their key risk factors lost weight, but even the obese lengthened their walking distance. Choosing a key risk factor improved the results independently of other factors.

The TULPPA program is a good example of cooperation between the public healthcare and heart associations, and it will also be introduced in other parts of the country. On the whole, this rehabilitation model has proven to be useful and suitable for healthcare centers. It was also cost-effective: The rehabilitation cost per patient was two-thirds that of a hospital day.

The Swiss Heart Foundation

A cardiac event or a cardiovascular disease requires life-long aftercare. This insight led to the establishment of the first training groups for heart patients (heart groups) in Switzerland in the early 1980s, which was driven by the private initiative of committed physicians and heart patients. Four years ago, the Swiss Heart Foundation started to take care of the heart groups with the aim of promoting the establishment of a nationwide network. Today, 85 heart groups for long-term rehabilitation exist in Switzerland.

The Heart Groups and Their Activities

The members of these local self-help groups jointly pursue their goal of reducing the risk factors of cardiovascular disease. They are determined to regain their physical and mental abilities and use the group to train behavior based on health awareness that they also practice in their daily lives. Under the supervision of experienced physiotherapists or PE (physical education) teachers, they meet for an exercise program of 60–90 minutes duration once to three times a week. In addition, most heart groups regularly offer nutritional, smoking cessation, and stress management consulting.

Organization and Quality of a Heart Group

A physician is responsible for medical matters. The cardiac therapist is in charge of the heart training program. The quality and safety of the programs is guaranteed by the "Swiss working group for cardiac rehabilitation" (SAKR) of the Swiss Society of Cardiology.[6]

This group has also defined a requirements specification for heart groups. One member, who has the role of a heart group leader, is usually responsible for organizational and administrative matters in most of the cases. The costs of participating in a heart group vary. Frequently, participants with an additional health insurance get a part of the costs reimbursed by their insurance company.

The Services Provided by the Swiss Heart Foundation

The role of the Swiss Heart Foundation is to provide coordination and information for the heart groups. When heart groups affiliate to the foundation, they are allowed to call themselves "Partner of the Swiss Heart Foundation." The aims of the foundation are:

- to establish a nationwide network of active, local heart groups
- to support the heart groups with help and advice and, if necessary, represent their interests in their dealings with authorities and insurers
- to enable the groups to exchange experiences among themselves
- to support a comprehensive education of heart group members and, thus, further improve the success of a long-term secondary prevention.

For this purpose, the Swiss Heart Foundation provides a variety of informative material including a practical, step-by-step manual on how to initiate and establish a heart group, including ideas for activities within the group, a CD and all templates for forms and data sheets needed for administration. In addition, brochures with easily understandable information on cardiovascular disease, rehabilitation, and secondary prevention are offered to the groups and their members. Furthermore, an educational manual covering healthy nutrition, smoking cessation, and stress management is in the pipeline.

With public events on the World Heart Day or by means of the health platform "Rendez-vous Heart" (educational seminars and risk of heart attack tests in the "Heart Bus"), the heart group members are encouraged to play the role of messengers for a healthy lifestyle and to increase public awareness regarding the heart groups and their activities. Both the internet platform[7] and the newsletter "mein Herz" (my heart) aim at improving the ties within the network of heart groups.[8]

Future Prospects

When those affected by the disease are willing to assume responsibility for their lives, one might assume that the authorities as well as social and health insurers would support and encourage the establishment of patient support groups, especially in times of constantly increasing healthcare costs. Unfortunately, these bodies did not provide funds to support this project, which were requested by the Swiss Heart Foundation. This is one of the reasons why the Swiss Heart Foundation with its 85 heart groups still falls short of its aim of 200 heart groups for a nationwide coverage.

Furthermore, the still insufficient number of (trained) heart therapists and physicians willing to commit themselves to heart groups is partly responsible for the slow progress made to date. In practice, doctors still lack the necessary resoluteness when pointing out to their patients the possibilities of long-term rehabilitation. Despite all these difficulties, the Swiss Heart Foundation will continue its commitment to the promotion of heart groups, because these groups offer, last but not least, also a strategic advantage. The Swiss Heart Foundation has no regional structures. Heart groups could partly make up for this shortcoming in the medium term by converting themselves into small heart foundations and improving the implementation of our information and prevention work on a local level.

References

1. http://europa.eu.int/comm/health/ph_overview/ Documents/key01_mobility_en.pdf.
2. COM(2004) 301 final.
3. EUROASPIRE I and II Group. Lancet 2001;357:995– 1001.
4. Feste C, Anderson RM. Empowerment: from philosophy to practice. Patient Educ Couns 1995;26:139–144.
5. Rodwell CM. An analysis of the concept of empowerment. J Adv Nurs 1996;23:305–313.
6. DiClemente CC, Prochaska JO. Self-change and therapy change of smoking behavior: a comparison of processes of change in cessation and maintenance. Addict Behav 1982;7:133–142.
7. www.swisscardio.com.
8. www.swissheartgroups.ch.

Further information about the European Heart Network can be found at:www.ehnheart.org, and about the national heart foundations at: www.ehnheart.org/content/ListMember.asp?level0=1453&level1=1460.

43
Long-Term Maintenance Programs

Miguel F. Mendes

In the meta-analysis on cardiac rehabilitation (CR) after myocardial infarction published by Oldridge and coworkers,[1] a reduction rate of 24% in all-cause death was found for CR as a whole. The rate was larger for programs with a duration of 36 or more months, where a 38% all-cause death reduction was found, higher than the reduction by programs below 12 weeks (8%) or between 12 and 52 weeks (24%).

Cardiac rehabilitation programs produce benefits through different pathways: an increase in physical working capacity, reduction of myocardial demands, increase in myocardial oxygen supply and risk factor control, protection against arrhythmias and blood coagulation, and modulation of autonomic nervous system (ANS) activity, among others. More recently, an ant-inflamatory effect of exercise training was described[2] and a near-normalization of endothelial function was detected which seems to be a very important mechanism to explain many exercise benefits and why myocardial perfusion gets better without any new collaterals or apparent regression of coronary stenosis.[3]

Although it is known that the increase in functional capacity and the trend for endothelial function normalization take around 4 to 6 weeks to emerge after the beginning of an exercise program, it is not known for how long it is sustained after discontinuation of the exercise program. The benefits may well subside within weeks.

Control of risk factors for atherosclerotic disease is a crucial component in decreasing the pace of coronary artery disease (CAD) progression. The need to keep the disease under control, with a healthy lifestyle (with an exercise program) and with medication, is the rationale behind maintaining participation in the different forms of cardiac rehabilitation for as long as feasible.

CR Maintenance Phase Difficulties

Today's patients with acute myocardial infarction (AMI) experience a lower physical limitation due to the early reperfusion strategy, anti-remodeling medication, complete revascularization frequently obtained by percutaneous coronary interventions (PCI), and short in-hospital stay. This is in contrast to former decades where large myocardial necrotic zones, frequent residual ischemia, and several weeks of immobilization were the rule. However, the present short in-hospital stay is less optimal for professionals teaching patients and relatives about secondary prevention measures as recommended in the guidelines.

These and other difficulties, such as lack of motivation, financial problems, the need for speedy job resumption or timetable conflicts, also prevent patients' participation in the earlier phases of a classical CR program which should be the first step in a lifetime intervention.

Health systems' and insurance companies' financial restrictions have lowered the payment and reimbursement for CR in the last decades, which has consequently shortened the intervention from the typical 3–6 months to some weeks, a time period insufficient to promote long-lasting behavior change.

EUROASPIRE II[4] showed, in real life clinical practice, that there is a large potential and need for secondary prevention implementation, because many patients are not taking the medications recommended in clinical guidelines, nor have they adopted the appropriate lifestyle.

Many CAD patients, frequently old people, sometimes with low educational and socioeconomic levels, may be reluctant to abandon unhealthy behaviors.

Cardiac rehabilitation, a comprehensive secondary prevention program, is considered to be the appropriate intervention to promote the adoption of a healthy lifestyle, stress management, and risk factor control in CAD patients.[5] Today's challenge is to promote a comprehensive long-lasting program, including exercise, education, and secondary prevention interventions, that is affordable and likely to be maintained in the long run.

Maintenance Phase – A Long-Term Approach

The maintenance phase follows the in-hospital and transition phases of CR. In this phase patients should be autonomous, being in charge of their own personal healthcare program as recommended by a cardiologist. This must include a clear definition of the usual medication, exercise program and the goals to be reached in terms of tobacco cessation, blood pressure, glycemia, lipids, body weight, waist circumference, and stress control.

The clinical priorities, the intermediate and ultimate targets, should be discussed between doctor and patient and every secondary prevention goal must be reached progressively after a previously agreed period of time – 6–12 months.[6] To maintain a healthy behavior for many years it is important that health professionals assist the patient and family using specific education and communication skills in order to commit and cope with the program. The patient's commitment to self-care can be achieved through the educational program, promotion of the feeling of belonging to a group with similar problems, and friendly and frequent contact with the CR staff.

During the early phases of the CR there is a structured approach with formal exercise and educational sessions led by the health staff. In the maintenance phase, the program becomes less structured and patients may be encouraged to return less frequently to the program (e.g. once a month). Exercise will be performed alone (at home or outdoors), in a group like a coronary club, a community program, a gymnasium, a swimming pool, a dancing group, a golf club, or in a walking or jogging program.[6,7]

During the maintenance phase program, the important issues are: an exercise program and its safety, education/risk factor control, and adherence to healthy life habits.

Exercise Program and Safety

The exercise program must be adapted to the patient's personal preferences, physical capacity, co-morbidities, and convenience in terms of costs, transportation, and timetable.[8] A total of 1000 kcal should be accumulated in 3–5 exercise sessions per week with at least two interpolated rest days to avoid fatigue and permit muscular recovery. This level of exercise is frequently insufficient to reach the 1000 kcal/week goal; thus an increase in physical activity in occupational and leisure-time activities must be promoted as larger benefits can be obtained with a global training volume of 2000 kcal/week.

Even in the maintenance phase exercise should be medically prescribed according to the patient's cardiovascular limitations and co-morbidities, balancing the need to provide effective training with the need of a low cardiovascular and orthopedic risk.[9,10]

Exercise prescription starts with a medical evaluation where the patient's clinical status should be considered stable in terms of symptoms (angina and/or heart failure), ECG (ischemia and arrhythmias), and LV function. The usual contraindications for exercise should be ruled out. Afterwards, a maximal symptom-limited graded exercise test, performed under the patient's ongoing medication, will be performed for training heart rate (HR) calculation, for the possible detection of an exercise risk threshold (myocardial ischemia, arrhythmias, or blood pressure drop), and for choosing modes of exercise.

Exercise intensity must be moderate, which means between 50% and 80% of peak VO_2 and always 10–20 beats/min below the risk threshold.

Besides aerobic training, all other aspects of physical training, like range of motion, flexibility, and muscular strength, should be promoted with the exception of speed in training.

Muscular strength or resistance training should be performed two to three times a week, after the aerobic training period, exercising the most important muscle groups of the upper and lower body for 20–30 min using elastic bands, small weight or weights machines, through one to three sets of 8–15 repetitions at 50% of the maximum tolerable load.

Program Safety

Direct medical or paramedical supervision is not the rule in the maintenance phase because it is a time to promote the individual's autonomy. The patient should be in a stable clinical situation, knowing from the previous program phases all the information needed to reduce the exercise risk and must be able to self-monitor exercise. In special situations, such as people with neuromuscular disabilities, the assistance of a physiotherapist or medical supervision may be needed.[6,7]

Exercise safety should be considered in cardiac and musculoskeletal terms. The appropriate session format should be respected, always respecting warm-up and cool-down periods of 5–10 min duration, keeping the duration of aerobic training under 45 minutes and offering resistance training two to three times weekly, both of moderate intensity. The probability of occurrence of ventricular fibrillation or tachycardia (VF/VT) should also be very low: if there is significant risk, training should be conducted under ECG monitoring and in the presence of personnel trained in cardiopulmonary resuscitation. In these cases high-intensity exercise is not advisable.

To lower the risk of program-induced musculoskeletal injuries, which can easily occur in older people engaged in high-intensity programs, certain activities may be avoided: running, basketball, volleyball, jumping, rope skipping, aerobic dancing, downhill skiing whereas walking, cycling, swimming, rowing, cross-country skiing can be promoted.[6,7,9,10]

Program safety, even in this phase, remains the responsibility of the program director although it is known that the usual rate of cardiac arrest in medical supervised programs is very low: 1/109,500 patient hours.[11] A larger risk may be expected for patients with:

- a history of prior myocardial infarction or ventricular fibrillation
- a history of heart failure and/or an ejection fraction below 40%
- residual myocardial ischemia and/or three-vessel disease, ST depression below 120 beats/min
- peak exercise systolic blood pressure <130 mmHg, exertional hypotension and/or functional capacity <5 METs
- non-adherence to prescribed exercise intensity and to recommended session format.

At the beginning of maintenance training, the probability of adverse events is very low as the patient previously has been exercising under supervision and has recently performed a maximal exercise test. However, as CAD progresses over time, the risk may increase at a later stage. To counteract the increased risk, periodical medical controls should be scheduled including blood tests and repeated stress-testing whenever deemed necessary. In some cases patients may be offered a visit to the cardiac rehabilitation center for supervised sessions and refreshment of secondary prevention measures on a more regular basis, though with larger time intervals.

The patient should be able to self-monitor his exercise intensity using the Borg scale, a heart rate monitor, or his own measuring of the heart rate. Any symptoms or signs suggestive of myocardial ischemia or cardiac arrhythmias should be observed and if they occur the patient should discontinue training and contact his doctor for a medical check-up. The program will only restart after the doctor's formal permission.

Long-Term Education and Risk Factor Control

The education started in the earlier program phases (risk factor control, healthy lifestyle, and stress management) needs to be periodically refreshed for patients and relatives. Regular personal meetings, phone contacts, and periodical evaluations performed by a cardiac nurse, dietician and cardiologist or general practitioner should only be tapered down gradually and adapted individually.

The patient, his family members (and the CR center staff) should be aware that maintenance is at least as important as the earlier phases of CR and needs reinforcement. An education program will never be finished because medical science is always developing. Furthermore, as time goes by patients may be prone to relapse to former unhealthy behaviors, reducing their physical activity and allowing themselves to consume less-advisable foodstuffs or beverages.

Adherence to Healthy Life Habits

The maintenance phase carries a significant risk of being quickly abandoned, being a long-lasting (years) intervention with significant financial and personal costs. Patients may be frequently asymptomatic, previously sedentary and not wishing to do any lifestyle change.[12] A progressive decay in program compliance has been reported by Dorn and coworkers[13] and by others. By 3 years after the start of the program only 13% of the participants were still exercising regularly!

To counteract the poor compliance rates it is recommended to identify patients at high risk for drop-out (Table 43-1). The patient and family should be informed about the benefits of CR and of the risk of poor adherence. The patient's decision to discontinue the program (as with any other treatment) is a "reasoned decision." It is based on a personal judgment weighing the costs and risks of the treatment against the benefits according to personal perceptions and using the available information.[12] A high quality professional relationship between the CR staff and patient and optimal program access in terms of transportation, time schedule, and fees are further important factors supporting compliance.[14,15]

Performing the exercise in groups might be preferred for the maintenance phase as the patient will benefit from psychosocial support within the group. Here, patient organizations, voluntary organizations, coronary clubs, etc. are available in many countries. For practical reasons, for some patients home-based or work-site training is an alternative. Yet, regular contact with the CR center staff, phone calls or even via the internet are all helpful in supporting a continued healthy lifestyle.[14]

References

1. Oldridge NB, Guyatt GH, Fischer ME, et al. Cardiac rehabilitation after myocardial infarction. Combined experience of randomized clinical trials. JAMA 1988;260:945–950.
2. Conraads VM, Beckers P, Bosmans J, et al. Combined endurance/resistance training reduces plasma TNF-alpha receptor levels in patients with chronic heart failure and coronary artery disease. Eur Heart J 2002;23:1854–1860.
3. Hambrecht R, Wolf A, Gielen S, et al. Effect of exercise on coronary endothelial function in patients with coronary artery disease. N Engl J Med 2000;342:454–460.
4. EUROASPIRE II Study Group. Lifestyle and risk factor management and use of drug therapies in coronary patients from 15 countries. Principal results from EUROASPIRE II. Euro Heart Survey Programme. Eur Heart J 2001;22:554–572.
5. Kotseva K, Wood DA, De Bacquer D, et al. On behalf of the EUROASPIRE II survey. Cardiac rehabilitation for coronary patients: lifestyle, risk factor and therapeutic management. Results from the EUROASPIRE II survey. Eur Heart J 2004;6 (suppl J):J 17–J32.
6. American Association of Cardiovascular and Pulmonary Rehabilitation. Guidelines for Cardiac Rehabilitation and Secondary Prevention Pro-

TABLE 43-1. Drop-out factors

Factors	
Patient	Smoker, female gender, overweight, low motivation, previous physical inactivity, symptoms, more than one MI or concomitant disease
Program	High intensity, poorly organized, unfriendly staff, inconvenient location or time schedule. Expensive
Other	Lack of social support (e.g. spouse) or work related. Transportation

grammes, 4th edn. Champaign, IL: Human Kinetics; 2004: 53–68.

7. Dafoe WA, Lefroy S, Pashkow FJ, et al. Programmes models for cardiac rehabilitation. In: Pashkow FJ, Dafoe WA, eds. Clinical Cardiac Rehabilitation. A Cardiologist's Guide, 2nd edn. Baltimore: Williams & Wilkins; 1999.

8. Vale MJ, Jelinek MV, Best JD, et al. COACH Study Group. Coaching patients on achieving cardiovascular health (COACH): a multicenter randomized trial in patients with coronary heart disease. Arch Intern Med 2003;163:2775–2783.

9. Giannuzzi P, Mezzani A, Saner H, et al. Physical activity for primary and secondary prevention. Position paper of the Working Group on Cardiac Rehabilitation and Exercise Physiology of the European Society of Cardiology. Eur J Cardiovasc Prev Rehabil 2003;10:319–327.

10. Giannuzzi P, Saner H, Bjornstad H, et al. Secondary Prevention Through Cardiac Rehabilitation. Position Paper of the Working Group on Cardiac Rehabilitation and Exercise Physiology of the European Society of Cardiology. Eur Heart J 2003;24:1273–1278.

11. VanCamp S, Peterson R. Cardiovascular complications of outpatient cardiac rehabilitation programmes. JAMA 1986;256:1160–1163.

12. Ockene IS, Hayman LL, Pasternak RC, et al. Task force #4 – Adherence issues and behavioral changes: achieving a long term solution. 33rd Bethesda Conference. J Am Coll Cardiol 2002;40:630–640.

13. Dorn J, Naughton J, Imamura D, et al. Correlates of compliance in a randomized exercise trial in myocardial infarction patients. Med Sci Sports Exerc 2001;7:1081–1089.

14. Donovan JL, Blake DR. Patient non compliance: Deviance or reasoned decision making? Soc Sci Med 1992;34:507–513.

15. Oldridge N, Pashkow FJ. Adherence and motivation in cardiac rehabilitation. In: Pashkow FJ, Dafoe WA, eds. Clinical Cardiology Rehabilitation. A Cardiologist's Guide, 2nd edn. Baltimore: Williams & Wilkins; 1999: 487–503.

44
New Models of Care and Support

Jill F. Pattenden and Robert J. Lewin

In many industrialized countries, the percentage of the population that is elderly is rising; more people are surviving with conditions that in the past were fatal, and obesity and a sedentary lifestyle are still increasing. As a result, the number of people living with a chronic illness is also rising rapidly. For example, in the UK the proportion of people living with a chronic condition has risen from 21% in 1972 to 35% in 2002; 17% of those with a chronic condition have a cardiovascular illness or hypertension. Approximately 25% have three or more chronic health problems. The healthcare systems designed over the 20th century faced different challenges, initially to eradicate and then to control infectious disease and also to manage acute events. There was less attention given to prevention and rehabilitation, and services are not well suited to caring for a large number of people living, often for decades, with a high level of disability or complex disease management regimes. As a result, across the world healthcare planners and providers are seeking new and more cost-effective models of care. Information technology in the form of the internet is also available and will affect how healthcare is delivered.

As yet these changes are in their infancy and this chapter will describe three of the emerging methods and their implications for secondary care and rehabilitation in cardiovascular disease (CVD). They are, firstly, care led by specialist nurses, secondly, care delivered by lay-people or fellow patients, and finally e-health and internet-led programs.

Nurse-Led Multidisciplinary Care

New models of care include the development of the specialist nurse role in cardiology. Several studies with nurse-led multidisciplinary team management have shown this to be effective in reducing readmissions and improving quality of life in patients with chronic heart failure (CHF) and in particular left ventricular systolic dysfunction (LVSD). A recent meta-analysis showed that comprehensive discharge planning plus post-discharge support for older patients with CHF significantly reduced readmission rates and may improve health outcomes such as quality of life without increasing costs.[1] These nurses are skilled and a relatively rare resource and it is important that they are used to the best effect.

A model of care that has been influential around the world is that developed by Kaiser Permanente where there are three "cutting points" for providing different levels of patient care.[2] The first, containing as many as 70–80% of patients, relies mainly on them providing their own self-management using simple educational materials provided by healthcare staff. The second, much smaller group comprises those requiring somewhat more individualized care, formal educational and disease management programs, or regular telephone prompting about self-management. At the top of the apex (5–8%) are those who have very complex care needs resulting in repeated admissions to care. They would be offered a great deal of individualized multidisciplinary care. In this model the specialist heart failure nurse would operate mainly in the second area, helping to transition patients from acute care to be discharged to the care of primary care or community nurses. A "case manager" would organize all aspects of care for the few complex patients with multiple co-morbidities at the apex of the triangle. However, these staff would need a great deal of training and support resources and the debate is still unfinished as to the actual cost-effectiveness of this method.[3,4]

We have recently evaluated the role of the heart failure specialist nurse and found that one of the needs expressed both by patients and the nurses was for better advice on being physically active and managing emotions (this report is available on the British Heart Foundation website www.bhf.org.uk). Although these issues should be addressed in a traditional cardiac rehabilitation (CR) program, as yet there are very few programs prepared to take patients with heart failure, especially those in class III and IV on the New York Heart Association scale. Also, many of these patients are elderly, have serious co-morbidities, mobility and transport problems, and little desire to visit hospital more than is absolutely necessary. A solution we are currently developing and evaluating is a cognitive behavioral home-based self-management program organized around a workbook and written material tailored to the individual patient's needs. This could be facilitated either by the specialist nurse or from the local rehabilitation center by phone.

Nurse-Led Self-Care Management Programs

Many chronic diseases lend themselves to self-management as long as patients have the requisite cognitive skills, mental health, and health literacy, and a number of programs have been developed and evaluated. A recent review suggests that the effectiveness of self-management educational programs varies but that patients with diabetes and hypertension gain small to moderate benefit as measured by improved glycosylated hemoglobin levels and systolic blood pressure.[5] It is clear that effective self-care management programs differ from traditional "patient education." Michael Von Korff has recently described the common features of effective chronic disease management programs, which include: a personalized written care plan; education in self-management tailored to the individual's age and circumstances; the monitoring of outcome and adherence to treatment; the targeted use of specialist consultation or referral. He also notes that to be effective staff facilitating the program must: recognize and manage anxiety and depression; use the cognitive behavioral principles of step-by-step change; develop with the patient collaborative problem definition and goal setting; use motivational techniques and monitor the

success using outcome measurement.[6]

Although good self-care management has been shown to increase positive outcomes, people with several co-morbidities may sometimes feel overwhelmed and be unable to perform self-care strategies without additional individual and family support[7] and it is important that the educational and emotional needs of a patient's family and caregivers are attended to. In the UK, two cognitive behavioral cardiac rehabilitation programs that meet these criteria and are facilitated by a health professional and carried out mainly at home have proved both successful and popular with staff and patients. These are the Heart Manual[8] and the Angina Plan.[9]

Lay-Led Self-Care Management Programs

There are a number of apparent benefits in involving lay-people in helping their peers. Firstly, they often work as volunteers or for relatively little remuneration, thus reducing health costs. Secondly, they are plentiful, and a number of countries are beginning to run short of trained healthcare staff. Thirdly, and most importantly, they are often more like the people they are trying to help than doctors and nurses. This is especially true when the lay-advisor also has the same chronic illness. It has been suggested that they may act as more credible role models than people who have not experienced the illness.

One model of a lay-led generic chronic-disease self-management program that has been adopted worldwide is known in the UK as the Expert Patient Programme, developed at Stanford University by Kate Lorig.[10] In this program, two specially trained lay-people who have a chronic illness, using a manual and a preordained script, lead a group of other patients with chronic illnesses through a 2 hours a week, 6-week program. It involves problem solving, decision making, and confidence building to increase self-efficacy; goal setting; relaxation techniques and educational sessions on managing pain; increasing activity levels; and dealing with medical personnel. Evaluations have shown that it reduced hospital admissions and use of healthcare resources, increased feelings of self-efficacy, knowledge about the illness, and self-management behaviors, and improved some aspects of health status such as depression. Others have reported no change in use of healthcare resources, pain, shortness of breath, anxiety, or exercise.[11] This program has not yet been tested with solely CVD patients and compared with the gains that can be obtained from the best examples of cardiac rehabilitation programs the advantages are still questionable.

A cardiac specific lay-led program, "Braveheart," has been developed and evaluated in Scotland. This also uses pairs of trained "senior health mentors" to run groups, every 3 weeks for a year. The study concluded that lay health mentoring is feasible, practical and inclusive, positively influencing diet, physical activity, and health resource utilization in older subjects with ischemic heart disease without causing harm.[12]

Lay Advice and Support

There is a good deal of evidence to support the use of peer mentors (also called lay advisors or buddies) with at-risk patients[13] and cardiac patients. For example, peer advisors can provide social support to decrease heart disease-related depression, encourage healthy recovery, and decrease hospital readmission rate.[14] Peer support for cardiac surgery patients reduced anxiety and led to increased activity post surgery.[15] Peer support groups for people 12 months after a cardiac event led to an increase in physical activity and smoking cessation.[16] Home visits to post-MI patients by trained lay volunteers, who had attended CR themselves, significantly increased the likelihood of attendance at CR. Peer support was also shown to be useful in promoting exercise in seniors,[17] and using peers as an extension to care by nurses to post-MI patients had positive outcomes for both patient and the peer advisor.[18]

Frequently the aim is to provide a network of mentors who will be effective self-management role models, and can act as friendly and supportive listeners, facilitators, and sign posters to community support. In most cases, peer mentors are people with the same disease, matched for age, gender, and socioeconomic similarity. There is evidence that brief interventions in healthcare settings are effective in promoting physical activity, and have longer-term impact when supported in the community by exercise advisors, written materials, and accessible facilities. Exercise buddies can help cardiac patients or those at risk of developing cardiac disease to find an activity that is enjoyable and fits into their life, is affordable and accessible, home based or in groups according to preference, and addresses psychosocial needs by combining fun and social activity with physical activity. The mentor can then motivate and support mentees, face to face or by telephone, through goal setting and provide motivational counseling to encourage people to be less sedentary, walk more and use stairs.

Lay workers and volunteers offering peer support must be carefully recruited, and ideally matched by age and gender to their mentees, have reliable good quality training, task descriptions and ongoing support through newsletters, supervision from healthcare staff, assessment of their work and constructive feedback. A toolkit, "Developing a buddy network," can be downloaded from www.bhf.org.uk/publications.

Internet and eHealth

The internet is a resource that many people already use to educate themselves about health (often called eHealth) and there is increasing interest in using it to provide more interactive health information. For example, computer-tailored nutrition education appears to be a promising way of motivating people to make healthy dietary changes. The individualized feedback it provides mimics face-to-face counseling, and is more effective than general nutrition information. Telephone, e-mail or web logs can also be used to monitor physiological status, review care needs, and monitor self-management behaviors.

Nguyen et al. provide an overview of eHealth applications for patients with cardiovascular disease.[19] Such interactive health communications can be used to relay information, enable informed decision making, and promote self-care through professionally facilitated education and support programs. Internet resources can also provide automated tailored patient education, accessed independently by patients. They can also provide the potential for peer support from a virtual community of cardiac patients. A study reported by Nguyen et al. suggests that combining all three elements may enhance success.

Home-based CR using written materials and workbooks with brief communication, often by phone, has been shown to be as effective as conventional rehabilitation and the same methods lend themselves to the Internet. There is much research currently underway into methods of providing CR via the internet and at least one study has already reported it to be as effective as more conventional methods.[20] Within a few years internet-based two-way high quality video communication will be common for domestic users, opening up the possibility of people receiving individual consultations or even joining group-based programs from their home.

Currently there are some drawbacks to this method, the most obvious being access. It is still the case that in most countries use of the internet is low amongst elderly and deprived groups and some people with language difficulties or visual impairment may find eHealth methods impossible. However, as the current generation of enthusiastic users of the internet develop CVD and require rehabilitation and disease management interventions, it seems likely that they will expect healthcare, like many of their other services, to be available in this convenient manner.

Conclusions

The pressure to provide good long-term care to an increasingly large and disabled proportion of the population is leading to the development of new methods of provision. Cardiac care and rehabilitation will be affected by these developments. Although some of these changes are mainly motivated by cost saving, they may also have intrinsic value in their own right.

Specialist nurses visiting elderly, very ill or disabled patients at home, or coordinating that care through other workers, could use suitably modified home-based rehabilitation programs to bring help to those currently excluded. Better protocols for the long-term management of CVD, triaging people according to need and integrating the healthcare among primary, secondary and social care can only benefit patients. Cardiac rehabilitation services should not neglect the possibility of taking a role in these developments as they have much knowledge and experience to offer.

Lay-led chronic disease management programs are being encouraged and adopted by many health providers. The most widely implemented is the Stanford Chronic Disease Self-Management Program. Although it provided some benefits, it is not disease specific and early evidence from a national evaluation in the UK suggests that many patients do not wish to take part. It is not clear how it "fits" with CR or other disease-specific programs. The best CR programs have powerful effects in reducing mortality (20%) and morbidity (quality of life, anxiety, depression, functional ability) and in cost saving that surpass the results so far demonstrated by generic lay-led programs. Theoretically, a cardiac-specific program staffed by enthusiastic fellow CVD patients who have changed to a healthy lifestyle, developed skills to manage living with their heart disease and found ways to enjoy life, may encourage better uptake than one staffed by people with whom the patients feel they have little in common, especially in deprived communities. To date we are aware of only one such program, Braveheart; this small-scale study produced some useful gains and requires further attention and replication ideally in comparison to a conventional CR program. A rapid review of the current state of knowledge regarding lay-led self-management of chronic illness conducted by the NHS National Institute for Health and Clinical Excellence[21] concluded that no real evidence of long term effectiveness exists for these lay-led programs in the management of chronic illnesses at community or population level, and they should be provided only as a part of a range of formal and informal resources.

Similarly, a review of disease management programs for patients with heart failure recommended that although telecare and telemonitoring are increasingly used as a cost effective way of patient management and support, they should only be part of a range of multidisciplinary disease management program in cardiac disease, where services provided are appropriate for each individual patient, many of whom gain reassurance and support from face-to-face contact with a practitioner.[22]

Lay advisors and buddies are already used in CR programs to encourage others to join or to help people prior to or after cardiac surgery. There is increasing evidence to support expanding their involvement. Properly trained and supported peer advisors, especially when matched on age, gender and years of education, may be at least as effective in helping patients change their health behavior and maintain those new behaviors as healthcare workers. Long-term maintenance of gains has been the Achilles heel of CR; lay-led schemes based in the community may help to solve this problem. These schemes could be individual or group based, offer telephone support, and supply motivation and social support to encourage individuals to take part in light- to moderate-intensity activities. These could include walking, resistance work and aerobic activity or activities already available in the community, such as line dancing, tea dances, yoga, or bowls. Lay workers may also have a role in primary prevention using volunteer advisers in individuals' homes, workplaces, church settings, and community centers, or by telephone coaching and support after an initial assessment and discussion with healthcare staff.

The possibilities of eHealth to deliver and support people making lifestyle changes are enormous and are already being used. It is already possible for people to take part in home-based rehabilitation and in the next few years we can expect a number of research programs to report results.

References

1. Phillips CO, Writht SM, Kern DE, et al. Comprehensive discharge planning with postdischarge support for older patients with congestive heart failure: A meta-analysis; JAMA 2004;291:1358–1367.
2. Dixon J, Lewis R, Rosen R, et al. Can the NHS learn from US managed care organisations? BMJ 2004; 328:223–225.
3. Murphy E. Editorial: Case management and community matrons for long term conditions. BMJ 2004;329:1251–1252.
4. Hutt R, Rosen R, McCauley J. Case-managing Long-term Conditions: What impact does it have in the Treatment of Older People? London: Kings Fund; 2004.
5. Warsi A, Wang PS, LaValley MP, et al. Self-management education programs in chronic disease: a systematic review and methodological critique of the literature. Arch Intern Med 2004;164:1641–1649.
6. Von Korff M, Glasgow RE, Sharpe M. Organising care for chronic illness. BMJ 2002;325:92–94.
7. Chriss PM, Sheposh J, Carlson B, et al. Predictors of successful heart failure self-care maintenance in the first three months after hospitalization. Heart Lung 2004;33:345–353.
8. Lewin B, Robertson IH, Cayol EL, et al. Effects of self-help post myocardial infarction rehabilitation on psychological adjustment and use of health services. Lancet 1992;339:1036–1040.
9. Lewin RJ, Furze G, Robinson J, et al. A randomised controlled trial of a self-management plan for patients with newly diagnosed angina. Br J Gen Pract 2002;52:194–196, 199–201 (see also www.anginaplan.org.uk).
10. Bodenheimer T, Lorig K, Holman H, et al. Patient self-management of chronic disease in primary care. JAMA 2002;288:2469–2475.
11. Writht CC, Barlow JH, Turner AP, et al. Self-management training for people with chronic disease: an exploratory study. Br J Health Psychol 2003; 8:465–476.
12. Coull AJ, Taylor VH, Elton R, et al. A randomised controlled trial of senior lay health mentoring in older people with ischaemic heart disease: The Braveheart Project. Age Ageing 2004;33:348–354.
13. Joseph DH, Griffin M, Hall RF, et al. Peer coaching: an intervention for individuals struggling with diabetes. Diabetes Educ 2001;27:703–710.
14. Cashen MS, Dykes P, Gerber B. eHealth technology and internet resources: barriers for vulnerable populations. J Cardiovasc Nurs 2004;19:209–214.
15. Parent N, Fortin F. A randomised, controlled trial of vicarious experience through peer support for male first-time cardiac surgery patients: impact on anxiety, self-efficacy expectation, and self-reported activity. Heart Lung 2000;29:389–400.
16. Hildingh C, Fridlund B. Participation in peer support groups after a cardiac event: a 12 month follow up. Rehabil Nurs 2003;28:123–128.
17. Resnick B, Orwig D, Magaziner J, Wynne C. The effect of social support on exercise behavior in older adults. Clin Nurs Res 2002;11:52–70.
18. Whittemore R, Rankin SH, Callahan CD, et al. The peer advisor experience providing social support. Qual Health Res 2000;10:260–270.
19. Nguyen HQ, Carrieri-Kohlman V, Rankin SH, Slaughter R, Stulbarg MS. Supporting cardiac recovery through eHealth technology. J Cardiovasc Nurs 2004;19:200–208.
20. Southard BH, Southard DR, Nuckolls J. Clinical trial of an Internet-based case management system for secondary prevention of heart disease. J Cardiopulm Rehabil 2003;23:341–348.
21. Bury M, Newbould J, Taylor D. A rapid review of the current state of knowledge regarding lay-led self-management of chronic illness. Evidence review December 2005, NHS National Institute for Health and Clinical Excellence. Available at www.publichealth.nice.org.uk.
22. Gohler A, Januzzi JL, Worrell SS, Osterziel KJ, Gazelle GS, Dietz R, Siebert U. A systematic meta-analysis of the efficacy and heterogeneity of disease management programs in congestive heart failure. J Card Fail 2006;12:554–567.

Section VIII
Adapted Programs for Special Groups

Cardiac rehabilitation programs are primarily designed to limit the physiological and psychological effect of cardiac illness but even more to reduce the risk of sudden death or infarction, to control cardiac symptoms, to prevent re-hospitalization, and to stabilize or reverse the atherosclerotic process. These goals of cardiac rehabilitation are perfectly appropriate for patients with atherosclerotic heart disease as the main cardiovascular problem. However, there are a growing number of patients with special needs in cardiac rehabilitation. The great progress and increased success of early surgery in children with congenital heart disease has led to a growing number of adolescents and younger adults needing cardiac rehabilitation, which sometimes poses a special challenge to the rehabilitation team in regard to exercise training and also psychological adjustment. Gender issues in cardiac rehabilitation have not been addressed sufficiently so far in cardiovascular research. Although we know that women are less likely to attend cardiac rehabilitation programs than men and that they have a higher drop-out rate during the programs, we are far away from good solutions to this problem. Research in this field is urgently needed. Rehabilitation in patients with heart failure has become a specific but rewarding challenge for cardiac rehabilitation specialists. Exercise testing and training has to be adapted to decreased cardiac performance and to peripheral muscular problems. A comprehensive approach including counseling in regard to drug treatment and weight control as well as control of salt and water intake, support to overcome anxiety and depression, and instructions to adapt physical activity to the reduced cardiac performance are of crucial importance. The need for specific psychological support in these patients is now recognized. Although rehabilitation of cardiac transplantation may be a rare challenge in regular programs due to the low number of patients, specific physiological aspects of the cardiovascular system have a major impact on exercise testing and training modalities. Furthermore, adjustment of the patient, his family and partner have to be supported.

Quality of life and psychosocial adjustment are often poor in patients after ICD implantation. Avoidance of physical activity due to fear of defibrillator shocks is often encountered. Comprehensive cardiac rehabilitation in this patient group can help to overcome this problem and therefore to increase quality of life considerably. The patient with peripheral arterial disease is often a poly-morbid patient with extensive atherosclerosis including heart, brain, and kidney. Comprehensive risk factor management is crucial to reduce the global cardiovascular risk in these patients. Exercise training with walking with moderate claudication pain is a recognized treatment with a great potential to improve pain-free walking distance. Finally, comprehensive cardiac rehabilitation should become a cornerstone in the corporate setting to form an integral part of a "seamless care" model. This type of care may even become a marker of success for companies in the corporate setting.

Main Messages

Chapter 45: Cardiac Rehabilitation in Congenital Heart Disease

With the progress in the treatment of congenital heart disease (CHD), more and more affected children reach adulthood. This causes morbidity within this population to be a growing problem which demands special expertise. We expect CHD to be accompanied by deficits in the fields of motor skills, cognition, and emotion (not only in the person affected but also in their social environment). Preventive diagnostics and treatment have to be initiated early, aiming to find deficits and alleviate them through the use of specific measures. This is the reason for rehabilitative intervention in CHD, targeting a long-tem reduction of morbidity and an enhancement of the patient's quality of life.

Chapter 46: Gender Issues in Rehabilitation

Little is known about the needs and experiences of women with regard to cardiac rehabilitation. Diabetes, lipid abnormalities, cigarette smoking, and probably also psychological factors seem to be of special importance. Symptoms and signs of myocardial ischemia and infarction may be different from those in men. Women are less likely to be referred to cardiac rehabilitation programs, are less interested, and have higher drop-out rates than men. Cardiac rehabilitation programs should be made more attractive for women. However, further research in this field is urgently needed.

Chapter 47: Rehabilitation in Elderly Patients

Special needs for the growing number of elderly patients in cardiac rehabilitation have to be considered. Decreased mobility and impaired cognitive functions make program attendance difficult for many patients. Co-morbidities have a considerable impact on exercise testing and training. Depression and social isolation are more prominent than in younger patients. However, elderly patients profit from structured cardiac rehabilitation to the same extent as younger patients. The main goals of cardiac rehabilitation in elderly patients are preservation of mobility and independence, preservation of mental function, prevention/treatment of anxiety and depression, encouragement of social readaption and reintegration to enable the patient to return to the same lifestyle as before the event.

Chapter 48: Cardiac Rehabilitation in Chronic Heart Failure

The complexity and progressive nature of chronic heart failure (HF) requires demanding and time-consuming multidisciplinary strategies that need to be integrated and coordinated in a flexible disease management system. Cardiac rehabilitation is the ideal comprehensive structured disease intervention since it best addresses the complex interplay of medical, psychological, and behavioral factors facing chronic HF patients and carers. Core components of cardiac rehabilitation include baseline clinical assessment and risk stratification, optimal pharmacological therapy, management of HF-related diseases, non-pharmacological therapy in the form of an integrated management system with a continuing program of physical activity, exercise training, counseling and education, and psychological support.

Chapter 49: Rehabilitation after Cardiac Transplantation

Multifaceted physical and mental problems are encountered pre- and postoperatively in patients after cardiac transplantation. There are anatomical and physiological reasons for limited exercise tolerance. Dynamic exercise and resistance training both contribute to the prevention of side-effects of immunosuppressive therapy and to the reduction of cardiovascular risk factors, thus improving quality of life. Support for psychological adjustment of the patient and his family are important. Family adjustment and stabilization of partner relationships pose a great challenge.

Chapter 50: Rehabilitation in Patients with Implantable Devices

The need of patients with implantable cardioverter defibrillators (ICDs) for structured exercise training and rehabilitation is increasingly recognized. Compared to the general population, quality of life and psychosocial adjustment are often poor. Recent studies report psychological benefits for patients with ICDs after psychological intervention or comprehensive cardiac rehabilitation. Maximal or symptom-limited exercise testing in patients with optimal pharmacological treatment is safe and feasible. However, exercise training and testing should be performed in a professional and medical environment with continuous emphasis on safety measures.

Chapter 51: Rehabilitation in Peripheral Vascular Disease

The patient with peripheral artery disease is a potential polyvascular patient. Thus, an integrated approach to prevention and treatment of atherothrombosis as a whole (smoking cessation, aggressive treatment of dyslipidemia, diabetes mellitus, and hypertension) is warranted.

Patients with claudication are characterized by marked impairments in exercise performance and overall functional capacity and exercise training is an effective treatment.

Exercise training should consist of short periods of treadmill walking with an intensity that produces moderate claudication pain within the first 5 minutes of walking, interspersed with rest, throughout a 50-minute exercise session, three times weekly.

Chapter 52: Cardiac Rehabilitation and Wellness in the Corporate Setting

For cardiac rehabilitation to be successful in the corporate setting it should form an integral part of a "seamless care" service model. This should include preventative strategies that focus on optimizing health and wellness, reducing and managing cardiovascular risk when present and rehabilitating post-cardiac populations. Clinicians and a team of multidisciplinary healthcare professionals, are ideally suited to deliver such a service.

The potential for this model being generated into a successful business within the corporate sector is enormous. The successful companies of the future will undoubtedly have a wellness plan to go alongside their business plan.

45
Cardiac Rehabilitation in Congenital Heart Disease

Birna Bjarnason-Wehrens, Sigrid Dordel, Narayanswami Sreeram, and K. Brockmeier

Congenital malformations of the heart and vessels occur in 5–8 per 1000 live births, resulting in an incidence of approximately 0.7%.[1,2] Some of these malformations (10–15%) do not require correction. Between 70% and 80% of defects can be corrected, and an increasing number of therapeutic procedures can be performed by interventional catheterization techniques, avoiding the need for open heart surgery.[3] Definitive therapeutic procedures are increasingly carried out in early infancy, to avoid long-term complications resulting from the hemodynamic burden, or from chronic cyanosis. With improved techniques and experience, procedure-related mortality has been substantially lowered.[4] In 2002, a total of 27,772 operations for the treatment of CHD were performed in Europe. Germany leads this statistic with 5868 operations for congenital heart defects in 2003; 4415 of those were performed using a heart–lung machine. Significantly, almost half of all operations were performed on neonates and infants. In addition, there were more than 2000 catheter interventions.[3] In Germany mortality from congenital cardiac malformations (operated or unoperated) has decreased by approximately 64% since 1980.[3] With improved survival, the focus of follow-up care has had to shift from assessment of procedure-related mortality towards assessment of long-term quality of life.

Congenital Heart Disease (CHD)

The spectrum of CHD is diverse. Defects can roughly be categorized into left-to-right shunt lesions, cyanotic lesions, obstructive lesions, and complex lesions associated with common mixing and single ventricle physiology.[1] Table 45-1 and Figure 45-1 provide a list of the most frequent lesions, comprising approximately 80% of all malformations. For further details, see Allen et al.[1]

The impact of a congenital cardiac malformation on the development of the affected child depends on the type and severity of the malformation, as well as the timing and success of therapeutic measures. For some complex malformations with single ventricle physiology, only palliative solutions are available. Lesions such as tetralogy of Fallot,[6] atrioventricular septal defect,[7] and transposition of the great arteries[8] can be successfully corrected in infancy with good long-term outcome. Regardless of the immediate procedural outcome, long-term follow-up of patients with the entire spectrum of lesions which have been corrected or palliated shows that several new problems may appear in later life including residual valvular obstruction or insufficiency, myocardial dysfunction, and new potentially life-threatening arrhythmias related to previous surgical scars. It is mandatory therefore that all patients receive some form of life-long supervision. Depending on the degree of myocardial dysfunction, persistent cyanosis or dysrhythmias, disabilities and handicaps may exist that can have grave consequences for psychosocial and cognitive development.[9]

Possible Complications

In complex cardiac defects with or without surgical intervention, there is a complication rate of

TABLE 45-1. The most frequently diagnosed congenital heart diseases

Acyanotic vitia		Cyanotic vitia	
Obstructions in valves or vessels	Primary left–right shunt	Right–Left shunt	Complex lesions
Pulmonary stenosis (PS) 6–13%	Ventricular septal defects (VSD) (isolated) 14–16%	Tetralogy of Fallot (ToF) 9–14%	Single ventricle physiology, e.g. hypoplastic left heart syndrome (HLHS) 4–8%
Coarctation of the aorta (CoA) 8–11%	Atrial septal defects (ASD) 4–10%	Transposition of the great arteries (TGA) 10–11%	
Aortic stenosis (AS) 6–9%	Persistent ductus arteriosus (PDA) 10–15%		

Source: American Heart Association[2] and Mennicken et al.[5]

1–5% affecting other organs (hypoxic impairments, infarcts, multiple organ failure), which can lead to multiple disabilities.[9] Neurological impairments caused by persistent low cardiac output, acidosis, and/or hypoxia[4] range from light, general, or specific failures in brain function to severe spastic tetraparesis.[9] Brain damage and neurodevelopmental disorders in children with CHD may also be genetically determined in addition to the possibility of congenital malformations of the brain, and ischemia related to surgery.[10] For example, the duration of circulatory arrest during surgery[11,12] as well as the duration of a persistent low output state requiring intensive medical care after surgery are associated with these phenomena.[13,14]

Disturbances of growth are a consequence of insufficient caloric intake and a simultaneous, significantly increased energy demand in infants, children, and adolescents with hemodynamically relevant cardiac defects. Even when appropriate caloric intake is offered, problems may exist with absorption and metabolism.[15] Furthermore, eating disorders in infants and toddlers may be observed following long-term, intensive medical care. Extracardiac factors such as disturbed parent–child interaction may enhance disturbances of growth.[16] Early definitive correction of cardiac defects provides optimum conditions for successful catch-up growth and a normalization of the physical development.[15] Another recently recognized, and frequently underdiagnosed problem relates to young teenagers, usually female, who present with eating disturbances associated with a disturbed body image.

Congenital heart defects are frequently found in connection with malformation syndromes and chromosomal disorders (including Williams syndrome, Down's syndrome, and microdeletion of chromosome 22q11), which are linked to multiple disabilities.[9] Accordingly, 3.2–12% of congenital heart defects are accompanied by additional chromosomal anomalies, while 5.4–9.5% of patients with CHD have Down's syndrome.[17] The special needs of these patients have to be taken into account in their long-term treatment and in rehabilitation efforts. A microdeletion in the short arm of chromosome 22 (22q11) has a variable penetrance and is very frequently linked to CHD. Typical, but not obligatory, are substantial cognitive impairments as well as psychologically and psychiatrically relevant disorders, which may be very hard to distinguish from possible damage related to the therapeutic process. Therefore, the diagnosis of some heart defects typically associated with microdeletion of 22q11 requires further genetic testing, so that necessary intervention methods can be applied in a timely fashion.

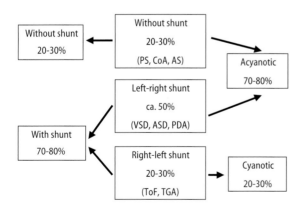

FIGURE 45-1. Classification of congenital heart defects according to defects with or without shunt and with or without cyanosis; see Table 45-1 for definitions of abbreviations. (Adapted and modified from Mennicken et al.[5])

Possible Consequences of Congenital Heart Disease

The consequences of cardiac lesions in children are diverse and can impose stress not only on the child but also on his or her social environment (Table 45-2).

Consequences for the Patient

Numerous studies have investigated the exercise tolerance of children with various forms of CHD. Depending on the severity of the defect, the success of corrective procedures, the presence and degree of residual sequelae, physical performance may be limited.[18] Even children with mild uncorrected lesions or without residual sequelae after previous surgery may reveal a substantial reduction in their physical performance. Overprotection and the resulting lack of physical activity may contribute to this. Thus far the scientific focus has predominantly been on children with complex heart defects.

Relatively few studies have focused on the motor abilities of children with CHD. Bellinger et al.[19] demonstrated a retardation of motor development for both gross and fine motor skills at 4-year follow-up after an uncomplicated neonatal arterial switch operation for transposition of the great arteries. The duration of total circulatory arrest (CA) was closely linked to gross motor skills, but not to fine motor skills. Distinctive limitations in fine motor skills and visual-spatial skills were observed at 8-year follow-up in the same patient cohort.[11] In their assessment of gross and fine motor skills of 5- to 14-year-olds, Stieh et al.[20] discovered significant deficits in motor development of children with cyanotic heart defects, as opposed to children with acyanotic CHD. In contrast to the data of Stieh, our study group found deficits in fine motor and gross motor skills for both cyanotic and acyanotic heart defects. In a study involving children with different diagnoses and varying levels of severity, 63.2% of the sample showed significant to grave deficits in gross motor skills.[21] Unverdorben et al.[22] demonstrated comparable results. They also made the interesting observation that, independent of the severity of the disease, children who were excused from physical education classes showed significantly reduced motor performance when compared to children participating in physical education in school.

Numerous studies report behavioral disorders in children and adolescents with CHD, especially – but not exclusively – in those with complex heart defects. Distinctive features became apparent on emotional, social, and cognitive levels, to varying degrees.[10] On the emotional level, predominantly internalizing disorders such as anxiety, low frustration tolerance, increased stress, and even depressions appeared. Disturbances of self-esteem, which may either be very low or extremely exaggerated, are also frequently observed. Particularly children who are not allowed to engage in exercise due to limited cardiac function or a perceived risk of sudden death are threatened by lowered self-esteem. Strong changes of mood, relapses to earlier stages of development, depression, and antisocial behavior have been observed especially in adolescents.[23–25] Additionally, children diagnosed with CHD reveal reduced social competence. Often their behavior is characterized by a tendency to retreat socially. This shyness makes building and maintaining relationships with children of the same age much harder. Numerous indicators of cognitive impairment are to be found in children with complex cardiac defects: significantly lower scores on IQ and achievement tests, learning disorders, reduced academic performance (reading, writing,

TABLE 45-2. Possible consequences of congenital heart disease for patients and their social environment

For the child:
Reduced physical performance
Restrictions in physical activity
Restricted participation in normal daily activities of healthy peers
Continuing dependence on care providers
Emotional disorders, mostly internalizing disorders such as anxiety, depression, etc.
Disturbances of social competence
Cognitive disorders

For parents and siblings:
Stress in parent–child relationship
Difficulties with education (for instance as a result of concerns over the child having a cardiac defect)
Stress on siblings (lack of attention)
Problems within the parents' relationship

Source: Adapted and modified according to Deutsche Gesellschaft für pädiatrische Kardiologie.[9]

mathematics), speech abnormalities, attention deficit disorders, disturbances in problem-solving behavior, etc.[10–12,14,19] These disorders may be caused by neurological damage, congenital malformation syndromes, and chromosomal anomalies. Yet, learning abilities of the child can also be affected by reduced perceptual abilities, lack of concentration, and attention deficits. These can either be caused by disturbed brain function or by adverse developmental conditions (situation within the family, reduced experience in regard to perception and physical activity). The lack of adequate academic education related to chronic illness may also have a negative impact.[4]

Quality of life studies have demonstrated contrasting outcomes. Some studies report no significant difference between CHD children and healthy peers while others demonstrate significantly lower quality of life, particularly in the areas of physical, social and overall function in CHD children compared to healthy controls. In a recent study where 182 parents of CHD children (54 having transposed great arteries, 55 a functionally single ventricle and 73 complex variants of functionally biventricular disease) completed a quality of life survey concerning their children, the parents reported a significantly lower quality of life than parents of healthy controls on all subscales of the instrument: overall, physical and emotional function, social and educational functioning. Quality of life did not correlate with socioeconomic status, number of open-heart operations, or the time since the last operation. Parents of children aged 8–12 years reported the lowest quality of life across all domains assessed. This span represents a time when surgical reintervention is common and also the time when children are first beginning to consider their own mortality and vulnerability. On comparing the diagnostic groups, parents of children with complex, functionally biventricular hearts reported the lowest scores for quality of life. Subjects reporting lowest quality of life were found to be significantly more likely to report functional disabilities.[25]

Consequences for the Family

The disease and the restrictions it causes (reduced physical performance, complications, continuing pharmacological treatment, operations, catheter interventions) in connection with hospitalization and frequent outpatient visits, and the overall worries about the child, impose grave stress on parents, siblings, and the entire family environment. Oftentimes, long-lasting separation of family members related to attending to the child in hospital, as well as emotional stress caused by the severe and often life-threatening heart defect of the child, also evoke psychological and somatic consequences and conflicts within the family.[26] Siblings suffer from lack of attention, often feel neglected, over-challenged, and misunderstood, and thus develop emotional disorders on their part. These may be eating disorders, sleeping disorders, regressive behavioral disorders, aggression, and/or problems in academic performance. It is crucial to approach such psychological burdens immediately and to counteract or solve conflict situations. At this point, the help of professionals (psychologists, social education workers, and social workers) who intervene at the psychosocial level is usually required.

Rehabilitation in Congenital Heart Disease

With the availability of long-term follow-up data for the entire spectrum of cardiac defects, it is becoming clear that life-long, qualified care – which may include rehabilitation measures – is required for affected children, adolescents, and adults. The decision on whether rehabilitation measures are required, and at which point and to what extent they are necessary, has to be made on an individual basis. Most frequently rehabilitation has to be initiated directly after surgery. However, rehabilitation measures may also be indicated several years after original intervention. While extensive rehabilitation is currently being offered for adult patients with coronary artery disease, such measures are not widely available to children with CHD.[27] Outpatient rehabilitation measures are often not accepted because of the long distances between patients' homes and the rehabilitation institutions. Inpatient care is very rarely offered and can only be carried out if at least one parent is present in order to avoid a painful and potentially long-term separation of the child from family.[23] However, a parent accompanying the child throughout inpatient rehabilitation significantly raises the costs of such therapy.

Rehabilitation for this group of patients has to be structured in three phases. Each phase involves somatic, educative, psychological, and social elements, which are managed by an interdisciplinary rehabilitation team.

Rehabilitation Goals

According to the WHO charter for children, every child has the right to an appropriate and undisturbed physical, mental, and emotional development. The main goals of rehabilitative measures are to eliminate or minimize impairments, disabilities, and handicaps linked to the disease and to prevent possible secondary effects. Other general rehabilitation goals are:

– Promotion of self-management and self-responsibility in terms of helping to self-help.
– Promotion of equal participation in social life and prevention or counteraction of possible discrimination. In this respect, it is particularly important to ensure and/or reestablish the affected person's integration into school, education, job, family, and society.
– Enhancement of the overall quality of life.
– Reduction of disease-related morbidity.

The specific rehabilitation goals are formulated from the patient's individual situation (age and stage of life, severity of the disease, time-span from the intervention, postoperative sequelae, co-morbidity, family and social situation, etc.). As a consequence of the diversity and complexity of cardiac defects and their effects on the whole life situation, the need for rehabilitation varies substantially, as do the corresponding rehabilitation goals. As an example, the general development of a child's personality is not only affected by medical and therapeutic interventions and/or improvement of physical fitness, but is also significantly influenced by emotional, psychosocial, and cognitive aspects of development. On the other hand, in adolescents education and coping strategies may be the main focus. This may involve providing extensive information about the cardiac defect, a personal history of the disease and its prognosis, past interventions and their consequences for heart and body, requirement for long-term medication, future

diagnostic or therapeutic procedures, and the necessity of hospital attendance for regular follow-up. Furthermore, support in terms of planning a future life independent from the parents, job training, choice of employment, sexuality, and family planning can be of great importance. Especially in adolescence, promoting acceptance of the disease can constitute an essential rehabilitation goal, as restricted acceptance may result in inefficient disease management.

A specific rehabilitation goal can also be catching up with family problems caused by the child's disease. Such problems may impact on the child/adolescent's development, their healing process, and/or their disease management. In some circumstances, this may require the integration of the whole family in the rehabilitation process.

Phases of Rehabilitation

The phase structure of rehabilitation in CHD is illustrated in Figure 45-2. Rehabilitation phase I includes treatment in a hospital or a cardiologic center for children. Here, the main focus is placed on somatic treatment including medical care and nursing. If surgery is performed on older children, adolescents, and adults, physiotherapeutic care is prioritized in order to achieve early mobilization. The most important goals are pain relief, thrombosis prophylaxis, stabilization of the circulatory system, as well as the management of existing neurological deficits.[28] In neonates, infants, and children, it is crucial for the attending doctor to provide information, counseling, and assistance to the family. Extensive information and advice offered to the parents constitutes the fundament of an adequate management of the child's heart defect. Hereby, parents also receive help in dealing with their unexpectedly difficult situation. Grief about the child being chronically ill, concerns about the future, fear of losing the child, and other worries should be addressed. Counseling by a psychological expert, a social education worker, and/or a representative of the appropriate religious society may be necessary or at least helpful, especially in severe and life-threatening diseases. Moreover, additional information and support offered by parents of other affected children contributes tremendously to the efficacy of these

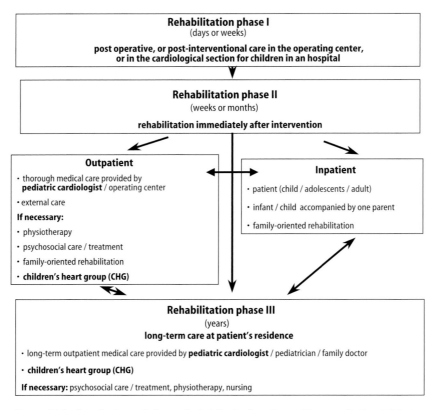

FIGURE 45-2. Organization and phases of rehabilitation in patients with congenital heart defects.

measures. Such self-help groups offer a great deal of emotional and social support, which is crucial at this point.[29] Many parent-support groups for children with specific cardiac lesions currently have their own internet websites, from which useful information concerning a particular therapeutic procedure, its outcome, and the possible complications are readily available. Encouraging parents to access these sites improves the quality of communication between parents and care providers, and also provides parents with a realistic view of the future, as seen from their perspective. Information and education about disease and rehabilitation should be provided to the parents in the course of several interviews, often going over ground which has previously been covered. At the time of diagnosis, the decision to have the child operated on and the operation itself are sources of great stress to the parents. At this point, they may not fully comprehend or accept detailed information. Therefore, it is crucial to take sufficient time and patience for parents' education. Communication

can furthermore be enhanced by means of information booklets. As parents are not only the most important persons for the child to relate to but are also responsible for their everyday care, they are an important part of the rehabilitation team.[29] For older children, adolescents, and young adults, age-appropriate information and education should be provided to the patients themselves. If needed, consultation with a (child-) psychologist and/or a social education worker should be available.

After surgical or interventional correction of a heart defect in a neonate or an infant, early rehabilitation is usually not necessary, as the patient is only discharged from hospital when it is evident that the parents are able to care for the child at home. As a result, rehabilitation phases I and II merge. After children are released from hospital, their further care is provided by a specialist. In this phase, external nursing services are recommended to support the parents. This may at first be used on a daily basis. With increasing time from the operation, the frequency and intensity of these services are reduced. Especially in regard to complex cardiac defects, extensive rehabilitation measures may become necessary at a later point in life. If early rehabilitation happens to be required after surgery (phase II), it is best pursued in a specifically designed and equipped in- or out-patient institution. Here, resources for all necessary therapeutic measures are available, ready to be employed by an interdisciplinary rehabilitation team. However, more frequently this phase is performed either in an outpatient setting or at the patient's home, directed by a children's heart center, pediatric cardiologist, or pediatrician. If needed, outpatient physiotherapy and/or psychosocial and psychomotor treatment are additionally integrated into the care program.

The transition to phase III rehabilitation is smooth. If necessary, it includes continuous, regular medical treatment at home, which is covered by a pediatric cardiologist sufficiently experienced in the care of grown-ups with CHD. If needed, these measures can be sustained through the promotion of psychomotor skills in a children's heart group and, at later ages, in an adult heart group.

The children's heart group (CHG) is a medically prescribed, supervised outpatient therapy option for children with heart defects and is led by a qualified exercise/sport therapist. Children in need of this therapy are given the opportunity to be physically active in a medically supervised, "protected area." Here, potentially existing psychomotor deficits can be identified and treated. Simultaneously, conditions for a thorough integration into physical activity of peers (as, for instance, physical education at school) are established. For most children, temporally limited participation (90–120 sessions or units) is sufficient. For children who, as a result of the severity of their disease, urgently require medical supervision during physical activity, longer participation (possibly for years) is desirable and practical in order to provide means for them to be physically active at all. CHGs meet once or twice a week for 60–90-minute sessions. To provide adequate individual attention, group sizes should be small (up to 10 children) and children should all be of approximately the same age. In the CHG, children gain knowledge about their physical limitations; they learn to become aware of their physical reac-

tions to high load and learn how to respond accordingly. The fun aspect of engaging in physical activity together with other children is particularly important. To the extent that the heart defect permits it, children ought to be encouraged to participate in physical activity with their peers, both in leisure time and at school. Participation in a CHG can also help to minimize parents' concerns and anxiety about their child being physically active and can thereby reduce overprotection. Consulting by the physician and the exercise/sport therapist along with the exchange of ideas with other parents can also provide valuable input and support for the family.

In both phase II and phase III, regular phone calls and/or email contact, along with visits from a health professional, may serve as means of continuing care for the patient and his family. Such measures could well be supported by continuous provision of information bulletins. The contact with the care team could further be improved through the implementation of a telephone hotline, which makes advice and assistance available for parents and patients. Such measures are primarily meant to serve as additional options within the care system. They are particularly important when circumstances do not allow for a patient's regular participation in therapy sessions and/or information meetings.

Need for Rehabilitation

It would be wrong to limit the need for rehabilitation to certain diagnoses and/or cardiac surgical interventions. In this respect, an urgent need for rehabilitation may as well exist due to behavioral disorders in children and adolescents with relatively mild heart defects. The need for rehabilitation can result from somatic, educative, and psychosocial, but also from family-related reasons, regardless of the patient's age or diagnosis[9] (Table 45-3). The indication for rehabilitation is provided by a pediatric cardiologist/pediatrician, possibly in association with a child neurologist and/or a child psychiatrist. The indication has to be determined and justified based on detailed medical diagnosis. If necessary, diagnostic data from other subspecialists (for instance child psychologists, social education workers, pediatric physiotherapists)

TABLE 45-3. Indications for rehabilitation

Independent of patients' age, need for rehabilitation may exist:
- after surgery with intra- or postoperative complications, or in case of extended convalescence
- for disturbed psychomotor development due to the severity of the defect or because of complex malformation syndromes
- for optimization or controlled reduction of pharmacologic therapy
- after heart transplantation
- for patients' and parents' education (for instance about medication use and individual dosage as, for example, with warfarin (Marcumar) after prosthetic valve replacement
- in case of inappropriately low (subjective) performance despite successful correction of the heart defect
- in case of insufficient acceptance and management of the disease
- to guide adolescents and adults regarding their future choice of education and career
- in special cases, especially in adolescents and young adults, as a means to prepare for future cardiac surgical or interventional procedures

Source: Adapted and modified according to Deutsche Gesellschaft für pädiatrische Kardiologie.[9]

must be considered. Only based on such detailed diagnostics can rehabilitation goals be formulated and recommendations for duration and setting (outpatient or inpatient) be given (Table 45-4). By means of an extensive interdisciplinary diagnostic approach, hidden deficits may be uncovered. Moreover, immediate intervention usually proves to be easier and less expensive than the treatment of avoidable long-term consequences.

Family-Oriented Rehabilitation

If possible, younger children should be accompanied by a parent while going through the rehabilitation process. This goes especially for inpatient care. For a chronically ill child, the relationship with the family is of utmost importance for positive management of the disease and constructive coping. However, as a consequence of the extraordinary amount of stress the chronic disease imposes on the family, a family-oriented rehabilitation including all family members may be indicated.

Regardless of the severity of the disease, family-oriented rehabilitation is required if:

- The family is unable to care for the child in a manner that will guarantee a successful healing process.
- The family cannot provide sufficient support, for instance as a result of anxiety, or if medical

and/or psychosocial factors affecting other family members negatively impact on the healing process of the primary patient.
- The disease has caused a breakdown in the family with resulting medical and psychosocial complications in other family members. This situation may occur in conjunction with life-threatening heart defects, multiple disabilities, or additional stressors.[9] The decision for family-oriented rehabilitation has to be made and justified on the basis of medical and/or psychosocial diagnostics, which include the entire family.

Family-oriented rehabilitation must be understood as medical/psychosocial care which aims at individual medical and psychotherapeutic measures for both the primary patient and other family members. The integration of the family into the medical care setting is required due to the complex somatic and psychosocial interaction, disturbed social behavior, anxiety, and/or learning disorders of the patient. In the best-case scenario, it is carried out as inpatient treatment.[30] As a consequence of specific developmental circumstances, inpatient treatment of children requires a duration of at least 4 to 6 weeks. For adolescents and adults, a minimum of 4 weeks is required.[9]

TABLE 45-4. Categories of support: patients (parents) of all categories need examination(s) by experts to investigate a potential benefit from rehabilitation. Patients from the first category may require repeated examination of their psychosocial status. Patients from categories two and three usually need only one examination of their psychosocial status

Rehabitation obligatory
Severe forms of congenital heart disease – complex congenital heart disease:
- palliative surgery (Fontan type palliation)
- congenital heart disease without possible definitive treatment
- after surgery/intervention with major residual defects
- severe congestive heart disease/cardiomyopathy
- after heart transplantation

Rehabilitation recommended
Less severe forms of congenital heart disease:
- after successful surgery
- after successful intervention
- with minor residual defects

Rehabilitation recommended under special, e.g. psychosocial, conditions
Congenital heart disease with marginal hemodynamic significance (e.g.):
- small left-to-right shunts
- insignificant semilunar valve stenosis

Content of Rehabilitation

The rehabilitation process has to be individualized, age-appropriate, and oriented to the specific needs. Great value is placed on the development and pro-motion of the patient's competence – and that of his family – in dealing with the disease and the resulting life situation. In this respect, the treatment is meant as an aid to self-help. Table 45-5 illustrates and differentiates the most important therapy areas.

TABLE 45-5. Differentiated illustration of therapy areas and the therapeutic team involved in rehabilitation measures for children and adolescents with congenital heart defects

Medical care-related, and physiotherapeutic area	Psychosocial area	Psychomotor area
Diagnosis:	*Diagnosis:*	*Diagnosis:*
– general physical examination	Psychological diagnosis:	Especially diagnosis of:
– laboratory diagnostics	– behavioral anomalies	– physical fitness
– ECG	– developmental delays	– motor skills
– spirometry	– emotional disorders	– perceptual skills, etc.
– 24-hour ECG	– inadequate disease	
– long-term measurement of blood pressure	management	*Personnel:*
– Sonography	– social nonconformism	– (child) physiotherapist**
– Echocardiography,	– family-related problems	– occupational therapist
– SaO$_2$ monitoring		– exercise/sport therapist
– incremental ergometry	*Personnel:*	– psychomotor therapist
– cycle- (spiro-) ergometry/treadmill-(spiro-) ergometry	– child psychiatrist**	
if necessary, including transcutaneus oximetry	– (child-) psychologist	*Therapy offers:*
	– social education workers	– ergotherapy
Personnel:	– educator (teacher)**	– perceptual training to promote
– pediatric cardiologist (in charge)	– art therapist	sensory development
– pediatrician	– music therapist*	– training of fine motor skills
– child neurologist**	– remedial teacher*	– concentration exercises
– (children's nurse)**		– training of social competence
– (child-)physiotherapist**	*Therapy offers:*	
– masseur and balneotherapist**	Counseling and group counseling,	Psychomotor and sport therapy, for
– dietary assistant**	for instance as a parents' circle	instance:
		– promotion of perception and
Therapy:	Family counseling and life-coaching:	movement
Nursing, medical treatment, and therapy are adjusted	– individual therapy	– improvement of body coordination,
to individual needs. Goals of all therapy subsequent	– couple therapy***	endurance, strength, speed and
to hospitalization are for instance:	– family therapy***	flexibility
– improvement of physical performance	– relaxation methods	– improvement of motor skills
– improvement of ventilation and lung function	– play therapy**	– development of a realistic self-
– optimization of antiarrhythmic therapy	– art therapy*	evaluation
– treatment of perioperative complications	– music therapy*	– improvement of social skills
– treatment of extracardiac complications	– social consulting, including	– advice for autonomous physical
– general recovery	school and job-related advice**	activity in daily life
	– age-specific pedagogical	– introduction to different sports
Physical therapy, for example:	attendance	– motivation for autonomous, life-long
– specific. neurophysiological/-kinesio-logical	– education in specific classes**	physical activity
physiotherapy (according to Bobath, Vojta,	– remedial pedagogy*	– parent–child gymnastics**
Brunkow, and others)**	– leisure pedagogy*	– advice for movement-oriented leisure
– ventilation therapy**		with the whole family
– inhalation therapy**		
– electrotherapy**		
– massages, medicinal baths**		
– dietary prescriptions/advice**		
– therapy for eating disorders**		

*Facultative, **by means of consulting services, if necessary, ***family-oriented therapy.
Source: Modified and completed according to Deutsche Gesellschaft für pädiatrische Kardiologie[9] and Rosendahl and van der Mei.[30]

The Impact of Physical Activity

Children have a basic need for physical activity. Their perceptual and motor experience not only determines their physical and motor development but also decisively impacts on their emotional, psychosocial, and cognitive development. In contrast, physical inactivity in childhood is abnormal – regardless of whether it is due to physical, emotional, psychosocial, or cognitive factors. Physical activity and sports should therefore be recommended and encouraged for all youth.[31]

Oftentimes, a cardiac disease means a restriction of the affected child's perceptual and motor experience. Complex and severe heart defects may – at least temporarily – cause reduced symptom-limited exercise tolerance, and therefore require a certain amount of rest. Times of inpatient examinations or corrective operations are always periods of more or less strict immobilization. Depending on their duration and the child's age and mental stability, they can lead to developmental stagnation or regression. Anxiety and worries about the ill child often cause parents to become overprotective. Anxiety, or at least great uncertainty, exists especially in regard to the danger one might expose a child to by allowing them to engage in physical activity. This is often –

unnecessarily – also the case with children whose physical capacities are grossly normal. An existing deficit could be easily compensated through specific motor training and would make further inactivity redundant. Figure 45-3 shows the network of possible causes and effects of physical inactivity in children with heart disease.

Considering the high relevance of physical activity and sports for current day social awareness, participation in physical activity together with healthy peers improves quality of life for children and adolescents. Particularly for them, physical activity and sports play an important social and socializing role. They experience an exclusion from sports and/or a restriction of their activity as extremely unpleasant. Accordingly, when asked about their disadvantages in comparison to peers, 62 children and adolescents with CHD put their physical restrictions in first place, even ahead of life expectancy and opportunities for employment.[32]

Recommendations for Physical Activity

With improved life expectancy, growing attention is given to the question of whether and to what extent physical activity should be

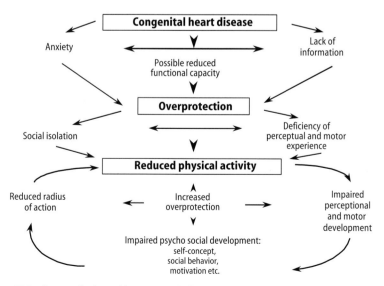

FIGURE 45-3. A network of possible causes and effects of physical inactivity in children with CHD.

recommended in order to improve the quality of life. Numerous groups of experts have provided recommendations concerning exercise for children with CHD.[33,34] Additionally, recommendations for the implementation of medically supervised heart groups have been published in Germany.[35] These recommendations can contribute to avoiding unnecessary exclusion of children and adolescents with heart disease from physical activity and sport. Moreover, they can minimize children's, parents', and teachers' insecurity in regard to the affected child's physical abilities.

In keeping with these recommendations, all young people with CHD who fulfill the necessary requirements should have the opportunity to participate in physical activity and, if needed, take part in specially adapted programs of physical education. For the assessment of aptitude and classification, the primary heart defect is less important than the current clinical status and potentially deleterious residual defects (Table 45-6).

For many of the affected children, no restriction of physical activity and sport is recommended.[33,34] This group includes all children and adolescents whose heart defects were definitively corrected in infancy or early childhood (patent ductus arteriosus, small atrial septal defect, ventricular septal defect), who do not have symptom-limited reduction of exercise capacity (group I.1). Even in patients with moderate residual defects (group I.2) (such as moderate aortic valve disease), normal load can be permitted in physical education and physical activities in leisure time. This also applies to children and adolescents whose cardiac defects do not require surgery (group II, for instance small septal defects or insignificant valvular stenosis).[35] Patient groups I.1, I.2, and II do need temporary participation in remedial programs and/or adapted physical education if a restriction of physical fitness and/or psychomotor deficits exists. In this context the indication for participation in special groups may also result from psychosocial reasons.[35]

Despite the reduction in mortality and improved hemodynamic outcomes of surgery and interventional catheterization, a considerable

TABLE 45-6. Classification according to current cardiac situation and postoperative clinical findings

Group I: patients after heart surgical/catheter interventional operations
1. No residual sequelae (complete correction)
2. With moderate residual sequelae
3. With significant residual sequelae
4. Patients with complex heart defects after palliative interventions:
   (a) such as the Fontan operation or the Mustard operation for TGA, where separation of systemic and pulmonary circulation has been achieved
   (b) patients in whom the two circulatory systems have not been separated (e.g. aortopulmonary shunt operation)

Group II: patients with heart defects not requiring operation
1. Shunt lesions with insignificant left-to-right shunt such as small atrial or ventricular septal defect
2. Insignificant valvular defects/anomalies such as congenital bicuspid aortic valve

Group III: patients with inoperable heart defects

Group IV: patients with chronic cardiomyopathy

Group V: patients with complex arrhythmia

Group VI: patients after heart transplantation

Source: Adapted and modified according to Deutsche Gesellschaft für Prävention und Rehabilitation von Herz-Kreislauferkrankungen.[35]

number of affected children and adolescents have hemodynamically significant residual defects, which may impair their expectancy and quality of life. For them, participation in special groups is most recommended. For patients with significant findings, complex heart defects subsequent to palliative interventions, inoperable heart defects, chronic cardiomyopathy, complex arrhythmia, or after heart transplantation, participation in physical activity cannot generally be advocated. Here, a decision for each individual patient has to be made in consultation with the attending pediatric cardiologist.

Patients with complex heart defects after palliative operations (I.4) represent a special group. In a great number of them (I.4a), a separation of the systemic and pulmonary circulations can be performed and thus no cyanosis persists. However, some patients remain cyanotic (I.4b). For these groups, and for children receiving anticoagulant therapy or with implanted devices (pacemakers, ICDs) or at a risk of sudden death, special and sometimes individual recommendations have to be made.[35]

Contraindications for participation in physical activity may result from the following:

- acute myocarditis
- children/adolescents with heart defects which acutely require surgery
- significant coarctation and/or heart failure NYHA class III/IV (preoperative)
- severe pulmonary hypertension
- severe cyanosis
- complex arrhythmia
- severe cardiomyopathy, obstructive hypertrophic cardiomyopathy.[35]

Required Preliminary Examinations

Prior to starting a physical training program, a thorough cardiological examination has to be performed in order to classify diagnosis and severity of the disease (Table 45-7). The objective of this examination is to determine the patient's individual symptom-limited cardiac capacity and the risk of exercise-related sudden cardiac death associated with the individual's specific disease.

Improvement of Motor Development

Improvement of physical activity in children with CHD should start as early as possible. In this way deficits in perceptual and motor experience and their negative consequences can be minimized. It is a special aim of motor interventions in children with CHD to develop individual perception of potential limitations and establish the boundaries of their exertional tolerance. In connection with acquiring age-appropriate knowledge about the disease-specific situation and the resulting symptom-limited capacity, this leads to a realistic self-estimation. In combination with this positive self-concept, emotional and psychosocial stability as well as a proper social integration, a realistic self-evaluation represents the most efficient protection from overload in daily life, physical activity and sport.

Children need to be provided with the opportunity to act out their basic need for physical activity and should only be stopped if there is a

TABLE 45-7. Required (preliminary) examinations prior to initialization physical training

Initial examination
Precise knowledge of patient's clinical history
General physical examination
ECG at rest
Echocardiography
Ergometry*(spiroergometry, if needed), especially in case of cyanotic vitia with transcutaneous O_2 measurement 6-minute running test, if needed with ECG monitoring (as an alternative for younger children)
Long-term ECG
Facultative: Stress echocardiography*
Control check-ups (at least yearly)
Clinical history
General clinical examination
ECG at rest
Echocardiography
Endurance testing*

*Starting at age 5 to 6.
Source: Adapted and modified according to Deutsche Gesellschaft für Prävention und Rehabilitation von Herz-Kreislauferkrankungen.[35]

specific danger of sudden death. They should participate in physical activity (indoors and outdoors) with their peers in an unrestricted fashion, as far as possible. This applies to play and guided activity in kindergarten, school, and/or sports clubs. Participation in specific, possibly medically supervised programs for the promotion of motor abilities can help to limit motor deficits and prepare and support the integration of children into their peer group.[35,36]

Results of empirical studies show that physical and motor performance of children and adolescents with CHD can be enhanced through regular engagement in autonomous or supervised physical activity. Furthermore emotional, psychosocial, and cognitive developmental processes can also be positively influenced.[37,38] Figure 45-4 illustrates how diverse, possibly negative consequences of CHD can be compensated through the improvement of motor abilities and skills.

The content of special motor training programs primarily aims at improvement of perceptual and motor development in order to compensate for existing deficits. Positive experience of one's own body, its functions, and capabilities constitutes the basis for developing a positive self-image, which in turn helps children with CHD to cope with their disease and the possible restrictions connected

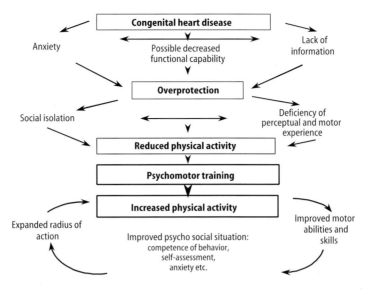

FIGURE 45-4. Compensation of negative consequences of CHD by means of goal-oriented improvement of motor development.

with it. Within the children's special group, based on differentiated body perception, children develop awareness of strain and learn to have the confidence to take breaks during group activities as often as needed.

Moreover, all age-appropriate forms of activity should be made available for children with CHD. At preschool and elementary school age, these are diverse coordinative tasks involving gross and fine motor skills. Specific resistance and endurance training is neither necessary nor efficient at the ages of 8 to 10. Improved strength and cardiovascular performance at this age result from improved motor coordination. Yet, should children exhibit muscular imbalance resulting from a lack of movement or unbalanced load (for instance frequent sitting), special compensation could be indicated.

Already at preschool and school age, but especially in adolescence, sport-specific skills are acquired and increasingly improved through diverse and varied physical activities depending on interests and available resources. An important goal is to offer insight into the diversity of physical activity and sports available to all young people. This will help them obtain specific skills and knowledge and thereby enable and motivate them to participate with their peers in physical activities and choose an appropriate lifetime-

sport. Special attention has to be given to the danger of abdominal strain. Already at preschool age, children with specific risk factors should learn to avoid breath-holding during exercise. The Valsalva maneuver can lead to dangerous blood pressure peaks. Lowered cardiac output during straining as well as post-pressor bradycardia may result in significant arrhythmia and even ventricular fibrillation. A rapid fall in blood pressure after straining at maximal workload sometimes leads to syncope, even in healthy persons.

The specific behavior patterns in youth often cause adolescents with CHD to consciously disregard their body signals in order to avoid the "embarrassment" that a necessary physical break would cause. By doing this, they expose themselves to potential danger. Prevention of this danger can – besides appeals to the adolescent's rationality – only be achieved through an early stabilization of personality and the improvement of self-responsibility and self-confidence.

Summary

Progress in the treatment of CHD has led to a dramatic reduction of mortality. More and more children with CHD reach adulthood, which causes morbidity within this population to be a growing problem that demands special expertise. Preventive diagnostics and treatment have to be initiated early, aiming to find deficits and alleviate them through the use of specific measures. We expect CHD to be accompanied by deficits in the fields of motor skills, cognition, and emotion (not only in the person affected but also in their social environment). However, even with less complex heart defects, deficits exist to a currently as yet unknown extent. This is the reason for rehabilitative intervention in CHD, targeting a long-tem reduction of morbidity and an enhancement of the patient's quality of life. Considering the financial outlay currently targeted towards invasive therapeutic measures, an increased expenditure of time and finances directed towards optimizing the quality of life of this patient group by institution of appropriate rehabilitation measures in a timely manner is justified.

References

1. Allen DH, Gutgesell HP, Clark EB, et al. Moss and Adams' Heart Disease in Infants, Children, and Adolescents. Including the Fetus and Young Adults, 6th edn, Vols 1 and 2. Philadelphia: Lippincott Williams & Wilkins; 2001.
2. American Heart Association. Cardiac Disease in Children: Statistics. Available at: http://www.americanheart.org/presenter.jhtml?identifier=4498.
3. Bruckenberger E. Herzbericht 2003. Hanover: Eigenverlag; 2004.
4. Deanfield J, Thaulow E, Warnes C, et al. Management of grown up congenital heart disease. The Task Force on the Management of Grown Up Congenital Heart disease of the European Society of Cardiology. European Heart Journal 2003;24:1035–1084.
5. Mennicken U, Franz Ch, Hirsch H. Angeborene Herzfehler. In: Siegenthaler W, Kaufmann H, Hornborste H, et al., eds. Lehrbuch der Inneren Medizin. Stuttgart: Thieme; 1992:99–130.
6. Norgaard MA, Lauridsen P, Helvind M, et al. Twenty-to-thirty-seven-year-follow-up after repair for tetralogy of Fallot. Eur J Cardiothorac Surg 1999;16:125–130.
7. Schaffer R, Berdat P, Stolle B, et al. Surgery of the complete atrioventricular canal: relationship between age at operation, mitral regurgitation, size of the ventricular septum defect, additional mal-

8. Hutter PA, Kreb DL, Mantel SF, et al. Twenty-five years' experience with the arterial switch operation. Thorac Cardiovasc Surg 2002;124:790–797.
9. Deutsche Gesellschaft für pädiatrische Kardiologie. Rehabilitation bei angeborenen und erworbenen Herzerkrankungen im Kindes- und Jugendalter. Leitlinien zur Diagnostik und Therapie in der Pädiatrischen Kardiologie (2003);1–7. AMWF online http:/www.uni-düsseldorf.de AWMF/11/pkard031.htm, 30.05.2005.
10. Wernovsky G, Newburger J. Neurologic and developmental morbidity in children with complex congenital heart disease. J Pediatr 2003;142:6–8.
11. Bellinger DC, Wypij D, duPlessis AJ, et al. Neurodevelopmental status at eight years in children with dextro-transposition of the great arteries: The Boston Circulatory Arrest Trial. J Thorac Cardiovasc Surg 2003;126:1385–1396.
12. Wypij D, Newburger J, Rappaport LA, et al. The effect of duration of deep hypothermic circulatory arrest in infant heart surgery on late neurodevelopment: The Boston Circulatory Arrest Trial. J Thorac Cardiovasc Surg 2003;126:1397–1403.
13. Newburger J, Wypij D, Bellinger DC, et al. Length of stay after infant heart surgery is related to cognitive outcome at age 8 years. J Pediatr 2003;143:67–73.
14. Dunbar-Masterson C, Wyoij D, Bellinger DC, et al. General health status of children with D-transposition of the great arteries after the arterial switch operation. Circulation 2001;104(Suppl I):I-138–I-142.
15. Singer H. Einfluss angeborener Herzfehler auf die Entwicklung von Kindern und Jugendlichen. In: Bjarnason-Wehrens B, Dordel S, eds. Motorische Förderung von Kindern mit angeborenen Herzfehlern. Sankt Augustin: Academiaverlag; 2001:9–25.
16. Abad-Sinden A, Sutphen JL. Growth and nutrition. In: Allen HD, Gutgesell HP, Eclard EB, et al., eds. Moss and Adams' Heart Disease in Infants and Adolescents, 6th edn, Vol 1. Philadelphia: Lippincott Williams & Wilkins; 2001:325–332.
17. Clark EB. Etiology of congenital cardiovascular malformations: epidemiology and genetics. In: Allen HD, Gutgesell HP, Eclard EB, et al., eds. Moss and Adams' Heart Disease in Infants and Adolescents, 6th edn, Vol 1. Philadelphia: Lippincott Williams & Wilkins; 2001:64–79.
18. Fredriksen PM, Ingjer F, Nystad W, et al. A comparison of VOpeak between patients with CHD and healthy subjects all aged 8–17 years. Eur J Appl Physiol 1999;80:409–416.

19. Bellinger DC, Wypij D, Kuban KC, et al. Development and neurological status of children at 4 years of age after heart surgery with hypothermic circulatory arrest or low-flow cardiopulmonary bypass. Circulation 1999;100:526–532.

20. Stieh H, Kramer HH, Harding P, et al. Gross and fine motor development is impaired in children with cyanotic congenital heart disease. Neuropediatrics 1998;30:77–82.

21. Dordel S, Bjarnason-Wehrens B, Lawrens W, et al. Efficiency of psychomotor training of children with (partly-) corrected congenital heart disease. Z Sportmed 1999;50:41–46.

22. Unverdorben M, Singer H, Trägler M, et al. Reduzierte koordinative Leistungs-fähigkeit – nicht nur ein medizinisches Problem? Herz/Kreisl 1997; 29:1881–1884.

23. Hassberg D, Döttling-Ulrich J. Psychologische Aspekte von Patienten mit angeborenen Herzfehlern und ihren Familien. In: Apitz J, ed. Pädiatrische Kardiologie. Darmstadt: Steinkopff; 2001: 803–807.

24. Kunick I. Die psychosoziale Situation des herzoperierten Kindes und Jugendlichen. In: Schmalz AA, Singer H, eds. Herzoperierte Kinder und Jugendliche. Ein Leitfaden zur Langzeitbetreuung in Klinik und Praxis. Stuttgart: Wissenschaftlich Verlagsgesellschaft; 1995:99–108.

25. Mussatto K, Tweddell J. Quality of life following surgery for congenital cardiac malformations in neonates and infants. Cardiol Young 2005;15(Suppl 1):174–178.

26. Lawoko S, Soares JJF. Distress and hoplessness among parents of children with congenital heart disease, parents of children with other diseases and parents of healthy children. J Psychosom Res 2002;52:193–208.

27. Calzolari A, Giordano U, Di Giacinto B, et al. Exercise and sports participation after surgery for congenital heart disease: the European perspective. Ital Heart J 2001;2:736–739.

28. Ammani Prasad S, Main E. Paediatrics. In: Pryor JA, Ammani-Prasad S. Physiotherapy for Respiratory and Cardiac Problems. Adults and Paediatrics, 3rd edn. Edinburgh: Churchill Livingstone; 2002: 425–455.

29. Kendall L, Sloper P, Lewin RJP, et al. The view of parents concerning the planning of services for rehabilitation of families of children with congenital cardiac disease. Cardiol Young 2003;13:20–27.

30. Rosendahl W, van der Mei SH. Family-orientated rehabilitation in patients with congenital heart disease. Kinder- und Jugendarzt 2000;31:665–671.

31. Sport and European Union, European Community, Administrative Department, January 2000:4–5.

32. Ratzmann U, Schneider P, Richter H. Psychologische Untersuchung bei Familien, Kindern und Jugendlichen nach Operation angeborener Herzfehler (Fallotsche Tetralogie und Aoertenisthmusstenose). Kinderärztl Praxis 1991;59:107–110.

33. Graham TP, Driscoll DJ, Gersony WM, et al. Task Force 2: congenital heart disease. J Am Coll Cardiol 2005;45:1326–1333.

34. Mitchell JH, Maron BJ, Epstein SE. Sixteenth Bethesda Conference: Cardiovascular abnormalities in the athlete: Recommendations regarding eligibility for competition. J Am Coll Cardiol 1985;6:29–30.

35. Deutsche Gesellschaft für Prävention und Rehabilitation von Herz-Kreislauferkran-kungen. Empfehlungen zur Leitung von Kinderherzgruppen (KHG). Herz/Kreisl 2000;32:414–418.

36. Longmuir PE, Tremblay MS, Goode RC. Postoperative exercise training develops normal levels of physical activity in a group of children following cardiac surgery. Pediatr Cardiol 1990;11:126–130.

37. Fredriksen PM, Kahrs N, Blaasvaer S, et al. Effect of physical training in children and adolescents with congenital heart disease. Cardiol Young 2000;10: 107–114.

38. Bjarnason-Wehrens B, Dordel S. Motorische Förderung von Kindern mit angeborenen Herzfehlern. Sankt Augustin: Academia; 2001.

46
Gender Issues in Rehabilitation

Karin Schenck-Gustafsson and Agneta Andersson

This is the story of a 37-year-old woman in her own words. She had no other cardiovascular risk factors than a history of smoking and being 3 months in the postpartum period.

I woke up with severe chest pain, my left arm was weak and heavy. I went to my general practitioner at the Primary Care Center. There, a nurse registered my ECG and a doctor came and asked me about my symptoms. I told him carefully about my severe chest pain and that my left arm felt weak. I told him that the pain prevented me from taking care of my 3-month-old baby. He told me that if you have a heart attack it would induce pain in my arm, not weakness and besides "you are too young to have a myocardial infarction." He sent me home with antacids for my stomach. Two days later I called my doctor and described a feeling of general chest discomfort and when walking rapidly chest pain was provoked. He told me not to worry but if the pain came back he recommended me to seek the Emergency Care Unit at the hospital. I stayed at home.

Two days later the same chest pain came back, now even worse than before and I went to the hospital. After two hours of waiting in the corridor an ECG was performed and the doctor told me that the ECG was normal. I got a paper bag to breathe in without any explanations (panic disorder?) or perhaps, as I was breastfeeding, it could be something with my breasts. I was sent to the gynecologist but he told me that this had nothing to do with gynecology and I was sent back to the emergency care unit. I still had my chest pain. Again I was sent home with antacids. The same day at home the chest pain was even worse. I went back to the emergency ward and a new ECG again revealed no changes. This time the pain radiated to my back and the doctor asked me to take a deep breath and did the pain increase? Perhaps.

The doctor said, we are going to send you home with something for the pain. After a while the doctor told me *that there was something wrong with my blood samples and I was sent immediately to the CCU. A coronary angiogram showed three-vessel disease and two days later CABG was performed. I felt ignored by the doctors and nurses and their little knowledge of female heart disease.*

Introduction

One important aim with cardiac rehabilitation is to reduce cardiovascular risk factors after a cardiac event. However, the risk factors are different and have a different impact in men than in women. Still, little is known about the needs and experiences of women with regard to cardiac rehabilitation. For example, lack of social support may be a more important risk factor in women for coronary heart disease (CHD) and for the rehabilitation process. Therefore, we might need specially designed programs for the female patients. There are obvious benefits of structured cardiac rehabilitation programs. However, so far, there are few or no trials of adequate size (especially not in women) to answer the question if and which type of cardiac rehabilitation programs are effective in reducing mortality or cardiac events and achieving a better quality of life. There is convincing evidence that physical activity reduces CHD morbidity and mortality among men but few studies have been carried out in women. Therefore, we might need specially designed programs for female patients. Questions emerge, like when after the cardiac event is the optimal time to start rehabilitation and for how long will the program last? We know that it is impossible to try to rehabilitate a patient with a deep depression, you have to treat the depression first. We also know that a standard 6–8-week training program with bicycle exercise twice a week after the myocardial infarction is not enough and does not cover the psychological part of the recovery process. Other questions: do certain patients need cardiac rehabilitation more than others do or could it be dangerous to expose some patients to cardiac rehabilitation? How to involve patients with a low quality of life, suffering from depression, anxiety, and negative stress?

Gender Differences in Coronary Heart Disease

Coronary heart disease is the leading cause of death and disability among men and women in Western countries. Of the 4 million people in Europe dying every year of cardiovascular disease, 53% are women. In recent decades CHD mortality rates have declined across all age groups among middle-aged and older persons, in a majority of Western countries; however, the overall decline rate has been slower in women than in men. The gender difference in CHD mortality has consequently been reduced. Women have a longer life expectancy than men and suffer from clinical manifestations of CHD about 10 years later than men. Younger women have a lower incidence of CHD compared with men the same age, but by age 70 the incidence of CHD is comparable for men and women. This gender differential in CHD incidence is not fully understood. A cardioprotective effect of endogenous estrogens has been hypothesized as the main pathophysiological explanation. In addition, a gender bias among physicians in recognizing CHD in women has been claimed. Until recently, knowledge about CHD regarding prevention, risk factors, clinical manifestations, therapy and prognosis was based on studies that involved predominantly or exclusively middle-aged men.[1] Also, earlier reports from the Framingham cohort fostered the perception that angina pectoris is a benign problem in women.[2] However, in the past several years the information about female CHD and the gender differential in CHD has expanded considerably.[3]

Although women and men share several conventional risk factors for CHD, both non-modifiable (age and genetic predisposition) and modifiable (cigarette smoking, hypertension, obesity, dyslipidemia, diabetes mellitus, sedentary life style, and psychological stress), their impact may be different in women.[4] Recently nine major risk factors were found to be responsible for 90% of the myocardial infarctions.[5] Diabetes mellitus, lipid abnormalities, cigarette smoking, and possibly also psychosocial factors, seem to be of special importance in women.[6] Diabetes mellitus seems to abolish the gender protection in women and is associated with a less favorable in-hospital and long-term prognosis in subjects with MI, with a greater adverse impact for women than for men. Low HDL cholesterol and elevated triglyceride levels may be particularly important in younger women and may better predict CHD in women than total and LDL cholesterol levels. Also the ApoB/ApoA1 ratio has been claimed to be of greater importance in women than in men. Cigarette smoking is one of the leading preventable causes of CHD in women, and although the percentage of smokers in the population has decreased over the past three decades in Western countries, an alarming increase in smoking among young women has been reported. Among middle-aged women in the Nurses Health study more than 50% of MIs were attributable to tobacco. Also, a recent study showed that the smoking association with CHD was much stronger in women than men.[7] The increased risk of CHD with smoking is dose-dependent, and smoking cessation decreased the risk within 3 to 5 years to the level of women who had never smoked.

It is also known that smoking women reach their menopause 2–3 years earlier probably because of the proposed lowering of endogenous estrogen levels induced by smoking.

A risk factor specific to women is ovarian hormone status, for example oral contraceptives, pregnancy, and menopause and hormone replacement therapy. Polycystic ovarian syndrome, gestational diabetes or hypertension, pregnancy toxicosis and birth complications are also claimed to be important hormonal cardiovascular risk factors. Menopause, including premature menopause, is associated with negative changes in several cardiovascular risk factors. Meta-analyses of observational studies, mostly conducted in the

United States, showed a risk reduction of CHD events of 35–50% with hormone replacement therapy. The epidemiological evidence was supported by clinical and experimental studies reporting beneficial effects of estrogens on lipids and lipoproteins, carbohydrate metabolism, hemostasis, vasomotor effects, and atheroma formation. However, there may be differential effects of estrogens on components of the inflammatory response. A major concern and criticism of the observational studies has been the selection bias. Recently, randomized, placebo-controlled trials (HERS) failed to show any beneficial effect of combined estrogens/progestin therapy on coronary events.[8,9] In 2002, the results of the first randomized primary prevention trial of HRT, the Women's Health Initiative (WHI), were reported,[10] and the finding of an increased risk of CHD after initiation of combined estrogens/progestin therapy was similar to HERS, and the trial was stopped early. The part of the trial comparing estrogens alone with placebo was discontinued because of the increased incidence of stroke and total cardiovascular disease, no effect on CHD incidence, and no overall benefit of estrogen use. Hence, to date, questions still remain regarding how estrogens and progestin modulate cardiovascular risk in women.

The symptoms of angina pectoris and MI are often not the same in men and women. Many women present with different ischemic symptoms, and have chest pain triggered by emotional stress.[11] As women are usually about 10 years older than men when they present with acute MI, the difference may be more related to age than sex. Some studies reported longer delay before seeking medical care and physician delay in recognizing signs of CHD in women. Fewer women were referred to a cardiologist, hospitalized and admitted to coronary care units. The initial MI was clinically unrecognized in a higher proportion of women than men in the Framingham cohort. Women are older and have more co-morbidity, especially hypertension, diabetes mellitus and congestive heart failure, when they present with clinical manifestations of CHD. Some studies suggest that unstable angina and non-Q-wave infarction occurs more frequently in women. Also, women with chest pain have a greater likelihood of normal coronary arteries on angiograms in selected patient populations. Diagnosis of CHD

poses a particular problem in women as the accuracy of many diagnostic techniques was validated in predominantly male populations. False-positive exercise tests are more prevalent in women than men, especially in younger women.[6] Modern imaging techniques such as exercise and pharmacological echocardiography can be useful for female CHD patients but have not solved the problems encountered. Gender differences in the use of diagnostic tests and therapeutic measures have previously been reported from several studies. Women were less likely than men to receive thrombolysis, to be referred to coronary artery angiography, to have revascularization procedures, to be prescribed aspirin, beta-blockers, ACE inhibitors. and lipid-lowering drugs,[11] and to be enrolled in cardiac rehabilitation.[12] In several, but not in all of these investigations, the sex differences were diminished or abolished after controlling for age and other baseline characteristics.

Although women have a lower mortality rate from CHD at a given age than men, this survival advantage is lost once CHD becomes clinically evident. The prognosis after MI in women is equal or even worse compared with men in several studies. Results from hospital-based studies have indicated that women have poorer short-term survival both in the US and in Europe. In a 26-year follow-up of the Framingham population, women had an excess relative risk for death, over men, during a coronary event in nearly every age group. Interestingly, after stratifying for age, Vaccarino et al. reported that younger women, but not older women, had higher in-hospital and long-term mortality rates after myocardial infarctions (MI), relative to men at the same age.[13]

Background Gender Differences in Cardiac Rehabilitation

One of the goals of cardiac rehabilitation should be to improve psychological health, restore self-confidence, relieve anxiety and promote the return to ordinary daily living and work.

It is well known that depression and low perceived support after MI are associated with higher morbidity and mortality. There is convincing evidence that improvements in lifestyle, which include smoking cessation, diet, exercise, and stress management, can reduce further heart problems. It is known that psychosocial intervention is beneficial in lowering blood pressure, improving lipid levels, and reducing negative stress and symptoms of depression. However, psychosocial intervention in patients with MI showed no objective evidence of improvement in anxiety, depression, morbidity or mortality in a British study.[14]

A large US study[15] with 1084 women and 1397 men with a minor or major depression were treated when indicated with an SSRI or cognitive behavioral therapy. The intervention did not increase event-free survival, but less depression and less social isolation occurred in the intervention group.

Despite the benefits of rehabilitation, many patients fail to participate in a rehabilitation program, especially women. Women are also less likely to be referred, are less interested, and have higher drop-out rates than men.

People with low social support do not attend cardiac rehabilitation. Social support and marital status are significantly related to attendance, especially in women. Married women and women in general tend to take more care of the family and their relatives than their own health. Patients with low education level will attend cardiac rehabilitation to a lesser extent than patients with higher education. Practical reasons such as long distance to course location will influence participation and women are more likely to have such difficulties because of small children or other social responsibilities or they lack a driver's license.[16–19]

Depressive disorders have a clear relationship with CHD. There is overwhelming evidence that major depressions are underdiagnosed and untreated in patients with CHD. Approximately one in five patients have a major depression at the time of a cardiac event.[20] Depression will also increase the risk of new cardiac events.[21] In patients with CHD, the prevalence of major depression is nearly 20% and for minor depression 27%.[22]

Depression will reduce attendance in CR programs. After an acute cardiac event women express greater shortness of breath, less activity tolerance, and more anxiety and depression.[23]

A randomized controlled trial with 1376 post-MI Canadian patients showed that there was no evidence of benefit for a supportive and educational home nursing intervention. The female patients had a poorer overall outcome after one year compared with the male patients. It has been speculated that one of the reasons for the negative outcome in women could be that the female patients were disturbed by the frequent visits of a nurse to their homes.[24]

It was concluded in a meta-analysis[25] that intervention trials designed to reduce psychosocial stress have been limited in size and number. Accordingly we need to identify patients who will benefit most from psychosocial rehabilitation programs and probably make the programs more attractive for women.

This underlines the need for further studies in this field and consequently we have started a heart rehabilitation program with stress management especially designed for women.

The Saltsjöbaden Program: A Model of Cardiac Rehabilitation for Women

At the Saltsjöbaden rehabilitation center (Sweden) we provide a CR service designed for women. This program, aiming at promoting and maintaining lifestyle changes, commences with a 2-week inpatient residential course; participants then return to the center 2 months later for 5 days, and subsequently for 2 days two times yearly over the next 5 years. The groups contain 6–10 mainly younger women with established CHD. The residential course contains theoretical lectures, discussions, and different physical activities. Relatives are invited to join over a weekend. The psychosocial rehabilitation is based on an interactive, self-instructional program called "Stress as an Opportunity," which involves self-assessments concerning different causes of stress, a book on measures to combat stress, "homework cards," and a tape with information on stress and relaxation techniques.[27] The program consists of three phases: a diagnostic phase, an educational phase, intervention and secondary prevention (Tables 46-1, 46-2, and 46-3).

The biannual follow-up sessions start with a group interview and each session has a specific topic including theory (e.g. burnout symptoms, type A behavior, assertiveness, how to handle

TABLE 46-1. Diagnostic phase

Aim:
- Identify previous and present stress factors.
- Detect stress symptoms.
- Diagnose states of depression and/or anxiety.

How:
- Workshop where women interview each other respectively, and subsequently present their companion to the group in order to create a feeling of belonging and openness in the group.
- In-depth interview with a psychologist. The interview is focused on present strains and symptoms in private life and at work, i.e. factors that are of immediate importance to deal with. Referral for individual therapy whenever needed.

TABLE 46-2. Educational phase

Aim:
- To increase the women's awareness and understanding of the impact of stress and psychological strain.
- To increase ability to distinguish heart symptoms from stress and/or anxiety symptoms.

How:
- Education on mechanisms of work-related strains: high demands and low control, role conflicts, under- or overstimulation.

And on: contribution of personality factors such as low self-esteem, internal demands and stress-evoking behavior, increased strain and decreased resistance to illness and disease.

TABLE 46-3. Intervention and secondary prevention

Aim:
- To initiate and support improvements in lifestyle and in the psychosocial environment at home and/or at work.

How:
- Learn to use the module "Stress as an Opportunity."
- Learn: different relaxation techniques, e.g.: mini relaxation, progressive muscle relaxation, diaphragmatic breathing, visualization, and repetition of thought or word.
- Identify individual stress factors (group discussions, the self-assessment forms).
- Make an individual "action plan" how to reduce stress and/or adverse health behaviors in daily life (under the surveillance of CR personnel).
- Staff support to maintain health-promoting abilities and behaviors.
- Five-year follow-up of the individual action plan.

manipulative behavior and criticism), practical exercises (e.g. role-play), group discussions and self-assessments with feedback. In the annual assessment using validated questionnaires, data are collected on lifestyle and behavior, self-rated health and symptoms, sick leave and early retirement, healthcare utilization, medical and psychological risk factors, and personality factors (e.g. the Life Ladder (Figure 46-1)). At present the outcome of the program is being established in a

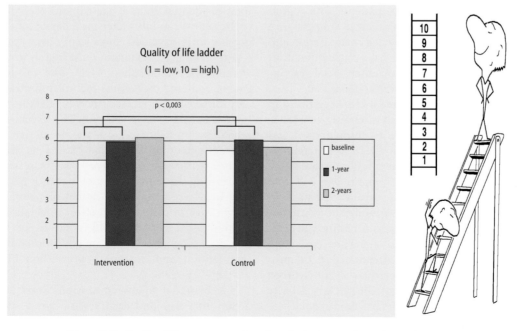

FIGURE 46-1. Quality of life measurement in patients in the intervention and control groups.

controlled study, where it appears that the typical patient is well-educated, often in administrative or other leading positions and highly devoted to their work; they are often smokers, divorced, and bringing up small children on their own with a low degree of social support and limited social network.

Conclusion

Do we need specially designed programs for the female heart patient? Risk factors and preventive actions to avoid risks differ between men and women. There is a difference in psychological and physiological reactions after a cardiac event and a gender difference in life conditions. The fact that depression and anxiety are more common in women may lead to different demands on cardiac rehabilitation.

Furthermore, women's increasing double work and multiple roles (now a recognized risk factor for CHD in both sexes) will increase the stress burden both at work and at home. There are obvious benefits of structured cardiac rehabilitation programs for women with special emphasis on psychosocial risk behavior.

References

1. Healy B. The Yentl syndrome. N Engl J Med 1991;325:274–276.
2. Kannel WB, Sorlie P, McNamara P. Prognosis after myocardial infarction: The Framingham Study. Am J Cardiol 1979;44:53–59.
3. Mosca L, Appel LJ, Benjamin EJ, et al. Circulation 2004;109:672–692.
4. Schenck-Gustafsson K. Risk factors for cardiovascular disease in women: assessment and management. Eur Heart J 1996;17(Suppl D):2–7.
5. Rosengren A, Hawken S, Ounpuu S, et al.; INTERHEART investigators. Association of psychosocial risk factors with risk of acute myocardial infarction in 11119 cases and 13648 controls from 52 countries (the INTERHEART study): case-control study. Lancet 2004;364(9438):912–914.
6. Ali-Khalili F. Coronary Heart Disease in women. Diagnostic and prognostic markers. Thesis 2000, Karolinska Institutet, Stockholm, Sweden.
7. Richey Sharrett A, Coady SA, Folsom AR, Couper DJ, Heiss G; ARIC Study. Smoking and diabetes differ in their association with subclinical atherosclerosis and coronary heart disease – the ARIC study. Atherosclerosis 2004;172:143–149.
8. Hulley S, Grady D, Bush T, et al., for the Heart and Estrogen/progestin Replacement Study (HERS) Research Group. Randomized trial of estrogen plus progestin for secondary prevention of coronary heart disease in postmenopausal women. JAMA 1998;288:605–613.
9. Grady D, Herrington D, Bittner V, et al., for the HERS research group. Cardiovascular disease outcomes during 6.8 years of hormone therapy: HERS II. JAMA 2002;228:49–57.
10. Writing Group for the Women's Health Initiative Investigators. Risks and benefits of estrogen plus progestin in healthy postmenopausal women: principal results from the Women's Health Initiative randomized controlled study. JAMA 2002;228:321–333.
11. Lundberg V, Wikström B, Boström S, Asplund K. Exploring sex differences in case fatality in acute myocardial infarction or coronary death events in northern Sweden MONICA Project. J Intern Med 2002;251:235–244.
12. Thomas RJ, Houston Miller N, Lamendola C, et al. National survey on gender differences in cardiac rehabilitation programmes. Patient characteristics and enrollment patterns, J Cardiopulmon Rehabil 1996;16:402–412.
13. Vaccarino V, Krumholz HM, Yarzebski J, Gore JM, Goldberg RJ. Sex differences in 2 years mortality after hospital discharge after myocardial infarction. Ann Intern Med 2001;134:173–181.
14. Jones DA, West RR. Psychological rehabilitation after myocardial infarction: multicentre randomised controlled trial. BMJ 1996;313:1517–1521.
15. The ENRICHD Investigators. JAMA 2003;289:3106–3116.
16. Gallagher R, McKinley S. Predictors of women's attendance of cardiac rehabilitation programmes. Prog Cardiovasc Nurs 2003;121–126.
17. Cooper AF, Jackson G. Factors associated with cardiac rehabilitation attendance: a systematic review of the literature. Clin Rehabil 2002;16:541–552.
18. Worcester MV, Murphy BM. Cardiac rehabilitation programmes: Predictors of non-attendance and drop out. Eur J Cardiovasc Prev Rehabil 2004; 11(4):328–335.
19. Lieberman L, Meana M, Stewart D. Cardiac rehabilitation: Gender differences in factors influencing participation. J Womens Health 1998;7:717–723.
20. Frasure-Smith N, Lesperance F, Juneau M, Talajic M, Bourassa MG. Gender, depression, and one year prognosis after myocardial infarction. Psychosom Med 1999;61:26–37.

21. Verrier RL, Dickerson LW. Central nervous system and behavioural factors in vagal control of cardiac arrhythmogenesis. In: Levy MM, Schwarz PJ, eds. Vagal Control of the Heart. Armonk, NY: Futura; 1994;557–577.

22. Carney RM, Rich MW, Tevelde AJ, et al. Major depressive disorders in coronary artery disease. Am J Cardiol 1987;60:1273–1275.

23. Frasure-Smith N, Lesperance F, Prince RH, et al. Randomised trial of home-based psychosocial nursing intervention for patients recovering from myocardial infarction. Lancet 1997;350(9076):473–479.

24. Rozanski A, Blumenthal JA, Kaplan J. Impact of psychological factors on the pathogenesis of cardiovascular disease and implications for therapy. Circulation 1999;99:2192–2217.

25. Eriksson I, Moser V, Unden A-L, Orth-Gomer K. Prevention of stress at work. Case study no 10. Condition of Work digest. ILO 1992; vol 11,2.

47
Rehabilitation in Elderly Patients

Hugo Saner

Introduction

The number of older people is growing rapidly worldwide. Today, more than 580 million people are older than 60 years and the number is projected to rise to 1000 million by 2020. The proportion of the population over 80 years, the so-called "old-old," is increasing most rapidly. Life expectancy at all ages is also increasing. At 65 years, life expectancy ranges from 14.9 to 18.9 years and at 80 years from 6.9 to 9.1 years for men and women, respectively. With the increase in life expectancy, the leading causes of death have shifted dramatically from infectious diseases to non-communicable diseases. Cardiovascular disease is the most frequent single cause of death in persons over 65 years of age, and most importantly it is responsible for considerable morbidity and a large burden of disease, particularly in the community.[1]

Age-Related Structural Changes

Cardiovascular pathologies such as hypertension and cerebrovascular diseases and heart diseases such as coronary artery disease, arrhythmias, and heart failure increase in incidence with increasing age.[2] Age per se is the major risk factor for cardiovascular diseases because specific pathophysiological mechanisms that underlie these diseases become superimposed on cardiac and vascular substrates that have been modified by the "aging process."[3–6] Age-related changes are most likely to be seen in the "old-old" who have escaped cardiovascular pathology earlier in life. This group demonstrates the dual processes, often interacting, of biological aging of the cardiovascular system and age-related pathology (Table 47-1). Age-related structural changes in the heart include increased left ventricular wall thickness independent of any increase in blood pressure,[3] increased fibrosis and calcification of the valves, particularly the mitral annulus and the aortic valve,[4,5] and loss of cells in the sinoatrial node.[5] The age-related vascular changes include increased stiffness of peripheral and central arteries,[6] increase in number of sites for lipid deposition, and more diffuse coronary artery changes.

Age-Related Functional Changes

Age-related functional changes are determined by heart rate, preload and afterload, muscle performance, and neurohormonal regulation, all of which may be influenced by age. There is little change in left ventricular systolic function with increasing age, although cardiac output may decrease in parallel with a reduction in lean body mass.[7] Increases in heart rate in response to exercise or stress caused by non-cardiovascular illnesses, particularly infections, are attenuated with increasing age.[8] Stroke volume increases only by "moving up" the Frank–Starling curve.[9,10] Thus end-diastolic volume increases. These age-related changes in cardiac response to exercise are mimicked by β-adrenergic blockade,[11] but β-adrenergic agonists do not reverse this aging process.[12] The decline in exercise performance with age may

TABLE 47-1. Cardiovascular adaptions in the elderly

– Increase in vascular stiffness and systolic blood pressure
– Left ventricular hypertrophy
– Diastolic dysfunction and relaxation abnormality
– Lower peak heart rate
– Slightly reduced cardiac output
– Increased peripheral vascular resistance
– Reduced peak oxygen consumption
– Lower plasma renin activity
– Reduced sensitivity to catecholamines
– Reduction in skin blood flow

additionally relate to peripheral factors, blood flow, and muscle mass rather than being solely the consequence of cardiac performance changes. Diastolic function is a major determinant of cardiac output in elderly persons. The rate and volume of early diastolic filling decreases with age.[13] The aged heart requires atrial contraction to maintain adequate diastolic filling, so atrial fibrillation being common in older people has a disproportionate effect on cardiac function.[7] Reduced ventricular compliance results in higher left ventricular diastolic pressure at rest and during exercise.[8,13] As a result, pulmonary and systemic venous congestion may occur in the presence of normal systolic function.[14] With increased afterload on the left ventricle, left ventricular hypertrophy occurs, even in the absence of hypertension or aortic stenosis. Diastolic dysfunction, at least in the early stages, may be a feature of normal aging. Later, however, it is a pathological process leading to significant left ventricular hypertrophy. At this stage, coronary heart disease, hypertension, or other pathologies are probably involved.

Complicating Factors in Elderly Patients with Heart Disease

Elderly patients constitute a high percentage of patients with myocardial infarction, heart surgery, and percutaneous transluminal coronary angioplasty (PTCA). Elderly patients are also at high risk of disability following a cardiovascular event (Table 47-2). The prevalence of diabetes and arterial hypertension is relatively high. There is also an increased incidence of complicated forms of coronary disease such as multi-vessel disease and left main coronary artery disease, severe and unstable angina as well as sinus node dysfunction, conduction disturbances, and heart failure. The risk of complications is increased in elderly patients after myocardial infarction, coronary angiography, PTCA, and surgery of the heart or the thoracic aorta. The duration of hospitalization is usually prolonged. Severe deconditioning may be a consequence of prolonged immobility. The risk of neurological complications and also of cognitive defects after heart surgery is increased. There is also a high incidence of co-morbidities. The rate of negative side-effects of medications is increased. Degenerative changes of the musculoskeletal system may add to the difficulties which may be encountered during follow-up and rehabilitation of such patients.

Cardiovascular Risk Factors

Regardless of predisposing factors, diet and lifestyle influence morbidity and mortality during the course of life. Because of the cumulative effect

TABLE 47-2. Complicating factors in elderly patients with cardiovascular disease

– Diabetes mellitus and arterial hypertension
– Complicated forms of coronary disease (multi-vessel disease, left main artery disease)
– Sinus node dysfunction, conduction disturbances
– Heart failure
– Increased complication rates after myocardial infarction, coronary arteriography, PTCA and heart surgery
– Prolonged hospitalization with severe deconditioning
– Mental disturbances and cognitive deficits after heart surgery
– Co-morbidities
– Increased rate of side-effects and dosage problems with medications
– Musculoskeletal problems

TABLE 47-3. Coronary risk profile in elderly cardiac patients

- Lower body mass index
- Lower triglycerides
- Higher HDL cholesterol
- Reduced exercise capacity
- More hypertension
- More diabetes
- Less smoking
- Less hostility, anxiety, and stress

of adverse factors throughout life, it is particularly important for elderly persons to adopt diet and lifestyle practices that minimize their risk of death from morbidity and maximize their prospects for healthful aging.

The cardiovascular risk profile in elderly patients differs considerably from that in younger patients (Table 47-3). There are fewer smokers but more patients with diabetes and arterial hypertension. The body mass generally decreases with age. The lipid profile shows generally lower triglycerides and a higher HDL cholesterol. Psychosocial risk factors such as hostility, anxiety, and stress are encountered with lower frequency compared to younger patients.[15–17]

The treatment of cardiovascular risk factors in elderly patients is as important as in younger patients. This is mainly due to the fact that cardiovascular disease is more prominent and the risk of acute complications is increased. The treatment includes a combination of lifestyle interventions with optimal medical therapy.

Nutrition

Although diet and lifestyle habits can change over time, generally they are characteristic of a person's way of living and reflect life-long health.[18] This is mainly true for dietary patterns. The risk of cardiovascular complications and death in relation to dietary habits has also been studied extensively in elderly patients.[19–22] Adherence to a Mediterranean type diet decreases the risk of cardiovascular events as well as cardiovascular and all-cause mortality and cancer. The strongest association was observed for coronary heart disease. In some Mediterranean diet scores alcohol has been included. However, moderate alcohol consumption is considered as a separate lifestyle factor because many studies observed an independent effect of alcohol on survival. This seems also to be true in elderly persons.[23] However, when interpreting the results of these studies it has to be kept in mind that the main focus of these studies is on primary prevention and that studies about the effects of dietary habits on cardiovascular events and mortality in the setting of secondary prevention are not yet based on solid scientific evidence.

Smoking Cessation

Smoking cessation has immediate positive consequences not only in younger, but also in elderly patients. Smoking cessation after aortocoronary bypass surgery in patients over 65 years of age decreases the mortality within a year after surgery by approximately 40%.[24] Smoking leads to an immediate increase in blood pressure, peripheral vascular resistance and heart rate and leads to a decrease in flow-mediated vasodilatation of the arteries with concomitant increase in clotting tendency and a decrease in HDL cholesterol.[25] This indicates that elderly smokers should be encouraged to stop smoking as is done in younger patients and they should also be offered nicotine replacement medications for suppression of craving if necessary. This recommendation is appropriate up to the age of 75–80 years; in old-old patients smoking cessation counseling becomes somewhat questionable, especially if patients are socially isolated after the loss of their friends and if they have the feeling that smoking is part of their quality of life.

Physical Activity

Physical activity is a key element for health in younger and in older people. There is good scientific evidence that physical training leads to improved cardiovascular fitness in elderly patients.[26–28] The risk of complications with physical exertion is acceptable if the training is preceded by screening for contraindications and followed by recommendations in regard to training intensity.[29,30] Furthermore regular physical activity helps to prevent important conditions in older age such as osteoporosis, non-insulin-dependent diabetes mellitus, hypertension, stroke, and perhaps even some cancers such as colon

TABLE 47-4. General benefits of physical training in elderly patients

- Emotional well-being, improved cognitive functions, and better mental health
- Physical well-being
- Functional abilities
- Endurance and strength (with decreased risk of falls)
- Decrease of blood pressure, blood glucose and blood lipids
- Prevention of osteoporosis
- Psychosocial benefits including prevention of social isolation

cancer (Table 47-4). Its function-preserving effects are also important.

Even healthy elderly people lose strength at a rate of 1–2% a year and power at a rate of 3–4% a year. The resulting weakness has important functional consequences for the performance of everyday activities. A similar argument applies for endurance capacity: 80% of women and 35% of men aged 70–74 years had an aerobic power to weight ratio so low that they would be unable to sustain comfortably a walk at 5 km/h.[29]

Regular exercise increases strength, endurance, and flexibility.[30–32] In percentage terms, the improvements seen in elderly people are similar to those in younger people. However, there is a larger variation due to patient selection in regard to gender, initial fitness and type, intensity, frequency, and duration of the training program. The maximal increase of aerobic capacity with training in elderly patients is about 35–40%. General training recommendations are similar in younger and in elderly patients. A stress test is mandatory before starting a physical training program in elderly patients. To achieve a sustained benefit from physical training this has to be performed at least 2–3 times a week for 20–30 minutes with a minimum heart rate of 50% of the maximal heart rate that has been achieved during a stress test on a treadmill or bicycle ergometer. An increase in training intensity up to 75–85% of the maximal heart rate that has been achieved during the stress test leads to a further improvement of aerobic capacity. These effects can be maintained through continuing training over months and years.

Physical training in elderly patients not only improves functional abilities, endurance, and strength but seems to have beneficial effects directly on the systolic function of the left ventri-

cle. It has been shown that regular physical training on 4 days a week over a time period of 12 months at 60–80% of maximal VO_2 leads to an increase of the left ventricular ejection fraction of up to 20% in healthy elderly persons.[33] The effects of physical training on diastolic left ventricular function are less clear.

A comprehensive exercise program for elderly patients includes activities to develop strength, endurance, flexibility, and coordination in a progressive and enjoyable way. It must use all major muscle groups in exercises that train through each individual's fullest possible pain-free ranges of movement. An exercise program for elderly patients must also aim to load the bones; target major functional, postural and pelvic floor muscles; include practice of functional movements; and emphasize the development of body awareness and balance skill. A combination of regular recreational walking and water gymnastics (both at an intensity that is comfortably challenging), preferably combined with specific exercises to improve strength and flexibility such as weight training, circuit training, step training, exercise to music, dancing, and Qi Gong,[34] will meet most of these criteria for most people.

Psychosocial Aspects

Psychosocial aspects and mental health can be seriously affected in elderly patients with cardiovascular disease. The impact of a cardiovascular event or intervention is usually more pronounced in elderly than in younger patients. Although personality factors such as anger and hostility may be encountered less frequently in elderly than in younger patients, a pre-existing tendency to anxiety and depression may be more prominent after an acute cardiovascular event or intervention or new symptoms of depression may evolve. Cognitive impairment after heart surgery with extracorporeal circulation may add to the psychosocial problems under such circumstances. Elderly patients often fear losing their independence by not being able to return to their own homes and the surroundings they are accustomed to. In such situations rehabilitative measures often contribute to a significant improvement of the physical and psychological deficiencies, increasing the chances that the patient may be able to return home to a life as independent as possible. Depression may lead to loneliness and a feeling of helplessness with the consequence of social isolation. Cardiovascular rehabilitation programs in elderly patients have to be targeted to help the patient during this difficult phase after an acute event by counseling, care, and physical training. Progress during physical training often leads to positive psychosocial changes including a decrease in anxiety and depression and improved social integration.[35,36] Elderly patients take particular advantage of group dynamics when participating in a physical training program that is offered in groups.

Pharmacological Interventions in Secondary Prevention

A study involving a large number of patients showed a 4.5% absolute risk reduction for cardiovascular events in high-risk patients aged 64 or older.[37] The patients in this study received different platelet aggregation inhibitors. However, positive results in these elderly men and women have only been achieved by using aspirin as monotherapy. The number needed to treat to prevent a cardiovascular event was 20 over a period of 2 years. The absolute risk of gastrointestinal bleeding with aspirin in those aged 70 years is about 3%, whereas the risk of a hemorrhagic cerebrovascular insult is increased by 40%. There is also an increased tendency with age to become anemic with aspirin use. However, despite the somewhat increased risk for bleeding complications there is consensus that aspirin should be recommended to elderly patients in secondary prevention of cardiovascular diseases.[38] There is emerging evidence that clopidogrel may become a valuable substitute if aspirin is not well tolerated. Clopidogrel leads to an even more pronounced decrease of cardiovascular events than aspirin with a similar incidence of hemorrhagic complications.

Beta-Blockers

A meta-analysis of three placebo-controlled studies with beta-blockers after myocardial infarction shows a 6% reduction in total mortality in patients aged 65–75 years compared to a reduction of 2.1% in younger patients.[39] This indicates that the use of beta-blockers in elderly patients is even more efficient than in younger patients.[40] The number needed to treat in patients aged 65–75 years is 20 to avoid one death within 2 years.[41] Despite these positive effects, elderly patients are less often treated with beta-blockers than younger patients. This is in part due to the fact that important contraindications for beta-blockers are more often encountered in elderly patients including asthma, chronic obstructive pulmonary disease, peripheral arterial disease, and the risk of hypoglycemia in patients with diabetes. Furthermore beta-blockers lead more often to hypotension, symptomatic bradycardia, and bronchospasm in elderly compared to younger patients. In patients older than 80 years there is no scientific evidence to use beta-blockers in secondary prevention.

ACE Inhibitors

There are four larger studies indicating that the use of ACE inhibitors in patients after myocardial infarction is also beneficial in the age group between 65 and 80 years.[40] The GISSI-3 study included 27% of patients older than 70 years; the absolute risk reduction for combined cardiovascular endpoints and mortality was 3.5 in this subpopulation; the number needed to treat for 6 weeks after infarction to prevent such an event was 30. The three other studies indicate an absolute risk reduction of mortality in all age groups between 4% and 6%. In conclusion, therapy with ACE inhibitors is indicated in most patients for secondary prevention after myocardial infarction, in particular in patients with decreased left ventricular function.

Statins

In the Heart Protection Study, 20,536 people with a total cholesterol of >3.5 mmol/L have been randomized to 40 mg simvastatin or placebo.[42] Sixty-five percent of these patients had coronary heart disease and 5860 patients were in the age group between 70 and 80 years at study entry. The risk reduction with statin therapy was 27% for coronary events and 25% for cardiovascular events. The risk reduction was 22% in the age group between 70 and 80 years. The risk reduction for a first coronary event was 20% in the age group between 70 and 80 years and 35% in the age group between 40 and 65 years. The PROSPER study included patients in the age group of 70 to 72 years with pre-existing cardiovascular disease and a total cholesterol between 4.9 and 9.0 mmol/L and triglycerides below 6.0 mmol/L.[43] Patients have been randomized to 40 mg pravastatin daily or placebo. A total of 5804 patients in the age group between 70 and 80 years have been included and followed over 3 years. There was a reduction of 90% for coronary events under statin therapy but no reduction in overall cardiovascular events. This indicates that the advantages of statin therapy in patients older than 80 years are not evident. In conclusion, most men and women aged less than 80 years should receive statin therapy for secondary prevention of coronary disease. However, the number needed to treat to prevent one cardiovascular event is 80 over a period of 5 years.

Cardiac Rehabilitation Programs

Data on exercise rehabilitation at elderly age are derived from one non-randomized controlled study and six observational studies, four of which compared older with younger coronary patients. Patients up to age 82 were included, and the elderly patients included a significant proportion of women. Rates of entry into cardiac rehabilitation were substantially lower among elderly patients than among younger patients,[44,45] and older women were even less likely to be referred for exercise rehabilitation than were older men.[46] The non-randomized controlled trial also documented statistically significant improvement in measures of exercise tolerance after exercise rehabilitation, with no significant difference between older and younger patients. Patients older and younger than 70 years of age had comparable responses to exercise training, and women and men showed comparable improvements.

The six observational studies documented statistically significant improvements in exercise tolerance in both older and younger patients[44–49] as well as comparable improvements in older men versus older women[50] and in patients aged 62–70 years versus patients older than 70 years. Elderly

TABLE 47-5. Main goals of cardiac rehabilitation in elderly patients

- Preservation of mobility and independence
- Preservation of mental function
- Prevention/treatment of anxiety and depression
- Encouragement of social readaption and reintegration
- Return to the same lifestyle as before the acute event

patients were less fit after a coronary event, in part because of lesser fitness prior to the event; a lower peak exercise capacity was characteristic of elderly patients. Adherence to exercise was 90%,[51] and significant reduction in coronary risk factors occurred in elderly patients who participated in multifactorial cardiac rehabilitation. No complications or adverse outcomes of exercise training at elderly aged were described in any study. Elderly patients of both genders should therefore be strongly encouraged to participate in exercise-based cardiac rehabilitation.

The main goals of cardiac rehabilitation in elderly patients are summarized in Table 47-5. The main focus is somewhat different to that in younger patients.

The provision of cardiac rehabilitation services for elderly patients can be home based and nurse led,[51,52] community based,[53,54] or hospital based in the setting of a multidisciplinary cardiac rehabilitation team. Elderly patients usually attend such cardiac rehabilitation programs two times a week and take advantage of the social integration in a group of patients of the same age. More treatment points should be given and should be repeated more often.

Physical Activity Programs

During physical activity more warnings of directional and step changes are necessary with emphasis on posture and technique. For endurance activities including gymnastics, walking and water gymnastics, 30 minutes of exercise two times a week seems appropriate and usually feasible. However, the older and frailer the participants, the greater the potential benefit from the inclusion of strengthening, stretching, balance and coordination activities and the greater the need for individually tailored exercise guidance from a trained specialist. As in younger patients, all sessions should start and finish gradually with a warm-up and cool-down. For frailer participants, many of the activities should be related closely to daily life and maintaining independence. Techniques of lifting, walking, transferring (moving from sitting to standing, standing to lying), and even crawling should be specifically taught and discussed. Information about the specific benefits of particular exercises is greatly appreciated; for example, shoulder mobility for reaching zips; stamina for "energy" and less breathlessness during exhaustion; or quadriceps, hand grip and biceps strengthening for carrying shopping or using the bus.

Above all, fitness must be fun. Important factors can be variety, the use of appropriate equipment, games, music and opportunities for socializing. A home exercise program can usefully complement the organized session. Provision must be made for a wide range of initial levels of habitual physical activity and for a variety of disabilities. If water training and swimming is considered, one has to be aware that a considerable percentage of patients suffer from incontinence and should therefore not participate in this type of training.

A symptom-limited stress test using either a bicycle or a treadmill ergometer is mandatory before training in patients with cardiovascular disease. Although it is not a primary goal to train with a particular intensity, one should keep in mind that the most efficient and still safe endurance training is performed with a heart rate of 50–80% of the maximal heart rate which has been achieved during the stress test without signs of ischemia or rhythm disturbances. The use of the Borg scale to rate perceived exertion is also advised in elderly patients. A target of Borg 13/14 corresponds well with a heart rate of 60–85% of the maximal heart rate achieved during stress testing and therefore indicates an efficient but safe training intensity.

Educational Programs

Besides exercise training, elderly patients should also attend classes with information about cardiovascular disease, treatment options and medication, nutrition counseling, psychosocial support, and smoking cessation if necessary. Team members should be aware that the type of information and the provision of the teaching is different to that in groups with younger patients. However, adherence to these teaching classes is high and the teaching atmosphere is usually pleasant and rewarding.

Benefits from Cardiac Rehabilitation Programs

A limited number of studies and publications are available in the field of exercise therapy and cardiac rehabilitation in elderly patients.[44–51,55–62] The benefits of exercise training and risk factor intervention have been described earlier in this chapter. Comparing the effects of different service provision of cardiac rehabilitation, either home-based or as outpatient hospital-based programs, Marchionni and colleagues found similar short-term effects in regard to total work capacity and quality of life in each age group. However, patients with home-based cardiac rehabilitation had more prolonged positive effects at lower costs.[63] The addition of cognitive behavior therapy may lead to greater improvements in self-reported physical function, particularly for patients with lower functioning at baseline.[64] Improvement in cardiovascular fitness may also lead to improved cognitive performance, as healthy older adults completing an exercise program showed significant gains in multiple cognitive domains.[65]

Cardiac rehabilitation programs have been shown to effective in elderly patients after myocardial infarction.[66] There is also some indication from a retrospective and non-randomized study that cardiac rehabilitation may improve outcome in elderly patients after percutaneous coronary intervention (PCI).[67] The authors found a lower incidence of major adverse cardiac events and restenosis when PCI patients are included in a cardiac rehabilitation program. Cardiac rehabilitation programs can also successfully be used to optimize recovery outcomes of older individuals after aortocoronary bypass surgery.[68]

There is evidence from one randomized controlled trial that cardiac rehabilitation offers an effective model of care for older patients with heart failure.[69] There were significant improvements in the NYHA classification and 6-minute walking distance at 24 weeks between the groups. Quality of life measured mainly by the Minnesota Living with Heart Failure questionnaire was improved with structured cardiac rehabilitation in elderly patients in several studies.[63,70] Finally, there is one study indicating that early rehabilitation in patients >65 years of age reduces consumption of medical care during the first year after myocardial infarction and that therefore this type of intervention may be cost-effective.[66]

References

1. Lye M, Donnellan CH. General cardiology; heart disease in the elderly. Heart 2000;84:560–566.
2. Ly EM, Donnellan CH. Heart disease in the elderly. Heart 2000;84:560–566.
3. Olivetti G, Melissari M, Capasso JM, et al. Cardiomyopathy of the aging human heart: myocyte loss and reactive hypertrophy. Circ Res 1991;68:1560–1568.
4. Fairweather DS, Aging of the heart and the cardiovascular system. Rev Clin Gerontol 1992;2:83–103.
5. Arrighi JA, Dilsizian V, Perronefilardi P, et al. Improvement of the age-related impairment in left-ventricular diastolic filling with verapamil in the normal human heart. Circulation 1994;90:213–219.
6. Wong WF, Gold S, Fukuyama O, et al. Diastolic dysfunction in elderly patients with congestive heart failure. Am J Cardiol 1989;63:1526–1528.
7. Luchi RJ, Taffet GE, Teasdale TA. Congestive heart failure in the elderly. J Am Geriatr Soc 1991;39:810–825.
8. European Study Group on Diastolic Heart Failure. How to diagnose diastolic heart failure. Eur Heart J 1998;19:990–1003.
9. Pitt B, Segal R, Martinez FA, et al. Randomised trial of losartan versus captopril in patients over 65 with heart failure (evaluation of losartan in the elderly study, ELITE). Lancet 1997;349:747–752.
10. Wei JY. Mechanisms of disease: age and the cardiovascular system. N Engl J Med 1992:327:1735–1739.
11. The Task Force of the Working Group on Heart Failure of the European Society of Cardiology. The treatment of heart failure. Eur Heart J 1997;18:736–753.
12. Rich MW, Beckham V, Wittenberg C, et al. A multidisciplinary intervention to prevent the readmission of elderly patients with congestive heart failure. N Engl J Med 1995;333:1190–1195.
13. Vasan RS, Benjamin EJ, Levy D. Prevalence, clinical features and prognosis of diastolic heart failure –
an epidemiologic perspective. J Am Coll Cardiol 1995;26:1565–1574.
14. Tresch DD. Management of the older patient with acute myocardial infarction: difference in clinical presentations between older and younger patients. J Am Geriatr Soc 1998;46:1157–1162.
15. Menotti A, Mulder I, Nissinen A, et al. Cardiovascular risk factors and 10-year all-cause mortality in elderly European male populations: the FINE study. Eur Heart J 2001;22:573–579.
16. Ruigomez A, Alonso J, Anto JM. Relationship of health behaviours to five-year mortality in an elderly cohort. Age Ageing 1995;24:113–119.
17. Haveman-Nies A, de Groot LP, Burema J, et al., for the SENECA Investigators. Dietary quality and lifestyle factors in relation to 10-year mortality in older Europeans: the SENECA study. Am J Epidemiol 2002;156:962–968.
18. Paffenbarger RS Jr, Hyde RT, Wing AL, Lee IM, Jung DL, Kampert JB. The association of changes in physical-activity level and other lifestyle characteristics with mortality among men. N Engl J Med 1993;328:538–545.
19. Trichopoulou A, Costacou T, Bamia C, Trichopoulos D. Adherence to a Mediterranean diet and survival in a Greek population. N Engl J Med 2003;348:2599–2608.
20. Trichopoulou A, Kouris-Blazos A, Wahlqvist ML, et al. Diet and overall survival in elderly people. BMJ 1995;311:1457–1460.
21. Haveman-Nies A, de Groot LP, Burema J, et al., for the SENECA Investigators. Dietary quality and lifestyle factors in relation to 10-year mortality in older Europeans: the SENECA study. Am J Epidemiol 2002;156:962–968.
22. Huijbregts P, Feskens E, Räsänen L et al. Dietary pattern and 20-year mortality in elderly men in Finland, Italy and the Netherlands: longitudinal cohort study. BMJ 1997;315:13–17.
23. Knoops KT, de Groot LC, Kromhout D, et al. Mediterranean diet, lifestyle factors, and 10-year mortality in elderly European men and women. JAMA 2004;292:1433–1439.
24. Hermanson B, Omenn GS, Kronmal RA, et al. Beneficial six-year outcome of smoking cessation in older men and women with coronary artery disease: results from the CASS registry. N Engl J Med 1998;319:1365–1369.
25. Sparrow D, Dawber T. The influence of cigarette smoking on prognosis after first myocardial infarction. J Chronic Dis 1978;31:425–432.
26. Paffenbarger RS Jr, Hyde RT, Wing AL, Lee IM, Jung DL, Kampert JB. The association of changes in physical-activity level and other lifestyle character-

istics with mortality among men. N Engl J Med 1993;328:538–545.

27. Bijnen FC, Caspersen CJ, Mosterd WL. Physical inactivity as a risk factor for coronary heart disease: a WHO and International Society and Federation of Cardiology position statement. Bull World Health Org 1994;72:1–4.

28. Wannamethee SG, Shaper AG, Walker M. Changes in physical activity, mortality and incidence of coronary heart disease in older men. Lancet 1998;351:1603–1608.

29. Young A, Dinau S. ABC of sports and exercise medicine: Activity in later life. BMJ 2005;330:189–191.

30. Ehsani AA. Cardiovascular adaptations to exercise training in the elderly. Fed Proc 1987;46:1840–1843.

31. Seals DR, Hagberg JM, Hurley BF, Ehsani AA, Holloszy JO. Endurance training in older men and women. I. Cardiovascular response to exercise. J Appl Physiol 1984;57:1024–1029.

32. Thomas SG, Cunningham DA, Rechnitzer PA, Donner AP, Howard JH. Determinants of the training response in elderly men. Med Sci Sports Exerc 1985;17:667–672.

33. Ehsani AA, Ogawa T, Miller TR, Spina RJ, Jilka SM. Exercise training improves left ventricular systolic function in older men. Circulation 1991;83:96–103.

34. Stenlund T, Lindstrom B, Granlund M, Burrel G. Cardiac rehabilitation for the elderly: Qi Gong and group discussions. Eur J Cardiovasc Prev Rehabil 2005;12(1):5–11.

35. Stern MJ, Clean P. National Exercise and Heart Disease Project. Psychosocial changes observed during a low-level exercise program. Arch Intern Med 1981;141:1463.

36. Ewart CK, Taylor CB, Reese LB, et al. Effects of early postmyocardial infarction exercise testing on self-perception and subsequent physical activity. Am J Cardiol 1983;51:1076.

37. Antiplatelets Trialists' Collaboration. Collaborative overview of randomized trials of antiplatelet therapy: prevention of death, myocardial infarction, and stroke by prolonged antiplatelet therapy in various categories of patients. BMJ 1994;308:81–106.

38. Silagy CA, McNeill JJ, Donnan GA, et al. The PACE pilot study: 12 month results and implications for future primary prevention trials in the elderly (prevention with lowdose aspirin of cardiovascular disease in the elderly). J Am Geriatr Soc 1994;42:643–647.

39. Rich MW. Therapy for acute myocardial infarction. Clin Geriatr Med 1996;12:141–168.

40. Dornbrook-Lavender KA, Roth MT, Pieper JA. Secondary prevention of coronary heart disease in the elderly. Ann Pharmacother 2003;37:1867–1876.

41. Gurwitz JH, Goldberg RJ, Chen Z, et al. Beta-blocker therapy in acute myocardial infarction: evidence for underutilization in the elderly. Am J Med 1992; 93:605–610.

42. Heart Protection Study Collaborative Group. MRClBHF heart protection study of cholesterol lowering with simvastatin in 20536 high risk individuals: a randomized placebo-controlled trial. Lancet 2002;360:7–22.

43. Shepard J, Blauw GJ, Murphy MB, et al. Pravastatin in elderly individuals at risk of vascular disease (PROSPER): a randomized controlled trial. Lancet 2002;360:1623–1630.

44. Ades PA, Hanson JS, Gunther PG, Tonino RP. Exercise conditioning in the elderly coronary patient. J Am Geriatr Soc 1987;35:121–124.

45. Lavie CJ, Milani RV, Littman AB. Benefits of cardiac rehabilitation and exercise training in secondary coronary prevention in the elderly. J Am Coll Cardiol 1993;22:678–683.

46. Ades PA, Waldmann ML, Gillespie C. A controlled trial of exercise training in older coronary patients. J Gerontol 1995;50A:M7–11.

47. Willliams MA, Maresh CM, Esterbrooks DJ, Harbrecht JJ, Sketch MH. Early exercise training in patients older than age 65 years compared with that in younger patients after acute myocardial infarction or coronary artery bypass grafting. Am J Cardiol 1985;55:263–266.

48. Stahle A. Effects of exercise training on fitness and quality of life in elderly patients. Eur Heart J 1999;20:1475–1484.

49. Ades PA, Waldmann ML, Poehlman ET, et al. Exercise conditioning in older coronary patients: submaximal lactate response and endurance capacity. Circulation 1993;88:572–577.

50. Ades PA, Waldmann ML, Polk D, Coflesky JT. Referral patterns and exercise response in the rehabilitation of female coronary patients aged ≥62 years. Am J Cardiol 1992;69:1422–1425.

51. Ashworth NL, Chad KE, Harrison EL, Reeder BA, Marshall SC. Home versus center based physical activity programs in older adults. Cochrane Database Syst Rev 2005 Jan 25.

52. Sinclair AJ, Conroy SP, Davies M, Bayer AJ. Post-discharge home-based support for older cardiac patients: a randomised controlled trial. Age Ageing 2005;34(4):338–343.

53. Lee S, Naimark B, Porter MM, Ready AE. Effects of a long-term, community-based cardiac rehabilitation program on middle-aged and elderly cardiac patients. Am J Geriatr Cardiol 2004;13(6):293–298.

54. Witt BJ, Jacobsen SJ, Weston SA, et al. Cardiac rehabilitation after myocardial infarction in the community. J Am Coll Cardiol 2004;44(5):988–996.

55. Aronow WS. Exercise therapy for older persons with cardiovascular disease. Am J Geriatr Cardiol 2001;10(5):245–249.

56. Shapira I, Fisman EZ, Motro M, Pines A, Ben-Ari E, Drory Y. Rehabilitation in older coronary patients. Am J Geriatr Cardiol 1995;4(6):48–55.

57. Lavie CJ, Milani RV, Cassidy MM, Gilliland YE. Benefits of cardiac rehabilitation and exercise training in older persons. Am J Geriatr Cardiol 1995;4(4):42–48.

58. Pepin V, Philips WT, Swan PD. Functional fitness assessment of older cardiac rehabilitation patients. J Cardiopulm Rehabil 2004;24(1):34–37.

59. Hardy SE, Gill TM. Strengthening the evidence base to support the use of cardiac rehabilitation with older individuals. J Cardiopulm Rehabil 2004;24(4):245–247.

60. Lavie CJ, Milani R. Benefits of cardiac rehabilitation in the elderly. Chest 2004;126(4):1010–1012.

61. Pasquali SK, Alexander KP, Peterson ED. Cardiac rehabilitation in the elderly. Am Heart J 2001;142(5):748–755.

62. Lavie CJ, Milani RV. Benefits of cardiac rehabilitation and exercise training programs in the elderly coronary patients. Am J Geriatr Cardiol 2001;10(6):323–327.

63. Marchionni N, Fattirolli F, Fumagalli S, et al. Improved exercise tolerance and quality of life with cardiac rehabilitation of older patients after myocardial infarction: results of a randomized, controlled trial. Circulation 2003;107(17):2201–2206.

64. Rejeski WJ, Foy CG, Brawley LR, et al. Older adults in cardiac rehabilitation: a new strategy for enhancing physical function. Med Sci Sports Exerc 2002;34(11):1705–1713.

65. Gunstad JG, MacGregor KL, Paul RH, et al. Cardiac rehabilitation improves cognitive performance in older adults with cardiovascular disease. J Cardiopulm Rehabil 2005;25:173–176.

66. Bondestam E. Effects of early rehabilitation and consumption of medical care during the first year after myocardial infarction in patients >65 years of age. Am J Cardiol 1995;75:767–771.

67. Dendale P, Berger J, Hansen D, Vaes J, Benit E, Weymans M. Cardiac rehabilitation reduces the rate of major adverse cardiac events after percutaneous coronary intervention. Eur J Cardiovasc Nurs 2005;4(2):113–116.

68. Dolansky MA, Moore SM. Effects of cardiac rehabilitation on the recovery outcomes of older adults after coronary artery bypass surgery. J Cardiopulm Rehabil 2004;24(4):236–244.

69. Austin J, Williams R, Ross L, Moseley L, Hutchison S. Randomised controlled trial of cardiac rehabilitation in elderly patients with heart failure. Eur J Heart Fail 2005;7(3):411–417.

70. McConnell TR, Laubach CA, Memon M, Gardner JK, Klinger TA, Palm RJ. Quality of life and self efficacy in cardiac rehabilitation patients over 70 years of age following acute myocardial infarction and bypass revascularization surgery. Am J Geriatr Cardiol 2000;9(4):210–218.

48
Cardiac Rehabilitation in Chronic Heart Failure

Ugo Corrà

Introduction

Chronic conditions are now the leading reason why people seek medical care.[1] The syndrome of heart failure (HF) is the final pathway for myriad diseases that affect the heart, and is a salient example of the challenge posed by chronic disease. Although the understanding of chronic HF pathophysiology has changed and therapeutic paradigms have been revolutionized,[2] a considerable burden of disability and unrelieved symptoms remains in optimally treated patients, with corresponding low quality of life, and poor prognosis which is worse than for many forms of cancer.[3] In addition, the existence of multiple medical co-morbid conditions, an aging population, potential interaction among multiple medications and psychological impact combine to aggravate the complexity of HF management. Thus, HF is a chronic, costly, and life-threatening disorder, and the need for adequate management strategies is clear.

Cardiac rehabilitation, as multifaceted and multidisciplinary intervention, has been proven to improve functional capacity, recovery, emotional well-being, and reduce hospital readmissions. Moreover, it is unique in educating patients and applying the appropriate medical therapy in addition to non-pharmacological treatment modalities.[4] A flexible, contemporary multidisciplinary intervention in a cardiac rehabilitation setting is a key medical option that emphasizes treating the patient with disease(s) rather than treating disease(s) in patients.

Core Components of Cardiac Rehabilitation in Chronic Heart Failure

All patients with established HF require a multifactorial seamless progressive approach, including baseline clinical assessment and risk stratification, optimal pharmacological therapy directed by national and international guidelines, management of HF-related diseases, non-pharmacological therapy in the form of an integrated management project with a continuing program on physical activity, exercise training, counseling and education, and psychological support (Table 48-1). A flexible, integrated management approach has been demonstrated to delay or prevent acute episodes of clinical deterioration, emergency department attendances, and hospital admissions.[5] To achieve these outcomes, it is necessary to ensure a continuum of care through an efficient, organized linkage between hospital and community including programmed referral procedures and controls. Finally, for all the above disease management stages and strategies, a multidisciplinary team of healthcare providers with specific interest, expertise and training, sharing the different areas of the program, is critically important and recommended.

Clinical Assessment of Patients with Established Heart Failure

Optimal medical management is the first step in ameliorating HF symptoms and survival. As the disease progresses and the HF population ages, medications directed at the underlying pathophysiology of HF may not completely relieve symptoms, and specific treatments of HF-related disease (and co-morbidities) directed toward comfort are needed alongside medical management. To guide a collaborative disease management, a more comprehensive assessment of precipitating factors and HF-related disease needs to be performed.

The 2001 American College of Cardiology/American Heart Association (ACC/AHA) Guidelines have developed a new classification of HF.[6] The evolution of HF has asymptomatic and symptomatic phases. In contrast to the NYHA classification, where a given NYHA class IV patient might rapidly improve to class III with diuretic therapy, the evolution from stage A to stage D in the individual patient has no reverse path. The new classification based on clinical (symptoms) and laboratory presentation (remodeling of left ventricular) underscores the progressive nature of HF and the fundamental preventive role of treatment strategies. The clinical manifestation of HF include several symptoms: dyspnea and fatigue during normal activities and/or those involving minimal effort; waking from sleep with breathlessness; swelling of ankles due to edema coupled with unexpected weight gain; muscular fatigue;

abdominal distension; and upper abdominal discomfort due to liver engorgement. Decreasing weight can also occur either from loss of appetite, nausea and abdominal discomfort on eating, or from dehydration. Weight loss might be associated with aspects of depression that may include blunted affect, sense of despair, and thoughts of death. Anxiety symptoms usually accompany the depression and may dominate the symptom presentation.

Nevertheless, symptoms alone cannot be relied on in defining severity of HF.[7] Careful history, physical examination, cardiac imaging and new biochemical assay, describing fluid status, functional capacity and cardiac rhythm, should be supplemented for the accurate assessment of HF severity. As regards physical examination, four hemodynamic profiles have been described in severe chronic HF patients.[8] These guide medical therapy with the goals of normal jugular venous pressure, resolution of orthopnea and edema, systolic blood pressure of at least 80 mmHg, stable renal function, and ability to walk the hospital ward without dizziness or dyspnea (Table 48-2). More detailed monitoring, including cognitive, psychological, and nutritional status definition, will be required if the patient has significant co-morbidity or has deteriorated since previous clinical review. Finally, specific evaluations (coronary angiography, invasive hemodynamic measurements, symptom-limited cardiopulmonary exercise testing, endomyocardial biopsy, sleep screening study) are necessary for selected HF patients or cardiac transplantation candidates.[6,7] Laboratory investigations will help not only to define the severity of HF but also to exclude the presence of contributing factors to worsening condition (arrhythmias, infection) and to identify co-morbidities and chronic HF-related diseases that can influence management.[6,7]

Chronic HF-Related Disease

Identification of factors that adversely affect quality of life or survival in HF may not only aid in better definition of prognosis but could also potentially provide new opportunities for novel

TABLE 48-2. Hemodynamic profile in heart failure and therapeutic strategies

Profile A	WARM and DRY NO evident elevated filling pressure and hypoperfusion	1. Maintaining stable volume 2. Prevention of disease progression
Profile B	WARM and WET Elevated filling pressure and NO hypoperfusion	1. Intravenous loop diuretics 2. Intravenous vasodilators
Profile C	COLD and WET Elevated filling pressure and hypoperfusion	1. Intravenous vasodilators 2. Inotropic infusions 3. Intravenous loop diuretics
Profile L	COLD and DRY NO elevated filling pressure and hypoperfusion	1. Inotropic infusions 2. Gradual introduction of Beta-blockers (BB)

therapeutic strategies. Several chronic HF-related conditions (and co-morbidities) have been commonly observed in patients not enrolled in clinical trials[9] and are generally ignored by cardiologists.

Depression

Depression is extremely common in the HF population. The wide range of prevalence rates across studies of chronic HF patients is likely due to the use of different diagnostic instruments and the inclusion of different patient population in terms of age, gender, and disease severity. Nevertheless, depression commonly goes undiagnosed.[10] Patients may be unwilling to disclose emotional distress to their physicians for fear of being stigmatized with the label of mental illness. On the other hand, physicians may not address depression because they have not been adequately trained to recognize both typical and atypical depressive symptoms, because of time constraints in high-volume settings, or because they do not know how to best treat the condition. Although an important barrier to the incorporation of depression management into the care of patients with chronic HF is evident, recent studies have documented that recognition and management of depression may be enhanced through the use of multidisciplinary team or disease management programs.[11] Treatment of depression is an important clinical strategy as this condition is associated with more frequent hospital admissions, decline in activities of daily living, worse NYHA functional classification, and increased medical costs.[12]

Anemia

Anemia is emerging as an important factor affecting HF progression.[13] The presence of anemia has been explained as an epiphenomenal marker of advanced heart failure (due to hemodilution due to volume overload, malnutrition from cachexia, or renal insufficiency), an index of high-dose ACE-inhibitor therapy that may inhibit hematopoietic cell proliferation or, finally, as cytokine-mediated bone marrow suppression in severe long-standing HF. A mild degree of anemia (<12.3 g/dL) is associated with worsened symptoms, functional status, and survival in chronic HF patients,[13] and subcutaneous erythropoietin and intravenous iron treatment have been found to improve health status and reduce hospitalizations.[14]

Renal Insufficiency

Measurement of renal function is integral to the management of chronic HF and it influences decision-making. Surprisingly, few studies have systematically evaluated the outcome significance of renal function: mortality is influenced either by increasing quartiles of estimated creatinine clearance,[15] or by a relatively small rise in serum creatinine,[16] irrespective of the patient's baseline renal function or peak serum creatinine. The prognostic impact of renal insufficiency is attributed, at least in part, to more advanced HF, excess co-morbidities, and/or therapeutic nihilism, due to the higher risk of drug toxicities. Moreover, renal insufficiency is associated with multiple changes in vascular pathobiology that may worsen cardiovascular outcome, including abnormalities in the coagulation/fibrinolytic systems, abnormal vascular calcification, hyper-homocystinemia, endothelial dysfunction, insulin resistance, elevated level of C-reactive protein, electrolyte perturbations, and hyperactivation of sympathetic nervous and renin–angiotensin systems.[17]

Cachexia

Cardiac cachexia is a serious complication of chronic HF. Although the definition of cardiac cachexia remains arbitrary,[18] its prevalence is increasing due to the prolonged life in patients with established HF and the mean age of populations with increasing longevity. The mechanism of the transition from HF to cardiac cachexia is not completely known: malabsorption and elevated resting metabolic rates, dietary deficiency, physical inactivity and deconditioning, insulin resistance, excessive inflammatory cytokine activation, and neuroendocrine abnormalities have been variously considered. This multifactorial syndrome is associated with a very high mortality rate.[19] A combination of medical treatment, dietary and physical activity may counteract the progression of cachexia.

Atrial Fibrillation

An important feature of atrial fibrillation (AF) and HF is their propensity to coexist, in part because they share antecedent risk factors, but also because one may directly predispose to the other. The prevalence of AF in various HF series ranges from 9.6% to 49.8%[20] and AF has been reported to have deleterious,[21] neutral,[22] or beneficial[23] impact on survival among chronic HF patients.

Sleep Disorders

Sleep-related breathing disorders are common in chronic HF and in patients with left ventricular systolic dysfunction.[24] Central sleep apnea (CSA) is an important factor that influences morbidity and mortality in HF.[25] The current debate is whether CSA is simply a reflection of severely compromised cardiac function with elevated filling pressure, or whether, for the same degree of cardiac dysfunction, CSA exerts unique and inde-

pendent pathological effects on the failing myocardium.[26] Moreover, at present, there is no consensus on whether CSA should be treated, and if so, what the optimum therapy of CSA in HF might be. Optimized drug therapy, pacing and cardiac resynchronization,[27] nocturnal supplemental oxygen, and various forms of noninvasive positive airway pressure have been investigated.

Pharmacological Approach

An optimal pharmacological approach is a fundamental part of the management strategy in chronic HF patients. Many options are available (Table 48-3) but few have been proven to be efficacious in improving symptoms and survival (Table 48-4). Treatment must be tailored according to the individual characteristics present in each patient: in the individual patient, coronary artery disease,

TABLE 48-3. Pharmacological therapeutic options for chronic heart failure patients with left ventricular systolic dysfunction

Inhibitors of RAS	ACE inhibitors
	Angiotensin receptor blockers
	Aldosterone antagonists
Inhibitors of SNS	Beta-blockers (carvedilol, bisoprolol, metoprolol)
	Antiadrenergic drugs (moxonidine, nolomirole)
Vasodilators	Calcium antagonist (amlodipine)
	Nitrates
	Hydralazine
Diuretics	Loop diuretics (furosemide, torasemide)
	Thiazides
	Potassium-sparing diuretics
Antiarrhythmic agents Inotropic agents	Amiodarone
	Digoxin
	Beta-agonists (xamoterol)
	Phosphodiesterase inhibitors
	Calcium-sensitizing agents (levosimendan)
Antithrombotic agents	Anticoagulant agents
	Antiplatelet agents
Investigational therapies	Anti-endothelin agents (enrasentan, bosentan, darusentan)
	Cytokine antagonists (etanercept)
	Matrix metalloproteinase inhibitors
	Arginine vasopressin antagonists (conivaptan)
	Adenosine agonists
	Metabolic agents (ranolazine)
	Statins
	Treatment of anemia (iron supplementation and erythropoietin)

RAS: renin–angiotensin system; SNS: sympathetic nervous system.

TABLE 48-4. Effects of drugs in chronic heart failure patients with left ventricular dysfunction

Agent	Symptoms	Worsening and hospitalization for HF	Mortality
ACE inhibitors	Improve	Decrease	Decrease in asymptomatic and in NYHA II to IV patients
Beta blockers (bisoprolol, carvedilol, metoprolol CR/XL)	Improve	Decrease	Decrease in NYHA II to IV patients
Angiotensin- receptor blocker (valsartan)	Improve	Decrease	May decrease in ACE-inhibitor-intolerant patients. May increase in patients taking both ACE inhibitors and beta-blockers
Aldosterone receptor antagonist (spironolactone)	Improve	Decrease	Decrease in NYHA III and IV patients
Hydralazine-isosorbide dinitrate	No effect	No effect	May decrease, especially in African Americans
Digoxin	Improve	Decrease	Neutral or may increase if SDC >1 ng/mL, or may decrease when SDC between 0.5 and 0.8 ng/mL
Loop diuretics	Improve	Decrease	May increase
Calcium antagonist (amlodipine)	May worsen	No effect	No effect
Inotropic agents	May improve	No effect	Increase
Systematic vasodilators (epoprostenol, flosequinan)	May improve	No effect	Increase

SDC: serum digoxin concentration.

hypertension, diabetes, atrial fibrillation, and valvular heart disease may coexist and contribute in various amounts to the clinical presentation of heart failure. Moreover, precipitating causes may further enhance the complexity of heart failure management. Keeping in mind the non-pharmacological therapeutic options (Table 48-5), medical therapy must be instituted according to guidelines, with adequate doses and modality of administration. Dosages of drugs prescribed should be equivalent to the dosage used in clinical trials: neither a lesser dose, which may be ineffective nor a higher dose, which may induce serious adverse effects, should be administered. Nevertheless, clinical trial

drug dosage is rarely achieved in the real world of the HF population,[28] particularly in older patients and in those with co-morbidity. A careful upward dosage titration is required in the introduction of both ACE inhibitors and beta-blockers. It is desirable to start with low-minimal dose, and gradually increase up to the target clinical trial dose: a "start low, go slow" policy is recommended. The up-titration schedule usually extends the convalescent period after the patient has been discharged from hospital.

Counseling and Education

Besides optimal pharmacological management, personal education and support of patient and family is imperative.[29] "Heart failure" has a strongly negative connotation for patients, who equate it with "cardiac arrest." A complete and continuous education program for treating chronic HF patients, including knowledge on causes of disease, drug regimen, dietary restriction, physical and work activities, lifestyle changes, and measures of self-management (Table 48-6), will empower patients (and their carers) to take a more active role in management. Understanding the information needs of patients and carers is vital, and good communication between healthcare professionals and patients/carers is essential

TABLE 48-5. Non-pharmacological therapeutic options for chronic heart failure patients with left ventricular dysfunction

Percutaneous and surgical myocardial revascularization
Exercise training
Education (general advice, dietary advice, advice on pharmacological treatment and on evolution of disease)
Treatment of sleep disorders (continuous positive airway pressure, oxygen supplementation)
Biventricular (multisite) pacing
Implantable cardioverter defibrillators
Ultrafiltration
Ventricular assist devices
Pumps and total artificial hearts
Heart transplantation
Gene therapy
Patient, family and hospital organization

TABLE 48-6. Non-pharmacological interventions for heart failure

General advice	Explanation of heart failure and its symptoms
	Causes of heart failure
	Identification and intervention in cases of worsening symptoms and signs
	Self-examination
Dietary advice	Sodium limitation
	Drinking
	Alcohol consumption
	Eating
Physical activity advice	Physical activity
	Traveling
	Work
	Sexual activity
Advice on pharmacological treatment	Explanation of drug effects
	Expected benefits
	Collateral and/or adverse effects
	Risk related to non prescribed suspension
Advise on disease progression	Prognosis
	Indication of heart transplantation

(Table 48-7). The content, style, and timing of information should be tailored to the needs of individual patients, and cognitive ability should be assessed when sharing information. Education should be delivered while the patient is in hospital and reinforced following discharge.

Lifestyle

Smoking

Cigarette smoking should be strongly discouraged in chronic HF patients. In addition to the well-established adverse effects on coronary artery disease, which is the underlying cause in a substantial proportion of patients, smoking has adverse hemodynamic effects in patients with chronic HF,[30] including increased heart rate and systemic blood pressure, mild increase in pulmonary artery pressure, ventricular filling pressure, and total systemic and pulmonary vascular resistance. Increased peripheral vasoconstriction may contribute to a mild reduction of stroke volume. In summary, smoking increases oxygen demand (double product) and decreases myocardial oxygen supply owing to reduced diastolic filling time (higher heart rate) and increases carboxyhemoglobin. In chronic HF patients, enhanced bronchopathic susceptibility and breathing problems precipitate or aggravate HF.[30]

Vaccination

Chronic HF predisposes the respiratory apparatus to infections and may, in turn, be exacerbated by this event. A preventive influenza and pneumococcus vaccine should be considered in all chronic HF patients.

Contraceptive Advice

Premenopausal women with severe chronic HF (NYHA III–IV) should be advised to use contraception to avoid a pregnancy, which would increase the risk of morbidity and mortality, both during pregnancy and delivery. Current hormonal contraceptive methods, with a low dose of estrogen and third-generation progestogen derivatives, are much safer than in the past, with a relatively low thromboembolic risk.[30]

Dietary Recommendations

Alcohol

In general, alcohol should be restricted to moderate levels given its myocardial depressant properties. High doses of alcohol intake predispose the patient to arrhythmias, particularly atrial fibrillation, and hypertension and may lead to important alterations in fluid balance. The prognosis in alcohol-induced cardiomyopathy is poor if consumption continues, and abstinence should be advised. Abstinence can result in substantial clinical benefit and improvement in left ventricular function.

TABLE 48-7. Recommendations for good communication

Listen to patients and respect their views and beliefs.

Give patients the information they ask for or need about their condition, its treatment and prognosis in a way they can understand. Use words that patients will understand. Repeat the information, if necessary.

Provide the most important information for the individual patient first.

Explain how each item will affect patients personally.

Make advice specific, detailed, and concrete.

Confirm understanding by questions.

Prepare diagrams, illustrative materials: use audio-visual means.

Share information with patient's partner and close relatives, if they ask you to do so.

Assess patient's cognitive ability.

Adopt an interactive approach with full participation of patient and carers.

Weight Reduction

Obesity has numerous adverse hemodynamic, cardiac structure and function effects, as well as a propensity for more ventricular arrhythmias. Almost one-third of morbidly obese patients have clinical evidence of HF and a significant increase in NYHA functional class can be achieved with weight reduction.[31] On the other hand, it has been documented that obese chronic HF patients have similar or improved prognosis compared to normal or underweight patients[32]: although these results are subject to debate, a lower body weight is likely to be associated with heightened metabolic state, and an involuntary weight loss, as in the cardiac cachexia syndrome, is associated with a poor outcome.[19] A liberalized fat intake is allowed for weight maintenance and adequate caloric intake in poorly nourished chronic HF patients, with normal or low levels of total and LDL cholesterol.

Physical Inactivity and Exercise Training

Following awareness of symptoms, the natural tendency for HF patients is to do whatever seems reasonable to avoid those symptoms: hence, recognition that effort induces undue dyspnea leads to progressive inactivity, contributing to muscular inefficiency and worsening of physical state that are responsible for further progression of disease. A sedentary lifestyle, with little or no physical activity during leisure time or at work, is a risk factor for the development and progress of cardiovascular disease.[33] Educational processes for chronic HF patients should emphasize the role of sedentary lifestyle as a risk factor, and the benefits of physical activity. Participation in a group exercise training program in a rehabilitation setting should be encouraged. Patients need to understand that they would be better being somewhat active. Advice regarding physical activity should be individualized, taking into account a patient's age, past habits, co-morbidities, preferences, and goals. Finally, patients should be reassured regarding the safety of the recommended protocol. As patients tend to revert to their previous sedentary habits over time, enjoyable activities and those undertaken in company should be recommended because they are more likely to be maintained in the long-term. Patients need to be forewarned of the risk of relapses. Therefore, education should underlie how benefits may be achieved and the need for its life-long continuation. If physical activity interruption has occurred, the physical, social and psychological origin should be investigated, barriers to attendance should be explored, and alternative approaches suggested.

Sexual Difficulties and Coping Strategies

Resumption of sexual activity may be dealt with during discussion of physical activity, and resumption of other activities of daily living. The time of resumption and safety are the main concerns and a delay in resuming sexual activity after HF onset or clinical instability is not uncommon, because of anxiety or depression. Specific advice for individual patients may vary, depending on the patient's age, clinical condition, physical status or other factors.

Medications: Indications, Dosing, Adverse Effects

Concerns about cost, compliance, and drug interactions have given polypharmacy a pejorative connotation, but chronic HF is a classic exception to the notion that "less is more." Few patients relish a regimen of multiple pill taking, but chronic HF is a typical disorder in which multiple drugs offer clear-cut advantages compared to monotherapy. The challenge, then, is making it work in real life. Educating patients about their condition and motivating their adherence to a course of therapy are steps towards success. A clear and comprehensible explanation of the basic purpose and action of each drug is a time-consuming process, even for expert and trained physicians and staff members. Patients' understanding of drug regimens should be periodically refreshed by delegated staff members (nurse coordinator, clinical nurse specialist, nurse practitioner, physician assistant) responsible for the educational monitoring of patients.

Prognosis: Life Expectancy, Advance Directives

Physicians may dislike discussing prognosis with patients, believing that patients expect too much certainty and will become angry if the prognosis is incorrect. Yet patients often think about their prognosis and may welcome opportunities to talk about it. Contrary to fears that discussions of prognosis will destroy patients' hope, such discussions can refocus hope more realistically and prevent false beliefs. A realistic understanding of prognosis allows patients to make informed decisions about their care and allows them to attend to legal and financial matters, complete advance directives, designate a medical decision-maker, emphasize participating in pleasurable activities, and focus on life closure and legacy issues.[34] Physicians in the outpatient and inpatient setting must communicate to each other the outcomes of discussions they have about patient preferences and ensure that patients do not incorrectly view discussions of advance directives and prognosis as signs of "giving up." The appropriate time to discuss prognosis and advance directives relies on patients' request, and can be discussed either during hospital stay or at an outpatient appointment.

Self-Monitoring

The regimens of care for chronic HF patients are often complex and demanding. Learning and retaining information is a considerable requirement and the response to such complex and demanding regimens may significantly influence outcome, particularly inability to control HF instability or progression. Family members and carers may face difficulties and therefore is important to involve them in the patient's education and to discuss any difficulties arising.

Weight

The need to weigh themselves daily is often poorly understood by patients. Weight gain is commonly due to fluid retention, which precedes the appearance of symptomatic pulmonary or systemic congestion. Hence, patients need to understand the sequence and the hazards. A gain of greater than 1.5 kg over 24 hours suggests developing fluid retention and an increase of greater than 2.0 kg over 2 days does likewise. This weight increase necessitates an increase in loop diuretic medication as a semi-urgent matter. Patients must be trained to respond by taking more diuretic: if an increased diuresis or an adequate weight loss is not achieved within 48 hours, an urgent appointment with the general practitioner is required.

Weight loss by patients should be reported: it may occur because of loss of appetite, induced by renal and hepatic dysfunction, hepatic congestion, or it may be a marker of psychological depression. Weight loss may foreshadow significant postural hypotension and falls.

Fluid Intake

Most guidelines have consensus views that fluid intake should be limited to 1.5 liters per day (or 2 liters in hot weather). Excess fluid intake which is not coupled with greater urinary output may tip a patient into acute HF.

Diuretic Therapy Management

With loop diuretics, the diuresis is usually considerable and lasts for a few hours. Hence, if the patient plans on being out during the day, the morning dose of the diuretic may not be taken, but, on the other hand, the evening dose is, not uncommonly, forgotten. As a result, fluid retention may occur.

Medication Adherence

To ensure adequate medication adherence and promote self-management, common patient beliefs should be addressed. Some patients consider that prescription represents a course of treatment, which is terminated when the supplied medication runs out. Other patients note that they feel well and hence consider medication is no longer required. Some cease taking medication because the drugs are too costly, and some reduce the dosage of prescribed medication. Finally, for patients with impaired cognitive function, a daily plan to assist memory, including with regard to medication dosage and times, may promote greater adherence by the patient.

Nutrition

With episodes of acute HF, appetite is much reduced and weight loss may occur. With recovery from clinical instability, recovery of appetite leads to regain of weight, usually slowly. Combined increases in saturated fat intake and weight, and increasing insulin resistance and blood pressure, may lead to further episodes of myocardial infarction or ischemia with severe adverse consequences. Salt restriction, in the form of no added salt at table and no added salt in cooking, tends to reduce fluid retention and decreases the incidence of congestion and worsening chronic HF.

Exercise Training

There has been extensive research into the positive protective effects of exercise training chronic HF patients. Principles of exercise physiology, practical aspects of initiating a training program in chronic HF patients, including patient selection, training methods, and adaptation of individual training intensities, and clinical results and prognostic implications of training interventions have been previously discussed in this book. Although to date, no large-scale, randomized trials that evaluate the long-term clinical efficacy or patient survival rates of exercise training in chronic HF have been reported, a systematic review of 81 published studies, including 2387 exercising patients,[35] and a meta-analysis of 9 randomized parallel controlled trials, including 395 exercising patients,[36] have recently concluded that properly supervised training programs are safe and associated with clear evidence of an overall reduction in mortality. In the last 25 years, the applicability and efficacy of exercise training and a long list of impressive physiological gains achieved have been substantiated in thousands of selected stable chronic HF patients, overwhelmingly advocating that exercise training can be a highly cost-effective resource in chronic HF in an increasingly competitive healthcare climate.

Organizational Aspects of Cardiac Rehabilitation in Chronic HF

Previous sections have examined the scientific evidence for the benefits of components of cardiac rehabilitation. This section will deal with the processes of effective organization and implementation of programs.

Multidisciplinary Programs

Cardiac rehabilitation services are available in a continuum that includes inpatient and outpatient rehabilitation (Table 48-8). Inpatient rehabilitation should begin as soon as possible after hospital admission: every eligible HF patient should receive appropriate strategies for optimal therapy and have access to an individualized program, and when possible, group education, according to clinical assessment and risk stratification. Education should be interactive with full participation of patient/carer: explanation should be given for each intervention and the early mobilization program should vary according to individual need and hospital protocols. Progression of mobilization should be developed according to the patient's clinical condition, functional capacity, age, and co-morbidity, with careful medical review and supervision. Education, reassurance and support, and mobilization should be part of routine daily care for every HF inpatient.

As the length stay for acute HF and procedures continues to decrease, patient and family attendance in outpatient cardiac rehabilitation assumes even greater importance. Structured outpatient cardiac rehabilitation is a crucial point for the development of a life-long approach to prevention. Attendance should start soon after discharge from hospital, ideally within the first few days. Outpatient cardiac rehabilitation may be provided in a range of settings, such as HF clinics, non-clinic settings (community health centers and general medical practices), or a combination of these.[37] Outpatient cardiac rehabilitation may also be provided on an individual basis at home, including a combination of home visits, telephone support (early telephone follow-up and continued telephone availability), telemedicine or specially developed self-education materials.[37] The main

TABLE 48-8. Continuum of cardiac rehabilitation services

Phases	Main elements
Inpatient cardiac rehabilitation	1. Assessment and risk screening
	2. Optimization of pharmacological therapy
	3. Identification and treatment of HF causative factors
	4. Management of HF-related diseases and competing co-morbidities
	5. Mobilization and initiate individualized activity program
	6. Address psychological issues
	7. Development of an action plan by patient and carer to ensure early response to symptom (problem recognition)
	8. Development of identification and modification of risk factor (patient and carer education)
	9. Discharge planning (referral to outpatient rehabilitation)
Outpatient cardiac rehabilitation	1. Individual assessment and regular review, with attention to physical, psychological and social parameters
	2. Referral to HF specialist, if required
	3. Supervised group or individual training
	4. Resistance training as appropriate
	5. Instruction on self-monitoring during physical activity and regular review of physical activity program
	6. Support skill development to enable behavior change and maintenance
	7. Management of psychological issues (depression), emotions, sleep disorders
	8. Self-management issues (management of symptoms, medications).
Continued care (disease progression prevention)	Home visits, telephone contacts, clinic/cardiologist/physician regular review, medications/weight checks, maintenance of understanding and physical activity, family support

elements of outpatient cardiac rehabilitation include assessment, review and follow-up, low- or moderate-intensity physical activity, exercise training, education, discussion, and counseling (Table 48-9). Although length, content, and type program can vary greatly, multidisciplinary HF clinics,[38] multidisciplinary teams providing specialized follow-up in a non-clinic setting,[39] telephone follow-up and attendance with primary care physicians if deterioration is evident,[40] and enhanced patient self-care activities,[41] have all demonstrated a persuasive reduction in all-cause hospital readmission and mortality. Moreover, the multidisciplinary approach has the potential to deliver substantial cost savings.[42]

In conclusion, HF management programs have substantial differences in intervention focus (e.g. patient self-management, medication management, and care coordination), mode (telephone, home, or specialty clinic visit), timing in relation to hospitalization discharge, intensity (frequency and duration of contacts), disease management training, cardiologist's involvement,

and nature, and extent of interaction with primary care physician.[41,42] Although a variety of disease management strategies with appropriate discharge planning and post-discharge support, in

TABLE 48-9. Key components of multidisciplinary intervention in outpatient cardiac rehabilitation in heart failure

Comprehensive discharge planning protocol (including written appointment with general practitioner, cardiologist, exercise group, community services)

Coordination of home care

Nurse-led education

Self-management guidelines for patients

Psychological support

Protocol-driven medication assessment and medication titration

Regularly scheduled visits, at clinic, or at home (medication review, review of health behaviors, activity review, review psychosocial functioning)

Follow-up visits at nurse-run clinic

Telephone follow-up (missed appointments, emergency patient needs, general practitioner attendance and reinforcement)

Telemonitoring of vital signs and clinical status

Communication with primary physician if deterioration or drug intolerance the hands of experienced healthcare professionals, can work in high-risk HF patients, patient education by enhanced self-care, follow-up monitoring by specially trained staff, and access to specialized HF clinics seem the most efficacious approaches.[37] Finally, the need for a continuum of care is clear and requires a lifetime program of self-care, prevention of lapses, recurrences and readmissions. Evaluation of ongoing cardiac rehabilitation program objectives on a regular basis is a key point for success.

Cardiac Rehabilitation Team

The recommended model for cardiac rehabilitation should be delivered by a multidisciplinary team (Tables 48-10, 48-11, 48-12). While many tasks can be shared by more than one team member, some tasks require specific skills and expertise and should be performed by the appropriate, designated health professional. Team

Table 48–11. Cardiac rehabilitation in heart failure: team staff and specific tasks (Part 2)

Heart failure nurse	1. Patient and family's education
	2. Ensuring long-term compliance
	3. Early detection of decompensation.
	4. Monitoring electrolyte balance and kidney function
	5. Implementation of management algorithms.
	6. Provide continuity for patients after discharge
Pharmacist	1. Drug–drug interaction
	2. Adjustment of dosing for renal or hepatic dysfunction
	3. Review all preparation and counseling to increase compliance with medications (especially for elderly patients)
Pyschologist	1. Open discussion of difficult situation
	2. Intervention to lessen depression and anxiety and stress management
	3. Behavioral strategies to help patient to acquire skills to change and maintain healthier behaviours
Dietitian	1. Deal with difficult concepts such as low sodium, reduced fat intake, and fluid restriction
	2. Assess caloric and protein requirements
	3. Incorporate dietary changes for co-morbidity conditions (diabetes, kidney dysfunction, etc.)

TABLE 48-10. Cardiac rehabilitation in heart failure: team staff and specific tasks (Part 1)

Cardiologist	1. Specialized training in heart failure and heart transplantation selection
	2. Knowledge in the pathophysiology of heart failure
	3. Knowledge in heart failure algorithms
	4. Knowledge in outcome indexes.
	5. Define the medical parameter of the program: review the medical content, timing of referral, modality of clinical assessment, ensure accurate information to general practitioners
	6. Encourage the patient to attend the program
	7. Coordinate and communicate with the team members, in order to minimize the amount of conflicting and inappropriate advice.
	8. Facilitate the roles of the other team members
	9. Support and review the program
	10. Supervise the discharge plan
Physiotherapist	1. Assess the physical needs of the patient
	2. Working closely with patient and the family, with the aim of improving ambulation, increasing independence, and improving flexibility
	3. Define exercise programs tailored to meets the requirements of the individual patient
	4. Establish appropriate exercise prescription
	5. Give instructions on exercise limitations
	6. Define timing and modality of exercise program monitoring
	7. Address emotional concerns of activities of daily living

members have different backgrounds and training and therefore different areas of expertise. To avoid overlapping of roles, it is important to determine in advance those tasks which should be undertaken by a designated team member and those which may be shared by several team members: failure to do so can create tension. Finally, team meetings are recommended to facilitate communication between team members and to provide regular opportunities to discuss patients who

TABLE 48-12. Cardiac rehabilitation in heart failure: team staff and specific tasks (Part 3)

Exercise physiologist	1. Provides exercise screening
	2. Provides exercise prescription
	3. Promotes exercise and physical activity counseling
	4. Supervises exercise activity: proficient assessment of patient's responses during exercise sessions
Social services	Direct patient to appropriate community program after hospital discharge
Primary care physician	1. Confirm referral to the program and encourage the patient toattend
	2. Reinforce the goals of the management program
	3. Responsible for long-term medical follow-up and education
	4. Assist and maintain lifestyle changes

have been recently enrolled or those who are experiencing problems. A designated program coordinator is essential to ensure efficient running of the rehabilitation program. The program and medical director should be a cardiologist with good organizational, management and interpersonal skills. The program coordinator organizes referrals, liaises with general practitioners, forwards discharge summaries to them when patients complete the program, convenes team meetings, and makes sure that all team members are familiar with the program. A good knowledge of each phase of each individual HF patient's cardiac rehabilitation process is required for this role. Team professionals from any of the disciplines included could undertake this role.

Performance Measures

Performance measures are standards of care for a particular illness or condition that are designed to assess and subsequently improve the quality of medical care. Performance measures are chosen on the basis of the knowledge or assumption that the particular item is linked to improved patient outcomes. In the field of HF, such measures might include documentation of the level of left ventricular function, medications used (prescription of ACE inhibitors and beta-blockers, at optimal doses, anticoagulant therapy in patients with AF) and monitored (digitalis monitoring) or patient education measures. These measures can be used either internally within an organization or publicly to compare the performance of providers, hospitals, and healthcare organizations.

Conclusions

In view of the complex progressive nature of HF, an increasing consensus supports the role of cardiac rehabilitation as an effective management system. Core components of cardiac rehabilitation include baseline clinical assessment and risk stratification, optimal pharmacological therapy, management of HF-related diseases, non-pharmacological therapy in the form of an integrated management project with a continuing program of physical activity, exercise training, counseling and education, and psychological support. Indeed, cardiac rehabilitation is a uniquely structured comprehensive multi-disciplinary intervention, with a flexible follow-up strategy, and easy access to a specialized HF team. All HF patients should attend a rehabilitation program as soon as they are discharged from acute care institutions to assure clinical stability and to prevent rehospitalization. The challenge for policy-makers is to develop strategies to increase participation in cardiac rehabilitation programs and to incorporate this management approach into the future healthcare planning to deal with the current epidemic of chronic HF patients being discharged from acute care institutions.

References

1. Anderson GF. Physician, public and policymaker perspective on chronic conditions. Arch Intern Med 2003;163:437–442.
2. Massie BM. 15 years of heart failure trials: what have we learned? Lancet 1998;352:si29–si33.
3. Stewart S, MacIntyre K, Hole DJ, Capewell S, et al. More "malignant" than cancer? Five-year survival following a first admission for heart failure. Eur J Heart Fail 2001;3:315–322.
4. Balady GJ, Ades PA, Comoss P, et al. AHA/AACVPR Scientific Statement. Core components of cardiac rehabilitation/secondary prevention programs. Circulation 2000;102:1069–1073.
5. Kimmelstiel C, Levine D, Perry K, et al. Randomized, controlled evaluation of short- and long-term benefits of heart failure disease management within diverse provider network. The SPAN-CHF. Circulation 2005;110:1450–1455.
6. Hunt SA, Baker DW, Chin MH, et al. ACC/AHA guidelines for the evaluation and management of chronic heart failure in the adult: a report of the American College of Cardiology/American Heart Association Task Force on Practice Guidelines. J Am Coll Cardiol 2001;38:2101–2113.
7. Guidelines for the diagnosis and treatment of chronic heart failure. Task force of European Society of Cardiology. Eur Heart J 2001;22:1527–1560.
8. Nohria A, Lewis E, Stevenson LW. Medical management of advanced heart failure. JAMA 2002;287:628–640.
9. Sharpe N. Clinical trials and the real world: selection bias and generalisability of trials results. Cardiovasc Drugs Ther 2002;16:75–77.

10. O'Connor CM, Joynt KE. Depression: are we ignoring an important comorbidity in heart failure? J Am Coll Cardiol 2004;43:1550–1552.

11. Luskin F, Reitz M, Newell K, et al. A controlled pilot study of stress management training in elderly patients with congestive heart failure. Prev Cardiol 2002;5:168–172.

12. Almeida OP, Flicker L. The mind of a failing heart: a systematic review of the association between congestive heart failure and cognitive functioning. Intern Med J 2001;31:290–295.

13. Horwich TB, Fonarow GC, Hamilton MA, et al. Anemia is associated with worse symptoms, greater impairment in functional capacity and significant increase in mortality in patients with advanced heart failure. J Am Coll Cardiol 2002;39:1780–1786.

14. Silverberg DS, Wexler D, Blum M, et al. The use of subcutaneous erythropoietin and intravenous iron for treatment of the anemia of severe, resistant congestive heart failure improve cardiac and renal function and functional class, and markedly reduce hospitalizations. J Am Coll Cardiol 2000;35:1737–1744.

15. Mahon NG, Blackstone EH, Francis GS, et al. The prognostic value of estimated creatinine clearance alongside functional capacity in ambulatory patients with chronic congestive heart failure. J Am Coll Cardiol 2002;40:1106–1113.

16. McAlister FA, Ezekowitz JA, Tonelli M, et al. Renal insufficiency and heart failure. Prognostic and therapeutic implications from a prospective cohort study. Circulation 2004;109:1004–1009.

17. McCullough PA. Why is chronic kidney disease the "spoiler" for cardiovascular outcomes? J Am Coll Cardiol 2003;41:725–728.

18. Anker SD, Sharma R. The syndrome of cardiac cachexia. Int J Cardiol 2002;85:51–66.

19. Anker SD, Coats AJS. Cardiac cachexia. A syndrome with impaired survival and immune and neuroendocrine activation. Chest 1999;115:836–847.

20. Ehrlich JR, Nattel S, Hohnloser SH. Atrial fibrillation and congestive heart failure: specific considerations at the intersection of two common and important cardiac disease sets. J Cardiovasc Electrophysiol 2002;13:399–405.

21. Middlekauff HR, Stevenson WG, Stevenson LW. Prognostic significance of atrial fibrillation in advanced heart failure: a study of 390 patients. Circulation 1991;84:40–48.

22. Carson PE, Johnson GR, Dunkman WB, et al. The influence of atrial fibrillation on prognosis in mild or moderate heart failure: the V-He FT VA Cooperative Studies Group. Circulation 1993;87:VI 102–VI 110.

23. Takarada A, Kurogane H, Hayashi T, et al. Prognostic significance of atrial fibrillation in dilated cardiomyopathy. Jpn Heart J 1993;34:749–758.

24. Lanfranchi PA, Somers VK, Braghiroli A, et al. Central sleep apnea in left ventricular dysfunction. Prevalence and implications for arrhythmic risk. Circulation 2003;107:727–732.

25. Lanfranchi PA, Braghiroli A, Bosimini E, et al. Prognostic value of nocturnal Cheyne-Stokes respiration in chronic heart failure. Circulation 1999;99:1435–1444.

26. Quan SF, Gersh BJ. Cardiovascular consequences of sleep-disordered breathing: past, present and future. Circulation 2004;109:951–957.

27. Sinha AM, Skobel EC, Breithardt OA, et al. Cardiac resynchronization therapy improves central sleep apnea and Cheyne-Stokes respiration in patients with chronic heart failure. J Am Coll Cardiol 2004;44:68–71.

28. Komajda M, Follath F, Swedberg K, et al. The Euro-Heart Failure Survey programme – a survey on the quality of care among patients with heart failure in Europe. Part 2: treatment. Eur Heart J 2003; 24:464–474.

29. Krumholz HM, Baker DW, Ashton CM, et al. Evaluating quality of care for patients with heart failure. Circulation 2000;101:e122–e140.

30. Colonna P, Sorino M, D'Agostino C, et al. Nonpharmacological care of heart failure: counselling, dietary restriction, rehabilitation, treatment of sleep apnea, and ultrafiltration. Am J Cardiol 2003;91(suppl):41F–50F.

31. Alpert MA, Terry BE, Mulekar M, et al. Cardiac morphology and left ventricular function in normotensive morbidly obese patients with and without congestive heart failure and effect of weight loss. Am J Cardiol 1997;80:736–740.

32. Horwich TB, Fonarow GC, Hamilton MA, et al. The relationship between obesity and mortality in patients with advanced heart failure. J Am Coll Cardiol 2001;38:789–795.

33. Giannuzzi P, Mezzani A, Saner H, et al. Physical activity for primary and secondary prevention. Position paper of the Working Group on Cardiac Rehabilitation and Exercise Physiology of the European Society of Cardiology. Eur J Cardiovasc Prev Rehabil 2003;10(5):319–327.

34. Pantilat SZ, Steimle AE. Palliative care for patients with hart failure. JAMA 2004;291:2476–2482.

35. Smart N, Marwick TH. Exercise training for patients with heart failure: a systematic review of factors that improve mortality and morbidity. Am J Med 2004;116:693–706.

36. Piepoli MF, Davos C, Francis DP, Coats AJ; ExTra-MATCH Collaborative. Exercise training meta-analysis of trials in patients with chronic heart failure (ExTraMATCH). BMJ 2004;328(7433):189.

37. McAlister FA, Stewart S, Ferrua S, et al. Multidisci-plinary strategies for the management of heart failure patients at high risk for admission. A recent systematic review of randomized trial. J Am Coll Cardiol 2004;44:810–819.

38. Cline CMJ, Israelsson BYA, Willenheimer RB, et al. Cost effective management programme for heart failure reduces hospitalization. Heart 1998;80:442–446.

39. Stewart S, Marley JE, Horowitz JD. Effects of a multidisciplinary home-based intervention on unplanned readmissions and survival among patients with chronic congestive heart failure: a randomized controlled study. Lancet 1999;354: 1077–1083.

40. Weinberger M, Oddone EZ, Henderson WG for the Veterans Affairs Cooperative Study Group on Primary Care and Hospital Readmissions. Does increased access to primary care reduce hospital readmissions? N Engl Med J 1996;334:1441–1447.

41. Krumholz HM, Amatruda J, Smith GL, et al. Ran-domized trial of an education and support inter-vention to prevent readmission of patients with heart failure. J Am Coll Cardiol 2002;39:83–89.

42. Phillips CO, Wright SM, Kern DE, et al. Compre-hensive discharge planning with postdischarge support for older patients with congestive heart failure. A meta-analysis. JAMA 2004;291:1358–1367.

49
Rehabilitation after Cardiac Transplantation

Carsten B. Cordes

Heart transplantation has been performed as definitive therapy for endstage heart failure since the early 1980s. According to the international registry the annual number of patients is probably well over 4000 worldwide. Any special rehabilitation program for this group will depend on sufficient local concentration of heart transplant recipients (HTRs). Since 60% of all patients are reported from centers with less than 30 patients per year, going without any formal rehabilitation is a reality for many.[1] On the other hand, one can hardly imagine a group of patients that is so obviously in need of rehabilitation because of the multifaceted physical and mental problems to be encountered pre- and postoperatively.

This chapter contains a concise overview of group-specific issues and can hopefully contribute to further improve rehabilitation of these patients, whose 5-year-survival is now close to 70%. Of all patients surviving the first year, 50% will live more than 12 years.[1] Since short-term survival is no longer the key issue for HTRs, a return to functional lifestyle with good quality of life becomes the desired outcome.

The core components of cardiac rehabilitation will be discussed with emphasis on the differing aspects in transplant recipients: baseline patient assessment, exercise training and physical activity counseling, risk factor management, nutritional counseling, psychosocial management, and vocational counselling.[2,3] Baseline assessment requires knowledge of the anatomical and physiological reasons for limited exercise tolerance, which will be described first.

Central Limitations to Exercise Tolerance

The denervated heart exhibits unique characteristics relevant to exercise performance. Resting heart rate is equal to or above 100 beats/min 6 weeks after surgery,[4] with a slow decrease over the years to the range of 80 to 90 beats/min. This intrinsic heart rate, in the absence of parasympathetic and sympathetic nerve fibers, is modulated almost entirely by circulating catecholamines. Thus rate response to exercise is typically sluggish, peak heart rate reaches only 70–80% of the value of age-matched controls and deceleration during recovery is delayed, as shown in Figure 49-1.

Interestingly, cardiac output as assessed via VO_2 during spiroergometry anticipates heart rate response. The limited chronotropic response seems to be compensated for by increased stroke volume due to augmented venous return. Thus the Frank–Starling mechanism is of much greater importance in transplanted hearts than usual.[5,6]

Heart rate reserve is limited to 20 to 30 beats/min in some patients, rarely exceeding 40–50% of resting heart rate.[7] The resulting *chronotropic incompetence* is the main contributor to exercise intolerance.[8] During the first year, peak heart rate increases according to Mercier et al.[9] from 58% of age-matched values at 1 month to 72% at 6 months. Givertz et al.[10] found no significant improvement in peak heart rate after the first year up to 5 years, which suggests the absence of functionally significant cardiac reinnervation during this time. Some HTRs, however,

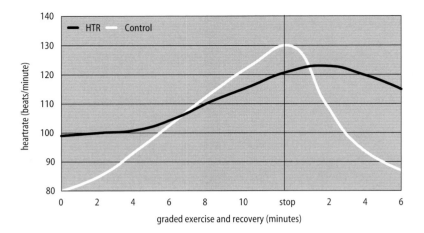

FIGURE 49-1. Typical heart rate response of HTRs early after operation with elevated resting pulse, delayed and flat increase towards a relatively low peak rate occurring after termination of exercise. Deceleration is slow and prolonged.

by performing strenuous long-term exercise programs are able to reach peak heart rate values close to age-matched controls.

For many years denervation of the donor heart was thought to be permanent. Nowadays it is generally accepted that in some HTRs there is partial reinnervation heterogeneously distributed in the myocardium and sometimes reaching the sinoatrial node.[11–13] This is supported by Bengel et al.,[14] who found improved heart rate response and contractile function in the group of HTRs with PET-demonstrated signs of sympathetic reinnervation. Nevertheless the functional significance, incidence, and time course of reinnervation are still not fully understood.

The second major contributor to exercise intolerance in HTRs is *diastolic dysfunction* due to altered left ventricular compliance with slower relaxation, probably linked to the absence of sympathetic innervation. Additional contributing factors may be mismatch between donor's heart size and the recipient's body size, molecular damage associated with brain death, number of rejection episodes, hypertension and myocardial ischemia from cardiac allograft vasculopathy. Cardiac output at rest is normal or only mildly reduced due to the fact that markedly reduced left ventricular end-diastolic volume and stroke volume (minus 20–40%) are compensated for by elevated resting heart rate.[8,12]

Pulmonary diffusing capacity (DLCO) is abnormal in chronic heart failure patients and persists after transplantation but is commonly not the limiting factor. Only when the measured value is 50% lower than predicted does it lead to relevant exercise-induced hypoxemia.

Peripheral Limitations to Exercise Tolerance

Chronic heart failure leads to muscle atrophy, decreased mitochondrial content, decreased oxidative enzymes, and a shift towards less fatigue-resistant type IIb fibers. These changes seem to persist for some time. In addition capillary/fiber ratio in skeletal muscle is reduced even late after transplantation by 27%.[15] Delayed oxygen recovery kinetics in mild heart failure are only partially reversed after heart transplantation.[16] Skeletal muscle strength as measured by knee extension of HTRs with a mean age of 50 is comparable to the values of untrained and sedentary 70- to 79-year-old volunteers.[8] Specific limitations arise from the use of corticosteroids promoting muscle atrophy and from ciclosporin, which leads to impaired NO synthesis by endothelial damage. So the characteristic high peripheral vascular resistance is due to the coaction of antecedent chronic heart failure and detrimental

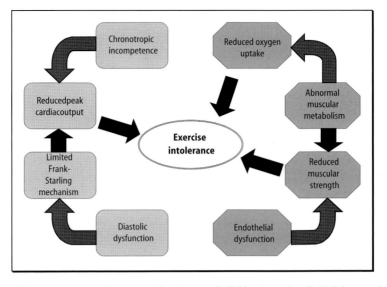

FIGURE 49-2. Summary of the most important factors contributing centrally (left) and peripherally (right) to exercise intolerance of HTRs.

side-effects of immunosuppression. Central and peripheral limitations lead to a higher rate of perceived exertion for HTRs at any given level of activity and peak VO$_2$ will not exceed 60% of the value of age-matched controls with similar level of physical activity.[12] Figure 49-2 summarizes central and peripheral limitations to exercise tolerance.

Exercise Training

The rationale for chronic dynamic exercise and resistance training is prevention of side-effects of immunosuppressive therapy and reduction of cardiovascular risk factors, thus improving quality of life. The former is directed against increasing body weight, insulin resistance, hypertension, and hypercholesterolemia. The latter may prevent glucocorticoid-induced osteoporosis and skeletal muscle myopathy. Both interact in increasing oxygen extraction by muscle, which decreases the need for cardiac output at a given level of muscular work,[17] whereas peak cardiac output itself is not significantly affected by exercise training.[18] Training programs have proved to be beneficial in the early postoperative period as well as 5 years after transplant. Kobashigawa et al.[19] could show in a randomized controlled trial that an individu-

alized 6-month program consisting of an average of 17 session of at least 30 minutes of muscular-strength and aerobic training at moderate intensity improved workload by 59% (35 W) compared to 18% (12 W) in the control group with no supervision. Also the relative increase in peak oxygen consumption (49%) was almost three times as high. Tegtbur et al.[20] started 5 years after transplant and instructed patients to use a computer-assisted cycle ergometer at home. After 12 months and an average of 114 training sessions with an intensity 10% below anaerobic threshold, continuous power output rose by 43% from 46 ± 12 to 66 ± 16 W. Quality of life improved and peak oxygen consumption increased by 12% whereas the control group lost 4%, which is consistent with Douard et al.[7] who found an annual decline of approximately 5% without exercise training after transplant.

Considering the fact that 60–80% of HTRs still have corticosteroids included in their immunosuppressive regime for a considerable period and that 30–50% of these will sustain osteoporotic fractures, effective countermeasures are definitely needed.[1] So far medical treatment has been disappointing. Only resistance exercise has been proved to restore bone mineral density to pretransplant level,[8] making this mode of training an

TABLE 49-1. Effects of exercise training

Parameter	Compared to normal	Change by training
Resting heart rate	+25–50%	Decreased
Peak heart rate	− 20–40%	Increased
Peak VO$_2$	− 30–40%	Increased 12–44%
Peak cardiac output	− 30–40%	None
Left ventricular ejection fraction at rest	Near normal	None
Left ventricular stroke volume at peak	− 20–30%	None
Pulmonary capillary wedge pressure (PCW) at peak	+25–50%	None
Right atrial pressure (RAP) at peak	+80–100%	None
Left ventricular end-diastolic pressure	Increased	Possibly reduced
Left ventricular end-diastolic diameter	−20–30%	None
Anaerobic threshold	Reduced	Increased 13–28%
Peak power output	Reduced	Increased 50–60%
Peak syst systolic arterial blood pressure (PR)	−20%	Increased
Rate of perceived exertion at given workload	Increased	Reduced
Lean body mass	Reduced	Increased 4%
Bone mineral density	Reduced	Restored to pre-transplant level
Muscular strength	Reduced	Increased
Muscular oxidative capacity	Reduced	Increased
Muscular capillary network	Reduced	None

indispensable part of any exercise prescription for HTRs.

A summary of effects of exercise training[8,12,18,21–23] is given in Table 49-1.

Effects of Exercise Training in Heart Transplant Recipients

Exercise intensity is best measured by rate of perceived exertion (RPE). Using the original Borg scale, RPE should be 12 to 14, which corresponds to the ventilatory threshold and a heart rate of usually between 60% and 80% of maximum. For testing protocols small increments of 10 W per minute are recommended to allow for the slow adaptation of heart rate in HTRs. Aerobic exercise may be started in the second or third week after transplant but should be discontinued during corticosteroid bolus therapy for rejection.

Resistance exercise should be added after 6 to 8 weeks. A practical approach to Aerobic exercise has been used by Kavanagh et al.,[21] who instructed patients with a mean age of 47 to start walking 1.6 km five times weekly at a pace that resulted in a perceived exertion of 13 to 14 on the Borg scale.

The pace should be increased over time to jogging with the objective to finally run 4.8 km in 36 minutes (8 km/h) within 6–8 months. This led to improvement of VO$_2$ from 22.2 to 27.9 mL/kg per minute and of peak power output from 107 to 161 W. Gains were equivalent to the reversal of the cumulative effects of 12 years' aging. Unfortunately these gains in physical fitness of HTRs cannot be preserved. They are lost over time despite training at a rate of normal aging. Activity counseling should emphasize the absolute necessity of regular exercise training of at least 30–40 min daily, including slowly progressing warm-up, closed-chain resistive activities (e.g. bridging, half-squats, toe raises, use of therapeutic bands) and walking/jogging/cycling in order to make up for the period of prolonged physical deconditioning, counteract some of the effects of immunosuppression, and maintain good quality of life.

Risk Factor Management

Mortality during the first year is 1.4 times that of the next 4 years combined.[1] Whereas rejection and infection dominate during the first months, mortality thereafter is mainly due to the development of cardiac allograft vasculopathy (CAV) and malignancies.

Measures Against Rejection

Basic medical therapy to reduce the incidence of acute rejection includes two or three of the following immunosuppressants: ciclosporin, azathioprine, corticosteroids. Ciclosporin, a calcineurin inhibitor, specifically acts on T-cell and B-cell activation and has markedly improved survival in the first 2 years after transplant. However, due to its negative effects on blood pressure, renal function, lipid and glucose metabolism, it had little positive impact on the determinants of long-term survival such as cardiac allograft vasculopathy (CAV). The patient may notice hypertrophic gingivitis, hypertrichosis, and tremor and headache. It decreases oxidative enzymes and may thus further limit oxidative capacity in HTR.[8] Tacrolimus, equally effective against acute rejection, is increasingly substituted for ciclosporin because of a lower incidence of hypertension and hyperlipidemia; however, there is a trend for more cases of new-onset diabetes.[24] Other side-effects are similar to ciclosporin, but it lacks the potential for hirsutism and gingival hyperplasia.[25] Azathioprine used to be the second pillar of immunosuppressive therapy. Its major side-effect is dose-dependent myelosuppression. Now it has widely been substituted by mycophenolate mofetil (MMF, CellCept), which acts more specifically on the lymphocytes and has shown to be more effective in reducing the number of rejection episodes.[1,24] It is usually well tolerated, but may sometimes lead to dose-dependent nausea, vomiting, or diarrhea. During the first year, 80% of HTRs are on a triple-drug-regime including corticosteroids gradually decreasing to about 60% in the fifth year with a maintenance dosage of usually 5 mg prednisolone per day.[1] Three days of high-dose prednisone (100–1000 mg) are the usual treatment for acute rejection grade 2 of the seven-grade biopsy-classification of the International Society of Heart and Lung Transplantation (ISHLT). Some long-term side-effects are well known. Osteopenia occurs in 100% of HTRs, osteoporotic fractures in 30–50%. There has been less focus on myopathy, but its impact on exercise intolerance because of muscular weakness of arms and legs should not be underestimated. Cosmetic effects like acne, hirsutism, moon face, and truncal obesity are particularly troubling to many patients.

Since quick, appropriate treatment is necessary to handle acute rejection, patients are instructed to practice self-monitoring. An unusually low blood pressure, a change of heart rate, unexplained weight gain or fatigue may be early signs of rejection even when there is no feeling of being sick. Adherence to the medical regime as well as careful self-monitoring including taking one's temperature twice daily is of vital importance.[26]

Measures Against Infection

During periods of increased immunosuppression within the initial 6 to 12 months, most centers prescribe medical prophylaxis against cytomegalovirus, herpes simplex reactivation, pneumocystis, aspergillus and candida species. It should be stressed, however, that the recipient of a transplant is expected to show an increased responsibility for himself by complying with the recommendations of his transplant center concerning personal hygiene and general measures to avoid those infections that are not due to latent viruses (Table 49-2). Medical personnel dealing with HTRs should be aware of the immunosuppression-induced impairment of the inflammatory response, which attenuates the signs and symptoms of invasive infection.

Active immunization with live virus is generally not recommended. Vaccination against flu and

TABLE 49-2. General measures to reduce the risk of infection

1. Good dental hygiene, no toothbrush older than 4 weeks
2. Frequent handwashing using liquid soap
3. Avoidance of close contact with people with infectious diseases (measles, chickenpox, mumps, mononucleosis, common cold, flu)
4. Avoidance of contact with persons having received oral polio vaccination for 8 weeks
5. If indispensable, pets in the household only under strict precautions limiting contact
6. No gardening without gloves
7. No contact with decaying plants, fruits, vegetables
8. No stay near construction work and compost heaps
9. No mold inside the home
10. Hydroculture (hydroponics) is better than potting compost in the home
11. Avoidance of swimming in public baths during the first months
12. Avoidance of hot tub, sauna, and whirlpool

pneumococcal pneumonia is deemed helpful by most centers to avoid serious infections.

Increasing numbers of transplant recipients are active intercontinental travelers. They should receive special counseling from their transplant center.[27] Female HTRs suffering from increased growth of facial and body hair are not advised to use the new method of electrolysis for permanent depilation because of the risk of infection.

Cardiac Allograft Vasculopathy

Cardiac allograft vasculopathy (CAV), the main determinant of long-term survival, is a rapidly progressive form of atherosclerosis that occurs uniquely in HTRs, characterized by concentric intimal proliferation in early stages (58% by one year), later developing diffuse narrowing in proximal and distal portions of the coronary tree (50% by 5 years). Occlusion of smaller arteries can go unnoticed, and chest pain is usually absent. Instead congestive heart failure, ventricular arrhythmias, and sudden death are the first clinical manifestations.

The published studies on cardiac rehabilitation for heart transplantation so far have not addressed CAV. Although exercise training would theoretically delay or prevent coronary artery disease progression in the transplanted heart, this still has to be studied.[17]

Risk factors for the development of CAV on the donor's side are hypertension and higher age, on the recipient's side coronary artery disease, number of rejection episodes in first year, symptomatic and asymptomatic cytomegalovirus infection, young age, hyperlipidemia, obesity, smoking, hypertension, and diabetes.. The latter five are amenable to lifestyle changes, exercise training, and adequate medication. Hypercholesterolemia is present in 52% by 1 year and 90% by 7 years.[1] Statins (pravastatin, simvastatin) not only lowered LDL cholesterol levels but also decreased the incidence of CAV and significantly improved survival. In addition, pravastatin reduced the number of rejection episodes.[28] Statins are now part of standard therapy, but dose-related myopathy and myolysis due to interaction with ciclosporin has not only been a theoretical danger. Most centers prefer pravastatin in doses up to 40 mg because its metabolism is less dependent on CYP3A4 and the risk of relevant drug interaction appears to be lower. Obesity can be controlled by daily exercise and a healthy diet. Cessation of smoking is a prerequisite for transplantation in most centers but psychological support may be needed not to resume old habits. Hypertension is linked to immunosuppressive therapy and denervation of cardiac volume receptors. It is very common and affects 73% by 1 year and 97% by 7 years.[1] It is sensitive to a low-sodium diet. Treatment with diltiazem and ACE inhibitors led to improved coronary artery diameter and less intimal thickening. Antihypertensive therapy is usually completed by diuretics. Beta-blockers should not be used as they hamper the already delayed chronotropic response of the denervated heart.

The cumulative incidence of new-onset diabetes after transplantation is 32% at 5 years. Risk factors are family history of diabetes, pre-transplant blood glucose level and post-transplant corticosteroid dose. There is mounting evidence that diabetes may play a pivotal role in the development of CAV. Regular screening, early diagnosis, and a stepwise therapeutic approach once A_{1C} exceeds 6.5% are recommended according to the International Consensus Guidelines.[29] Target blood pressure is 130/80 mmHg.

Malignancies

Whereas the incidence of solid organ malignancy is similar to that in the general population, skin cancer is increased by a factor of 20. It occurs in 18% of 7-year survivors. Next are lymphoproliferative disorders, bringing the overall cumulative incidence of post-transplant malignancies to 24%.[1] Since etiology is linked to immunosuppression, there is no prevention available other than reducing sun exposure. Early detection of any suspicious skin changes as well as of enlarged lymph nodes or any swelling beneath the skin is important.

Pharmacology of the Denervated Heart

Pharmacological distinctions due to denervation of the heart[30] that should be known to all medical personnel dealing with HTRs are listed in Table 49-3.

TABLE 49-3. Pharmacology of the denervated heart

Digitalis	Positive inotropic effect preserved
	No vagus-dependent dromotropic effect
	Not helpful to control ventricular rate in atrial fibrillation
Beta-blockers	Slows heart rate response to exercise even further
	Due to antagonism of circulating catecholamines
Verapamil	Dromotropic effect preserved due to direct action on atrioventricular node
	Helpful in atrial fibrillation
Chinidin	No vagolytic effect
	Helpful in atrial fibrillation
Atropine	No vagolytic effect
	Rare paradoxical effect with complete heart block and sinus arrest
Vasodilators	No reflex tachycardia
Epinephrine (adrenaline), norepinephrine (noradrenaline)	Positive inotropic and chronotropic effect

Nutritional Counseling

There are four major goals regarding nutrition after heart transplantation: avoidance of overweight, balancing of side-effects of immunosuppressants, limitation of classical cardiovascular risk factors, and avoidance of infection.

Overweight is a risk factor for diabetes, hypertension, hyperlipidemia, and CAV. A history of pre-transplant obesity or the correction of prior malabsorption by transplant may contribute to its development. Excessive caloric intake can be caused by an increased appetite due to corticosteroids. Patients have to be aware of the need to accept strict calorie control in relation to their energy consumption. Corticosteroids also lead to salt and fluid retention as well as elevation of blood sugar and cholesterol. Post-transplant nutrition should therefore contain low sodium, low total fat (<30% of calories), low saturated fat

TABLE 49-4. Dietary infection prophylaxis – food to be avoided

1. Raw meat
2. Raw seafood
3. Unpasteurized milk
4. Cheese from unpasteurized milk
5. Moldy cheese
6. Raw eggs
7. Soft ice

(<10% of calories) replaced by monounsaturated fat (oleic acid as in olive oil and rapeseed oil), no concentrated carbohydrates, and a wide variety of healthy fresh food. There are good reasons to follow this Mediterranean style diet,[31] even though controlled studies in HTRs to assess the influence of nutrition on CAV or survival have not been published.

To prevent infection with toxoplasma, listeria, salmonella, staphylococci and fungi to name the most important agents, a list of foods to be avoided as far as possible is given in Table 49-4. The level of evidence is of course rather limited and regional conditions have to be taken into account, which explains the considerable variance between centers in this regard. Fresh fruit and salad should be cleaned very carefully, especially during the first 6 months. For different reasons grapefruit juice should be avoided. It may decrease ciclosporin metabolism to an unpredictable extent.

Psychosocial Management

Cardiac transplantation is a process, not an event. It continues for the remainder of the recipient's life and it means a new set of problems in place of the old ones. There are some typical stages of adjustment.[32] A postoperative phase of euphoria usually comes to an end with the first rejection or other setback, conveying a feeling of vulnerability. Depression and anxiety may follow, after which the patient eventually settles into a more realistic acceptance of opportunities and limits. In our early experience with HTRs between 20 and 60 days after surgery we found that well-meaning medical information and advice on life after transplant had often turned into enduring concern and apprehensiveness as detected by the choice of topics HTRs discussed with psychologists.[4] This showed that careful presentation of recommendations is necessary, leaving the choice up to the patient and offering every possible support he or she may need to adjust. Subsequent to initial postoperative recovery poor medical compliance may account for significant morbidity and for up to 25% of deaths occurring. Risk of CAV was elevated 5-fold by persistent depression, 7-fold by medication non-compliance, 8-fold by persistent anger–hostility, and 10-fold by obesity within 3 years after transplant.[33] Therefore educational and psychotherapeutic interventions should be incorporated into the transplant team's comprehensive care and follow-up of HTRs.

Family adjustment and stabilization of partner relationships pose a great challenge. Whereas during the pre-transplant period spouses, children and other relatives may have relieved the patient from daily responsibilities, when the patient returns home in better physical condition, roles have to be carefully re-established. Trying to live up to high expectations may pose emotional stress on the HTR. Recently, however, more focus has been put on the suffering of family and spouses, with the provision of partner-groups at rehabilitation clinics and follow-up centers being recommended.[34]

Return to work rates vary widely from as low as 21% to as high as 79%. Obviously more factors are involved than successful surgery and good quality of life. In the United Kingdom, Kavanagh et al. reported 69% employment at 5 years and 57% at 12 years post transplant.[35] In the German series by Hetzer et al., 34% of survivors of 9 to 13 years were employed.[36] To interpret this one has to understand the national differences in social security with different thresholds for benefits of unemployment, partial disability, and permanent disability. Other important predictors are length of pre-transplant disability, employment history, education, and state of the economy. HTRs below the age of 65 are generally encouraged by the transplant team to resume work with very few exceptions (like construction work). Social workers should assist in reducing misconceptions about employment of HTRs on the part of the former or prospective employer.

References

1. Taylor DO, Edwards LB, Boucek MM, et al. The registry of the international society for heart and lung transplantation: Twenty-first official adult heart transplant report – 2004. J Heart Lung Transplant 2004;23:796–803.
2. Balady GJ, Ades PA, Comoss P, et al. Core components of cardiac rehabilitation programs. A statement for healthcare professionals from the American Heart Association and the American Association of Cardiovascular and Pulmonary Rehabilitation Writing Group. Circulation 2000;102: 1069–1073.
3. Giannuzzi P, Saner H, Björnstad H, et al. Secondary prevention through cardiac rehabilitation. Eur Heart J 2003;24:1273–1278.
4. Cordes C, Bertram R, Rosenblatt K, et al. Stationäre Rehabilitation nach Herztransplantation. Präv Rehab 1992;4:89–96.
5. Shepard RJ, Kavanagh T, Mertens DJ, et al. Kinetics of the transplanted heart. J Cardiopulm Rehabil 1995;15:288–296.
6. Banner NR. Exercise physiology and rehabilitation after heart transplantation. J Heart Lung Transplant 1992;11:237–240.
7. Douard H, Parrens E, Billes MA, et al. Predictive factors of maximal aerobic capacity after cardiac transplantation. Eur Heart J 1997;18:1823–1828.
8. Braith RW, Edwards DG. Exercise following heart transplantation. Sports Med 2000;30:171–192.
9. Mercier J, Ville N, Wintrebert P, et al. Influence of post-surgery time after cardiac transplantation on exercise responses. Med Sci Sports Exerc 1996;28:171–175.
10. Givertz MM, Hartley H, Colucci WS. Long-term sequential changes in exercise capacity and chronotropic responsiveness after cardiac transplantation. Circulation 1997;96:232–237.
11. Schwaiblmair M, von Scheidt W, Ueberfuhr P, et al. Functional significance of cardiac reinnervation in heart transplant recipients. J Heart Lung Transplant 1999;18:838–845.
12. Marconi C, Marzorati M. Exercise after heart transplantation. Eur J Appl Physiol 2003;90:250–259.
13. Gallego-Page JC, Segovia J, Alonso-Pulpon L, et al. Re-innervation after heart transplantation: a multidisciplinary study. J Heart Lung Transplant 2004; 23:674–682.
14. Bengel FM, Ueberfuhr P, Schiepel N, et al. Effect of sympathetic reinnervation on cardiac performance after heart transplantation. N Engl J Med 2001;345: 731–738.
15. Lampert E, Mettauer B, Hoppeler H, et al. Structure of skeletal muscle in heart transplant recipients. J Am Coll Cardiol 1996;28:980–984.
16. Nanas SN, Terrovitis JV, Charitos C, et al. Ventilatory response to exercise and kinetics of oxygen recovery are similar in cardiac transplant recipients and patients with mild chronic heart failure. J Heart Lung Transplant 2004;23:1154–1159.
17. Stewart KJ, Badenhop D, Brubaker PH, et al. Cardiac rehabilitation following percutaneous revascularization, heart transplant, heart valve surgery, and for chronic heart failure. Chest 2003;123:2104–2111.

18. Kavanagh T, Yacoub MH, Mertens DJ, et al. Cardiorespiratory responses to exercise training after orthotopic cardiac transplantation. Circulation 1988;77:162–171.

19. Kobashigawa JA, Leaf DA, Lee N, et al. A controlled trial of exercise rehabilitation after heart transplantation. N Engl J Med 1999;340:272–277.

20. Tegtbur U, Busse MW, Jung K, et al. Phase III Rehabilitation nach Herztransplantation. Z Kardiol 2003;92:908–915.

21. Kavanagh T, Mertens DJ, Shepard RJ, et al. Long-term cardiorespiratory results of exercise training following cardiac transplantation. Am J Cardiol 2003;91:190–194.

22. Squires RW. Cardiac rehabilitation issues for heart transplantation patients. J Cardiopulm Rehabil 1990;10:159–168.

23. Keteyian S, Ehrman J, Fedel F, et al. Heart rate – perceived exertion relationship during exercise in orthotopic heart transplant patients. J Cardiopulm Rehabil 1990;10:287–293.

24. Keogh A. Calcineurin inhibitors in heart transplantation. J Heart Lung Transplant 2004;23:S202–S206.

25. Lindenfeld J, Miller GG, Shakar SF, et al. Drug therapy in the heart transplant recipient. Circulation 2004;110:3858–3865.

26. Körfer R, Tenderich G, Schulz U. Informationen zur Herztransplantation. Lengerich: Pabst Science Publishers; 2004.

27. Kotton CN, Ryan ET, Fishman JA. Prevention of infection in adult travelers after solid organ transplantation. Am J Transplant 2005;5:8–14.

28. Valantine H. Cardiac allograft vasculopathy after heart transplantation: risk factors and management. J Heart Lung Transplant 2004;23:S187–S193.

29. Marchetti P. New-onset diabetes after transplantation. J Heart Lung Transplant 2004;23:S194–S201.

30. Scheld HH, Deng MC, Hammel D. Leitfaden Herztransplantation – interdisziplinäre Betreuung vor, während und nach Herztransplantation, 2nd edn. Darmstadt: Steinkopff; 2001.

31. Salen P, De Lorgeril M, Boissonnat P, et al. Effects of a French Mediterranean diet on heart transplant recipients with hypercholesterolemia. Am J Cardiol 1994;73:825–827.

32. Shapiro PA. Life after heart transplantation. Prog Cardiovasc Dis 1990;32:405–418.

33. Dew MA, Kormos RL, Roth LH, et al. Early post-transplant medical compliance and mental health predict physical morbidity and mortality one to three years after heart transplantation. J Heart Lung Transplant 1999;18:549–562.

34. Bunzel B, Laederach-Hofmann K, Schubert MT. Patients benefit – partners suffer? The impact of heart transplantation on the partner relationship. Transpl Int 1999;12:33–41.

35. Kavanagh T, Yacoub MH, Kennedy J, et al. Return to work after heart transplantation: 12-year follow-up. J Heart Lung Transplant 1999;18:846–851.

36. Hetzer R, Albert W, Hummel M. Status of patients presently living 9 to 13 years after orthotopic heart transplantation. Ann Thorac Surg 1997;64:1661–1668.

50
Rehabilitation in Patients with Implantable Devices

L. Vanhees, S. Beloka, M. Martens, and A. Stevens

Implantable devices were introduced as life-saving equipment for millions of people suffering from coronary heart disease. Nowadays, not only traditional antiarrhythmic pharmacological therapy has been shown to decrease sudden cardiac death, but also pacemakers and cardioverter defibrillators have proved their value in the treatment of life-threatening rhythm disorders. In heart failure, cardiac resynchronisation therapy (CRT) and assist devices have recently demonstrated their importance, but no published data regarding physical exercise or training are available yet. This chapter will mainly deal with physical exercise and rehabilitation in patients who have received an implantable cardioverter defibrillator. Cardiac rehabilitation in patients with assist devices or pacemakers will be discussed only briefly.

Assist and Pacemaker Devices

Non-pharmacological approaches to improve the morbidity and mortality in patients with moderate to severe heart failure have been sought for several decades. A solution has been found in cardiac resynchronization therapy (atrial-synchronized biventricular pacing), which was designed to stimulate the ventricle at multiple sites to improve the coordination of the contractions, and thus improve cardiac performance. In the numerous clinical trials, consistent benefits have been reported in quality of life, exercise capacity, and functional status. Up to now, no data on the effect of exercise training in CRT has been published, but the first randomised controlled trials, proving the additional gain in exercise tolerance after a physical training program, have been recently presented at 2 international meetings, EuroPRevent – Athens 2006 and at the World Congress of Cardiology – Barcelona 2006.[1-3] However, the long-term benefit of this treatment regarding hospitalization and mortality has still to be established.[4,5]

Quality of life and impact on survival after implantation of the assist device were described by Grady et al.[6] Quality of life is rather good and stable from 1 month to 1 year after the implantation. Items in the physical domain of quality of life (walking and dressing oneself) are associated with the risk of dying.

Improvements in exercise capacity as an immediate effect of the implantation of the device have been reported, but as yet no training studies have been performed in this relatively new patient population.

The advanced current pacemaker devices treat brady- and tachyarrhythmias, sinus arrhythmias, and conduction disturbances by altering the lead wire of the pulse generator to supply adequate electricity for continuing the metabolic and physical stimuli of the myocardial activity.

Research has documented that pacemaker therapy may reinstate regular exercise capability, reduce symptoms or abnormalities, and improve quality of life and survival.[7] Pacemakers must be considered as implanted devices which may influence the reaction of heart rate. This is the major concern when developing basic guidelines for exercise programs. Cardiac rehabilitation for patients with a pacemaker is feasible when the rate-response setting of each patient is adapted correctly, avoiding functional destruction by insufficient pacing rates. Greco et al. described the use of the oxygen pulse reserve (mL O_2/beat, measured during an exercise test) and the pacing rate, in patients with pacemakers, in order to tailor the rate response in a cardiac rehabilitation program. After a period of 2–7 months, there was an average improvement in peak oxygen consumption of 23%.[8]

No general guidelines for physical training and rehabilitation have been described yet for the population of patients with a pacemaker.

Implantable Cardioverter Defibrillators

The implantable cardioverter defibrillator (ICD) has evolved to be the golden standard therapy for patients at high risk for malignant ventricular arrhythmias or sudden cardiac death (SCD). These patients include those who have survived a life-threatening dysrhythmic event (secondary prevention) and those who suffer from cardiac disease who are symptomless but at risk for such arrhythmias (primary prevention). In addition, new ICDs also provide full featured dual chamber pacing, and could treat atrial arrhythmias and congestive heart failure by means of biventricular pacing.[9]

The ICD is an external device implanted in the recipient's chest, designed to deliver pacings and shocking pulses to the myocardium. By delivering an electric shock, ventricular tachycardia/fibrillation and SCD can effectively be aborted. The AVID (Antiarrhythmics Versus Implantable Defibrillators) trial was the first large trial that showed the superiority of the ICD compared to antiarrhythmic drugs in terms of increasing overall survival in patients who had survived a previous event.[10]

Psychosocial Aspects and Quality of Life

It is logical to think that the implantation of a life-saving device would make the patient confident of the improved life expectancy and relieve the fear of sudden death. But living with the possibility of receiving a defibrillating shock at any time can be emotionally devastating. Compared to the general population, quality of life and psychosocial adjustment are poor in patients with ICDs.[11,12] According to Sears et al., ICD-specific fears and symptoms of anxiety are the most common symptoms experienced by patients with ICD.[11] Moreover, 13–38% of these patients experience diagnosable levels of anxiety. ICD-specific fears include fear of shock, fear of device malfunction, fear of death, and fear of embarrassment. The health-related quality of life is also negatively associated with fear of exercise.[12]

Social and working life can also be negatively influenced as there is limitation of action, due to the fear that stress or emotions might alert the device. Others may worry about their body image or avoid exercise and sexual activity because of fears of arrhythmias and discharge of the ICD.[13] In some countries, driving is even, at least temporarily, prohibited.[14,15]

Also partners of ICD patients report feelings of helplessness and uncertainty about what to do if, or when, the ICD discharges. They worry about the reliability of the ICD and about their own position if their partner should die.[16] This may commonly result in overprotection of the ICD patient, and partners often restrict or restrain them from doing physical activities.

The importance of involving, educating, and equipping partners with the relevant information and skills so that they can empower and support the patient to reach informed decisions should not be underestimated. In the absence of such interventions, the potential for misconceptions, misguided beliefs, and marital conflicts can increase, perpetuating further uncertainty, fear, and loss of control as well as precipitating physical symptoms.[17]

Recent studies report the psychological benefits for patients with ICDs after psychological intervention or comprehensive cardiac rehabilitation. Kohn et al. studied cognitive behavioral therapy in patients with ICDs in a randomized controlled trial. They concluded that cognitive behavioral therapy was associated with decreased levels of depression and anxiety, and increased adjustment, particularly among those patients who received a shock.[18] Fitchet et al. reported decreased anxiety scores after 12 weeks of comprehensive cardiac rehabilitation, including psychosocial counseling, in a randomized controlled trial.[19]

These data demonstrate the importance of planning and organizing psychosocial support for patients with ICDs in comprehensive cardiac rehabilitation.

Exercise Testing

The design of an exercise program should always be preceded by a maximal or symptom-limited exercise test.[20] Despite the fear of patients with an ICD and the risk of harmful and threatening symptoms, the exercise test has a key role in the evaluation of arrhythmias, the ICD device, peak heart rate and exercise tolerance, and medical therapy.

The testing protocol should be a standard graded exercise tolerance test on a motor driven treadmill or cycle ergometer with assessment of ECG, blood pressure, and oxygen uptake. The assessed peak oxygen uptake is the most accurate measure of functional capacity. It can also be estimated by exercise hemodynamic data or the external workload that was achieved. A submaximal test (terminating the test at a given percentage of predicted maximum heart rate) is not recommended because medications affect the age-predicted maximum of the heart rate, it would only give an estimate of the actual exercise tolerance, and it would not give the opportunity to evaluate the reactions of cardiac rhythm and the ICD on maximal exercise.

The participant elicits a maximum cardiorespiratory response by continuing the exercise test till exhaustion or fatigue. In some studies, the point when the patient reached a heart rate threshold of cut-off point minus 10 to 30 beats was one of the endpoints of the test, in order to avoid discharge of the ICD.[19,21,22] However, Lampman and Knight state that when the cut-off point is situated below the age-predicted maximum, the ICD should be temporarily switched off during the exercise test.[20] This way, the patient can reach his or her true maximum without being at risk for inappropriate shocks. It seems more logical to perform a maximal exercise test with the ICD activated, because that way you can gather information about the reaction of the cardiac rhythm and the ICD to exercise. The result of the exercise test can give confidence that exercise at a predetermined level is safe and can be performed in the controlled environment of cardiac rehabilitation (consistent with the report[19] of Fitchet et al.).

Some sources are available for exercise testing in patients with an ICD[23-25] or in patients with malignant ventricular arrhythmias.[26-28] There are few studies that give accurate data about the results of exercise testing and complications in patients with ICDs or ventricular arrhythmias.[19,21,22,26,27] A summary can be found in Table 50-1. From this table, it can be concluded that there were few complications during exercise

TABLE 50-1. Exercise testing in patients with malignant ventricular arrhythmias or ICD

Authors	Patients	Exercise testing	Endpoints	Complications during the test
Young et al., 1984	263 – arrhythmias	Maximal ET (treadmill) *stage 1*: 1 mph at 0 degrees (↑ elevation/2 min) *stage 6*: 3.0 mph at 14 degrees	Exhaustion	24 arrhythmias 17 prolonged VTs
Allen et al., 1988	64 – arrhythmias	Maximal ET (treadmill) Maximal exercise test (86%) Modified low-level (14%)	Fatigue Dyspnea Symptomatic arrhythmia	5 sustained VTs
Vanhees et al., 2001	8 – ICD	Maximal ET (bicycle) 20 W + 30 W/3 min	Exhaustion HR threshold (= detection rate − 30 beats)	1 VT without ICD intervention or adverse clinical manifestations
Fitchet et al., 2003	34 – ICD	Symptom-limited ET (treadmill) 1.6 km/h + 0.8/2 min until 7.2 km/h Constant gradient 10%	RPE = 7/10 = hard effort HR = 75% of the age-adjusted maximum HR threshold (= detection rate − 10 beats)	No discharges during ET
Vanhees et al., 2004	92 – ICD	Maximal ET (bicycle) 20 W + 20 W/min	Exhaustion: 100% HR threshold (= detection rate − 20 beats): 0%	1 VT requiring over-pacing

ET: exercise test; HR: heart rate; RPE: rate of perceived exertion scale; VT: ventricular tachycardia.

testing in patients with ICDs. In the last and largest study in patients with ICDs,[19] all patients stopped the exercise test because of exhaustion and the predetermined target heart rate of cut-off minus 20 beats was not reached. Most of the patients received drugs with negative chronotropic properties.

In conclusion, it can be stated that maximal or symptom-limited exercise testing in ICD patients with optimal pharmacological treatment is safe and feasible, but should only be performed in a professional and medical environment with continuous emphasis on safety measures.

Exercise Training

Three reports described general experiences and some guidelines for exercise training. Two of them discussed exercise training in patients with malignant ventricular arrhythmias,[24,25] and one publication described the prescription of exercise training specifically for patients with an ICD.[23] To the present, there are only three studies with accurate published data that have examined the influence of exercise training in ICD patients.[19,21,22] The components and results of the exercise programs in these studies are presented in Table 50-2.

Taking these results into account, some adapted recommendations for exercise training can be

formulated. An ambulatory, supervised exercise training program should contain three training sessions a week for at least 12 weeks. The sessions should have a duration of 90 minutes and consist of a warming up, the main exercise part, and a cooling down. The warming up is a period of calm physical activity of 5–10 minutes, inducing the patient into cardiovascular adjustments and limiting the risk of arrhythmias or other cardiovascular complications. It can include low-intensity aerobic exercise and flexibility exercises. The cooling down is a mild exercise or relative rest of 5–10 minutes, protecting the patient from possible complications in the early recovery period and to help the cardiovascular system to return slowly to a resting condition.

The main part of the training session can contain aerobic exercises like walking, jogging, cycling, arm ergometry, rowing, predominantly isotonic callisthenics. The exercise intensity is individually determined for every patient, based on the participant's clinical status and the initial exercise tolerance assessed by the baseline exercise test. The interval for training heart rate (HR) is calculated, using the formula of Karvonen: $HR_{training} = HR_{rest} + 60–90\% (HR_{peak} – HR_{rest})$. Furthermore, ICD patients are instructed not to surpass the upper heart rate threshold, which was determined in the studies mentioned above as

TABLE 50-2. Components and results of exercise programs for patients with an ICD

Author	Study plan	No	Training characteristics	Exercise tolerance	Complications during training
Vanhees et al., 2001	3 months comprehensive CR with aerobic exercise training	8	TF: 3 sessions/week TD: 90 min/session TI: (HRrest + 60–90% (HRmax − HRrest)) with upper limit of HR = detection rate − 30 beats	Peak VO$_2$: +24%	1 asymptomatic VT with ICD intervention
Fitchet et al., 2003	12 weeks comprehensive CR with exercise training	16	TF: not specified TD: not specified TI: HR of 60–75% of age adjusted maximum with upper limit of HR = detection rate − 10 beats	Exercise time: +16%	No ICD discharges
Vanhees et al., 2004	3 months comprehensive CR with aerobic exercise training	92	TF: 3 sessions/week TD: 90 min/session TI: Leuven: (HRrest + 60–90% (HRmax − HRrest)) with upper limit of HR = detection rate − 20 beats TI: Leiden: 50–80% max intensity	Peak VO$_2$: +17%	3 ICD discharges after VT: patients dropped out of the study 1 ICD discharge after VT 1 VT without intervention 1 inappropriate shock

CR: cardiac rehabilitation program; TF: training frequency; TD: training duration, TI: training intensity; HR: heart rate; VT: ventricular tachycardia.

detection rate minus 10, 20 or even 30 beats. The cut-off rate is determined for each individual depending on the slowest ventricular tachycardia and the exercise physiologist is responsible for knowing the cut-off rate for the device of each patient who participates in the rehabilitation program. It is recommended to increase the exercise intensity progressively, based on feedback from the patient and on the results of further exercise tests.[29] Based on our experience, we recommend an upper heart rate threshold during exercise training of the detection rate minus 20 beats/min.

Patients with a history of ventricular arrhythmias provoked by ischemia or heart failure exacerbations should also pay attention to the body position. It is recommended to perform exercise in an upright position rather than prolonged supine activities, because of lower left ventricular filling pressures in the upright position.[23]

The possibility of ECG monitoring should be available in the training room. During the first training sessions, the ECG monitoring assures confidence, freedom of movements, and safety from shocks that may occur during exercise. It can give valuable information about heart rhythm, and it can make the patient confident in the safety of exercise. When there are no problems during the first sessions, other heart monitoring devices (e.g. Polar) give enough information to train safely. In the absence of a heart rate monitor, patients should palpate their peripheral pulse regularly during and after the exercises, in order to determine if the pulse is within the limits of the target heart rate.[23]

The rehabilitation environment should be light and airy and adequately equipped in order to encourage exercise. Although there is a specific need for close supervision and electrographic monitoring during exercise activities, the same safety measures should be taken as in cardiac rehabilitation programs for a general population of cardiac patients. These safety considerations are already well described.[20]

Exercise training may provoke limited ventricular tachycardia in patients with ICDs during training and/or at the end of the training exercise program. The diagnosis of ventricular tachyarrhythmia occurs when the heart rate exceeds the programmed cut-off rate and consequently

the therapy is delivered by the ICD. After a shock has been delivered, the ICD is interrogated for the next 24 hours in order to locate the reason and to make adaptations to the ICD therapy program. The rehabilitation program should be continued, if necessary with an adapted exercise prescription, as soon as the patient is clinically stable and feels confident to restart training.

There is great emphasis on the individualization of risk factor management, a multidisciplinary approach to ensure provision of optimal care and the need for life-long exercise participation. Cardiologists, physicians, exercise physiologists, dietitians, psychologists, and other professionals should collaborate to manage risk reduction through follow-up techniques, including office or clinic visits, attendance of cardiac rehabilitation sessions and mail or telephone contact to show interest in the patient and to keep the patient motivated for participation in the program.

References

1. Tan Lip-Bun. Contractile reserve and cardiac circulatory power. Presentation at Europrevent – Athens 2006.
2. Courrelongue M, Bordachar P, Brette S, et al. Additional benefit of exercise training in patients with cardiac resynchronisation therapy. Presentation at Europrevent – Athens 2006.
3. Conraads V, Vanderheyden M, Paelinck B, et al. Endurance training potentiates exercise capacity in patients with chronic heart failure referred for cardiac resynchronisation therapy. Presentation at the World Congress of Cardiology – Barcelona 2006.
4. Boehmer JP. Device therapy for heart failure. Am J Cardiol 2003;91(suppl):53D–59D.
5. Abraham WT, Hayes DL. Cardiac resynchronization therapy for heart failure. Circulation 2003;108: 2596–2603.
6. Grady KL, Meyer PM, Dressler D, et al. Longitudinal change in quality of life and impact on survival after left ventricular assist device implantation. Ann Thorac Surg 2004;77(4):1321–1327.
7. Sharp CT, Busse EF, Burgers JJ, Haennel RG. Exercise prescription for patients with pacemakers. J Cardiopulm Rehabil 1998;21(3):421–31.
8. Greco EM, Guardini S, Citelli L. Cardiac rehabilitation with rate responsive pacemakers. Pacing Clin Electrophysiol 1998;21(3):169–194.

9. Glikson M, Friedman PA. The implantable cardioverter defibrillator. Lancet 2001;357(9262):1107–1117.

10. A comparison of antiarrhythmic-drug therapy with implantable defibrillators in patients resuscitated from near-fatal ventricular arrhythmias. The Antiarrhythmics versus Implantable Defibrillators (AVID) Investigators. N Engl J Med 1997;337:1576–1583.

11. Sears SF, Todaro JF, Urizar G, et al. Assessing the psychosocial impact of the ICD: a national survey of implantable cardioverter defibrillator health care providers. Pacing Clin Electrophysiol 2000;23(6):939–945.

12. van Ittersum M, de Greef M, van Gelder I, Coster J, Brugemann J, van der Schans C. Fear of exercise and health-related quality of life in patients with an implantable cardioverter defibrillator. Int J Rehabil Res 2003;26(2):117–122.

13. Fetzer SJ. The patient with an implantable cardioverter defibrillator. J Perianesth Nurs 2003;18(6):398–405.

14. Petch MC. Driving and heart disease – task force report. Eur Heart J 1998;19:1165–1177.

15. Epstein AE, Miles WM, Benditt DG, et al. Personal and public safety issues related to arrhythmias that may affect consciousness: implications for regulation and physician recommendations – a medical/scientific statement from the American Heart Association and the North American Society of Pacing and Electrophysiology. Circulation 1996;94:1147–1166.

16. Lewin RJP, Frizelle DJ, Kaye GC. A rehabilitative approach to patients with internal cardioverter-defibrillators. Heart 2001;85:371–372.

17. Albarran JW, Tagney J, James J. Partners of ICD patients – an exploratory study of their experiences. Eur J Cardiovasc Nurs 2004;3:201–210.

18. Kohn CS, Petrucci RJ, Baessler C, Soto DM, Movsowitz C. The effect of psychological intervention on patients' long-term adjustment to the ICD: a prospective study. Pacing Clin Electrophysiol 2000;23(4 Pt 1):450–456.

19. Fitchet A, Doherty PJ, Bundy C, Bell W, Fitzpatrick, Garratt CJ. Comprehensive cardiac rehabilitation programme for implantable cardioverter-defibrillator patients: a randomised controlled trial. Heart 2003;89:155–160.

20. Vanhees L, McGee H, Dugmore LD, Vuori I, Pentilla U-R, on behalf of the Carinex Working group: The Carinex Survey: Current Guidelines and Practices in Cardiac Rehabilitation within Europe. Acco Leuven/Amersfoort; 1999.

21. Vanhees L, Schepers D, Heidbuchel H, Defoor J, Fagard R. Exercise performance and training in patients with implantable cardioverter defibrillators and coronary heart disease. Am J Cardiol 2001;87:712–715.

22. Vanhees L, Kornaat M, Defoor J, et al. Effect of exercise training in patients with an implantable cardioverter defibrillator. Eur Heart J 2004;25:1120–1126.

23. Lampman RM, Knight BP. Prescribing exercise training for patients with defibrillators. Am J Phys Med Rehabil 2000;79:292–297.

24. Kelly TM. Exercise testing and training of patients with malignant ventricular arrhythmias. Med Sci Sports Exerc 1996;28:53–61.

25. Pashkow FJ, Schweikert RA, Wilkoff BL. Exercise testing and training in patients with malignant arrhythmias. Exerc Sport Sci Rev 1997;25:235–269.

26. Allen BJ, Casey TP, Brodsky A, Luckett CR, Henry WL. Exercise testing in patients with life-threatening tachyarrhythmias: Results and correlation with clinical and arrhythmia factors. Am Heart J 1988;116:997–1002.

27. Young DZ, Lampert S, Graboys B, Lown B. Safety of maximal exercise testing in patients at high risk for ventricular arrhythmia. Circulation 1984;70(2):184–191.

28. Weaver WD, Cobb LA, Hallstrom AP. Characteristics of survivors of exertion- and nonexertion-related cardiac arrest: value of subsequent exercise testing. Am J Cardiol 1982;50:671–676.

29. LaFontaine T, Gordon N. Comprehensive cardiovascular risk reduction in patients with coronary artery disease. In Resource Manual for guidelines for exercise testing and prescription (edited by ACSM), 4th edn. Baltimore: Williams & Wilkins; 2001.

51
Rehabilitation in Peripheral Vascular Disease

Jean-Paul Schmid

Intermittent Claudication: Clinical Aspects

Definition

The term claudication is derived from the Latin word claudicatio, translated as "to limp." In vascular disease nomenclature, claudication describes the symptom of exercise-induced muscle ischemia, most commonly due to peripheral artery disease (PAD). The patient with intermittent claudication typically describes leg pain that is caused and reliably reproduced by a certain degree of exertion. The pain is sufficiently intense to stop the activity and is promptly relieved by rest, usually within minutes. A given degree of exercise, commonly measured in pain-free distance able to walk, consistently reproduces symptoms. The Fontaine stages are commonly used to rate symptom severity (Table 51-1).

Ankle–Brachial Index

The Doppler evaluation adds to the physical examination after a careful pulse examination. The calculation of the ankle–brachial index (ABI) is easy to perform and provides a widely used and well-accepted instrument in the assessment of flow limitation. The brachial, posterior tibial, and dorsal pedis pressures are measured using an appropriately sized blood pressure cuff placed on the arms and above the ankles. Using a handheld continuous-wave Doppler probe, the systolic pressure in each artery is determined when flow resumes after gradual cuff deflation. The ABI is calculated by dividing the highest pressure obtained at the ankle by the higher of the arm measurements.

Table 51-2 presents the clinical classification of PAD based on ABI value. Values >90 are considered normal, whereas those between 0.40 and 0.90 fall into the claudication range, between 0.20 and 0.40 into the ischemic rest pain range, and those <0.20 are consistent with tissue necrosis. Values <0.90 are thought to represent >50% vessel stenosis and, independently of the presence or absence of symptoms, serve as a marker for systemic atherosclerosis. ABI values >1.25 are considered falsely elevated, most commonly from vessel wall rigidity due to medial calcinosis associated with diabetes. This rigidity may be so severe that pressures cannot be obtained, in which case the result is recorded as non-compressible.

Intermittent Claudication: Part of a Multisite Atherothrombosis

A complete medical history beyond that elicited specifically for claudication is a sine qua non for proper patient evaluation and management. Given the association of PAD with systemic atherosclerosis, detailed information on the signs and symptoms of coronary and cerebrovascular disease should be elicited. Existing risk factors, as well as plans for their subsequent modification and systemic therapy, should be noted.

Atherosclerosis is a systemic disease and PAD is part of this multisite disease. Epidemiological

TABLE 51-1. Classification of peripheral artery disease: Fontaine stages

I	Pathological finding at physical examination; patient without symptoms also during exercise
II	Intermittent claudication: symptoms during exercise
IIa	Pain-free walking distance: >200 m
IIb	Pain-free walking distance: <200 m
III	Pain at rest: mostly during the night, relief of pain by position change or getting up
IV	Acral lesion, gangrene

evidence for involvement of multiple arteries in patients with PAD was found in the San Diego artery study.[1] At the time of presentation, a history of acute myocardial infarction or stroke, or related surgery, was detected in 29.4% of male and 21.2% of female patients with PAD, whereas the corresponding figures for matching males and females without PAD were 11.5% and 9.3%, respectively. Conversely, among patients presenting with coronary artery or cerebrovascular disease, 32.3% of men and 25% of women also had peripheral arterial involvement. Thus, the association between coronary artery disease and PAD or cerebrovascular disease and vice versa were two to three times those in the respective control groups, irrespective of the presence or absence of PAD symptoms.

In the Atherosclerosis Risk in Communities (ARIC) study (15,000 subjects),[2] an ankle–brachial index below 0.9 served as a conventional marker of PAD. The probability of these PAD patients having previous or associated coronary artery disease or cerebrovascular disease was 3- to 5-fold higher than in non-PAD patients adjusted for sex and race. Moreover, asymptomatic carotid plaques and/or an increased intima–media thickness of the common carotid artery were often found in asymptomatic PAD patients. Thus, low

TABLE 51-2. Ankle–brachial index values and clinical classification

Clinical presentation	Ankle–brachial index
Non-compressible	≥1.30
Normal	0.91–1.30
Claudication	0.41–0.90
Rest pain	0.21–0.40
Tissue loss	≤0.20

and subnormal ABI values suggest the presence of generalized atherothrombosis, even if the patient is asymptomatic.

The concept of multiterritory atherothrombosis was also supported by Aronow and Ahn in a prospective study of 1886 elderly patients.[3] Of this population, 5% had symptomatic atherothrombosis in all three main arterial regions and 20% in two of the main arterial regions.

Modification of Risk Factors

The patient with PAD should be regarded as an actual or potential polyvascular patient. It should be recalled that the reaction of the plaque to rupture, which leads to symptoms, appears to be a consistent, individual feature, irrespective of the arterial site primarily involved. Thus besides organ-specific therapeutic measures to be used during the different clinical events, an integrated approach to prevention and treatment of atherothrombosis as a whole is highly desirable.

Smoking Cessation

Peripheral artery disease is particularly high in the smoking male population. To stop smoking therefore is of paramount importance. Smoking cessation slows the progression to critical leg ischemia and reduces the risks of myocardial infarction and death from vascular causes. Although the authors of a meta-analysis of published data concluded that smoking cessation alone did not improve maximal treadmill walking distance,[4] smoking cessation programs, nicotine replacement therapy, and the use of antidepressant drugs such as bupropion should be encouraged.

Treatment of Hyperlipidemia

Several large clinical trials have determined the benefits of lowering cholesterol concentrations in patients with coronary artery disease. In patients with PAD, therapy with a statin not only lowers serum cholesterol concentrations, but also improves endothelial function, as well as other markers of atherosclerotic risk. In PAD, several trials have shown beneficial effects of therapy on disease progression, and the severity of claudication. Lipid-lowering therapy has also shown its benefits in patients with PAD, who often have coexisting coronary and cerebral arterial disease. The current recommendation for patients with peripheral arterial disease is to achieve a serum LDL cholesterol concentration of less than 100 mg/dL (2.6 mmol/L) and a serum triglyceride concentration of less than 150 mg/dL (1.7 mmol/L). A statin should be given as initial therapy, but niacin and fibrates may play an important role in patients with low serum HDL or high serum triglyceride concentrations.

Treatment of Diabetes Mellitus

Intensive control of blood glucose prevents the microvascular complications of diabetes, but its effect on macrovascular complications is less certain. The Diabetes Control and Complications Trial comparing intensive and conventional insulin therapy in 1441 patients with type 1 diabetes showed an association of intensive therapy with a trend toward a reduction in cardiovascular events ($P = 0.08$) but no effect on the risk of peripheral arterial disease was noted.[5] The results were similar in 3867 patients with type 2 diabetes in the United Kingdom Prospective Diabetes Study, which compared intensive drug treatment using sulfonylurea or insulin with dietary therapy.[6] Intensive drug therapy was associated with a trend toward a reduction in myocardial infarction ($P = 0.05$) but had no effect on the risk of death or amputation due to peripheral arterial disease (relative risk 0.6; 95% confidence interval, 0.4 to 1.2). These data suggest that intensive blood glucose control in patients with either type 1 or type 2 diabetes may not directly affect PAD.

Treatment of Hypertension

Hypertension is a major risk factor for PAD, but data are not available to clarify whether treatment will alter the progression of the disease or the risk of claudication. Beta-adrenergic-antagonist drugs have been thought to have unfavorable effects on symptoms in patients with PAD. This concern arose from several early case reports of worsening claudication and decreases in blood flow in the legs in patients taking these drugs. A meta-analysis and a critical review of different studies, however, concluded that beta-adrenergic antagonists are safe in patients with PAD, except in the most severely affected patients, in whom the drugs should be administered with caution.[7,8]

The use of angiotensin-converting enzyme inhibitors in patients with peripheral arterial disease may confer protection against cardiovascular events beyond that expected from lowering of blood pressure. In the Heart Outcomes Prevention Evaluation Study,[9] 4051 of the 9297 patients (44%) had evidence of peripheral arterial disease (ankle–brachial index values of <0.90). In the entire study population, the primary endpoint of death from vascular causes, nonfatal myocardial infarction, or stroke occurred in 17.7% of the placebo group, as compared with 14.1% of the ramipril group. The efficacy of ramipril did not differ significantly between patients with PAD and those without it. This study suggests that angiotensin-converting enzyme inhibitors reduce the risk of ischemic events in PAD patients.

Non-Pharmacological Therapy for Claudication

Goals of Therapy

Patients with claudication have marked impairment in exercise performance and overall functional capacity. Their peak oxygen consumption measured during graded treadmill exercise is 50% of that of age-matched normal subjects, indicating a level of impairment similar to that among patients with New York Heart Association class III heart failure. In addition, patients with claudication typically report great difficulty in walking short distances, even at a slow speed. Reduced walking capacity is associated with impairment in the performance of activities of daily living and in health-related quality of life. Improving mobility and improving quality of life are important treatment goals for patients with PAD.

Exercise Therapy

The primary non-pharmacological treatment for claudication is a formal exercise training program, as demonstrated in over 20 randomized trials (albeit many with small samples).[10] Exercise improves not only maximal treadmill walking distance, but also health-related quality of life and community-based functional capacity (i.e., the ability to walk at defined speeds and for defined distances). A meta-analysis of randomized trials found that exercise training increased maximal treadmill walking distance by 179 m (95% CI 60 to 298). This degree of improvement should translate into longer walking distances on level ground.[4]

Although exercise-induced improvement in walking ability is well established, the magnitude of the responses to training across studies has varied. Such variability may be explained by study-specific differences in the intensity, duration, and frequency of the exercise prescription and the methods of measuring exercise capacity. One meta-analysis that examined both non-randomized and randomized trials showed that exercise training improved pain-free walking time in patients with claudication by an average of 180% and improved maximal walking time by an average of 120%.[11] The greatest improvements in walking ability occurred when each exercise session lasted more than 30 minutes, when sessions took place at least three times per week, when the patient walked until near-maximal pain, and when the program lasted 6 months or longer. A meta-analysis from the Cochrane Collaboration that considered only randomized controlled trials concluded that exercise improved maximal walking time by an average of 150% (range 74–230%). It would appear that the exercise-induced increases in maximal walking ability exceeded those attained with medication, which has been estimated to result in improved maximal walking distance (20–25% with pentoxifylline and 40–60% with cilostazol).

Exercise-induced improvement in walking ability results in improvement in routine daily activities. Such increases in activity, if associated with improvements in cardiovascular risk factors, might also reduce the risk of adverse cardiovascular events, thereby potentially improving the poor prognosis with respect to survival in this population.

The time course of the response to a program of exercise has not been fully established. Clinical benefits have been observed as early as 4 weeks after the initiation of exercise and may continue to accrue after 6 months of participation.[12] Improvements in walking ability after 6 months of supervised exercise rehabilitation three times per week were sustained when patients continued to participate in an exercise maintenance program for an additional 12 months.[13]

Exercise Prescription

The key elements of a therapeutic exercise program are summarized in Table 51-3. Because of the frequently concomitant clinical or occult coronary artery disease, it is prudent to perform treadmill or bicycle exercise testing with 12-lead electrocardiographic monitoring before an exercise program is initiated, so that ischemic symptoms, ST–T wave changes, and arrhythmias may be identified.

TABLE 51-3. Key elements of a therapeutic exercise training program for rehabilitation from PAD in patients with claudication[14]

Exercise guidelines for claudication
Warm-up and cool-down periods of 5–10 min each.

Types of exercise
Treadmill and track walking are the most effective exercises for claudication.
Resistance training has benefit for patients with other forms of cardiovascular disease, and its use, as tolerated, for general fitness is complementary to walking but not a substitute for it.

Intensity
The initial workload of the treadmill is set to a speed and grade that elicits claudication symptoms within 3 to 5 min.
Patients walk at this workload until claudication of moderate severity occurs, then rest standing or sitting for a brief period to permit symptoms to subside.

Duration
The exercise–rest–exercise pattern should be repeated throughout the exercise session.
The initial session will usually include 35 min of intermittent walking; walking is increased by 5 min each session until 50 min of intermittent walking can be accomplished.

Frequency
Treadmill or track walking 3 to 5 times per week.

Role of direct supervision
As the patient's walking ability improves, the exercise workload should be increased by modifying the treadmill grade or speed (or both) to ensure that the stimulus of claudication pain always occurs during the workout.
As walking ability improves, and a higher heart rate is reached, there is the possibility that cardiac signs and symptoms may appear. These symptoms should be appropriately diagnosed and treated.

Although this group of patients will, by definition, have claudication-limited exercise (and therefore will not achieve a true maximal exercise performance), the findings from the exercise test can be used to determine that there are no untoward cardiovascular responses at the exercise level reached. The exercise test also provides information about claudication thresholds and heart rate and blood pressure responses for use in establishing an exercise prescription. Enrollment of the patient in a medically supervised exercise program with electrocardiographic, heart rate, blood pressure, and blood glucose monitoring is encouraged. Many cardiac rehabilitation exercise programs can accommodate patients with claudication, providing an environment conducive to the lifestyle change that underlies long-term compliance with exercise and risk factor modification.

The methods of exercise prescription include establishing a training intensity that produces moderate claudication pain within the first 5 minutes of treadmill walking (Table 51-3). Each training session consists of short periods of treadmill walking interspersed with rest throughout a 50-minute exercise session, three times weekly. Many patients with claudication also have reduced muscle mass, as well as a lack of muscle strength and endurance, which exacerbates their physical impairment. Resistance training, when appropriately prescribed, is generally recommended for most patients with other manifestations of cardiovascular disease, because of its beneficial effects on strength and endurance, cardiovascular function, metabolism, coronary risk factors, and psychosocial wellbeing. Nevertheless, in patients with claudication, resistance training does not directly improve walking ability, whereas walking itself is most effective in increasing claudication-limited walking capacity.

Clinicians should recognize that there are no data to support the efficacy of the informal "go home and walk" advice that is still the most typical exercise prescription for patients with claudication. In contrast, a supervised hospital- or clinic-based program, which ensures that patients are receiving a standardized exercise stimulus in a safe environment, is effective.

Mechanisms of Action

The occurrence of the classical symptoms of PAD, such as intermittent or, at later stages, rest pain is only weakly related to the extent of peripheral atherothrombosis. Occurrence and severity of symptoms are influenced by many factors, including the following: development of an efficient collateral circulation; microcirculatory response; walking and exercise requirements of the individual; and the adjunctive effect of continued smoking, poor control of diabetes and hypertension, and occasional inflammatory episodes that lead to superimposed acute or subacute arterial thrombosis.

Exercise-induced increases in functional capacity and lessening of claudication symptoms may be explained by several mechanisms, including measurable improvements in endothelial vasodilator function, skeletal muscle metabolism, blood viscosity, and inflammatory responses. Exercise training is not associated with substantial changes in blood flow to the legs, and the changes that occur do not predict the clinical response. Therefore these mechanisms are unlikely to account for the large improvements in pain-free walking that can be achieved. Improvements in the biomechanics of walking also contribute to increased walking ability.

Although exercise training has multiple beneficial effects, current knowledge does not permit accurate estimation of the relative contribution of each mechanism. Exercise training has additional benefits that go beyond improvements in functional capacity and claudication symptoms. Exercise-induced enhancement of endothelial function may also improve systemic cardiovascular health. Additional potential benefits of exercise include reduced blood pressure, an improved lipid profile, better glycemic control in patients with diabetes, and reduced central obesity, although the magnitude and durability of these effects have yet to be studied prospectively in patients with claudication.

Although exercise training is effective as a single intervention, it may augment the effects of other treatments for claudication. Revascularization by either bypass surgery or angioplasty can be effective for the relief of claudication symptoms and the improvement of walking ability in patients with progressively worsening claudication in whom initial conservative management has failed. In one randomized study, the combination of revascularization procedures and exercise was more effective than either intervention alone.

References

1. Criqui MH, Denenberg JO, Langer RD, Fronek A. The epidemiology of peripheral arterial disease: importance of identifying the population at risk. Vasc Med 1997;2(3):221–226.

2. Zheng ZJ, Sharrett AR, Chambless LE, et al. Associations of ankle-brachial index with clinical coronary heart disease, stroke and preclinical carotid and popliteal atherosclerosis: the Atherosclerosis Risk in Communities (ARIC) Study. Atherosclerosis 1997;131(1):115–125.

3. Aronow WS, Ahn C. Prevalence of coexistence of coronary artery disease, peripheral arterial disease, and atherothrombotic brain infarction in men and women > or = 62 years of age. Am J Cardiol 1994; 74(1):64–65.

4. Girolami B, Bernardi E, Prins MH, et al. Treatment of intermittent claudication with physical training, smoking cessation, pentoxifylline, or nafronyl: a meta-analysis. Arch Intern Med 1999;159(4):337–345.

5. Effect of intensive diabetes management on macrovascular events and risk factors in the Diabetes Control and Complications Trial. Am J Cardiol 1995;75(14):894–903.

6. Intensive blood-glucose control with sulphonylureas or insulin compared with conventional treatment and risk of complications in patients with type 2 diabetes (UKPDS 33). UK Prospective Diabetes Study (UKPDS) Group. Lancet 1998; 352(9131):837–853.

7. Heintzen MP, Strauer BE. Peripheral vascular effects of beta-blockers. Eur Heart J 1994;15(Suppl C):2–7.

8. Radack K, Deck C. Beta-adrenergic blocker therapy does not worsen intermittent claudication in subjects with peripheral arterial disease. A meta-analysis of randomized controlled trials. Arch Intern Med 1991;151(9):1769–1776.

9. The HOPE (Heart Outcomes Prevention Evaluation) Study: the design of a large, simple randomized trial of an angiotensin-converting enzyme inhibitor (ramipril) and vitamin E in patients at high risk of cardiovascular events. The HOPE study investigators. Can J Cardiol 1996;12(2):127–137.

10. Nehler MR, Hiatt WR. Exercise therapy for claudication. Ann Vasc Surg 1999;13(1):109–114.

11. Gardner AW, Poehlman ET. Exercise rehabilitation programs for the treatment of claudication pain. A meta-analysis. JAMA 1995;274(12):975–980.

12. Gibellini R, Fanello M, Bardile AF, Salerno M, Aloi T. Exercise training in intermittent claudication. Int Angiol 2000;19(1):8–13.

13. Gardner AW, Katzel LI, Sorkin JD, Goldberg AP. Effects of long-term exercise rehabilitation on claudication distances in patients with peripheral arterial disease: a randomized controlled trial. J Cardiopulm Rehabil 2002;22(3):192–198.

14. Stewart KJ, Hiatt WR, Regensteiner JG, Hirsch AT. Exercise training for claudication. N Engl J Med 2002;347(24):1941–1951.

52
Cardiac Rehabilitation and Wellness in the Corporate Setting

L. Dorian Dugmore

Healthcare systems throughout Europe are feeling the strain due to the ever increasing demands made upon them to provide treatments and solutions for many cardiovascular related diseases (CV). The corporate setting provides an ideal location for delivering both cardiac rehabilitation and preventative strategies that can help combat the ever increasing burden that cardiovascular illness is placing upon society.[1]

For cardiac rehabilitation to be successful in the corporate setting, it is highly desirable that it becomes an integrated part of a comprehensive cardiovascular and lifestyle intervention program. The focus of such a program should be to provide a "seamless care" model that provides clients with a choice of interventions depending upon their health profile. These should range from:

- Guidelines to maintain optimum health because no discernable CV risk factors are present (prevention)
- When CV risk factors are identified, the delivery of a lifestyle management program to control and reduce them
- Upon the clinical diagnosis of CV disease, the delivery a comprehensive cardiac rehabilitation program

Certain aspects of these interventions may be combined depending on individual circumstances and ideally all of the above should be capable of delivery within the same surroundings.

Employees who have suffered a cardiovascular event and/or intervention may not wish to receive attention through programs that solely highlight their plight. In contrast, such individuals may feel more comfortable and amenable to being involved in an ongoing scheme for all employees, which attempts to look at a continuum that moves from prevention to rehabilitation (Figure 52-1). Positioning an employee's rehabilitation following a cardiac event/intervention so that there is a perception of moving back along the wellness continuum towards optimum health may also offer a more attractive proposition.

Providing such a service in the corporate setting can potentially offer great benefits to all employees and not just the cardiac patient. In order for such models to be successful "upstream medicine" should be the main focus where prevention (primary/secondary/tertiary) is the constant goal.[1] Such an approach will also encourage traditional models of "corporate occupational medicine" to move alongside "wellness" and prevention in order to create new models of healthcare.

Background to Corporate Wellness/Cardiac Rehabilitation

There are many corporations that have developed effective work site health promotion, fitness, wellness, and cardiac rehabilitation programs. The Johnson & Johnson "Live for Life" program has been made available to more than 25,000 employees at 43 locations in the US, Puerto Rico, Canada, and Europe.[2] The long-term aim of the program was to help contain healthcare costs attributable to unhealthy lifestyles that are amenable to modification in the work setting.[2] Specific program objectives were to improve health knowledge, physical fitness, and nutrition, to control weight, stress, blood pressure, and alcohol con-

Optimum Health	Some CV Disease Markers present	CV Disease Diagnosed (with/without surgery)

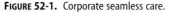

No Risk Factors = Prevention	Lifestyle/Risk Factor Management	Cardiac Rehabilitation

FIGURE 52-1. Corporate seamless care.

sumption, to stop smoking, and to use medical supplies appropriately.[2] This program proved to be one of the few that attempted to compare the effectiveness of selected cardiovascular/lifestyle risk reduction interventions through a randomized control study. Preliminary findings, after 12 months, indicated that, compared with the control groups, the "Live For Life" group showed statistically significant improvements in weight reduction, exercise tolerance, and blood pressure control.[2] Healthcare savings of $224.66 per employee were also found from the "Live For Life" Health and Wellness program.[3]

Other schemes based in the US and Canada have developed programs that focused on health promotion, fitness, and wellness. For example, Motorola's wellness and disease management programs saved $3.93 for every dollar invested through reduced healthcare costs.[4] This amounted to $6.5 million annual savings in medical expenses for lifestyle-related diagnoses (obesity, hypertension, and stress).[4] Northeast Utilities' "Well Aware" program, in its first 24 months, reduced lifestyle and behavioral claims by $1,400,000.[5] Caterpillar's "Healthy Balance" program was also projected to result in long-term savings of $700 million by 2015.[6] Pfizer's Health and Wellness program in the US and Puerto Rico together with Daimler Chrysler's program in the US have produced similar results, the latter placing greater importance on health risk assessment as an effective tool for reducing healthcare costs.[7]

We must be cautious when citing healthcare savings data from the US and making comparisons with European countries with the expectancy of similar benefits. National healthcare systems in many European countries often cover much of the cost when treating illness, whereas in the US, the cost of healthcare falls on the individual.

There are, however, a growing number of corporate organizations in Europe who are investing in corporate prevention, rehabilitation, and well-ness programs. Within the UK, adidas have funded the development a dedicated wellness center that provides both preventive and rehabilitative programs for employees and other corporate agencies. The following case study represents early findings from the wellness center in 1998 (unpublished data).

Case Study 1 (Corporate CV Risk – "An Early Cause for Concern")

Two hundred and one employees initially signed up voluntarily to receive full cardiorespiratory and cardiovascular risk profiling following the inception of the "Adifit for LIFE" program launched in 1998. The mean age of adidas employees from this first cohort study was 31.4 years. Early results revealed 152 employees (76%) to be in physically inactive jobs, 104 employees (52%) were overweight with a mean body fat score of 28.7%, 102 employees (51%) ate an elevated fatty diet (greater than 30% total fat); 72 employees (36%) recorded raised total cholesterol levels with a mean of 5.8 mmol/L, and 26 of these employees (13%) were at 2–3 times the risk for heart disease due to markedly elevated cholesterol scores (NCEP Guidelines); 45 employees (22%) recorded mild to severe diastolic blood pressures with a mean score of 95 mmHg; 18 employees recorded positive stress tests; 10 were referred for further cardiac investigations and 2 subsequently received coronary artery by pass grafts. Consequently, adidas UK strongly supported the development of their Wellness Centre and its program in the light of these findings. The company encouraged employees to participate in this wellness scheme, which focused on cardiovascular risk reduction and lifestyle management. As a result of the success of this program, the company was awarded European and International Best Practice Awards from the IHRSA International Institute of Exercise and Health for "creating outcome based programs including initial testing data on compliance and follow up testing."

Goldman Sachs, the international investment bank, has invested substantial monies in creating a comprehensive wellness center in London and has similar centers in New York and Frankfurt. This company is also developing similar wellness initiatives in their Far Eastern branches. Unilever, Marks & Spencer, and other European based companies are also developing programs focused on preventing and treating disease. In Holland, Achmea, a large insurance group, have recently taken a significant interest in linking fitness centers with wellness initiatives that ultimately will reduce cardiovascular risk and healthcare costs.[8]

There are also a number of corporate based cardiac rehabilitation programs. The US based Coors Brewing Company opened their Wellness Center in 1981 and shortly afterwards opened a phase II early post-hospitalization cardiac rehabilitation program for employees, spouses, dependents, and retirees. This program contained exercise and conditioning, vocational, educational, psychosocial and follow-up components.[7] Direct savings on healthcare costs plus replacement employee cost avoidance produced annual savings of $325.000.[7] The goals of the program were to keep the employee in a job, to provide them with an opportunity to learn secondary prevention strategies, and to make appropriate work site changes to accommodate the employee when necessary. Corporate cardiac rehabilitation programs have also been developed at the Boeing Company, in Seattle, dating back to 1974, which were a development from the original CAPRI cardiac rehabilitation community programs in 1968.[8] Their corporate experience shows that while cardiac arrest and myocardial infarction were prominent in those early years, these have been replaced by problems with early angioplasty closure and chronic heart failure with atrial fibrillation.[8] Many employees had already experienced phase I and II programs and were subsequently looking for phase III and/or phase IV schemes that focus on cardiac/lifestyle risk factor management. Such approaches clearly mirror the "seamless care" model discussed previously and show a growing interest in corporate wellness that includes both prevention and rehabilitation.

Lifestyle/Exercise Studies and Their Application to the Corporate Setting

The SCRIP trial (Stanford Coronary Risk Intervention Project) in 1994 showed the effectiveness of intermittent tracking on cardiac risk factor reduction in cardiac patients.[9] Significantly less progression of heart disease in the experimental group (29% progression) was noted when compared with those patients who were not treated (41% progression). Low-fat diets, moderate-intensity exercise (15–45 minutes every other day), smoking cessation/relapse prevention, weight management, and lipid therapy were the main interventions used. This home-based program used tracking led by nurse healthcare professionals to follow up patients at 2–3-month intervals and has since been successfully used by the Stanford group in the corporate setting.[9]

Using methods employed in the SCRIP trial, the Health Education and Risk Reduction Training (HEAR[2]T) program was developed to target risk reduction in the workplace and healthcare setting.[10] Some of the methods/instruments used in the HEAR[2]T program have been implemented into the corporate setting at adidas. Using this approach, recent unpublished data from the UK based "Adifit for LIFE" program revealed the top four highest cardiovascular risk appraisal scores all belonged to women within the company! This highlighted the urgency of promoting the "Adifit for LIFE" program to women within the company, and was accomplished through health promotion, tracking, and follow-up. It succeeded in achieving a higher enrollment of women onto the "Adifit for LIFE" program. Add to this, recent research findings from the Diabetes Prevention Project where medication (metformin) helped to improve glycemic control, reducing diabetic risk by 31%, but not as effectively as intensive lifestyle interventions (exercise and diet) which reduced the development of diabetes by 58%.[11] Such findings from "lifestyle-related studies" increasingly suggest the potential effectiveness of "lifestyle change" programs if they are successfully applied and tracked.

Corporate Cardiac Rehabilitation

Within cardiac rehabilitation we are concerned with "return to work" following myocardial infarction and coronary artery surgery. The next logical step must be to increase the provision for corporate programs that deal with cardiac rehabilitation. The most successful models should not deal with this in isolation, bringing attention solely to the cardiac patient, but in combination with preventive and wellness strategies that are offered to the entire workforce. If achieved effectively such approaches should only benefit the return of the cardiac patient into the workforce with minimum disruption to the patient, their family, and the work setting.

The following represents a case study of cardiac rehabilitation within the workplace using the "Adifit for LIFE" program.

Case Study 2 (Client X, Adidas Employee)

A 52-year-old male, body mass index, 32. First visit to the adidas Wellness Centre, May 2003, with symptomatic retrosternal chest pain. Resting ECG normal, blood pressure elevated at 210/140 mmHg. Immediate medication to lower blood pressure recommended. Client X returned within 3 to 4 days of this initial visit where blood pressure was extremely elevated at 278/168 mmHg. Further urgent medicated blood pressure control was recommended and immediately supplied with the full approval/cooperation of the patient's own family physician. Subsequent cardiorespiratory stress testing following effective blood pressure control revealed significant ECG changes (inferolateral ST-segment depression) at fairly light treadmill exercise (Borg scale of Perceived Exertion Rating: 11). Significant risk factor modification program recommended and undertaken. April 2004, coronary angiography revealed significant coronary artery stenosis (70% in all three major coronary arteries). Client X was recommended immediate coronary angioplasty. He began a "prehabilitation" program at the adidas Wellness Centre to further reduce risk factors and prepare himself for surgery. A clinically super-

vised treadmill ECG-monitored walking program was also undertaken daily, at intensity levels below the ischemic threshold. July 2004 saw Client X receive four drug eluting stents to his right coronary artery followed by daily cardiac rehabilitation at the adidas Wellness Centre. March 2005 saw Client X receive a further four drug eluting stents to his left main coronary artery followed by a second course of intensive cardiac rehabilitation. Following his successful rehabilitation by July 2005, Client X was exercising on the treadmill completely free of symptoms within the adidas activity center. After a gradual increase in working hours over a 6-week period, Client X is back in full-time work.

In review, it is essential that an initial close liaison is established between the cardiologist/medical team/health insurers and family of the cardiac patient returning to the corporate workplace. The role of a corporate healthcare professional as a cardiac liaison link cannot be overestimated in this situation. Graded exercise testing prior to entry into a corporate wellness/rehabilitation scheme with full cardiorespiratory analysis is desirable, especially if the patient is going to be given an "exercise prescription" and is taking medications that will modify heart rate response to exercise (e.g. beta blockade).

Preferentially a full lifestyle/cardiovascular risk reduction program should be tailored to each employee. Getting an individual to contract into a cardiac rehabilitation and/or cardiovascular risk reduction/preventative program also helps adherence to goals that have been set. All employee records should be stored in a confidential/secure area preferably within the Wellness Centre. Also a close relationship with an employee's family physician, regularly supplying them with updated clinical documentation/information, will help promote more effective "case management." Having a registered doctor/cardiologist linked with corporate wellness programs also offers a distinct advantage here. Similarly, such links should be generated with corporate human resource (HR) departments but only with the employee's signed consent to share information and with complete confidentiality guaranteed.

Program components should include those recognized as essential to the effective delivery of cardiac rehabilitation services and those recommended by the appropriate national/international cardiac rehabilitation organizations (i.e. the European Society of Cardiology Guidelines on Cardiac Rehabilitation and Secondary Prevention), notably: exercise/conditioning, nutritional/dietary counseling, cardiac risk factor management, smoking cessation/relapse prevention, stress management, vocational, educational and psychosocial aspects, quality of life measurements specific to cardiac populations, and evaluation/outcome measures for the program. In addition, it is highly desirable that a behavioral counseling approach is taken when delivering cardiac rehabilitation/wellness/preventive services to employees, promoting a client-centered approach towards lifestyle change and cardiovascular risk reduction/management.

The Wellness/Cardiac Rehabilitation Corporate Facility

Ideally such a facility should be multipurpose in design and cater for both wellness/preventive and cardiac rehabilitation programs. In an ideal setting the following may be envisaged; a resting metabolism measurement laboratory, a stress testing/clinical evaluation laboratory, essential cardiac resuscitation/life support equipment, lifestyle counseling facilities, a physical activity center, and health education/resource facilities. Consequently new and innovative models for corporate wellness/cardiac rehabilitation service provision should be created. These should include comprehensive "needs assessment profiling" detailing a company's specific requirements before final programs are designed. In addition, together with creating data-based programs that cover health profiling and economic benefits (e.g. reduced absenteeism, reduced employee turnover, improved productivity), efforts to make such programs increasingly cost-effective in terms of capital investment and revenue generation over the medium to long term are essential for corporate wellness to develop and reach its true potential.

Case Study 3 (the "Adidas/Wellness International Model For Corporate Wellness")

This model uses a "seamless care" approach to provide both cardiac rehabilitation and preventive medicine services within the corporate setting (Figure 52-2). Initially adidas UK, one of the

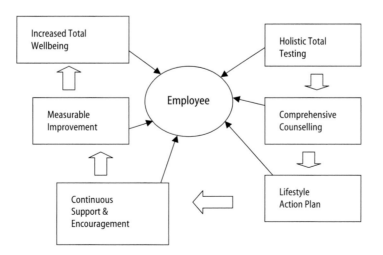

Proactive; Prediction, Intervention, Prevention & Improvement

Figure 52-2. The adidas/Wellness International model for corporate wellness.

world's leading sporting goods brands, provided substantial funding to create a unique wellness center in their Area North headquarters in Stockport, England. Following substantial capital investment and an initial "lead in" time to create the center, and its programs, adidas entered into a strategic partnership with Wellness International. The latter were contracted to provide wellness/preventive and cardiac rehabilitation services to adidas employees. The success of the center and its programs has attracted other corporate and sporting agencies to purchase the services of Wellness International using its international staff of healthcare professionals. Through a profit share arrangement, adidas are now able to recover a significant proportion of the costs for providing wellness/cardiac rehabilitation services to their employees and work strategically with Wellness International to further develop their programs. This has resulted in close links with several international partners including the HEAR²T program at Stanford University, Palo Alto, California and the "Life Wellness Institute" in San Diego, California. This example serves to demonstrate an innovative approach to making wellness work in the corporate setting and fits perfectly into the adidas philosophy of being a world leading sports brand and "the performance company."

The New Wellness/Cardiac Rehabilitation Professional

With the development of new "seamless" care corporate wellness/rehabilitation programs, there is an emerging need to create a new "brand" of healthcare professional. It would be highly desirable that such a "wellness professional" develops a "skills set" that combines the essential elements of clinical medicine, cardiac rehabilitation, nutrition, health/fitness, and behavioral counseling. This mirrors, but on a broader scale, the "nurse/healthcare practitioner" model already used in family practice in both North America and certain areas of Europe. Corporately this has already been recognized in the UK, with adidas, Wellness International and Technogym (Italy) all taking an interest in promoting the emergence of this new "Wellness Professional." Most recently, a new and innovative

Master of Science (MSc) university degree course in Preventative Medicine and Wellness has been launched in the Northwest of England, its inspiration coming to a large degree from the success of the adidas/Wellness International corporate programs.

This new "Wellness Professional", in addition to the skills described previously, should be competent and certified in basic/intermediate cardiac life support, phlebotomy and have attended/received training in clinical ECG interpretation and behavioral counseling techniques. As corporate wellness grows, exciting opportunities are on the horizon for this new "wellness professional."

Summary

To emphasize the potential need for a "seamless care" corporate wellness model that includes cardiac rehabilitation, the following comment relating to the WHO MONICA Project and cardiovascular disease is very apt:

In the light of shrinking resources for healthcare worldwide, the preventative approach is the only way to stop the growing epidemic and deal with the problem in future generations.

(Dr Ingrid Martin, Head, WHO Cardiovascular Diseases Programme, February 2000)

Add to this comment, recent findings from the last 3 years of the UK *Sunday Times* review to find the top 100 companies in Britain.[12] This reported a worrying and consistent finding from employees who work for these companies, notably, "work interferes with my health" (Jonathan Austin, CEO Best Companies). The picture is becoming clearer, the workplace represents a captive arena to cater for people's health and deal with cardiovascular risk and/or disease. Corporate organizations should be encouraged to look at the "profit and loss" of their employees' health together with the profit and loss of their company's financial performance. "If a corporate business places a great emphasis on the performance of its people, it follows, that helping to look after their health makes perfect sense" (Neil Snowball, International Director of Wellness for Goldman Sachs).

However, convincing corporate organizations to provide wellness/cardiovascular risk management interventions for their employees still remains a significant challenge. There is still a paucity of real data on a large scale to substantiate such programs, especially in Europe. There is certainly a need to develop corporate wellness/cardiovascular strategies that match the philosophy of the business world in that they make "good business sense." Fading rapidly are the days when corporate organizations provide wellness interventions in the workplace to "feel good about themselves." In such situations these interventions are so often the first things to go, when in business terms "the going gets tough." In other words, they may have been perceived as a business luxury and not an essential. However, if they start to pay for themselves with data to prove it, then the climate will hopefully change and they will become "essential" to the business.

There are still many challenges and unanswered questions. What about smaller companies who simply cannot afford corporate wellness programs and/or facilities? Can they combine with other smaller companies to purchase these services on a periodic basis? Can government agencies be persuaded to consider tax relief for companies that provide wellness "upstream" initiatives for their employees? Can insurance premiums be reduced for companies and employees who demonstrate improved cardiovascular risk profiles? Especially when private healthcare costs are rising in Europe and more employees at senior/management levels expect this cover as part of an employment benefits package.[13]

Perhaps we should realize that "health promotion" in the workplace is no longer a sufficient label under which to provide cardiovascular risk reduction and management programs and health intervention should be incorporated into a new and improved "corporate wellness concept."

The potential for corporate wellness and cardiovascular risk factor management in the workplace is enormous, hence the forecast by many experts that "wellness" is the next "trillion dollar" business.[1] Equally many business leaders are recognizing that "successful companies of the millennium will have a wellness plan to go alongside their business plan."

References

1. Pilzer PZ. The Wellness Revolution. New York: John Wiley; 2002.
2. Goetzel RZ, Ozminkowski RJ, Ling D, Rutter KB, Isaac F, Wang S. The long term impact of Johnson and Johnson's health and wellness programme on employee health risks. J Occup Envir Med 2002;44:417–424.
3. Opatz JP. Economic Impact of Worksite Health Promotion. Champaign, IL: Human Kinetics; 1994.
4. US Department of Health and Human Services: Prevention Makes Common "Cents". Washington DC: US Dept of Health and Human Services; Sept 2003.
5. National Cholesterol Education Program (NCEP). Executive Summary of the third report of the Expert Panel on Detection, Evaluation and Treatment of High Blood Cholesterol in Adults (Adult Treatment Panel III). JAMA 2001;285:2486–2497.
6. Leisure Data base Company. "State of the Industry, Europe 2003", Health Club Management, Oct 2003. Hertfordshire, England: Leisure Media Company Ltd.
7. Henritze J, Brammell HI. Phase II cardiac wellness at the Adolph Coors Company. Am J Health Prom 1089;4:25–31.
8. Pashkow FJ, Defoe WA. Clinical Cardiac Rehabilitation, 2nd edn. Baltimore: Williams & Wilkins; 1999:446–479.
9. Haskell WL, Alderman EL, Fair JM, et al. Effects of intensive multifactor risk reduction on coronary atherosclerosis and clinical cardiac events in men and women with coronary artery disease: The Stanford Coronary Risk Intervention Project. Circulation 1994;89:975–990.
10. Berra K. The effect of lifestyle interventions on quality of life and patient satisfaction with health and health care. J Cardiov Nurs 2003;18:319–325.
11. Diabetes Prevention Program Research Group, Reduction in the incidence of type 2 diabetes with lifestyle intervention or metformin. N Engl J Med 2002;346:393–403.
12. Sunday Times Business Supplement. 100 Best Companies to Work For. London: Sunday Times Publishing; March 6, 2005.
13. Pronk N. A sense of urgency to improve employee health: The bottom line and the role of worksite health promotion. ACSM Health Fitness J 2003; 7:6–11.

Section IX
Pharmacotherapy, Organization, Evaluation

In the final section of the book we have gathered contributions on organizational aspects of cardiac rehabilitation, such as rehabilitation options, referral to the program, safety aspects, and training of the staff. It is concluded with models for program evaluation.

Which modalities can be offered, which patients might benefit most from low-cost non-supervised programs based upon individual home training and for whom would a more costly admission to a specialized residential model be preferable?

Good professional competence of the cardiac rehabilitation (CR) staff is a prerequisite for the quality of the service but in what ways can this be achieved, maintained, and further developed? Here, experience from staff training in Ireland may be seen as an educational example.

In the early days of exercise training, telemetric ECG monitoring was used widely but over the years this practice has been questioned and remains under debate, the argument in favor being the numbers of elderly patients with heart failure who may develop significant rhythm disturbances, the argument against being that in modern cardiology fewer patients are enrolled with persistent residual coronary ischemia. Does safety call for ECG surveillance? What are the principal safety demands for CR?

Referring eligible patients to CR remains a main obstacle in the access to the service. Are there "easy way out" solutions? Standardized models? A well-functioning method of computer-assisted referral from the Netherlands is described.

Regular outcome control and quality assurance of comprehensive CR is remarkably seldom used, yet this is greatly needed if CR is to defend its position in competition with other more resource-demanding therapies. Guidelines recommend that both an individual patient assessment at completion of the program is provided and that an annual service assessment is compiled. In this chapter we propose a basic audit model, a standard model based upon the EuroCardioRehab concept, and an extended version including an economic evaluation.

In the field of economic evaluation a cardiologist or CR staff worker may be less experienced. However, an insight into the different methods of economic analysis is valuable when designing a program that is built upon an effective use of available means. The last contribution in this section gives a concise overview of the common methods of economic evaluation.

Main Messages

Chapter 53: Pharmacotherapy in Prevention and Rehabilitation

A number of classes of drugs have demonstrated efficacy in the prevention and rehabilitation of cardiovascular disease. We review in brief lipid-lowering, antihypertensive, antiplatelet, anti-ischemic, and antiarrhythmic drugs as well as drugs for smoking cessation, weight control, and prevention of diabetes.

Chapter 54: Rehabilitation Modalities

Comprehensive cardiac rehabilitation (CR) can be provided on different levels of care varying from a home-based program for the low-risk patient to residential care in a specialized center for the patient at high risk. This chapter concerns risk stratification before enrollment in CR and the quality demands for the different rehabilitation modalities.

Chapter 55: Developing Cardiac Rehabilitation Services: From Policy Development to Staff Training Programs

The development of cardiac rehabilitation services requires the active involvement of cardiologists both in their clinical capacity and as patient advocates. This, when coupled with national and or regional strategic policy and policy implementation frameworks, can be a potent stimulus in assisting the development of secondary prevention strategies such as cardiac rehabilitation.

Multidisciplinary teams provide an excellent model for the currently evolving concept of the cardiac care team. The increasing burden of interventional cardiology can be obviated by the provision of appropriately trained cardiac rehabilitation personnel possessing an in-depth knowledge of the relevant aspects of cardiological practice. To this end a specially designed training program is described herein, which has yielded an excellent cadre of individuals capable of supporting the cardiologist in the provision of cardiac rehabilitation.

Chapter 56: Safety Aspects of Cardiac Rehabilitation

Cardiac rehabilitation programs including physical training can be recommended to a wide range of cardiac patients. The beneficial effects on physical capacity, psychological well-being and on cardiac risk factors can be obtained at very low risk of adverse events.

Adverse events can be prevented if there is a risk stratification of the individual patient, if contraindications for enrollment are observed and if the training is conducted by well-trained staff (e.g. specialized physiotherapist or exercise therapist).

Supervised training with continuous ECG monitoring is indicated only for a minority of patients, mainly for those with an implantable cardioversion device.

Chapter 57: Communication: Automatic Referral to Phase II Cardiac Rehabilitation

Referral to a phase II cardiac rehabilitation program requires complete data and precise information for the cardiac rehabilitation team. Yet the referral should be an effective instrument, not an obstacle in communication between acute cardiac care, referring physicians, and rehabilitation services. This chapter gives an example of a standard manual referral model and of a new computer-based system that gives an automatic rehabilitation proposal based upon individual patient data and existing national guidelines.

Chapter 58: Future Developments in Preventive Cardiology: The EUROACTION Project

EUROACTION is a demonstration project with the aim to raise standards of preventive cardiology in Europe by demonstrating that the recommended European and national lifestyle, risk factor and therapeutic goals in cardiovascular disease prevention are achievable and sustainable in everyday clinical practice.

Chapter 59: Outcome Measurement and Audit

Quality assurance and outcome measurements of cardiac rehabilitation should be an integral part of the service and include an individual patient assessment and an annual service assessment. Based upon the EuroCardioRehab concept, this chapter describes three levels of audit: a basic outcome report, the standard EuroCardioRehab audit, and an extended version with focus on health economy.

Chapter 60: Economic Evaluation of Cardiac Rehabilitation

Cost-effectiveness will be an increasingly important part of decision-making in specific healthcare service as well as for treatment efficiency purposes. Cardiac rehabilitation has been shown to be an effective use of healthcare resources. Yet cardiac rehabilitation services will need to recognize and acknowledge the importance of documenting the efficiency of their program for their managers in light of the competing demands from other healthcare services for limited and finite healthcare resources.

53
Pharmacotherapy in Prevention and Rehabilitation

Dan Atar and Serena Tonstad

Primary Prevention

Lipid-Lowering Drugs

Recent European guidelines for cardiovascular disease (CVD) prevention in clinical practice recommend the use of preventive strategies based on the identification of individuals at high absolute risk for CVD.[1] To identify high-risk individuals these guidelines have chosen the Systematic Coronary Risk Evaluation (SCORE) risk model as a tool in clinical practice.[2] Lipid-lowering drugs are recommended in individuals with a 10-year risk of fatal CVD of ≥5%. These guidelines should be adapted to reflect practical, economic, and medical circumstances in each country. Therapy with inhibitors of HMG CoA reductase (statins) reduces risk across a wide baseline range of cholesterol values and risk levels of CVD in several primary prevention trials including the West of Scotland Coronary Prevention Study (WOSCOPS),[3] the Air Force/Texas Coronary Atherosclerosis Prevention Study (AFCAPS/TexCAPS),[4] and the Anglo-Scandinavian Cardiac Outcomes Trial-Lipid Lowering Arm (ASCOT-LLA)[5] study. An overview of the effect of statins on cardiovascular disease morbidity and mortality is presented below in the section on secondary prevention, as these results pertain both to primary and secondary preventive lipid-lowering therapy.

Individuals who may have genetic lipid disorders such as familial hypercholesterolemia or, more commonly, familial combined hyperlipidemia should, when available, be referred to a specialist evaluation. This evaluation should include an assessment of the family history and other risk factors, previous lipid values and values in other family members, and molecular genetic diagnosis, if relevant. These patients may require two or more drugs for lowering of their LDL cholesterol level to <3 mmol/L. Thus, statins may be combined with bile acid sequestrants, including colesevelam hydrochloride, nicotinic acid and ezetimibe, and, in individuals with hypertriglyceridemia, with fibrates to achieve optimal lipid levels. Even so, achieving optimal LDL cholesterol levels in this group may be difficult. Encouragingly, the reduction of LDL cholesterol by at least 50% has been shown to lead to the regression of atherosclerosis[6] and is feasible in most patients. The combination of fibrates or nicotinic acids with statins may potentiate the risk of myopathy and requires special vigilance.

Antihypertensive Drugs

Blood pressure lowering therapy should be considered in individuals with repeated measures of systolic blood pressure >140 mmHg and/or diastolic blood pressure >90 mmHg. Guidelines recommend that the overall cardiovascular risk should be considered.[1] Treatment directed at lowering blood pressure should include lifestyle change encompassing smoking cessation, moderation of alcohol consumption, weight reduction, physical exercise, reduction of high salt intake and other dietary changes. When these measures fail, pharmacological treatment is indicated.

A number of large clinical trials have investigated differences in the efficiency of older versus newer antihypertensive drug strategies. In general, no clear-cut differences are detectable between the various classes of antihypertensive drugs, although this statement is a matter of ongoing dispute. In initiating drug treatment, therapy should always be started gently, and target blood pressure will not generally be achieved within the first months. An important modern principle of drug treatment is to attempt combination therapy early on. Many experts recommend a low dose of a single drug as the primary approach, and if blood pressure control is not achieved, to add a low dose of a different agent, rather than increasing the dose of the first compound. The reason for this strategy is to diminish the possibility of eliciting adverse effects of the drugs. It is essential to keep in mind that antihypertensive therapy must remain operational for many years, even decades, in most patients. Classes of antihypertensive drugs that are currently available are shown in Table 53-1.

In general contemporary treatment allows for almost all combinations of the various drug classes. Combinations that are particularly effective include:

- diuretics and beta-blockers
- diuretics and ACE inhibitors
- diuretics and angiotensin receptor blockers
- calcium antagonists and beta-blockers
- calcium antagonists and ACE inhibitors
- calcium antagonists and angiotensin receptor blockers
- calcium antagonists and diuretics
- alpha-blockers and beta-blockers

Nevertheless, in the presence of certain conditions, the so-called "compelling indications," the

TABLE 53-1. Classes of antihypertensive drugs that are currently available

Diuretics
Beta-blockers
Alpha-1-blockers
ACE inhibitors
Angiotensin receptor blockers
Calcium antagonists
Centrally active receptor-antagonists

use of specific antihypertensive classes is mandated, as shown in Table 53-2.

Antiplatelet Drugs

Primary prevention with antiplatelet agents is focused almost solely on acetylsalicylic acid (ASA).[7] The effect of ASA has been scrutinized in six large primary prevention trials (Table 53-3).[8-13]

Although some of these trials investigated high-risk patients with one or more risk factors, the yearly cardiovascular event rate was rather low in all of these studies. The reduction in the odds ratio for adverse cardiovascular events in favor of ASA was in the range of 0–29%, which translates into an absolute reduction of ischemic events in the range of 0–3 per 1000 treated patients/year. This effect is countered by 1–2 serious gastrointestinal bleeds per 1000 patients/year. Hence even in the two trials that achieved a reduction of 2–3 ischemic events per 1000 patients/year the overall gain appears to be quite minuscule when the risk of serious bleeding is taken into account.

On the basis of these data, an expert panel organized under the auspices of the European Society of Cardiology has issued a consensus report in 2004 on the use of antiplatelet agents[7]. In this report primary prophylaxis with ASA is recommended in a daily dose of 75–100 mg only in asymptomatic individuals who have an estimated risk for ischemic events that is greater than 3%/year. However, it must be recognized that the following points of uncertainty remain.

- Whether diabetes should be included in the risk assessment. The PPP study[12] surprisingly showed that diabetics did not attain the same preventive benefit conferred by ASA as non-diabetics.
- Whether the use of ASA for primary prevention should be limited to individuals under the age of 70.[14] Increased age may heighten the predisposition for gastrointestinal bleeding,[15] and possibly be associated with severe generalized bleeds.[16]
- Whether the expert recommendations are applicable to women as well to men, given that five of the published trials have predominantly focused on men. The Women's Health Study[13] recently provided pertinent information.

TABLE 53-2. List over so-called "compelling indications," as well as contraindications in different classes of antihypertensive drugs

Class	Conditions favoring the use	Contraindications	
		Compelling	Possible
Diuretics (thiazides)	Congestive heart failure Elderly hypertensives Isolated systolic hypertension	Gout	Pregnancy
Diuretics (loop)	Renal insufficiency Congestive heart failure		
Diuretics (antialdosterone)	Congestive heart failure Post-myocardial infarction	Renal failure Hyperkalemia	

Beta-blockers	Angina pectoris
	Post myocardial infarction
	Congestive heart failure (up-titration)
	Pregnancy
	Tachyarrhythmias
		Asthma
		Chronic obstructive
		   pulmonary disease
		Atrioventricular block
		   (grade 2 of 3)
			Peripheral vascular disease
			Glucose intolerance
			Athletes and physically
			   active patients

Calcium antagonists (dihydropyridines)	Elderly patients Isolated systolic hypertension Angina pectoris Peripheral vascular disease Carotid atherosclerosis Pregnancy		Tachyarrhythmias Congestive heart failure

Calcium antagonists (verapamil,
   diltiazem)
	Angina pectoris
	Carotid atherosclerosis
	Supraventricular tachycardia
		Atrioventricular block
		   (grade 2 or 3)
		Congestive heart failure	

ACE inhibitors	Congestive heart failure LV dysfunction Post myocardial infarction Non-diabetic nephropathy Type 1 diabetic nephropathy Proteinuria	Pregnancy Hyperkalemia Bilateral renal artery stenosis	

Angiotensin II receptor antagonists
   (AT1 blockers)
	Diabetic nephropathy
	Diabetic microalbuminuria
	Proteinuria
	Left ventricular hypertrophy
	ACE inhibitor cough
		Pregnancy
		Hyperkalemia
		Bilateral renal artery
		   stenosis	

Alpha-blockers	Prostatic hyperplasia (BPH) Glucose intolerance Hyperlipidemia	Orthostatic hypotension	Congestive heart failure

Source: Reprinted from Guidelines Committee. 2003 European Society of Hypertension-European Society of Cardiology Guidelines for the Management of Arterial Hypertension. Heart Drug 2004;4:6–51. © 2004 S. Karger AG, Basel, with permission.

TABLE 53-3. Overview over the major primary prevention trials for ASA

Trial name	Investigated subjects	No.	Follow-up (years)	Odds ratio	Prevented events/patient year (% year)
BDT: British Doctors Trial[8]	Healthy men	5.139	5.8	1.3	0
PHS: Physicians Health Study[9]	Healthy men	22.071	5.0	0.82	1.2
TPT: Thrombosis Prevention Trial[10]	"High-risk" men	5.085	6.3	0.83	2.7
HOT: Hypertension Optimal Treatment Study[11]	Hypertensive men and women	18.790	3.8	0.85	1.6
PPP: Primary Prevention Project[12]	"High-risk" men and women	4.495	3.6	0.71	2.6
WHS: Women Primary Prevention Study[13]	Healthy women	39.876	10.1	0.91	0

Among 39,876 healthy women who were randomized to 100 mg of ASA every second day versus placebo and followed up for 10 years, a significant 20% reduction in the incidence of stroke was observed, but no reduction in acute myocardial infarction. On the other hand, four of the five previous studies in men resulted in a significant reduction in myocardial infarction, but not in ischemic stroke.

In regard to other antiplatelet compounds, the recent CHARISMA trial[17] failed to show any benefit of a combination of ASA and clopidogrel as a primary prevention strategy.

Taken together, the available evidence does not support a systematic use of ASA or any other antiplatelet drug as a primary prevention strategy. This does not preclude the well-established indication for antiplatelet therapy in patients with acute or chronic ischemic heart disease, and patients with other atherosclerotic manifestations, as described below.

Secondary Prevention

Ischemic Heart Disease and Systemic Atherosclerosis Including Stroke and Post-AMI Therapy

Lipid-Lowering Drugs

The central role of cholesterol in atherosclerosis is based on epidemiological studies, molecular biology, and randomized clinical trials. The first pharmacological intervention studies achieving cholesterol reduction manifested unequivocally the tight correlation between the achieved LDL cholesterol reduction on the one hand, and the reduction in cardiovascular events on the other hand. In general for every 1 mmol of reduction in LDL cholesterol an approximately 21% risk reduction in cardiovascular events is observed in the course of the observation period. This extrapolation is based on a wide array of pharmacological and other cholesterol-lowering studies, including the Lipid Research Clinics, the Scandinavian Simvastatin Survival Study (4-S),[18] WOSCOPS,[3] Cholesterol and Recurrent Events (CARE),[19] AFCAPS/TexCAPS,[4] Long-Term Intervention with Pravastatin in Ischaemic Disease (LIPID),[20] Heart

Protection Study (HPS),[21] ASCOT-LLA,[5] and Collaborative Atorvastatin Diabetes Study (CARDS) trials.[22] These trials represent some of the most comprehensive scientific assessments of drug treatments that have ever been performed. All of these studies have one common feature: they compared a lipid-lowering intervention to placebo.

The publication of the HPS[21] performed in over 20,000 high-risk patients provided further important evidence. This study compared simvastatin with placebo and found the same degree of benefit, in relative terms, of lowering LDL cholesterol from about 3 to 2 mmol/L as from 4 to 3 mmol/L. Observationally, treatment with simvastatin resulted in a 24% risk reduction for cardiovascular events, regardless of whether the baseline LDL cholesterol value was >3.5 mmol/L, between 3.0 and 3.5 mmol/L, or <3.0 mmol/L.

Against this background, a new era in cholesterol intervention research began, namely, the principle of head-to-head comparisons between different statins. The three most important studies performed with this aim were the PROVE-IT,[23] Treating to New Targets (TNT),[24] and the Incremental Decrease in End Points Through Aggressive Lipid Lowering (IDEAL)[25] studies. In the PROVE-IT trial[23] more than 4000 patients with acute coronary syndrome were randomized to pravastatin 40 mg daily or atorvastatin 80 mg daily, and followed for 2.5 years. While the group treated with pravastatin achieved a mean LDL cholesterol reduction to about 2.5 mmol/L, the atorvastatin group achieved a mean LDL cholesterol level of 2.0 mmol/L. Notably, after only 30 months of follow-up, the study showed that the risk of death or cardiovascular events in the atorvastatin group was significantly reduced by 16% compared to the pravastatin group.

The next pivotal study is the TNT trial,[24] which investigated over 10,000 patients randomized to low- or high-dose atorvastatin. While the group given atorvastatin 10 mg daily attained a mean LDL cholesterol level of 2.6 mmol/L, the high-dose atorvastatin group (80 mg daily) achieved an LDL cholesterol level of 1.9 mmol/L. After 6 years of follow-up there was a significant 22% relative risk reduction in cardiovascular events in the group that received 80 mg of atorvastatin compared to the group that received 10 mg. This did not result in a reduction of overall mortality; however, such a reduction was not expected given that the entire study population received active treatment. Furthermore, the protocol specified the inclusion of patients with relatively low baseline cholesterol levels, in contrast to previously conducted studies of statins.

Amidst this intriguing development came the publication of the IDEAL study,[25] culminating more than one decade of intense cholesterol research. This study randomized 8888 patients with established coronary disease to simvastatin 20–40 mg daily or atorvastatin 80 mg daily in an open label (with blinded endpoints) design. The primary endpoint was cardiovascular death, myocardial infarction, or cardiac arrest. Over 50% of the subjects had been treated with simvastatin prior to enrollment, while approximately 11% were treated with atorvastatin, and 14% received different statins. Analyses after 5 years of follow-up showed a trend towards a more favorable outcome in the atorvastatin-group, i.e. an 11% risk reduction that did not, however, achieve conventional statistical significance ($P = 0.07$). However, in regard to a key secondary endpoint (cardiovascular death, myocardial infarction, cardiac arrest and stroke), which was equivalent to the primary endpoint in the TNT study, the achieved reduction in relative risk was 13%, a reduction that was statistically significant. The side-effect profiles of the two compounds were very similar, and there was no increase in rhabdomyolysis or myopathy in any of the groups. However, the atorvastatin group experienced an elevation of liver enzymes slightly more frequently than the simvastatin-group. On the whole, the main hypothesis of the study, "the lower the LDL cholesterol, the better," was confirmed. When the effect of further LDL cholesterol lowering as shown in the IDEAL study is superimposed on the regression line between cardiac events and reduction in LDL cholesterol computed by the Cholesterol Treatment Trialists collaboration, the IDEAL study results are consistent with previous studies.

Taken together, these studies show that the achievable gains due to intensive cholesterol-lowering therapy in low-risk populations such as the IDEAL and TNT study populations do not include a reduction in all-cause mortality, but do include a reduction in cardiovascular events. There results justify aggressive cholesterol lower-

ing in relatively young patients with very high cardiovascular risk (primary prevention) and/or already established cardiovascular disease or diabetes. These results may lead to reconsideration of international guidelines for cardiovascular prevention.

Antihypertensive Drugs

The pharmacotherapy of arterial hypertension is discussed in the section on primary prevention above.

Antiplatelet Drugs

All cases of acute cardiovascular disease including acute coronary syndrome, i.e., unstable angina, acute myocardial infarction including non-ST-elevation myocardial infarction (non-STEMI) and ST-elevation myocardial infarction (STEMI), as well as in ischemic stroke, are an indisputable indication for antiplatelet treatment. As a starting dose, 300 mg of ASA is recommended, either by oral or intravenous administration, and subsequently a daily dose of 75–100 mg.[26]

Treatment with ASA results in a 30–50% reduction in adverse cardiovascular events in acute coronary syndromes, and a somewhat less impressive, yet still significant reduction of approximately 10% in acute ischemic stroke. One reason for this lesser effect in stroke could be due to uncontrollable bleeding from increased instability of the cerebral artery in acute cerebral infarction. In absolute terms, 40–50 ischemic events are prevented per 1000 patients with acute coronary syndromes and 10 events are prevented per 1000 patients with acute ischemic stroke treated for one year.

ASA in a dose of 75 mg daily is also indicated as secondary prophylaxis in all patients with known ischemic heart disease, that is, patients with a history of myocardial infarction, stable angina pectoris, ischemic stroke, or cerebral transient ischemic attack (TIA).[26] The same holds true for patients with a history of percutaneous coronary intervention (PCI) or coronary artery bypass graft operation (CABG), as well as patients with peripheral artery disease. The latter group includes both symptomatic and asymptomatic patients, including those with a decreased peripheral (i.e., ankle) perfusion pressure, aortic aneurysm, or any other form of atherosclerosis. In this patient population the odds ratio for an ischemic event is reduced by about 20–30% for a given study period.[27] Hence this strategy translates into 10–20 prevented events per 1000 patients per year. The number needed to treat is 5–10 patients per 10 patient-years. The treatment reduces all forms of new ischemic events, and applies equally to men and women. Clopidogrel is indicated for patients who do not tolerate ASA.

Serious side-effects, predominantly major gastrointestinal bleeds, occur with a frequency of 1–2 cases per 1000 treated patients/year during long-term prophylaxis with 75 mg of ASA.[15,16] While an incidence of this magnitude can be regarded as a relatively minor problem compared to the prophylactic gain that is achieved, the frequency of gastrointestinal bleeds increases with age. In the age group of 70–80 years, major bleeds may occur in 7 per 1000 treated patients/year.[14]

In patients with cerebral TIA or ischemic stroke (of non-cardiogenic etiology), combined preventive pharmacological treatment consisting of ASA 75 mg daily and a depot (retard) formulation of dipyridamole 200 mg twice a day is recommended. According to the ESPS-2 study,[28] this preventive treatment reduces the risk of new cerebral events by about 35%.

The effects of the ADP receptor blocker clopidogrel in patients with atherosclerotic manifestations have been investigated extensively in the CAPRIE[29] and more recently, the CHARISMA trials.[17] The CAPRIE trial[29] found a slight advantage of clopidogrel over ASA in a population of patients with chronic ischemic heart disease, cerebrovascular disease or peripheral artery disease, but the achieved gain was so small that clopidogrel has not replaced ASA on a large-scale basis in clinical practice. This is certainly due to differences in cost between the two drugs. Likewise the CHARISMA trial,[17] while failing to show any benefit of a combination of ASA and clopidogrel on the primary endpoint, found a slight advantage of combined treatment with ASA and clopidogrel in the subgroup of patients with established cardiovascular disease. The practical and clinical consequences of these findings remain to be established; however, dual antiplatelet therapy will probably not replace ASA on a broad scale for secondary prevention

in patients with stable atherosclerotic disease in the current climate of increasing cost/benefit awareness.

In contrast to the situation in primary prevention, the addition of clopidogrel to ASA is indicated in all cases of acute coronary syndrome, including unstable angina, non-STEMI and STEMI. There is comprehensive scientific evidence to support this indication, e.g. the CURE,[30] CREDO,[31] CLARITY,[32] and COMMIT[33] studies. Clopidogrel is given orally at a starting dose of 300 to 600 mg, and continued at a dose of 75 mg daily. This treatment is usually given for 9 to 12 months in survivors of non-STEMI or STEMI. Treatment with clopidogrel is mandatory in all patients who have undergone a stenting procedure, whether electively or acutely. In elective cases, the CLASSICS study[34] has documented the benefit of combined clopidogrel and ASA therapy for at least 4 weeks.

Anti-Ischemic Drugs

Despite impressive advancements in catheter-based and surgical revascularization therapy for chronic ischemic heart disease, pharmacological treatment of angina pectoris remains a cornerstone in cardiovascular prevention and rehabilitation. It has become clear that while lipid-lowering and platelet-inhibiting drugs are mainstays of this treatment, drugs for symptom relief also play an important role. This is due to the observation that even fully revascularized patients may experience recurrent coronary stenoses over time. Furthermore, vascularization may not be achieved for all lesions, for example due to non-accessible or peripheral anatomic locations.

The three main classes of drugs that ameliorate chronic unstable angina are the nitrates, beta-blockers, and calcium antagonists.[35] All of these agents are effective in increasing myocardial perfusion and/or decreasing the myocardial demand for oxygen. Nitrates are either given as sublingual formulations, or as delayed release compounds. The first group acts very rapidly, with an onset of symptom relief within 10–60 seconds. Nitrates precipitate a systemic venous dilatation, leading to a pre- and afterload reduction, as well as causing a powerful coronary artery dilatation.[36] One of the problems with nitrates is the need for a nitrate-free interval between dosing, in order to prevent the nitrate tolerance or nitrate idiosyncrasy.[37] In practice, a minimum of 8 hours of a drug-free interval per day is required. This may be achieved by administration of the drug in the morning and at midday. Even though no large-scale trial evidence has proven the effect of nitrates in patients with stable angina pectoris, the use of this old and well-proven class of drugs is well established in modern medicine. The most important side-effect of nitrates is headache, which can occur in up to 10% of patients. In some patients, continued use diminishes the frequency of headache over time.

Beta-blockers are the most effective antianginal drugs available.[38] Their pharmacological action is directed toward the beta-1 receptor of the cardiomyocytes in the myocardium. This leads to a slowing of the heart rate and a reduction in myocardial contractility (i.e. negative chronotropic and negative inotropic effects). Thus an efficient reduction of myocardial oxygen demand is achieved, alleviating this trigger of ischemia.[39] Cardioselective compounds are generally preferred in patients who have partial contraindications against beta-blockers, such as asthma, peripheral artery disease, and insulin-dependent diabetes mellitus. In addition to providing efficient relief of anginal symptoms, beta-blockers exert an antiarrhythmic and myocardial-protective effect, and are therefore also indicated in post-myocardial infarction patients.[38]

Calcium antagonists are also useful in chronic angina pectoris. They work at the vessel wall, causing coronary and peripheral vessel dilatation.[35] Calcium antagonists (or calcium-channel blockers) are divided into a dihydropyridine and a non-dihydropyridine class. The latter comprises verapamil and diltiazem, compounds that effectively delay atrioventricular excitation (i.e., a negative dromotropic effect).[40,41] Together with the negative inotropic effect of the class, these agents are effective in reducing the angina threshold. The dihydropyridines, on the other hand, such as nifedipine or amlodipine, are neutral in terms of chronotropy. They cause a more dominant smooth muscle relaxation leading to a powerful blood pressure reduction. All calcium antagonists should be used with care in patients with heart failure, due to their negative inotropic effect.

In addition to these three classes of drugs, the agent molsidomine can also be utilized as an antianginal compound. The compound's action is similar to that of the nitrates, but no known idiosyncratic (i.e., tolerance-generating) effects have been observed. Finally, nicorandil, a K^+-channel opener, has shown to be an effective drug for refractory angina pectoris.[42]

All of these drugs can easily be combined for optimization of treatment. Care should be exerted when combining non-dihydropyridine calcium channel blockers (verapamil, diltiazem) with beta-blockers, due to the inherent risk of atrioventricular conduction delays and atrioventricular blockade.

Antiarrhythmic Drugs

Many drugs of different classes have been studied for their antiarrhythmic effects in ischemic heart disease. None of these attempts have been successful, and – except for beta-blockers after myocardial infarction – there is no general therapeutic indication for this type of therapy in cardiovascular prevention and rehabilitation.[43] Of cause, this picture changes entirely in patients with syncope due to arrhythmias or in survivors of cardiac arrest. In these patients comprehensive antiarrhythmic therapy, including radiofrequency ablation and/or the implantation of an intracardiac cardioverter defibrillator (ICD), may be indicated.[44]

Congestive Heart Failure

Congestive heart failure is increasingly prevalent and its pharmacotherapy has changed substantially over the last two decades.[45] The comprehensiveness and complexity of heart failure therapy justifies its management through skilled specialized heart failure teams that are trained in handling multifaceted pharmacological regimens. The major classes of drugs indicated for chronic heart failure are:

– diuretics
– ACE inhibitors/angiotensin receptor blockers
– beta-blockers
– aldosterone antagonists
– digitalis

Diuretics

Diuretics are essential for treating and counteracting the "congestive" aspect of congestive heart failure, that is, the tendency toward the development of chronic fluid overload.[46] This is particularly the case in patients with peripheral edema, general overhydration, or manifest pulmonary edema. The pathophysiological mechanism for this fluid accumulation is the result of a decreased perfusion of the kidneys, due to a compromised cardiac output. As a result of this hypoperfusion, the endohormonal renin–angiotensin axis is activated, leading to sodium and fluid retention and ultimately fluid overload. Even though no controlled randomized trial has demonstrated the effect of diuretics in heart failure, their routine use is mandatory. Both loop diuretics, thiazides and metolazone, as well as potassium-sparing diuretics, should be considered for this indication, depending on how powerful an anticongestive effect is required.

ACE Inhibitors

ACE inhibitors are indicated both in asymptomatic and symptomatic heart failure. These drugs improve survival, diminish symptoms such as shortness of breath, and increase functional capacity.[47] In general, ACE inhibitors should be given with care in patients with renal failure and/or hyperkalemia. Side-effects include cough, hypotension, and rarely angioedema. In clinical trials an initial side-effect has been reported to occur in up to 10% of all patients. In these cases angiotensin receptor blockers may safely replace ACE inhibitors. Because various ACE inhibitors have been assessed in large-scale clinical trials to date, it appears that they share a class-effect, and that the earliest ACE inhibitors on the market (enalapril, captopril) as well as the newer, once-daily agents, are indicated in heart failure.

Beta-Blockers

These agents are indicated in patients who are in a stable stage of their disease, regardless of whether the underlying ventricular systolic dysfunction is mild, moderate, or severe. Beta-blockers have shown to improve functional class, reduce symptoms (except during the initial run-in period of one to two weeks when symptoms may slightly worsen), and substantially decrease mortality. Four compounds have been shown to confer these beneficial effects, namely bisoprolol, metoprolol succinate, and nebivolol, as well as the combined alpha- and beta-blocker carvedilol.[48–51] Side-effects are described in the section on anti-ischemic drugs. Therapy with beta-blockers as well as ACE inhibitors should be initiated with the lowest available dose, and should encompass slow, incremental up-titration over time. Based on knowledge gained through the CIBIS-3 study, it is entirely at the physician's discretion to decide whether ACE inhibitors or beta-blocker therapy should be started initially in chronic heart failure patients. In clinical practice, an up-titration scheme will usually be able to encompass both classes of drugs simultaneously.

Angiotensin II Receptor Blockers

This family of drugs can replace ACE inhibitors in the case of ACE inhibitor intolerance.[52] They exert the same beneficial effects as the ACE inhibitors but with a significantly lower rate of side-effects. Because these drugs were developed relatively recently, they cost much more than ACE inhibitors, and as a result do not replace ACE inhibitors as the first drug of choice. These drugs may be considered in combination with ACE inhibitors in patients who continue to be symptomatic (the so-called "dual blockade"). However, care must be given not to elicit renal failure by this combination.

Aldosterone Receptor Antagonists

Aldosterone receptor antagonists are also indicated in congestive heart failure, but only in patients with more severe symptoms (functional NYHA class III or IV).[53,54] The indication extends to patients who have left ventricular systolic dysfunction after myocardial infarction. This class of drugs includes spironolactone and eplerenone. Eplerenone is only indicated in post-infarction patients.

Digitalis Glycosides

This class of drugs, derived from the purple foxglove (*Digitalis purpurea*), is the oldest among all currently used medications. Its first use in heart failure was described in 1775. Digitalis preparations are indicated in those patients with heart failure who have concomitant atrial fibrillation, or who are persistently symptomatic despite all the above pharmacological approaches. Digoxin and digitoxin both decrease atrioventricular conductance, thus diminishing ventricular heart rate. Even though digitalis has no effect on mortality, its salutary actions lead to reduced hospitalizations and amelioration of symptoms.[55] Any form of cardiac block, dysfunction of the atrioventricular or sinus node and bradyarrhythmia are important contraindications to digitalis.

A variety of positive inotropic agents direct their effects against decreased ventricular contractile function. Although these compounds represent a conceptually straightforward principle to counteract the mechanisms of reduced ventricular contractility, their use in clinical practice has unfortunately shown that they actually increase mortality in heart failure. Accordingly, none of the existing inotropic stimulants (except for digoxin) are indicated in patients with chronic heart failure.

Arrhythmias Including Atrial Fibrillation

Atrial fibrillation is the most common cardiac arrhythmia. Its prevalence in populations over 75 years may be as high as over 10%.[56] The two major challenges in managing patients with atrial fibrillation are the rhythm disturbances on one hand and the prevention of systemic thromboembolism on the other.

There are two fundamental approaches to managing the inherent arrhythmia linked to atrial fibrillation: either aiming toward the re-establishment and maintenance of sinus rhythm, or the acceptance of chronic (permanent) atrial fibrillation and regulation of atrioventricular conduction, such that the ventricular heart rate is adequate. These two strategies are called "rhythm control" and "frequency control." As a rule of thumb, rhythm control and frequency control have similar prognoses in regard to longevity, survival, and quality of life.[57]

The initial approach to patients with new-onset atrial fibrillation is usually re-establishing and maintaining sinus rhythm. The advantages of this approach include a total restoration of the physiologic excitation pathway of the heart, as well as retaining the hope of avoiding long-term anticoagulation therapy. These advantages, however, must be balanced against the disadvantages of using antiarrhythmic drugs in order to maintain sinus rhythm. These drugs are generally considered less safe than drugs directed at pure frequency control.[58]

Rhythm control may require cardioversion, that is, an electrical or pharmacological short-term stimulation aiming at terminating the paroxysm of atrial fibrillation, converting it into sinus rhythm. Several drugs can be utilized to achieve pharmacological cardioversion. Although pharmacological cardioversion is doubtless less effective than electrical cardioversion, the possibility of succeeding with an intravenous injection and no anesthesia, such as is required in electrical cardioversion, is clearly attractive. In addition, electrical cardioversion is often perceived by the public as a particularly unpleasant event, reminiscent of electrical convulsion therapy for severe mental depression. Nevertheless, the risk of thromboembolism and stroke is similar whether a pharmacological or electrical tactic is chosen.[59]

Successful pharmacological cardioversion is well documented for the antiarrhythmic agents dofetilide, flecainide, ibutilide, or propafenone. In addition, substances such as amiodarone, quinidine, and sotalol are occasionally utilized. The mechanisms of these agents differ according to the known variability at the cellular level (Table 53-4).[60] According to the Vaughan Williams classification, the most effective cardioversion is achieved by either class III or class Ic antiarrhythmics. The major problem with all of these drugs is their potential for pro-arrhythmic effects, including the risk of torsades-de-pointes ventricular tachycardia or other life-threatening arrhythmias or conduction delays.

Notably, standard drugs used for frequency control, such as beta-blockers and certain calcium channel antagonists (verapamil and diltiazem), are surprisingly efficient in restoring sinus rhythm.

Both in paroxysmal and in permanent (chronic) atrial fibrillation, long-term anticoagulation is indicated.[61] The level of anticoagulation should be directed to maintaining an

Table 53-4. Vaughan Williams classification of antiarrhythmic drug action

Type 1A
   Disopyramide
   Procainamide
   Quinidine
Type 1B
   Lidocaine
   Mexiletine
Type 1C
   Flecainide
   Moricizine
   Propafenone
Type II
   Beta-blockers (e.g. propranolol)
Type III
   Amiodarone
   Bretylium
   Dofetilide
   Ibutilide
   Sotalol
Type IV
   Calcium-channel antagonists (e.g. verapamil and diltiazem)

Source: Reprinted from ACC/AHA/ESC practice guidelines. Eur Heart J, Vol. 22, issue 20, October 2001 with permission from The European Society of Cardiology. Original source: Vaughan Williams EM. A classification of antiarrhythmic action as reassessed after a decade of new drugs. J Clin Pharmacol 1984;24:129–147, 1984, © Sage Publications Inc.

international normalized ratio of 2.0–3.5. This does not apply to patients under the age of 60 years in whom no structural heart disease has been documented (the so-called lone fibrillators). In these patients treatment with ASA in a dose of 160–325 mg daily is an alternative. In general, the protective effects of ASA against systemic emboli is far inferior to that conferred by vitamin K antagonists.[62] The indication for all oral anticoagulation should be evaluated and examined regularly. In patients over the age of 80–85 years, the benefits of anticoagulant protection against stroke must be balanced against the increased risk of bleeding.

Valvular Heart Disease

Pharmacotherapy in prevention and rehabilitation applies also for patients with valvular heart disease. The main purpose is the prevention of infective endocarditis. This is a disease of valves and neighboring endovascular/intracardiac structures due to infection with microorganisms. The primary preventive principle is a prophylactic antibiotic course in all patients at risk in whom bacteremia is expected.[63] These include patients with prosthetic heart valves, patients with surgically corrected congenital cardiac abnormalities, and patients with moderate to severe congenital or acquired valvular heart disease. This includes patients with mitral valve prolapse if substantial mitral incompetence is present, patients with bicuspid aortic valves, as well as patients with a previous history of infective endocarditis.

A wide variety of invasive diagnostic or therapeutic procedures may cause bacteremia. The list includes dental procedures, tonsillectomy, any biopsy or uroscopic investigation in the urinary tract, colonoscopy, gynecological procedures, and gastrointestinal interventional procedures.[64]

The prophylactic antibiotic regimens depend on the location of the index procedure.[65] For example, in dental procedures amoxicillin 2.0 g is recommended orally one hour before the scheduled dental treatment. In gastrointestinal or urinary procedures, the recommendation is ampicillin or amoxicillin 2.0 g intravenously or amoxicillin together with a bodyweight-adjusted dose of gentamicin (at 1.5 mg/kg intravenously). Alternative regimens are available if there is a history of allergic reactions to penicillin derivatives.

Gender Differences

As discussed recently,[66] the effectiveness and side-effect profile of drugs for cardiovascular disease in women is less well-studied than among men. Gender differences should be taken into account during therapy with beta-blockers, ACE inhibitors, digitalis, and antiarrhythmic drugs.

Pharmacotherapy for Smoking Cessation

Quitting smoking is one of the primary lifestyle changes that reduce the risk of cardiovascular disease in primary and secondary prevention. However, the addictive nature of nicotine makes smoking cessation difficult to initiate, and withdrawal symptoms, including cravings for cigarettes, make continued abstinence difficult to maintain. Studies show that the majority of serious quit attempts will fail within 1 year.[67] This is understandable in the light of evidence showing that cigarette dependence produces long-lasting structural and functional changes in the central nervous system.[67,68] Fortunately a number of drug therapies have been established as first-line therapies to aid smoking cessation. Fewer therapies have been shown to be effective in the maintenance of cessation.[69]

Nicotine replacement therapy (NRT) and bupropion are two pharmacotherapeutic options that are recommended as first-line treatments for motivated smokers trying to quit.[67,70] The recommended duration of therapy for bupropion (Zyban) is 7 to 12 weeks; for NRTs, treatment duration ranges from 4 weeks to 6 months. NRT has been shown to be effective in the form of gum, transdermal patches, nasal spray, inhaler, lozenges, and sublingual tablets. NRT and bupropion can be combined. A medical model for the prescription and follow-up of bupropion has been described.[71] The choice of medical therapy should be based on patient preference, history of previous use, contraindications, adverse effects, and physician experience.[71]

Recently, varenicline, a highly selective $\alpha 4\beta 2$ nicotinic receptor partial agonist, has been developed specifically for smoking cessation. Knockout and knock-in studies in mice have shown that the $\alpha 4\beta 2$ nicotinic acetylcholine receptors are necessary and sufficient for dopamine release and nicotine addiction to be established.[72,73] Studies have shown an increased odds ratios for continuous abstinence from cigarettes with varenicline compared to placebo or bupropion.[68]

Although these therapies have demonstrated efficacy in the acute stages of quitting, the duration of treatment that is currently recommended may not be sufficient for smokers to maintain abstinence from smoking.[74,67] In one trial, smokers who quit after 7 weeks of treatment with open-label bupropion were randomized to bupropion or placebo for a further 45 weeks.[75] A significant benefit from continued therapy was evident at the end of the randomized phase and at 6 months thereafter, though not at 1 year. In a study published as an abstract to date, an additional 12 weeks of treatment with varenicline improved cessation rates 6 months after the end of treatment in subjects who had quit smoking with the aid of an initial 12-week course of varenicline.[68] These results suggest that for some smokers, the use of long-term treatment may be beneficial.

Pharmacotherapy for Weight Management and Prevention of Diabetes

Weight reduction for the prevention of cardiovascular disease is an imperative in the current environment of epidemic obesity and metabolic syndrome. However, the failure rate is 70–95% within 1–2 years of weight loss. Weight loss is followed by a number of adaptations including decreased thyroid and immune function and changes in signaling in the central nervous system that result in weight regain. Thus, the treatment of obesity, which is the common denominator underlying the variable symptoms of the metabolic syndrome, remains a challenge in cardiovascular rehabilitation and prevention. Programs should emphasize a moderate weight loss of 5–10% that is achievable by lifestyle change, rather than dieting, and that is maintainable over time. Drugs may assist with this goal, but no studies that demonstrate a reduction in cardiovascular morbidity or mortality as a result of drug-assisted weight reduction have been done. Promisingly, treatment with a number of drugs may reduce the incidence of type 2 diabetes. This is important in light of the high risk of fatal and nonfatal macrovascular events in patients with type 2 diabetes.

Orlistat and sibutramine are two pharmacotherapeutic options to assist weight reduction and prevent weight regain. Orlistat is a lipase inhibitor, causing partial malabsorption of dietary fat. The XENDOS study showed that the additional weight loss induced by orlistat compared to placebo, though small, reduced the development of type 2 diabetes by 37% in a large group of obese patients treated for 4 years.[76] The attrition rate in this trial was 57%, which is similar to that observed in most large-scale obesity trials, but limits the representativeness of the results. Sibutramine induces weight loss by inhibiting the neuronal reuptake of norepinephrine and serotonin at the receptor sites that affect food intake, and preventing the decline in energy expenditure during weight loss. The SCOUT study is currently examining the effect of sibutramine on cardiovascular morbidity and mortality.[77] Recently rimonabant, a selective cannabinoid-1 receptor blocker, was approved for the treatment of overweight and obesity. Studies have shown that combined with lifestyle intervention, a dose of 20 mg of rimonabant effectively reduces body weight and waist circumference and improves some cardiovascular risk factors.[78]

A number of other drug classes have been studied in regard to preventing type 2 diabetes. These include oral antidiabetic agents (metformin, acarbose, sulfonylureas, and thiazolidinediones), antihypertensive drugs, and lipid-lowering drugs. Of these only oral antidiabetic drugs have been studied in randomized controlled clinical trials with the incidence of diabetes as the primary endpoint. Decreases in diabetes incidence have been shown with metformin, acarbose, and troglitazone; however, it is unknown whether these drugs prevent or only delay the onset of diabetes.[79] Studies of the effect of antihypertensive and lipid-lowering drugs on diabetes incidence have all been post-hoc analyses of trials with other primary endpoints; however, several ongoing trials will be able to provide more evidence on the pharmacological prevention of type 2 diabetes.[79]

Finally, it must be noted that metformin and pioglitazone are two oral antidiabetic drugs that may reduce cardiovascular events in patients with type 2 diabetes.[80,81]

References

1. De Backer G, Ambrosioni E, Borch-Johnsen K, et al. European guidelines on cardiovascular disease prevention in clinical practice. Third Joint Task Force of European and Other Societies on Cardiovascular Disease Prevention in Clinical Practice. Eur Heart J 2003;24:1601-10.
2. Conroy RM, Pyorala K, Fitzgerald AP, et al. Estimation of ten-year risk of fatal cardiovascular disease in Europe: the SCORE project. Eur Heart J 2003; 24:987–1003.
3. Shepherd J, Cobbe SM, Ford I, et al. Prevention of coronary heart disease with pravastatin in men with hypercholesterolemia. West of Scotland Coronary Prevention Study Group. N Engl J Med 1995;333(20):1301–1307.
4. Downs JR, Clearfield M, Weis S, et al. Primary prevention of acute coronary events with lovastatin in men and women with average cholesterol levels: results of AFCAPS/TexCAPS. Air Force/Texas Coronary Atherosclerosis Prevention Study. JAMA 1998;279(20):1615–1622.
5. Sever PS, Dahlof B, Poulter NR, et al. ASCOT investigators. Prevention of coronary and stroke events with atorvastatin in hypertensive patients who have average or lower-than- average cholesterol concentrations, in the Anglo-Scandinavian Cardiac Outcomes Trial-Lipid Lowering Arm (ASCOT-LLA): a multicentre randomised controlled trial. Lancet 2003;361(9364):1149–1158.
6. Nissen SE, Tuzcu EM, Schoenhagen P, et al. Effect of intensive compared with moderate lipid-lowering therapy on progression of coronary atherosclerosis. JAMA 2004;291:1071–1080.
7. ESC Expert Consensus Document on the Use of Antiplatelet Agents. Eur Heart J 2004;25:166–181.
8. Peto R, Gray R, Collins R, et al. Randomised trial of prophylactic daily aspirin in British male doctors. BMJ 1988;296(6618):313–316.
9. The Steering Committee of the Physicians' Health Study Research Group. Belanger C, Buring JE, Eberlein K, et al. Preliminary Report: Findings from the aspirin component of the ongoing Physicians' Health Study. N Engl J Med 1988;318: 262–264.
10. Thrombosis prevention trial: randomised trial of low-intensity oral anticoagulation with warfarin and low-dose aspirin in the primary prevention of ischaemic heart disease in men at increased risk. The Medical Research Council's General Practice Research Framework. Lancet 1998;351(9098):233–241.
11. Hansson L, Zanchetti A, Carruthers SG, et al. Effects of intensive blood-pressure lowering and low-dose aspirin in patients with hypertension: principal results of the Hypertension Optimal Treatment (HOT) randomised trial. HOT Study Group. Lancet 1998;351(9118):1755–1762.
12. Sacco M, Pellegrini F, Roncaglioni MC, et al. (PPP Collaborative Group). Primary prevention of cardiovascular events with low-dose aspirin and vitamin E in type 2 diabetic patients: results of the Primary Prevention Project (PPP) trial. Diabetes Care 2003;26(12):3264-1372.
13. Ridker PM, Cook NR, Lee I-M, et al. A Randomized Trial of Low-Dose Aspirin in the Primary Preven-

tion of Cardiovascular Disease in Women. N Engl J Med 2005;352:1293–1304.

14. Elwood P, Baigent C. Aspirin for everyone older than 50?: FOR and AGAINST. BMJ 2005;330;1440–1442.

15. Hernández-Díaz S. Incidence of serious upper gastrointestinal bleeding/perforation in the general population: review of epidemiologic studies J Clin Epidemiol 2002;55:157–639.

16. Patrono C, Coller B, Dalen JE, et al. Platelet-active drugs: the relationships among dose, effectiveness, and side effects. Chest 2001;119:39S–63S.

17. Bhatt DL, Fox KAA, Hacke W, et al. Clopidogrel and aspirin versus aspirin alone for the prevention of atherothrombotic events. N Engl J Med 2006; 354(16):1706–1717.

18. Scandinavian Simvastatin Survival Study (4S) Group. Randomized trial of cholesterol- lowering in 4444 patients with coronary-heart-disease: the Scandinavian Simvastatin Survival Study (4S). Lancet 1994;344:1383–1389.

19. Sacks FM, Pfeffer MA, Moye LA, et al. The Cholesterol and Recurrent Events Trial Investigators: The effect of pravastatin on coronary events after myocardial infarction in patients with average cholesterol levels. N Engl J Med 1996;335:1001–1009.

20. Simes RJ, Marschner IC, Hunt D, et al. (On Behalf of the LIPID Study Investigators). Relationship Between Lipid Levels and Clinical Outcomes in the Long-Term Intervention With Pravastatin in Ischemic Disease (LIPID) Trial. To what extent is the reduction in coronary events with pravastatin explained by on-study lipid levels? Circulation 2002;105:1162–1169.

21. Collins R, Armitage J, Parish S, et al. (Heart Protection Study Collaborative Group). MRC/BHF Heart Protection Study of cholesterol-lowering with simvastatin in 5963 people with diabetes: a randomised placebo-controlled trial. Lancet 2003;361(9374): 2005–2016.

22. Colhoun HM, Betteridge DJ, Durrington PN, et al. Primary prevention of cardiovascular disease with atorvastatin in type 2 diabetes in the Collaborative Atorvastatin Diabetes Study (CARDS): multicentre randomised placebo-controlled trial. Lancet 2004;364 (9435):685–696.

23. Cannon CP, Braunwald E, McCabe CH, et al. Intensive versus moderate lipid lowering with statins after acute coronary syndromes N Engl J Med. 2004;350:1495–1504.

24. Larosa JC, Grundy SM, Waters DD, et al. Intensive lipid lowering with atorvastatin in patients with stable coronary disease. N Engl J Med. 2005;352: 1425–1435.

25. Pedersen TR, Faergeman O, Kastelein JJP, et al. High-dose atorvastatin versus usual-dose simvastatin for secondary prevention after myocardial infarction: the IDEAL study: a randomized controlled trial. JAMA 2005;294:2437–2445.

26. Antithrombotic Trialists' Collaboration. Collaborative metaanalysis of randomised trials of antiplatelet therapy for prevention of death, myocardial infarction, and stroke in high risk patients. BMJ 2002;324:71–86.

27. Patrono C, Rodríguez LAG, Landolfi R, et al. Low-dose aspirin for the prevention of atherothrombosis. N Engl J Med 2005;353:2373–2383.

28. Diener HC, Cunha L, Forbes C, et al. European Stroke Prevention Study 2: dipyridamole and acetylsalicylic acid in the secondary prevention of stroke. J Neurol Sci 1996;143:1–13.

29. CAPRIE Steering Committee. A randomised, blinded trial of clopidogrel versus aspirin in patients at risk of ischaemic events (CAPRIE). Lancet 1996;348:1329–1339.

30. The Clopidogrel in Unstable Angina to Prevent Recurrent Events Trial Investigators. Effects of clopidogrel in addition to aspirin in patients with acute coronary syndromes without ST-segment elevation. N Engl J Med 2001;345:494–502.

31. Steinhubl SR, Berger PB, Mann JT, et al. for the CREDO Investigators. Early and sustained dual oral antiplatelet therapy following percutaneous coronary intervention. A randomized controlled trial. JAMA 2002;288:2411–2420.

32. Sabatine MS, Cannon CP, Gibson CM, et al. (for the CLARITY–TIMI 28 Investigators). Addition of clopidogrel to aspirin and fibrinolytic therapy for myocardial infarction with ST-segment elevation. N Engl J Med 2005;352:1179–1189.

33. Chen ZM, Jiang LX, Chen YP, et al. (COMMIT (ClOpidogrel and Metoprolol in Myocardial Infarction Trial) collaborative group). Addition of clopidogrel to aspirin in 45,852 patients with acute myocardial infarction: randomised placebo-controlled trial. Lancet 2005;366(9497):1607–1621.

34. Bertrand ME, Rupprecht HJ, Urban P, et al. (CLASSICS Investigators). Double-blind study of the safety of clopidogrel with and without a loading dose in combination with aspirin compared with ticlopidine in combination with aspirin after coronary stenting: the clopidogrel aspirin stent international cooperative study (CLASSICS). Circulation 2000;102(6):624–629.

35. Fox KM, Davies GT. Pathophysiology, investigation and treatment of chronic stable angina. In: Julian

DG, Camm AJ, Fox KM, Hall RJC, Poole-Wilson PA, eds. Diseases of the Heart. London: Saunders; 1996;1000–1026.

36. Ferdinand KC. Isosorbide dinitrate and hydralazine hydrochloride: a review of efficacy and safety. Expert Rev Cardiovasc Ther.2005;3(6):993–1001.

37. Parent R, Leblanc N, Lavallee M. Nitroglycerin reduces myocardial oxygen consumption during exercise despite vascular tolerance. Am J Physiol Heart Circ Physiol 2006;290(3):H1226–3124.

38. The Beta-Blocker Pooling Project Research Group. The Beta-Blocker Pooling Project (BBPP): subgroup findings from randomized trials in post infarction patients. Eur Heart J 1988;9:8–16.

39. Savonitto S, Ardissiono D, Egstrup K, et al. Combination therapy with metoprolol and nifedipine versus monotherapy in patients with stable angina pectoris. Results of the International Multicenter Angina Exercise (IMAGE) Study. J Am Coll Cardiol 1996;27:311–316.

40. Gibson RS, Boden WE, Theroux P, et al. Diltiazem and reinfarction in patients with non Q-wave myocardial infarction: results of a double-blind, randomized, multi-center trial. N Engl J Med 1986;315:423.

41. Danish Study Group on Verapamil in Myocardial Infarction. Effect of verapamil on mortality and major events after acute myocardial infarction (the Danish Verapamil Infarction Trial II – DAVIT II). Am J Cardiol 1990;66:779.

42. IONA Study Group. Effect of nicorandil on coronary events in patients with stable angina: the Impact Of Nicorandil in Angina (IONA) randomised trial. Lancet 2002;359(9314):1269–1275.

43. Huikuri HV, Mahaux V, Bloch-Thomsen PE. Cardiac arrhythmias and risk stratification after myocardial infarction: results of the CARISMA pilot study. Pacing Clin Electrophysiol 2003;26(1 Pt 2):416–419.

44. Brignole M, Alboni P, Benditt DG, et al.; Task Force on Syncope, European Society of Cardiology. Guidelines on management (diagnosis and treatment) of syncope – update 2004. Europace 2004; 6(6):467–537.

45. Cleland JG, Khand A, Clark A. The heart failure epidemic: exactly how big is it? Eur Heart J 2001;22(8):623–626.

46. Follath F. Do diuretics differ in terms of clinical outcome in congestive heart failure? Eur Heart J 1998;19(Suppl P):P5–8.

47. Flather MD, Yusuf S, Kober L, et al. Long-term ACE-inhibitor therapy in patients with heart failure or left-ventricular dysfunction: a systematic overview of data from individual patients. ACE-Inhibitor Myocardial Infarction Collaborative Group. Lancet 2000;355(9215):1575–1581.

48. Flather MD, Shibata MC, Coats AJ, et al. (SENIORS Investigators). Randomized trial to determine the effect of nebivolol on mortality and cardiovascular hospital admission in elderly patients with heart failure (SENIORS). Eur Heart J 2005;26(3): 215–225.

49. Packer M, Coats AJ, Fowler MB, et al. (Carvedilol Prospective Randomized Cumulative Survival Study Group). Effect of carvedilol on survival in severe chronic heart failure. N Engl J Med 2001;344(22):1651–1658.

50. The Cardiac Insufficiency Bisoprolol Study II (CIBIS-II): a randomised trial. Lancet. 1999; 353(9146):9–13.

51. MERIT-HF Investigators. Effect of metoprolol CR/XL in chronic heart failure: Metoprolol CR/XL Randomised Intervention Trial in Congestive Heart Failure (MERIT-HF). Lancet 1999;353 (9169):2001–2007.

52. Pfeffer MA, Swedberg K, Granger CB, et al. (CHARM Investigators and Committees). Effects of candesartan on mortality and morbidity in patients with chronic heart failure: the CHARM-Overall programme. Lancet 2003;362(9386):759–766.

53. Pitt B, Zannad F, Remme WJ, et al. The effect of spironolactone on morbidity and mortality in patients with severe heart failure. Randomized Aldactone Evaluation Study Investigators. N Engl J Med 1999;341(10):709–717.

54. Pitt B, Remme W, Zannad F, et al. (Eplerenone Post-Acute Myocardial Infarction Heart Failure Efficacy and Survival Study Investigators). Eplerenone, a selective aldosterone blocker, in patients with left ventricular dysfunction after myocardial infarction. N Engl J Med 2003;348(14):1309–1321.

55. Rich MW, McSherry F, Williford WO, et al. (Digitalis Investigation Group). Effect of age on mortality, hospitalizations and response to digoxin in patients with heart failure: the DIG study. J Am Coll Cardiol 2001;38(3):806–813.

56. Furberg CD, Psaty BM, Manolio TA, et al. Prevalence of atrial fibrillation in elderly subjects (the Cardiovascular Health Study). Am J Cardiol 1994;74: 236–241.

57. Hohnloser SH, Kuck KH, Lilienthal J. Rhythm or rate control in atrial fibrillation: Pharmacological Intervention in Atrial Fibrillation (PIAF): a randomised trial. Lancet 2000;356:1789–1794.

58. Hamer ME, Blumenthal JA, McCarthy EA, et al. Quality-of-life assessment in patients with paroxysmal atrial fibrillation or paroxysmal supraventricular tachycardia. Am J Cardiol 1994;74:826–829.

59. Planning and Steering Committees of the AFFIRM study for the NHLBI AFFIRM investigators. Atrial fibrillation follow-up investigation of rhythm management: the AFFIRM study design. Am J Cardiol 1997;79:1198–1202.

60. Vaughan Williams EM. A classification of antiarrhythmic actions reassessed after a decade of new drugs. J Clin Pharmacol 1984;24:129–147.

61. Stroke Prevention in Atrial Fibrillation Investigators. Predictors of thromboembolism in atrial fibrillation, I: clinical features of patients at risk. Ann Intern Med 1992;116:1–5.

62. Hart RG, Pearce LA, McBride R, et al. (for the Stroke Prevention in Atrial Fibrillation (SPAF) Investigators). Factors associated with ischemic stroke during aspirin therapy in atrial fibrillation: analysis of 2012 participants in the SPAF I-III clinical trials. Stroke 1999;30:1223–1229.

63. Durack DT. Prevention of infective endocarditis. N Engl J Med 1995;332(1):38–44.

64. Fowler VG, Durack DT. Infective endocarditis. Curr Opin Cardiol 1994;9(3):389–400.

65. Horstkotte D, Follath F, Gutschik E, et al.; Task Force Members on Infective Endocarditis of the European Society of Cardiology; ESC Committee for Practice Guidelines (CPG); Document Reviewers. Guidelines on prevention, diagnosis and treatment of infective endocarditis executive summary; the task force on infective endocarditis of the European Society of Cardiology. Eur Heart J. 2004;25(3): 267–276.

66. Jochmann N, Stangl K, Garbe E, et al. Female-specific aspects in the pharmacotherapy of chronic cardiovascular diseases. Eur Heart J 2005,26: 1585–1595.

67. Fiore MC, Bailey W, Cohen SJ, et al. Treating tobacco use and dependence. US Department of Health and Human Services: Agency for Healthcare Research Quality, Rockville, MD; 2000.

68. Gonzales D, Rennard SI, Nides M, et al. For the varenicline phase 3 study group. Varenicline, an a4b2 nicotinic acetylcholine receptor partial agonist, vs sustained-release bupropion and placebo for smoking cessation: a randomized controlled trial. JAMA 2006;296:47–55.

69. Jorenby DE, Hays JT, Rigotti NA, et al. For the varenicline phase 3 study group. Efficacy of varenicline, an a4b2 nicotinic acetylcholine receptor partial agonist vs placebo or sustained-release bupropion for smoking cessation: a randomized controlled trial. JAMA 2006;296:56–63.

70. Tonstad S, Tønnesen P, Hajek P, et al. For the varenicline phase 3 study group. Effect of maintenance therapy with varenicline on smoking cessation. A randomized controlled trial. JAMA 2006;296:64–71.

71. Tonstad S, Johnston JA. Does bupropion have advantages over other medical therapies in the cessation of smoking? Expert Opin Pharmacother 2004;5:727–734.

72. Piciotto MR, Zoli M, Rimondi R, et al. Acetylcholine receptors containing the b2 subunit are involved in the reinforcing properties of nicotine. Nature 1998;39:173–177.

73. Tapper AR, McKinney SL, Nashmi R, et al. Nicotine activation of a4 receptors: sufficient for reward, tolerance, and sensitization. Science 2004;306:1029–1032.

74. Sims TH, Fiore MC. Pharmacotherapy for treating tobacco dependence: what is the ideal duration of therapy? CNS Drugs 2002;16:653–662.

75. Hays JT, Hurt RD, Rigotti NA, et al. Sustained-release bupropion for pharmacologic relapse prevention after smoking cessation: a randomized, controlled trial. Ann Intern Med 2001;135: 423–433.

76. Torgerson JS, Hauptman J, Boldrin MN, et al. Xenical in the prevention of diabetes in obese subjects (XENDOS) study: a randomized study of orlistat as an adjunct to lifestyle changes for the prevention of type 2 diabetes in obese patients. Diabetes Care 2004;27:155–161.

77. James WPT. The SCOUT-study: risk-benefit profile of sibutramine in overweight high-risk cardiovascular patients. Eur Heart J 2005;7(Supplement L):L44–48.

78. Pi-Sunyer FX, Aronne LJ, Heshmati HM, et al. Effect of rimonabant, a cannabinoid-1 receptor blocker, on weight and cardiometabolic risk factors in overweight or obese patients: RIO-North American: a randomized controlled trial. JAMA 2006;295: 761–775.

79. Padwal R, Varney J, Majumdar SR, et al. A systematic review of drug therapy to delay or prevent type 2 diabetes. Diabetes Care 2005;28: 736–744.

80. UK Prospective Diabetes Study (UKPDS) Group. Effect of intensive blood-glucose control with metformin on complications in overweight patients with type 2 diabetes (UKPDS 34). Lancet 1998;352: 854–865.

81. Dormandy JA, Charbonnel B, Eckland DJA, et al. Secondary prevention of macrovascular events in patients with type 2 diabetes in the PROactive Study (PROspective pioglitAzone Clinical Trial in macroVascular Events): a randomised controlled trial. Lancet 2005;366:1279–1289.

54
Rehabilitation Modalities

Pantaleo Giannuzzi

Background and Rationale

Cardiac rehabilitation (CR) programs were first developed in the 1960s when the benefits of ambulation during prolonged hospitalization for coronary events had been documented. Exercise was the primary component of these programs. They were predominantly offered to survivors of uncomplicated myocardial infarction and initiated at a time remote from the acute event. Concern about the safety of unsupervised exercise after discharge led to the development of highly structured rehabilitation programs that were supervised by physicians and included electrocardiographic monitoring. The safety and benefits of moderate-intensity exercise training programs were intensively investigated in supervised programs. More recent data clearly indicate that unsupervised or home-based programs are also safe and effective in appropriately selected patients.[1-11] Furthermore, favorable effects of exercise training have also been demonstrated in patients with large myocardial infarctions, left ventricular dysfunction, and even heart failure.[12-22]

During the past three decades, changes in the delivery of rehabilitative care for cardiac patients have reflected changes in demography and characteristics of the patients, and predominantly reflect changes in clinical care. In the early years of CR, most patients enrolled in exercise training programs were those who had recovered from uncomplicated myocardial infarction. In subsequent years, post-infarction patients with complications were also included and considered for more limited and gradual exercise rehabilitation. Many patients who currently receive rehabilitation services are recovering from CABG, PCI or other forms of myocardial revascularization. With aging of the population, cardiac rehabilitative care is now provided to a sizeable number of older patients, many of whom have severe and complicated coronary illness and serious associated pathologies.[3,4,5,12] Furthermore, many patients once considered to be too high risk for structured rehabilitation programs, such as patients with residual myocardial ischemia, compensated heart failure, serious arrhythmias, and implanted cardiac devices (pacemaker, ventricular resynchronization, ICD), currently derive benefit from more gradual and more protracted and often supervised exercise training.[3,4,7,9,10,12,22] This is combined with education, counseling, behavioral strategies and other psychosocial interventions and vocational counseling strategies to assist the patient to achieve coronary risk reduction and other cardiovascular health-related goals.[4,12]

CR is now considered a multifactorial process that includes clinical assistance and optimized therapy to relieve symptoms and achieve clinical stability, exercise training, education and counseling regarding risk reduction and lifestyle changes, the use of behavioral interventions, vocational counseling, and adequate follow-up. These services are an essential component of the contemporary management of patients with multiple presentations of coronary heart disease and with heart failure and should be integrated into a long-term comprehensive care of all cardiac patients.

The progressive aging of the population, the increasing accuracy of diagnostic procedures, and the spreading use of potent cardiovascular drugs for the treatment of acute coronary syndromes and heart failure will lead to an estimated increase in the prevalence of ischemic heart disease of about 30%, even with a predicted decrease in incidence rate of 25%. The population is clearly becoming older and sicker, and the prevalence of serious co-morbid conditions such as diabetes mellitus and cerebrovascular diseases among patients admitted for acute coronary syndromes is striking. The demographics of patients undergoing surgical coronary revascularization and valvular interventions are changing rapidly as well. This population is characteristically older, more commonly female, advanced in age, likely to have three-vessel disease or abnormal left ventricular (LV) function, co-morbidity, and more complications. In addition, because of the aging of the population, the number of patients with chronic heart failure and the healthcare impact of this syndrome is growing. All of these patients have a great need for cardiac care, clinical assistance, and psychosocial support after the acute phase.

Importantly, with continuing shortening of length of stay, the amount of time spent in the hospital during the acute event is no longer adequate to verify clinical stability, to perform a comprehensive risk stratification, to promote functional recovery, and to acquire the skills required to monitor exercise activity or to cover the educational material adequately. For these reasons, we see a greater need for structured residential CR programs, especially for high-risk patients and those more incapacitated, to facilitate the transition to an independent life at home and the adherence to an individualized, long-lasting outpatient program for clinical monitoring, lifestyle changes, and effective secondary prevention.

Risk Stratification for Appropriate Modality of CR

Authoritative, detailed documents addressing the organizational structure, delivery, and management approaches to CR services highlight the value of *risk stratification* of cardiac patients as a basis for *individual* therapeutic interventions, prescription of exercise training and appropriate exercise supervision, educational and behavioral interventions.

Medical evaluation of the patients, including complications during the acute event and present clinical status, and assessment of their level of risk are the first steps of CR. This stratification should include the evaluation of the risk of progression of coronary artery disease (namely known coronary risk factors and inappropriate lifestyle) and the risk of cardiovascular events. Risk stratification of cardiac events is based on the assessment of clinical stability, of ventricular dysfunction, functional capacity, myocardial ischemia and arrhythmias. The initial assessment should incorporate the patient's educational, psychosocial status, lifestyle and social needs as a basis for recommending interventions.

Patients are classified as at low, intermediate or high risk level (Table 54-1).

TABLE 54-1. Risk stratification

Low risk
- Uncomplicated in-hospital course during the acute phase
- Preserved left ventricular function (i.e. ejection fraction ≥50%)
- No detectable residual ischemia or complex arrhythmias
- Functional capacity >6 METs on graded exercise

Intermediate risk
- Left ventricular ejection fraction between 31% and 49% or below 40% with preserved functional capacity
- Myocardial ischemia at intermediate level or exercise ST-segment depression below 2 mm, or reversible defects during stress echocardiography or nuclear radiography
- No sustained ventricular arrhythmias

High risk
- Survivors of sudden cardiac arrest or acute phase complications: cardiogenic shock, heart failure, severe arrhythmias, respiratory insufficiency, recurrent ischemia
- Persistent clinical instability: decompensation, respiratory distress, renal insufficiency, infections, marked deconditioning
- Severely depressed LV function (i.e. ejection fraction ≤30%) or below 40% with low functional capacity
- Marked induced myocardial ischemia with ST-segment depression >2 mm, extensive ischemia occurring at low threshold (<6 METs or <100 watts), or severe reversible perfusion defect
- Complex ventricular arrhythmias at rest or during exercise, a drop in systolic blood pressure of ≥15 mmHg during effort or failure to rise during graded exercise testing, with high level of disability

CR Services and Patterns of Rehabilitative Care

The WHO classifies CR facilities into three categories depending on the qualifications of staff members, on the equipment, and on the complexity and specialization of interventions: (a) basic facilities, delivering care and interventions at the community level (using schools, gymnasiums, clubs); (b) intermediate facilities developed within a city hospital; (c) advanced facilities in a major CR center, where high levels of medical services are available.

Basic facilities should be reserved for low-risk patients, mainly directed towards stable, chronic patients, in order to maintain them at the highest level of independence, to promote appropriate lifestyle changes for effective secondary prevention, and to reduce the risk of subsequent cardiac events. Intermediate or advanced CR facilities should be reserved for patients in the early phase of their disease and for those with high- or intermediate-risk stratification. Different patterns of rehabilitative care are currently delivered by specialized hospital-based teams: residential CR for more complicated, disabled patients; and outpatient CR for more independent, low-risk and clinically stable patients requiring less supervision. There may be variations of individual or group programs and center-based or home-based programs.

While the objectives are identical to those of the outpatient CR programs, residential rehabilitation programs are specifically structured to provide more intensive and/or complex interventions, and have the advantage being able to start early after the acute event, to include more complicated high-risk or clinically unstable patients, to include more severely incapacitated and/or elderly patients (especially those with co-morbidity), and thus, to facilitate the transition from the hospital phase to a more stable clinical condition which may allow the maintenance of an independent life at home. One major disadvantage of residential programs is the relatively short duration of intervention with regard to risk factor management and lifestyle changes. Therefore, residential

CR programs should be followed up by a long-term outpatient risk reduction and secondary prevention program, with appropriate clinical and functional monitoring. Home-based rehabilitation programs directed by physicians and coordinated by nurses have also been developed as a way of expanding the delivery of secondary prevention services.

The former ESC Working Group on Cardiac Rehabilitation and Exercise Physiology (at present European Association for Cardiovascular Prevention and Rehabilitation)[3] strongly emphasizes that CR programs should consist of a multifaceted and multidisciplinary approach to overall cardiovascular risk reduction, and that programs that consist of exercise training alone are not considered CR. It should be also recognized that exercise is often the vehicle for facilitating other aspects of CR, including coronary risk reduction and optimization of psychosocial support. Thus, evaluation of the overall quality of life impact should become an integral part of outcome measures of rehabilitation.

Core components of cardiac rehabilitation/secondary prevention programs are: baseline patient assessment, physical activity counseling and exercise training, nutritional counseling, risk factor management (lipids, hypertension, weight, diabetes, and smoking), psychosocial management, vocational counseling, and optimized medical therapy. The way CR is delivered varies depending on national circumstances and resources. The provision of these services by specialized hospital-based teams in an outpatient setting is recommended, and a period of 8–12 weeks is considered adequate to cover the core components of cardiac rehabilitation/secondary prevention programs appropriately. Shorter programs may be considered under special circumstances but their efficiency is not proven in the literature. All patients after an acute cardiovascular event should be entered into a comprehensive, multidisciplinary intensive CR program. On completion of this "introductory" program of secondary prevention, they should be oriented to a long-term maintenance regimen with the use of support systems such as coronary clubs, gymnasia or other facilities to promote long-term prevention strategies in the community.

Indications for Residential CR

Generally, residential CR, either in a city hospital or in a major CR center, is preferable for intermediate- and high-risk patients, especially for those with a complicated in-hospital course during the acute phase or persistent clinical instability, to promote more stable clinical conditions and a more rapid functional recovery.

Residential CR programs are reserved for the following categories of patients:

(a) patients with severe in-hospital complications after myocardial infarction, cardiac surgery, or percutaneous transluminal coronary angioplasty

(b) patients with persistent clinical instability or complications after the acute event, or serious concomitant diseases at high risk of cardiovascular events

(c) clinically unstable patients with advanced heart failure (class III and IV), particularly those who are candidates for heart transplantation, and/or those needing intermittent or continuous drug infusion and/or mechanical support

(d) patients after a recent heart transplantation.

In addition,

(e) patients discharged very early after the acute event, even uncomplicated, particularly if they are older, females, or at higher risk of progression of coronary artery disease, and

(f) patients unable to attend a formal outpatient CR program for any logistic reasons should also be considered for residential CR programs.

Programs and Staffing for Residential CR

Residential CR at an intermediate level should assure basic clinical care and ability to cope with any possible emergencies; noninvasive prognostic and functional evaluation for comprehensive risk stratification; controlled exercise training with appropriate supervision; health education programs and counseling regarding risk reduction and lifestyle changes; psychosocial status assessment and the use of behavioral interventions. Therefore, in addition to cardiologists, the staff must include nurses, rehabilitation therapists, a dietitian, and a psycholoist in consultation with an occupational health specialist.

Advanced residential CR is provided in highly specialized major CR centers, where a high level of medical services, well-qualified staff members, multidisciplinary care, assistance and interventions are available. They should offer sophisticated noninvasive diagnostic techniques (including nuclear cardiology); invasive procedures and monitoring (right-heart hemodynamics); ergometric and occupational evaluation with appropriate interventions; a deep screening for known and less well-known coronary risk factors, including genetic determinations particularly for patients with premature coronary artery disease; specific educational and behavioral interventions and psychosocial support for selected patients.

An intermediate care unit or heart failure unit is also required for treatment and monitoring of more complicated, clinically unstable patients, especially those with advanced heart failure, and those potential candidates or in a waiting list for heart transplantation. In these patients, multidisciplinary clinical and psychosocial support, appropriate health educational and vocational interventions, together with adequate follow-up in collaboration with the family physician should be provided.

After the residential interventions, CR should be continued and integrated into a long-lasting outpatient program either at an intermediate or advanced CR service, depending on the patient's needs.

Conclusion

Although the objectives are identical to those of the outpatient cardiac rehabilitation (CR) programs, residential rehabilitation programs are specifically structured to provide more intensive and/or complex interventions, and have the advantage being able (1) to start earlier after the acute event, (2) to include high-risk, more complicated or clinically unstable patients, (3) to include more severely incapacitated and/or elderly patients (especially those with co-morbidity), and thus, (4) to facilitate the transition from the hospital phase to a more stable clinical condition and the maintenance of an independent life at home. Ideally, residential CR programs should be followed up by a long-lasting outpatient risk reduction and secondary prevention program, with appropriate clinical and functional monitoring.

References

1. Recommendations by the Working Group on Cardiac Rehabilitation of the European Society of Cardiology. Longterm comprehensive care of cardiac patients. Eur Heart J 1992;13(Suppl C):1C–45C.
2. Rehabilitation after cardiovascular diseases, with special emphasis on developing countries: report of a WHO Committee. World Health Organ Tech Rep Ser 1993;831:1–122.
3. Giannuzzi P, et al. Position Paper of the Working group on Cardiac Rehabilitation and Exercise Physiology of the European Society of Cardiology. Eur Heart J 2003;24:1273–1278.
4. Ades PA. Cardiac rehabilitation and secondary prevention of coronary heart disease. N Engl J Med 2001;345:892–902.
5. Pasquali SK, Alexander KP, Peterson ED. Cardiac rehabilitation in the elderly. Am Heart J 2001; 142(5):748–755.
6. EUROASPIRE II Study Group. EUROASPIRE II. Lifestyle and risk factor management and use of drug therapies in coronary patients from 15 countries. Eur Heart J 2001;22:554–572.
7. Wenger NK, Froelicher ES, Smith LK, et al. Cardiac rehabilitation. Clinical practice guideline. No. 17 Rockville, MD: US. Department of Health and Human Services, Public Health Service, Agency for Health Care Policy and Research and the National Heart, Lung, and Blood Institute. AHCPR No. 96-0672. October 1995.
8. Fletcher GF, Balady G, Blair SN, et al. Statement on exercise: benefits and recommendations for physical activity programs for all Americans. A statement for health professionals by the committee on exercise and cardiac rehabilitation of the council on clinical cardiology, American Heart Association. Circulation 1996;94:857–862.
9. Cobelli F, Tavazzi L. Relative role of ambulatory and residential rehabilitation. J Cardiovasc Risk 1996;3: 172–175.
10. Effective Health Care: Cardiac rehabilitation. Effective Health Care Bulletins 1998;4(4):1–12.
11. Monpere C. Cardiac rehabilitation: guidelines and recommendations. Dis Manage Health Outcomes 1998;4:143–156.
12. Balady GJ, Ades PA, Comoss P, et al. Core components of cardiac rehabilitation/secondary prevention programs. A statement for healthcare professionals from the American Heart Association and the American Association of Cardiovascular and Pulmonary Rehabilitation. Circulation 2000; 102:1069–1073.
13. Smith SC, Blair SN, Bonow RO, et al. AHA/ACC guidelines for preventing heart attack and death in patients with atherosclerotic cardiovascular disease: 2001 update. Circulation 2001;104:1577–1599.
14. Fletcher GF, Balady GJ, Ezra A, et al. AHA scientific statement: exercise standards for testing and training. Circulation 2001;104:1694–1740.
15. Jolliffe JA, Rees K, Taylor RS, et al. Exercise-based rehabilitation for coronary heart disease. The Cochrane Library, Issue 3, 2001.
16. Dugmore LD, Tipson RJ, Phillips MH, et al. Changes in cardiorespiratory fitness, psychological well-being, quality of life, and vocational status following a 12 month cardiac exercise rehabilitation programme. Heart 1999;81:359–366.
17. Oldridge NB, Guyatt GH, Fischer ME, et al. Cardiac rehabilitation after myocardial infarction. Combined experience of randomized clinical trials. JAMA 1988;260:945–950.
18. O'Connor GT, Buring JE, Yusuf S, et al. An overview of randomized trials of rehabilitation with exercise after myocardial infarction. Circulation 1989;80: 234–244.
19. Vanhees L, Mc Gee HM, Dugmore LD, Schepers D, Van Daele P; Carinex Working Group: Cardiac Rehabilitation Information Exchange. A representative study of cardiac rehabilitation activities in European Union Member States: the Carinex survey. J Cardiopulm Rehabil 2002;22(4):264–272.
20. Hambrecht R, Gielen S, Linke A, et al. Effects of exercise training on left ventricular function and peripheral resistance in patients with chronic heart failure: A randomized trial. JAMA 2000;283:3095–3101.
21. Belardinelli R, Georgiou D, Cianci G, et al. Randomized controlled trial of long-term moderate

exercise training in chronic heart failure: effects on functional capacity, quality of life, and clinical outcome. Circulation 1999;99:1173–1182.

22. Giannuzzi P, Tavazzi L, Meyer K, et al. for the Working Group on Cardiac Rehabilitation and Exercise Physiology and Working Group on Heart Failure of the European Society of Cardiology. Recommendations for exercise training in chronic heart failure patients. Eur Heart J 2001;22:125–135.

55

Developing Cardiac Rehabilitation Services: From Policy Development to Staff Training Programs

John H. Horgan

Introduction

The provision of multifactorial cardiac rehabilitation and secondary prevention strategies requires a range of skills and knowledge which, while understood by cardiologists, are delivered only in part by them. The role of the cardiologist in the initiation of cardiac rehabilitation programs is self-evident. As patient advisors, cardiologists are in an ideal position to recommend the benefits of cardiac rehabilitation to the individual patient. They are also in a prime position within the health services and individual medical institutions to espouse the establishment and appropriate financial support of such services. However, most cardiologists today, while appreciating the value of secondary prevention as an essential follow-up to cardiovascular interventions including surgery, are not in a position to provide personally the advice and supervision of the individual patient's activities that is required, due to the time demands of the greatly expanded application of new technologies in cardiovascular services.

There are thus a number of distinct challenges to ensuring the provision of cardiac rehabilitation services.[1] Firstly, cardiologists must work at the policy and health service level to promote the establishment and ongoing provision of cardiac rehabilitation services. In tandem with this "top down" approach, cardiologists must ensure that as resources become available, they can ensure the provision of high quality cardiac rehabilitation programs for their patients. This needs to be achieved through the provision of appropriately trained cardiac rehabilitation staff. In this era of

rapid scientific development, cardiologists must start with their own training. Leading a cardiac rehabilitation team requires academic and team management skills. Alongside this there needs to be training for other health professionals who will work with the cardiologist to deliver the program for patients. This "bottom up" approach of providing staff appropriately trained to deliver services is an essential counterpoint to the more "top down" activities necessary to deliver policy and resource change in the provision of cardiac rehabilitation services. These three issues are dealt with in the next sections with illustrations of how that can be addressed.

Health Policy Changes to Promote Cardiac Rehabilitation Service Delivery

It is essential that cardiac rehabilitation services are identified and supported in national strategic, policy and policy implementation documents if these services are to be established and maintained and not subject to budgetary or other influences in the health or wider economic systems. Having clear commitments to service delivery is the most important protection that cardiac rehabilitation services can have. It allows individuals and centers or regions to look for the services that are committed and to resist efforts to dismantle services in the interests of other priorities, for example removing or reducing space or redeploying staffing already committed to cardiac rehabilitation services. Thus it is worth a lot of investment of time by individuals to this higher order aim, as when there is policy level protection, the debates can be about "how" to provide services rather than about "will you" provide services.

A number of countries have developed explicit national policies on cardiac rehabilitation services. Two examples are the Republic of Ireland and the United Kingdom. The UK's strategy – *A National Service Framework for Coronary Heart Disease* (2000) – has 12 sets of standards with one dedicated to cardiac rehabilitation.[2] The Republic of Ireland's first national cardiovascular strategy – entitled *Building Healthier Hearts* (1999) – identified cardiac rehabilitation as a key aspect of services, devoted a whole chapter to it and produced 10 specific recommendations.[3] These recommendations endorsed the need to expand cardiac rehabilitation services to all hospitals treating patients with heart disease; to have these programs supervised by a cardiologist/physician with a special interest in cardiology; to have programs run by a specially trained cardiac rehabilitation coordinator; to ensure a system of rehabilitation starting from phase I in hospital to phase IV in long-term community maintenance; to ensure adequate funding for staff training, equipment and facilities; and to develop a national audit system for cardiac rehabilitation. The impact of a national strategy on cardiac rehabilitation service development has been significant. A review before the strategy commenced showed that only 29% of relevant hospitals had a cardiac rehabilitation program in 1998.[4] The first recommendation of the strategy in relation to cardiac rehabilitation was that "every hospital that treats patients with heart disease should provide a cardiac rehabilitation service." Five years later, in 2003, a repeat survey showed that 77% had programs, with the remainder in advanced stages of planning.[5]

The benefits to cardiac rehabilitation service development are evident following a focused health service strategy in which cardiac rehabilitation was prioritized. Thus collective efforts across centers to encourage the prioritization of cardiac rehabilitation in national health policy initiatives can be a very efficient method of supporting development. The next challenge in the Irish system, as in others, is to ensure optimum levels of service uptake among cardiac patients. A recent study estimating the total number of patients referred to and completing cardiac rehabilitation programs in the UK in 2000 found that only 45–67% of patients were referred while just 27–41% attended.[6] On a more European-wide front, a 1996 survey found levels never exceeding 50% across 13 of the then 15 EU member states.[7] Another "top down" recommendation of the Irish strategy was the development of a national audit system. This has been achieved and is currently being rolled out nationally. It is also forming a basis for European initiatives in this area. These have been developed with current European guidelines in mind.[8] Only in this way can the real gap between service availability and universal service delivery be achieved. The CARINEX project demonstrated that service uptake was a particular challenge across all of the EU states surveyed.[7] While centers could produce numbers in terms of program throughput, particularly at phase III, very few could say what proportion of eligible patients were being serviced and why others were not invited or did not attend. These examples given here of the Irish system are to illustrate how individuals, centers, regions or national groups such as cardiac rehabilitation associations or professional bodies such as national cardiac societies can use "top down" approaches. Documentation may prove beneficial so that those interested in this approach do not have to undertake development de novo.

In terms of moving to "bottom up" approaches, specific training for professionals is considered next.

Professional Training for Cardiac Rehabilitation: Training for Cardiologists

Countries that have put in place policies to review the provision of cardiac rehabilitation services have uniformly recommended the involvement of a cardiologist or a cardiovascular physician as an essential requirement for the establishment of programs. At present, however, the training of most cardiologists does not include a mandatory requirement to obtain experience in the areas of rehabilitation or secondary prevention although the acquisition of knowledge in this area is recommended. It can no longer be assumed that the knowledge required to impart appropriate advice in terms of secondary prevention strategies can be obtained during the clinical rotations which form part of most cardiology training programs. Given the importance of national guidelines, with their emphasis on primary and secondary prevention, it is essential that future cardiology training programs worldwide should obligate trainees to acquire experience of the broad area of secondary prevention and rehabilitation, the value of which is becoming increasingly obvious and is supported by a growing literature as outlined in great detail elsewhere in this book. The European Society of Cardiology has made significant developments in this field with a core curriculum now established. This will be an important mechanism to ensure cardiac rehabilitation has effective leadership in the coming decades.

Professional Training for Cardiac Rehabilitation: Training for Other Health Professionals

The multifactorial nature of cardiac rehabilitation requires the expertise of a range of non-medical heath professionals including nurses, physiotherapists, occupational therapists, physical educationalists, nutritionist, pharmacists, vocational counselors, and psychologists. The exact combination in a team may differ from country to country depending on the resources available in terms of staffing and roles among different professional groups. While not every team will require the input of each of the above, many of the areas of special expertise peculiar to these professional groups are of particular value in designing and/or delivering cardiac rehabilitation programs. The education of these individuals, however, will have been confined to the core focus of their specialty and no in-depth training in cardiovascular disease is generally provided, even in the case of nurses. The rapid advances in

our understanding of cardiovascular pathology means that staff working in this area must have a basic familiarity with cardiovascular medicine and its treatments.

While it is unreasonable to expect all professionals in these other disciplines who interact with cardiac patients to have an extensive knowledge of modern cardiovascular medicine and surgery, those entrusted with the coordination of rehabilitation programs should have a mechanism by which such an overall knowledge can be obtained. Such individuals can provide a valuable link between the cardiologist, other members of the cardiac rehabilitation team, and the patient. To address this need for specialist education of those who will coordinate cardiac rehabilitation programs in the Irish context, an educational program was established with emphasis on the provision of a broad general training in cardiac rehabilitation program delivery. It is characterized by its multidisciplinary approach to cardiac rehabilitation and the combination of clinical and academic training. The aim is to produce cardiac rehabilitation coordinators who practice their profession in a way that combines attention to best practice from clinical and research evidence with sensitivity to the needs of individual patients. Such training can help promote cohesion among cardiac rehabilitation centers and promote acceptable standards of service to patients. In recognition of the course coverage and standard, the program now leads to a Masters in Cardiac Rehabilitation (MSc Cardiac Rehab) through the National University of Ireland and the Royal College of Surgeons in Ireland. The course outline has been published[9] and is briefly outlined here.

The aim of the course is to provide professional training for health professionals to qualify them to develop and coordinate cardiac rehabilitation programs within the healthcare services. The objective is to ensure that through the integration of theoretical and clinical training, graduates will be able to promote the delivery of multifactorial cardiac rehabilitation services. Trainees are provided with the knowledge and skills to coordinate the activities of a multidisciplinary cardiac rehabilitation team. The course is based on a scientist-practitioner model with the practice of cardiac rehabilitation grounded on scientific research. The course has both an academic and skills-based component. It produces graduates who will practice their profession in a way that combines attention to best practice from clinical and research evidence with sensitivity to the needs of individual patients. The course is run over an academic year. The first component is an intensive course of both formal lectures and practical sessions in physiology, exercise training, exercise stress testing, and psychological counseling The second component is an intensive course of both formal lectures and practical sessions in psychology, exercise training, and exercise stress testing. This includes off-site visits to other cardiac rehabilitation centers for further training. The final component comprises attendance at formal lectures on research methodology followed by individual completion of a course-related research thesis.

Trainees are assigned to the various components of a multidisciplinary cardiac rehabilitation service to learn the skills of various team members. Staff include cardiologists, nurses, medical staff, ECG technicians, exercise physiologists, anatomists, psychologists and a dietician, pharmacist and vocational officer. All trainees must possess Basic Life Support (BLS) and Advanced Cardiac Life Support (ACLS) certification before completion of the program. Academic content is summarized in Table 55-1.

The total number of contact teaching hours are 360, with a further 300 hours of directed learning.

The clinical training aims to ensure that trainees are competent in planning and supervising multifactorial cardiac rehabilitation classes. Training in planning and design of cardiac rehabilitation programs is provided, for example choice of safe and appropriate locations for

exercise and other components, report writing, referral letters, class planning, and coordination with other disciplines. Trainees are assigned to the various components of the cardiac rehabilitation setting to learn the skills and activities of the various team members. Trainees acquire practical experience with ECG technicians, psychologists, and a dietitian, pharmacist and vocational officer. Trainees are required to successfully run both psycho-educational and exercise classes. These classes are graded by the supervising professionals and contribute to course grades.

It has been an important principle of the course that students can be from any of the health professional disciplines (since the training is not in service delivery but in service coordination and management). In practice, since in many situations the coordinator will fulfil this and other roles in a program, they have mostly been experienced cardiac nurses with some physiotherapists and physicians. The course has unseen written exams, a course planning project, grades for practical/clinical work, a research dissertation, and an oral examination, all overseen by an external examiner. For those who opt not to do the research dissertation component (since this may not be of interest to or a personal strength of the professional involved), a diploma is available on successful completion. To date, having started in 1992, 51 students have graduated with diplomas from the program with 11 undertaking research dissertations for MSc qualifications.

The development of this training program in the early 1990s was undertaken to bridge the gap between aspiration and action for busy cardiologists committed to the concept. It has proven to be the enabler for national development of programs. Some cardiologists have been able to have selected staff released for training in order to run programs in the hospital which are cardiologist led but coordinator provided and managed. Training was supported by hospitals and also importantly by the national heart association – the Irish Heart Foundation. Staff training also meant that as soon as there was a national commitment to providing cardiac rehabilitation through

TABLE 55-1. MSc program: theory-based and competency-based components (allocated hours)

	Theory-based	Competency-based	Total
Physiology	40	17	57
Clinical cardiology	40	–	40
Cardiac rehabilitation	88	155	243
Research methodology	20	–	20

the national strategy in 1999, there was a cadre of highly trained and motivated professionals to undertake this work. Some of the graduates also took up health service management positions to implement the cardiovascular strategy when it was launched and thus the message of the value of cardiac rehabilitation services was communicated to a much wider and different audience within the health system. This shows how bottom up and top down approaches can be very complementary in promoting cardiac rehabilitation development.

Conclusion

The rehabilitation system as it has evolved can be seen as the prototype of the concept of the cardiac care teams now utilized in the provision of acute chest pain and heart failure clinics. The establishment of such teams has already begun to mitigate to some extent problems arising from the interventional burden which has devolved on cardiologists. The financial implication of the sharing of clinical responsibility between physicians and non-physician members of cardiac teams may be seen by third party payers as a mechanism by which costs of care can be reduced and availability enhanced. It is critical, therefore, that outcomes are evaluated so that decisions concerning the sharing of specific responsibilities can be based on evidence that these changes have brought about improved outcomes. A trans-national agreed system would be of great importance in facilitating international comparisons. The strategies outlined here can go a long way towards achieving the desired goal.

References

1. Horgan JH, McGee HM. Cardiac rehabilitation: future directions. In: Jones D, West R, eds. Cardiac Rehabilitation. London: BMJ Publishing; 1995.
2. Department of Health. A National Service Framework for Coronary Heart Disease. London: Department of Health; 2000.
3. Department of Health. Building Healthier Hearts. The report of the Cardiovascular Health Strategy Group. Dublin: Government Publications; 1999.
4. McGee HM, Hevey D, Horgan JH. Cardiac rehabilitation service provision in Ireland. Ir J Med Sci 2001;170:159–162.
5. Lavin D, Hevey D, McGee HM, De la Harpe D, Kiernan M, Shelley E. Cardiac rehabilitation services in Ireland: the impact of a coordinated national development strategy. Ir J Med Sci 2005;174(4): 33–38.
6. Griebsch I, Brown J, Rees K, et al. Is provision and funding of cardiac rehabilitation appropriate for the achievement of national service framework goals? Proceedings from the Society of Social Medicine 47th Annual Scientific Meeting, Edinburgh, 17–19th Sep 2003.
7. Vanhees L, McGee HM, Dugmore LD, Schepers D, Van Daele P. A representative Study of Cardiac Rehabilitation Activities in European Union Member States. The Carinex Survey. J Cardiopulm Rehabil 2002;22:264–272.
8. Giannuzzi P, Saner H, Bjornstad H, et al. Secondary prevention through cardiac rehabilitation: position paper of the Working Group on Cardiac Rehabilitation and Exercise Physiology of the European Society of Cardiology. Eur Heart J 2003;24: 1273–1278.
9. Hevey D, McGee, Cahill A, Newton H, Horgan, JH. Training cardiac rehabilitation co-ordinators. Coronary Health Care 2000;4:142–145.

56
Safety Aspects of Cardiac Rehabilitation

Bo Hedbäck

In a comprehensive cardiac rehabilitation program, the different forms of physical training may put patients at risk, although a review of the literature has shown that cardiac or orthopedic events rarely occur. This may be further limited through adequate safety precautions. The risk is fully outweighed by the benefits of participation, independent of the indication for enrollment: after myocardial infarction (MI), percutaneous coronary intervention, coronary artery bypass grafting, in patients with chronic heart failure or in patients with implantable cardioversion devices (ICD).[1-3]

Dynamic Exercise Training

There are few reports on the risks for cardiac patients of participating in physical training programs and these concern mainly dynamic exercise training.[4-7]

Collecting data by means of a questionnaire or a telephone interview, Haskell reported in 1978 from the United States a rate of one cardiac arrest per 111,996 patient-hours of physical exercise.[4] Van Camp and Peterson found in 1986 a cardiac arrest rate of one per 32,593 training hours.[5] Data from Cantwell showed in 1993 a major event rate of one per 31,226.[6]

More recently, VanHees et al. published a hospital-based program from Belgium with a rate of one cardiac arrest per 29,214 patient-hours. The use of antiarrhythmic agents and the presence of ST depression at baseline were predictive of complications requiring resuscitation in the course of the program. During an observation period of 20 years two patients suffered an acute myocardial infarction and four patients developed ventricular tachycardia with temporary loss of consciousness.[7]

According to the author's experience from a Swedish program, four cardiac arrests occurred during high-intensity physical training from 1980 to 1995, which were successfully resuscitated. This indicates a larger cardiac arrest rate of approximately one per 10,000 training hours, which may be explained by the inclusion of patients at high risk (large size MI with persisting moderate heart failure).[8]

Resistance Training

Over the years, training modalities have been extended from mainly dynamic exercise for coronary patients at low risk to more extensive models combining dynamic exercise with resistance training[9] or even exercise in swimming pools at a thermoneutral water temperature (32–35°C). Patients at higher risk, for example with moderate chronic heart failure, patients waiting for cardiac transplant and post-transplant patients, and patients with an ICD, are more often enrolled in adapted physical training.[10,11]

Resistance training is widely utilized and appears to be safe: there is one report of more than 26,000 maximal dynamic strength assessments done without a single cardiovascular event.[12] However, resistance training may be hazardous for a small percentage of the population. Haykowsky et al.[13] reported three cases of nonfatal subarachnoid hemorrhage associated with weight-lifting training. This was probably due to a previously innocuous intracranial aneurysm which ruptured in response to a marked increase in intracerebral pressure caused by the effort. For the estimated 1% of the population with an undetected intracranial aneurysm, resistance training may be inappropriate but at present most cases remain undiagnosed.

Resistance training may even cause injuries from the musculoskeletal system. Shaw et al.[14] have proposed a standardized questionnaire to evaluate injuries and complaints of muscular soreness which cause the individual to alter or stop the physical training.

Hydrotherapy

Physical training in water may lead to hemodynamic adaptations which might be clinically relevant for heart failure patients,[15] but when training is restricted to patients with mild to moderate heart failure the benefits may well be obtained. This type of training may be an attractive alternative for elderly patients, in whom arthritic joint and osteoporotic complaints limit conventional physical exercise.[16] However, special safety precautions must be taken as cardiopulmonary resuscitation in a wet environment may be dangerous.

The Risk Today?

No study covers the last decade in which the acute management of the coronary patient has changed the clinical picture of the participant in cardiac rehabilitation. On the one hand, if fewer patients have residual ischemia after a cardiac event, this would result in a lower level of risk of complications during exercise. On the other hand, the early studies included mainly patients at low risk. Today more elderly and high-risk patients are enrolled in the physical training programs, for example patients with chronic heart failure, ICD or with transcutaneous epidural analgesia (TEDA). Even if this may increase the risk of adverse events one might assume that the landwinnings of modern cardiology will lead to a considerably lower event rate than one per 30,000 patient-hours of training.

Contraindications

Even though most patients are eligible for physical training programs, there are still contraindications for participation: the presence of unstable angina, symptomatic ventricular arrhythmia, and/or insufficiently stabilized or severe heart failure.

Patients with unstable angina should be referred immediately to cardiological care for further investigation. Therefore we recommend that the cardiac rehabilitation (CR) staff inquire about the state of health of patients before the training session starts in order to detect signs of angina or other significant symptoms (heart failure, infectious disease, side-effect of medication).

Patients with symptomatic ventricular arrhythmias (dizziness or fainting) should not be allowed to participate in exercise training. A referral to a cardiologist is needed and after adequate medication or if needed an ICD, they may join or re-enter the program.

Patients with chronic heart failure should be stable and on optimal medication. They should be informed to contact a physician before joining the program if symptoms of worsening heart failure occur during daily activities.

Safety Precautions

Safety in a physical training program commences with an adequate risk stratification of the patient independent of the type of exercise training that will be provided. All relevant data from the patient's medical history, the acute care period, the ongoing medication, and planned therapy should be available for the CR team. Information to the participants on the content of the program must be given, the patient should be reassured about the risks of exertion but at the same time be encouraged to report any symptoms before, during and directly after exercise. An individually targeted training intensity and duration is needed to reduce the risk of overstraining the patient.

ECG telemetry monitoring remains a controversial issue, as monitoring will have a considerable economic impact on the program, which can not be motivated by health-economic gains. Yet, if telemetry monitoring is available, patients with a low left ventricular ejection fraction (<30%), with an increase of arrhythmia during exercise (ventricular extrasystole, occurrence of atrial fibrillation), and patients with known severe coronary artery disease and/or signs of residual ischemia during exercise testing (≥ 2 mV) may be candidates for ECG surveillance.

Furthermore, the number of patients with implantable defibrillators is now increasing and a considerable rise in ICD patients participating in exercise training is noted. These patients need continuous ECG monitoring and supervision by a physician during the training sessions because of the risk of arrhythmias causing appropriate or even inappropriate shocks. Reports in the literature demonstrate that exercise training for ICD patients is safe, feasible and produces favorable results if carefully supervised by qualified staff. Even ICD malfunctions and other technical problems can be detected early.[10,11]

A well-trained staff is essential for safety and we refer to earlier chapters in this book that address this issue. The head of the CR unit is responsible for safety management and control. If this is not a cardiologist, a named cardiologist should be included in the CR team in order to assure the medical quality of the program and its safety.

An automatic or semi-automatic DC-converter should be available at the training sessions during a phase II program as well as an emergency kit with medication that may be needed. In the unlikely event of a cardiac arrest, the patient should undergo immediate DC-conversion and be transported to the nearest coronary care unit.

All staff members should be trained in cardiopulmonary resuscitation and retraining should be performed at least once yearly. This should include fast transport of the patient to the coronary care unit. If the training facility is situated outside the hospital, emergency equipment should be available at the premises and emergency medical care available at short notice.

Phase III programs (maintenance programs) are usually located outside medical facilities in training halls, sports clubs, gymnasia, etc. Here we recommend basic knowledge in resuscitation among the leaders, a plan for alerting acute medical support and, if funds are available, access to automatic DC-converting equipment.

In summary we recommend careful risk stratification before a cardiac patient enters the program, complete referral documentation from acute care, an individually targeted exercise program with a choice of training options, well-trained and attentive staff, resuscitation training with regularly tested equipment, and ECG monitoring in restricted cases. Provided these conditions are fulfilled, the cardiac rehabilitation program will provide a safe and effective service.

References

1. Ades PA. Cardiac rehabilitation and secondary prevention of coronary heart disease. N Engl J Med 2001;345:892–902.
2. Gianuzzi P, Saner H, Bjornstad H, et al. Secondary prevention through cardiac rehabilitation: position paper of the Working Group on Cardiac Rehabilitation and Exercise Physiology of the European Society of Cardiology. Eur Heart J 2003;23:1273–1278.
3. Hedbäck B, Perk J, Wodlin P. Long-term reduction of cardiac mortality after myocardial infarction: 10-year results of a comprehensive rehabilitation programme. Eur Heart J 1993;14:831–835.
4. Haskell WL. Cardiovascular complications during exercise training of cardiac patients. Circulation 1978;57:920–924.
5. Van Camp SP, Peterson RA. Cardiovascular complications of outpatient cardiac rehabilitation programs. JAMA 1986;256:1160–1163.
6. Cantwell JD. Cardiac complications of exercise. In: Broustet JP, ed. Proceedings of the 5th World Congress on Cardiac Rehabilitation. Andover: Intercept; 1993:139–149.
7. Vanhees L, Stevens A, Schepers D, Defoor J, Rademakers F, Fagard R. Determinants of the effects of physical training and of the complications requiring resuscitation during exercise in patients with cardiovascular disease. Eur J Cardiovasc Prev Rehabil 2004;11:304–312.
8. Hedbäck B, Perk J. Can high-risk patients after myocardial infarction participate in comprehensive cardiac rehabilitation? Scand J Rehab Med 1990;22:15–20.
9. McCartney N, McKelvie RS. The role of resistance training in patients with cardiac disease. J Card Risk 1996;3:160–166.
10. Kamke W, Dovifat C, Schranz M, Behrens J, Völler

H. Cardiac rehabilitation in patients with implantable defibrillators, feasibility and complications. Z Kardiol 2003;92:869–875.

11. Vanhees L, Schepers D, Heidbüchel H, Defoor J, Fagard R. Exercise performance and training in patients with implantable cardioverter-defibrillators and coronary heart disease. Am J Cardiol 2001;87:712–715.

12. Gordon NF, Kohl III HW, Pollock ML, Vaandrager H, Gibbons LS, Blair SN. Cardiovascular safety of maximal strength testing in healthy adults. Am J Cardiol 1995;76:851–853.

13. Haykowsky MJ, Findlay JM, Ignaszewski AP. Aneurysmal subarachnoid hemorrhage associated with weight training: three case reports. Clin J Sports Med 1996;6(1):52–55.

14. Shaw CE, McCully KK, Posner JD. Injuries during the one repetition maximum assessment in the elderly. J Cardiopulm Rehabil 1995;15:283–287.

15. Tei C, Horikiri Y, Park JC, et al. Acute hemodynamic improvement by thermal vasodilation in congestive heart failure. Circulation 1995;91(10): 2582–2590.

16. Cider A, Schaufelberger M, Sunnerhagen KS, Andersson B. Hydrotherapy – a new approach to improve function in the older patient with chronic heart failure. Eur J Heart Fail 2003;5(4): 527–535.

57
Communication: Automatic Referral to Phase II Cardiac Rehabilitation

P.J. Senden

Comprehensive cardiac rehabilitation (CR) is beneficial for a wide variety of coronary patients: after a myocardial infarction (MI), following percutaneous transluminal coronary angioplasty (PCI), coronary artery bypass grafting (CABG), implantable cardiac defibrillators, cardiac rhythm surgery and ablation techniques, stable angina pectoris, and chronic heart failure.[1,2] Yet in several countries CR is underused due to multiple factors, not least the unsatisfactory referral practices.

Patients and health insurance companies require tailor-made, cost-effective models. Physicians or other allied health workers need simple, straightforward but concise referral routines, not a time-consuming and complicated practice.[3-5] In this chapter, a model for automatic referral based upon experience from the Netherlands is proposed to increase utilization and promote equity in CR access.

Automatic Referral

Automatic referral is defined as the enrollment of all eligible cardiac patients (based on practice guidelines), which includes authorization from the referring physician and transfer of relevant medical data in order to facilitate intake in the program and tailoring individual components. There are two modes of automatic referral: a systematic manual approach by health workers as has been practice over the past years or a fully standardized system and computer-based system. Independent of method, the encouragement by the referring physician is of key importance for

the patient's willingness to attend. The cardiologist plays an important role in motivating coronary patients to join CR.

In the manual mode, a cardiac nurse (or other allied health worker) serves as a liaison and informs all eligible cardiac patients prior to discharge about CR and provides them with an intake appointment. An example of a modified flow diagram is shown in Figure 57-1.

In the computer-based format, electronic patient records are utilized to ensure referral for all eligible cardiac patients. According to the Dutch guidelines, cardiac rehabilitation should offer several options: an information module, an exercise program, a lifestyle program, or a combination of these elements (www.cardss.nl).[6]

When designing a program, for the individual patient the use of a specific decision tree (Figure 57-1, Table 57-1) is recommended in which all questions can be answered by a nurse, physiotherapist, or CR coordinator. For the use of the decision tree a computer-based decision support system has been developed in concordance with the national guidelines. This system provides identification of goals and methods of the CR program based upon the patient's condition, history, and needs. In addition, it creates an electronic patient record and provides information for management services.

The decision support system is user-friendly and can be used from early rehabilitation even before the start of phase II to the later part of the recovery phase. The system allows for entering patient data at different occasions and by different users. Once all patient data have been entered,

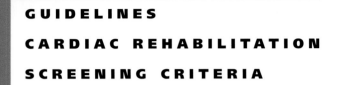

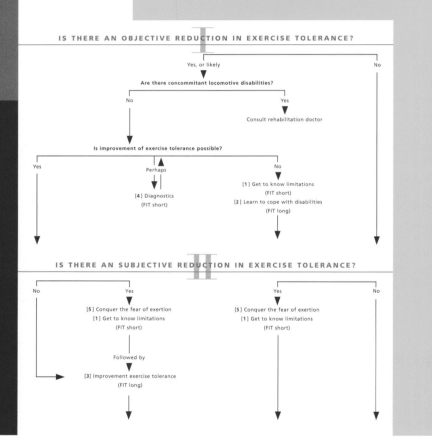

FIGURE 57-1. Decision tree for cardiac rehabilitation.[6]

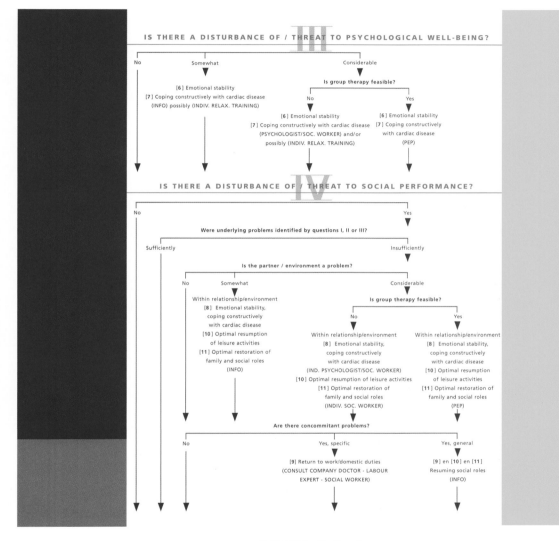

FIGURE 57-1. *Continued*

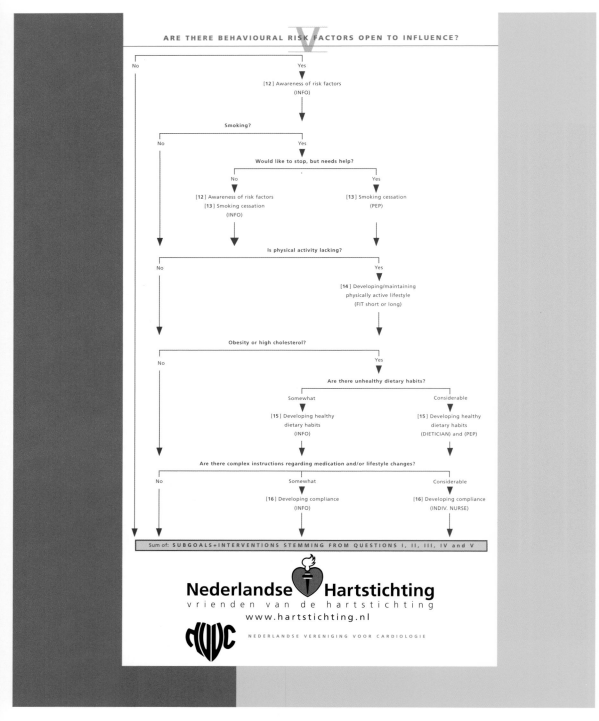

FIGURE 57-1. *Continued*

TABLE 57-1. Intake cardiac rehabilitation for postoperative and myocardial infarction patients

Clinical information: Date discharge hospital: / Tel. nr. after discharge: / X-test yes/no d.d.: / reason for admission: postoperatively/myocardial infarction / Authorization (ward)physician:

Information Cardiac Rehab: / Date intake CR: / Follow up visit with: / Intake done by: / date.

Info from	nr	Question	Fill in at hospital		Referral CR?	Fill in by cardiac rehabilitation	
			Answer fill in, if → precedes			Situation at intake	delayed intake
Physio/ Physician*	1	**Is there an objective decrease of exercise capacity due to the symptoms at the moment of discharge?**	○ Yes–probably ○ No				
Physio/ Physician*	1a	Is increase of the exercise capacity necessary for future (job/ housekeeping/ leisure time)	○ Yes–probably→ ○ No	For:			
Physio/ Physician*	1b	Are there physical limitations not compatible with group training? (like CVA, spinal cord lesion, serious joint problems, amputations)	○ Yes → ○ No/more or less	Like: / Physio level:			
Physician	1c	Are there cardiac contraindications known at discharge for contribution to a physical training program? (Serious rhythm disorders, valve disease, unstable angina pectoris)	○ Yes → ○ No	What: →	No		
Physician	1d	Has cardiologic treatment been completed?	○ Yes ○ No →	Treatment plan→	No		
Physio/ Physician*	2	**Does the patient show a real judgment of his exercise capacity?** (knows the limitations, not frightened to exercise)	○ No → ○ Yes	Namely:			
Nurse/ Social worker*	3	**Is there a more than usual disturbance/ or threat of psychological behavior seen or expected** (psychological imbalance, dysfunctional coping with the disease)	○ No ○ Yes →	Namely:			
Nurse/ Social worker*	4	**Is there any disturbance of social function expected in relation to**	○ No				
	4a	Family situation or partner relation (restarting tasks / to fill in role pattern and expectations)	○ Yes →	Camellia			

(Continued)

TABLE 57-1. *Continued*

Clinical information: Date discharge hospital: X-test yes/no d.d.:   Authorization (ward)physician:
Tel. nr. after discharge: reason for admission: postoperatively/myocardial infarction

Information Cardiac Rehab: Date intake CR: Intake done by:
Follow up visit with: date.

Info from	nr	Question	Answer fill in, if → precedes		Fill in by cardiac rehabilitation		
			Fill in at hospital		Referral CR?	Situation at intake	delayed intake
	4b	Job related (expected problems with return to work)	○ No ○ Yes →				
	4c	Other	○ Yes →	Namely Like:			
Nurse.	**5**	**Are there modifiable risk factors:**					
	5a	• Smoking before admission	○ Yes ○ → No	Attempt to quit? ○ Yes ○ No			
	5b	• Overweight due to insufficient exercise and/orunhealthy nutrition?	○ Yes ○ No				
	5c	• Insufficient exercise (less than 3X / week, 30 minutes with at least 50% maximal heart rate = brisk walking, cycling)	○ Yes ○ No				
	5d	• Unhealthy nutrition	○ Yes ○ No				
	5e	• Poor compliance	○ Yes ○ No ○ Unknown				
	5f	• Is the environment stimulating for the desired change in behavior? (smoking, eating and exercise pattern)	○ Yes ○ No ○ Unknown				
Nurse.	6a	**Has the patient been informed that CR will contact him/her?** (Not valid in case of contra indications)	○ Yes ○ No ○ NVT (contraindicated)				
	6b	**Did the patient receive the brochure about CR?**	○ Yes ○ No				
Nurse.	7	**Fill in who performed the consultation** ○ physiotherapist – ○ social worker – ○ dietitian – ○ clinical psychologist					

*Answers are primarily given by the first or second discipline. At discharge the nursing staff checks the sheet is complete and the referral is authorized by the ward physician.
If there at least a "**no**" in the first column due to contraindications there will be no intake scheduled and no direct contact with CR. There remains the possibility that the cardiologist will refer the patient later on.
•, All other patients will receive an invitation for the intake and X-test.

TABLE 57-2. Referral data to primary care at the end of phase II CR: check list

---

· **Cardiovascular history:**
Coronary heart disease: MI, CABG, PCI, other cardiac surgery
Cerebrovascular disease: TIA, stroke
Heart failure, peripheral artery disease

· **Cardiovascular risk profile:**
Gender, age, CHD among first line relatives (men <55 years, women <65 years)
BMI, waist circumference, smoking, blood pressure, alcohol intake, level of physical exercise, presence of the metabolic syndrome and/or diabetes mellitus

· **Ongoing medication**

· **Results of recent laboratory tests:**
P-glucose, blood lipids: total cholesterol, LDL cholesterol, HDL cholesterol, triglycerides, other relevant tests, e.g. electrolytes (sodium, potassium), creatinine, and proteinuria

· **CR recommendations for patient:**

Stop smoking	○	More exercise	○
Lower blood pressure	○	Weight reduction	○
Lower blood lipids	○	Lower blood glucose	○
Reduce alcohol intake	○	Other:	○

Specific agreements with the patient: ....

---

the software proposes an individually adapted set of rehabilitation goals and methods according to the Dutch guidelines. The rehabilitation staff may accept these recommendations, or adjust them manually if deemed necessary and appropriate. Thereafter the final result of the recommendation should be authorized by the physician in charge of the care of the patient. In our experience, the decision support system has shown to be an improvement compared to standard practice and is now in regular use in CR centers around the country.

Communication

After the phase II CR program, patients will be referred to the family doctor and if needed to a dietitian or a physiotherapist. Maintenance of physical activity should be encouraged; sports clubs or specific phase III maintenance programs in the community (patient organizations, coro-nary clubs etc.) are often valuable in supporting the patient.

For a minority it may be recommended to have access to centers with a more specific experience in dealing with coronary patients and where patients may experience a sense of comfort and safety. In referring the patient to the family doctor and/or other health program, providers' relevant data must be available (Table 57-2). These may include data regarding exercise capacity, the outcome of the physical training program including specific performance data, results of risk factor intervention such as dietary counseling, smoking cessation, stress management, and promotion of an active lifestyle.

For the primary care physician, information must be made available on the cardiovascular history, risk profile, relevant blood tests, recommendations for continued patient care and medication (Table 57-2).

References

1. Taylor RS, Brown A, Ebrahim S, Jolliffe J, et al. Exercise-based rehabilitation for patients with coronary heart disease: systematic review and meta-analysis of randomized controlled trials. Am J Med 2004;116: 682–692.
2. Sears SF, Kovacs AH, Conti JB, Handberg E. Expanding the scope of practice for cardiac rehabilitation: managing patients with implantable cardioverter defibrillators. J Cardiopulm Rehabil 2004;24:209–215.
3. King KM, Teo KK. Cardiac rehabilitation referral and attendance: not one and the same. Rehabil Nurs 1998;23:246–251.
4. Daly J, Sindone AP, Thompson DR, Hancock K, Chang E, Davidson P. Barriers to participation in and adherence to cardiac rehabilitation programmes: a critical literature review. Prog Cardiovasc Nurs 2002;17:8–17.
5. Jackson L, Leclerc J, Erskine Y, Linden W. Getting the most out of cardiac rehabilitation: a review of referral and adherence predictors. Heart 2005;91:10–14.
6. Goud R, Peek N, Strijbis AM, de Clercq PA, Hasman A. A computer-based guideline implementation system for cardiac rehabilitation screening. Computers in Cardiology 2005 (CinC), Lyon, September 2005.

58
Future Developments in Preventive Cardiology: The EUROACTION Project

David A. Wood

Although there is substantial scientific evidence that professional lifestyle intervention on smoking, diet and physical activity, together with control of blood pressure, cholesterol and glycemia, and selective use of cardioprotective drug therapies can reduce cardiovascular morbidity and mortality, the translation of that evidence into everyday clinical practice remains a challenge. The joint European Societies guidelines on prevention of cardiovascular disease (CVD) define priorities for preventive cardiology in clinical practice, thresholds for treatment, and treatment goals.[1] The priorities are firstly patients with established atherosclerotic cardiovascular disease; coronary disease, and all other manifestations of atherosclerosis. The second priority is apparently healthy individuals in the general population who are at high risk of developing CVD because of hypertension, dyslipidemia, diabetes, or a combination of these and other risk factors. The third is the families (first degree blood relatives) of both coronary patients and high-risk individuals.

Cardiac rehabilitation traditionally focused on physical rehabilitation but this specialty has gradually evolved into more comprehensive professional lifestyle programs – smoking cessation, making healthy food choices, and becoming physically active – based on behavioral models of change. Risk factor management in terms of controlling blood pressure, lipids and glucose to defined targets, and the use of prophylactic drug therapies, is also now an integral part of this approach. Finally, the psychosocial and vocational support required to help patients lead as full a life as possible is also provided. This evolution in cardiac rehabilitation is reflected in the current World Health Organization definition:[2]

The rehabilitation of cardiac patients is the sum of activities required *to influence favourably the underlying cause of the disease*, as well as the best possible physical, mental and social conditions, so that they may, by their own efforts preserve or resume when lost, as normal a place as possible in the community. Rehabilitation cannot be regarded as an isolated form of therapy but must be integrated with the whole treatment of which it forms only one facet.

The important change to this definition was the addition of the words highlighted in italics; namely "to influence favourably the underlying cause of the disease" – in short, all aspects of CVD prevention. The overall preventive objective for patients who present with symptoms of coronary artery disease – stable angina, unstable angina, or acute MI – is to reduce the risk of a further nonfatal event or death from cardiovascular disease. Cardiac rehabilitation was originally provided only for patients recovering from a myocardial infarction (MI) and those who had coronary artery bypass graft (CABG) surgery (or other forms of cardiac surgery). With the more recent emphasis on influencing the underlying causes of atherosclerotic disease, patients presenting with all forms of coronary artery disease, including unstable and stable angina, are now being included in cardiovascular prevention and rehabilitation programs. By addressing lifestyle and risk factor management, and prescribing prophylactic drug therapies, the risk of cardiovascular events can be reduced in all these patients.

Unfortunately, risk factor management in patients with CHD in Europe is far from optimal. Surveys of clinical practice such as EUROASPIRE I and II (European Action on Secondary and Primary Prevention by Intervention to Reduce Events) have shown that integration of cardiovascular disease prevention into daily practice is inadequate.[3–5] There is still considerable potential to further reduce cardiovascular risk in patients with established CHD as many are not achieving the recommended lifestyle and risk factor goals. The majority of coronary patients in the EUROASPIRE II survey in 15 countries were not advised to follow a cardiac rehabilitation program, and less than a third of all patients attended such a program.[6] The traditions and practice of cardiac rehabilitation in Europe differ substantially between countries, ranging from intensive residential rehabilitation through to ambulatory hospital-, community- and home-based programs. They also differ in their patient populations, staffing, management protocols, duration, and follow-up. According to the EUROASPIRE II data, whatever form of cardiac rehabilitation was provided for the coronary patients who reported attending such programs, the majority still did not achieve the lifestyle, risk factor, and therapeutic goals.[6] In families with premature CHD (men <55 years and women <65 years) it is recommended that all first degree relatives are assessed for CVD risk. Yet, the second EUROASPIRE study, which surveyed the relatives (siblings and offspring) of patients with premature CHD, found that only 1 in 10 of these relatives had had any form of CVD risk assessment as a result of premature disease occurring in their families.[7] Looking beyond coronary patients and their families to those apparently healthy individuals in the general population who are at high risk of developing CVD, the clinical challenge is even greater. The first issue is how to identify those at high risk of CVD. The traditional medical model of measuring and classifying risk factors in isolation, for example hypertension, is gradually being replaced with an integrated approach based on the principle of total CVD risk. Instead of classifying a person as having hypertension or not, the total risk approach requires an assessment of all CVD risk factors – age, sex, smoking habit, blood pressure, lipids – and then integrating these data to

estimate the total risk (percentage chance) of developing CVD over a defined time period. In Europe the CVD risk charts based on SCORE are used to estimate total risk of developing CVD.[8] A SCORE of ≥5% for fatal CVD over 10 years is the recommended threshold for more intensive lifestyle intervention and appropriate use of drug therapies. Compared to the number of people with CVD the number of people at high risk of developing CVD is considerably greater. Just like EUROASPIRE, other international audits of clinical practice show that management of these high-risk people is even poorer than that of patients with established CVD.[9]

So the challenge for preventive cardiology at all levels – for coronary patients, the relatives of patients with premature disease, and for people at high total risk of developing CVD – is considerable. What is required is innovative models of preventive care which can be integrated with everyday clinical practice to help patients and their families achieve a healthier lifestyle, modify their other risk factors, and reduce their total risk of developing or having recurrent atherosclerotic disease.

EUROACTION

EUROACTION is a European Society of Cardiology demonstration project in preventive cardiology (www.escardio.org/Euroaction) led by specialists from the European Association for Cardiovascular Prevention and Rehabilitation working together with the Working Group on Cardiovascular Nursing. The aim of EuroAction is to raise standards of preventive cardiology in Europe by demonstrating that the recommended European and national lifestyle, risk factor and therapeutic goals in cardiovascular disease prevention (Table 58-1) are achievable and sustainable in everyday clinical practice.[10]

Objectives

The objectives of the EUROACTION project are:

1. To demonstrate the process of care and immediate impact of a 16-week specialist nurse-led multidisciplinary hospital-based cardiovascular prevention and rehabilitation program on

TABLE 58-1. European lifestyle and risk factor targets

- Giving up smoking
- Eating a healthy diet
- Becoming physically active
- Achieving and maintaining a healthy shape (waist circumference below 94 cm (37 inches) for men and below 80 cm (31.5 inches) for women) and weight (body mass index below 25 kg/m^2)
- Blood pressure *below* 140/90 mmHg (and for those with diabetes *below* 130/80 mmHg)
- Cholesterol *below* 4.5 mmol/L (175 mg/dL) (LDL cholesterol *below* 2.5 mmol/L (100 mg/dL))
- Blood glucose *below* 6.1 mmol/L (110 mg/dL) and good glycemic control in all persons with diabetes

lifestyle, risk factors, and therapeutic management of coronary patients and their families.

2. To demonstrate the process of care and impact of a hospital-led preventive cardiology program for all first degree relatives of coronary patients with premature disease.

3. To demonstrate the process of care and the longer-term impact of this program for all coronary patients, partners, and first degree relatives at 1 year.

4. To demonstrate the process of care and impact of a specialist nurse-led preventive cardiology program in general practice on management of high-risk individuals and their partners at 1 year.

5. To follow up all patients with coronary disease, high-risk individuals and their partners, and first degree relatives of patients with premature coronary disease for cardiovascular nonfatal events and cardiovascular and all-cause mortality in order to determine the relationship between intervention and event-free survival.

EuroAction is being conducted in eight European countries: Denmark, France, Italy, Poland, Spain, Sweden, the Netherlands, and the United Kingdom.

Study Design

EUROACTION is a cluster randomized controlled trial with clinical follow-up at 16 weeks and 1 year (hospital arm) and at 1 year only (primary care arm). A summary of the scientific protocol has been published.[10] In each of six countries, two district general hospitals (France, Italy, Poland, Spain, Sweden, and the United Kingdom) and two general practices (Denmark, Italy, Poland, Spain, the Netherlands, and the United Kingdom) have been recruited from different geographical areas. Comparable pairs of hospitals and comparable pairs of general practices have been randomized, within their respective country pairs, to intervention or usual care.

Priority Patients and Families

Hospitals

In each hospital the following patients and their families are prospectively identified when they are admitted as inpatients or seen as outpatients:

1. Consecutive patients (men and women) <80 years presenting for the first time (incident cases) as inpatients or outpatients with a consultant diagnosis of coronary artery disease:
   (a) acute myocardial infarction
   (b) unstable angina
   (c) stable angina.
2. Partners of all patients.
3. First degree relatives (siblings and offspring >18 years) of patients with premature CHD (men <55 years and women <65 years) living in the same household or elsewhere.

General Practices

In each general practice the following patients and their families are prospectively identified when they attend their general practitioner for whatever reason:

1. Consecutive patients (men and women) >50 years and <80 years with no history of cardiovascular disease who are:
   (a) at high total cardiovascular risk (HeartScore ≥5% over 10 years, either now or when projected to age 60 years)[8] and on no medical treatment for blood pressure, lipids, or diabetes
   (b) on treatment with antihypertensive and/or lipid-lowering drug therapies started in the last year but with no diabetes
   (c) diagnosed with diabetes mellitus (treated by diet alone or with oral hypoglycemic

drug therapy and/or insulin) within the last 3 years.
2. Partners of all patients.

The Preventive Cardiology Programs

The Cardiovascular Prevention and Rehabilitation (CVPR) Program (Hospital Arm)

Aim

The EUROACTION CVPR program is a nurse-led comprehensive, multidisciplinary, hospital-based 16-week program for coronary patients and their families. The aim of the program is to help coronary patients and their partners, and first degree relatives of patients with premature coronary disease, to achieve the European lifestyle, risk factor, and therapeutic goals as defined in the 1998 Joint European Societies' guidelines (Table 58-1).[11]

The partners of coronary patients, together with first degree blood relatives of patients with premature coronary heart disease (men <55 years and women <65 years) living in the same household, are also identified. They are also invited to attend the cardiovascular prevention and rehabilitation program in order to help them achieve the same lifestyle, risk factor, and therapeutic goals.

The program is coordinated by a specialist cardiac nurse. In each hospital, the team is made up of two nurses, a dietitian, and a physiotherapist supported by a lead cardiologist. These core disciplines facilitate lifestyle change in relation to smoking, diet, and physical activity. However, other disciplines are involved as required, for example pharmacists, clinical psychologists, and occupational therapists. The lead cardiologist works closely with the specialist nurses to ensure patients and families achieve the blood pressure, cholesterol, and diabetes targets. The cardiologist prescribes and up-titrates cardioprotective medications.

Family Approach

The nurse proactively identifies newly diagnosed coronary patients and recruits them to the CVPR program (Figure 58-1). As the program is family based, the partners of all coronary patients, and first degree relatives of patients with premature

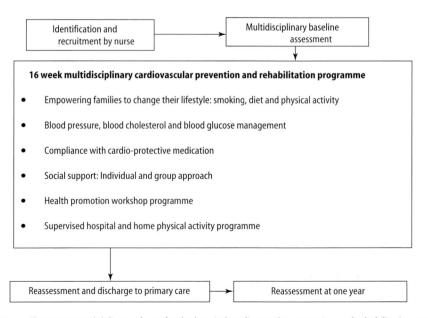

FIGURE 58-1. The process and delivery of care for the hospital cardiovascular prevention and rehabilitation program.

coronary disease (men <55 years and women <65 years), are also recruited to the program. Partners of patients who present with coronary disease are at higher risk of developing cardiovascular disease than the general population,[12,13] because of a common lifestyle and shared cardiovascular risk factors. In addition, first degree relatives of patients with premature coronary disease are at particularly high risk, in part for the same reasons, but also because some families have inherited dyslipidemias, for example familial hypercholesterolemia, resulting in premature atherosclerotic disease. So when coronary disease develops, it is appropriate to offer lifestyle and risk factor management to the whole family, not just the coronary patient. Those first degree blood relatives of patients with premature coronary disease not living in the same household are supported through a postal relatives pack.

Initial Family Assessment

The initial assessment of the family is by the whole multidisciplinary team and forms the starting point for the intervention. The nurse explains the nature of the diagnosis and the causes of atherosclerosis, and the three disciplines carry out a full family assessment of cardiovascular risk, and discuss a plan to work together to reduce that risk. This assessment of patients, partners, and relatives includes smoking habit, diet and physical activity; measurement of body mass index (BMI), waist circumference, blood pressure, cholesterol, and glucose. Medications are recorded and compliance is assessed. Health beliefs, anxiety and depression, illness perception and mood are also assessed with self-administered questionnaires.

Each patient and family member is given a Personal Record Card (www.escardio.org/EURO ACTION), which is pocket sized but opens out to an A4 sheet. Lifestyle and risk factor goals are summarized and progress is recorded as well as medications and appointments. All families are given a Family Support Pack (www. escardio.org/EUROACTION), which reinforces the information provided by the team at the initial assessment and at the subsequent health promotion workshop and exercise sessions. It provides contact details of the nurse, describes the family

approach to the program, and contains information cards on smoking, diet, physical activity and weight management, blood pressure, cholesterol, and diabetes. The pack provides information about coronary disease, cardiac investigations and procedures and cardioprotective medications.

The Lifestyle Intervention

Coronary patients and their families require integrated, multidisciplinary support to achieve appropriate lifestyle change: quitting smoking, making healthier food choices, achieving a healthy weight and shape, and increasing physical activity – based on behavioral models of change. Families work together to achieve lifestyle changes and support each other in sustaining them over a lifetime. Involving the patient's partner, and other family members sharing the same household, in making behavioral change is more likely to be successful than treating the patient in isolation.[13]

The multidisciplinary team use a common approach to lifestyle change in patients and families. This is based on the stages of change model proposed by Prochaska and DiClemente,[14] which recognizes that individuals are not equally ready to change their behavior at a given point in time. Those who are ready and motivated are more likely to change. The team draws on various methods to increase motivation, overcome barriers, and develop strategies. For example, motivational counseling[15] can provide a way to work with ambivalence, to increase motivation and self efficacy, to set goals, and to create a management plan.

The program provides both group and one-to-one support, which comes from three sources: the family; other people attending the program; and from the health professionals.

Smoking Cessation

The aim is to help patients and families stop smoking completely.

The nurse assesses current smoking status, health beliefs regarding tobacco smoking, history of tobacco smoking, and previous quit attempts in patients, partners and relatives. Breath carbon monoxide is recorded. The person's stage of change is assessed in relation to smoking behavior and the level of dependence on nicotine. This informs the level of support and follow-up required, and the need for pharmacological therapy to manage nicotine withdrawal. The nurse helps the person to prepare for a quit attempt, sets a quit date, and makes contingency plans in the event of a relapse. The cardiologist is asked to prescribe nicotine replacement therapy or other drug therapy if appropriate.

In summary, the nurse motivates and helps those who are ready to quit, monitors the precontemplators and contemplators who are not yet ready, provides maintenance and follow-up to those who are attempting to quit, and ensures pharmacological support where appropriate.

Dietary Intervention

The aim is to give professional advice on food and food choices to compose a diet associated with the lowest risk of cardiovascular disease (Table 58-2).

The dietitian assesses knowledge and attitudes to diet, and measures weight and height and waist circumference in patients and their families. Body mass index (BMI) is calculated from the weight

TABLE 58-2. The European recommendations for dietary intake

a. Goals for which scientific evidence is strong and public health gain large
  1. Saturated fat and *trans* fats:
    i. Less than 10% of dietary energy from saturated fat
    ii. Less than 2% of energy from *trans* fats
  2. Fruit and vegetables:
    i. More than 400 g/day
  3. Salt:
    i. Less than 6 g/day
  4. Obesity and overweight:
    i. BMI < 25 kg/m^2
    ii. PAL of more than 1.75 PAL
b. Goals for which scientific evidence is moderate and public health gain moderate
  1. Total fat
    i. Less than 30% of total energy
  2. Polyunsaturated fat
    i. n-6 polyunsaturated fat: 4–8% energy
    ii. n-3 polyunsaturated fat: 2 g/day of linolenic acid and 200 mg/day of very long chain fatty acids
c. Goals for which scientific evidence is weaker and public health gain smaller
  1. Dietary fiber: more than 25 g/day (or 3MJ) of dietary fiber and more than 55% of energy from complex carbohydrates
  2. Folate from food: more than 400 μg/day
  3. Sugary foods: four or fewer occasions per day

and height measurements. As the lifestyle intervention is family based, the dietitian addresses the main person in the household responsible for buying and preparing food, and advises the whole "family" rather than an "individual" on their own. The dietitian translates the recommendations in Table 58-2 into practical advice which is individualized to family members. Advice is given in terms of food (not nutrients) and patterns of eating. This advice is adapted for the specific needs of each individual by taking account of factors such as weight, raised blood pressure, dyslipidemia, and diabetes.

Dietary goals are set which are realistic and achievable depending on stage of change. For example, for weight management, the dietitian sets an initial goal of 5–10% weight loss, if achieving the healthy BMI range is unrealistic in the short term.

The dietitian sees patients and families on a weekly basis. By attending the weekly health promotion workshop and exercise sessions, the dietitian is available to provide advice as required. The dietitian organizes the healthy eating and weight management workshop. The dietitian also advises on local facilities available in the community to provide support to families.

Physical Activity Intervention

The aim is to help patients and families to increase their physical activity safely to the level associated with the lowest risk of CVD. The advice is to choose enjoyable activities which fit into people's daily routine, preferably 30 to 45 minutes, four to five times weekly at 60–75% of the average maximum heart rate.

The physiotherapist assesses habitual physical activity, functional capacity, and other factors in patients and families. The physiotherapist develops an individual physical activity plan with realistic goals for each family member based on stages of change. Every week for 8 weeks, the physiotherapist leads a progressive endurance exercise training program, which is group based. This exercises individuals at between 60% and 75% of a predetermined asymptomatic maximum heart rate. The program is intentionally not equipment based so it can be used at home. Patients gain the ability to sustain and self-regulate safe and effective physical activity levels. The individualized physical activity plan developed by the physiotherapist for each family member follows the hospital-based exercise prescription. In addition, the step-counter (Digi-walker 200 pedometer) is used as a motivational tool. Targets are set and reviewed every week.

The total physical activity prescription aims to achieve the European recommendations for each individual as well as equipping families with the necessary knowledge and skills to maintain their physical activity levels safely and effectively in the longer term.

Managing Patients and Families to Target Blood Pressure, Cholesterol, and Glucose

The aim is to bring the blood pressure, blood cholesterol and blood glucose of all patients, partners and first degree relatives to below target levels.

The nurse and cardiologist are responsible for the management of blood pressure, cholesterol, and glucose.

The European target for blood pressure is <140/90 mmHg (130/85 mmHg in diabetes). The blood pressure is measured at the initial assessment, and the nurse consults the cardiologist if it is above target level. The cardiologist initiates or up-titrates medication as appropriate. The nurse measures the blood pressure at weekly intervals during the program. Once drug treatment is started, weekly monitoring continues until the blood pressure is reduced below target.

The European target for total cholesterol is <5.0 mmol/L (190 mg/dL). The total cholesterol is measured at the initial assessment. If the cholesterol is above the target level, a statin is prescribed if it has not already been started. The blood cholesterol is monitored monthly until the target is reached. The cardiologist up-titrates treatment if required.

The European target for fasting blood glucose is <6.1 mmol/L (110 mg/dL). A fasting and random glucose are measured at the initial assessment. An oral glucose tolerance test is performed if the fasting glucose is ≥6.1 mmol/L (110 mg/dL) to diagnose diabetes or impaired glucose tolerance. Patients and other family members diagnosed with diabetes or impaired glucose tolerance are managed according to the diabetic target for blood pressure, the cholesterol target as well as the glycemic target. People who are diagnosed with diabetes are also referred to the diabetologist.

The nurse checks that all appropriate cardioprotective medications are prescribed: antiplatelet therapy, beta-blockers, ACE inhibitors/angiotensin II receptor blockers, and lipid-lowering drugs. The nurse checks the dose of these drugs to make sure they are evidence based. The nurse liaises with the cardiologist to initiate a prescription or up-titration of these medications. The nurse also provides education and information to patients and families about their medications to facilitate compliance.

The Health Promotion Workshop Program

The nurse coordinates an 8-week rolling program of workshops which include the topics listed in Table 58-3. The workshops are part of the weekly meetings which bring patients and families together. They are an important part of the group support provided by the program. The workshops are designed to be interactive, informative and to provide an open forum for discussion.

Reassessment

On completion of the program, the patient and family are reassessed for lifestyle, risk factor, and therapeutic management. The results of this 16-week assessment are sent to the person's own physician to encourage continuation of appropriate

TABLE 58-3. Health promotion workshop topics in the hospital cardiovascular prevention and rehabilitation program

1. Information about coronary heart disease and cardiac procedures
2. Understanding cardiovascular risk
   a. Adopting healthy lifestyle habits to reduce cardiovascular risk
      i. Smoking and cardiovascular disease
      ii. Healthy eating: choosing the right foods
      iii. Benefits of physical activity
   b. Other risk factors: Blood pressure, blood cholesterol and blood glucose: how lifestyle change and medication help.
3. Understanding cardioprotective medications
4. Living with coronary heart disease
   a. Recovering from cardiac events and procedures
   b. Sexual activity and CHD
   c. Returning to work
5. Coping emotionally with coronary heart disease
   a. Managing stress and learning how to relax
   b. Anxiety and depression – positive thinking

treatment in the long term. A final reassessment takes place one year after identification.

The Personal Support Pack: for First Degree Relatives of Patients with Premature Coronary Disease

The first degree relatives (siblings or offspring over the age of 18) of patients who present with premature coronary disease (men who present with CHD before the age of 55 and women before the age of 65) are identified by the nurse. Relatives who live in the same household as the index patient are recruited to the program. Those relatives who do not live in the same household as the patient are sent a Personal Support Pack (www.escardio.org/EuroAction) in the post. This pack comprises a covering letter, an education booklet, a questionnaire, and a letter to the relative's own physician. The booklet provides information on coronary disease and cardiovascular risk, and advice on how to adopt a healthy lifestyle. The questionnaire has two sections. Section 1 is completed by the relative and includes questions on their current lifestyle regarding smoking, diet, and physical activity. Section 2 is for the relative's physician, who is asked to measure and record body mass index, waist measurement, blood pressure and blood cholesterol, and to record medications. The physician is requested to manage the relative to the lifestyle and risk factor targets.

A follow-up questionnaire is sent to relatives one year later to evaluate lifestyle, risk factor, and therapeutic management.

The Cardiovascular Prevention (CVP) Program (Primary Care Arm)

Aim

The EUROACTION CVP primary care program is based on the same principles as the hospital CVPR program, particularly in relation to the family-based approach and lifestyle management. It is a nurse-led multidisciplinary cardiovascular prevention program for individuals at high risk of developing cardiovascular disease and for their partners. The aim of the program is to help high-risk individuals and their partners to achieve the European lifestyle, risk factor, and therapeutic

targets as defined in the Joint European Societies' guidelines (Table 58-1).[11]

Individuals at high cardiovascular risk are identified opportunistically in the following way:

1. Men and women 50 years of age or older, but less than 80 years who are found to be at high total (multifactorial) risk: Men with at least 1 (women with at least 2) cardiovascular risk factor(s) (smoking and/or raised blood pressure, i.e. $\geq$140/90 mmHg, and/or raised total cholesterol, i.e. $\geq$5 mmol/L (190 mg/dL) currently on no medication for arterial hypertension and/or dyslipidemia, who are screened by the nurse and found to be at high multifactorial risk: CVD risk $\geq$5% over 10 years (now or projected to age 60 years), according to the HeartScore risk estimation system[8] (www.escardio.org/HeartScore).

2. Men and women in the same age range, who have been started on treatment in the last year with antihypertensive and/or lipid-lowering therapies but with no diabetes.

3. Men and women, in the same age range, who have been diagnosed in the last 3 years with diabetes and are under treatment with diet, oral hypoglycemics, and/or insulin regardless of treatment for hypertension and dyslipidemia.

In intervention general practices a cardiovascular prevention (CVP) program is delivered by specialist nurses supported by the HeartScore risk assessment tool and the EUROACTION educational materials. (www.escardio.org/HeartScore) The object is to achieve national and European lifestyle, risk factor, and therapeutic targets for cardiovascular disease prevention. The partners of high-risk individuals living in the same household are identified and supported through the same program and screened at the end of the program.

The program is coordinated by a specialist nurse. In each practice, the team is made up of one cardiac specialist nurse, and the general practitioners (GP) working in the practice. The nurse is specially trained to address smoking, diet, and physical activity. However, the nurse can refer to other disciplines as required. The GPs work with the specialist nurse to ensure that patients and their partners achieve the blood pressure, cholesterol, and glucose targets. The GPs prescribe and up-titrate cardioprotective medications.

Family Approach

The nurse proactively identifies high-risk individuals and recruits them to the CVP program along with their partners (Figure 58-2).

Initial Family Assessment

The initial assessment of the family by the nurse is the starting point for the intervention. The nurse explains the concept of cardiovascular risk, carries out a full assessment of risk, and discusses a family plan for reducing risk. This assessment of patients and their partners includes smoking habit, diet and physical activity; measurement of BMI, waist circumference, blood pressure, cholesterol, and glucose. Medications are recorded and compliance is assessed. Health beliefs, anxiety and depression, illness perception and mood are also assessed.

Each family member is given a Personal Record Card and a Family Support Pack (www. escardio.org/EUROACTION).

The Lifestyle Intervention

The family approach to lifestyle intervention is the same as the hospital CVPR program. The nurse is trained to address all three elements of lifestyle change: stopping smoking, making healthier food choices, achieving a healthier weight and shape, and increasing physical activity, based on a behavioral model of change. The nurse does not lead a formal exercise training program, but encourages a home physical activity program, and the use of appropriate facilities in the community.

Managing Patients and Families to Target Blood Pressure, Cholesterol, and Glucose

The aim is to bring the blood pressure, blood cholesterol, and blood glucose of all patients and partners to below target levels. The nurse and GP are responsible for management of blood pressure, cholesterol, and glucose according to defined protocols.

The nurse checks that all appropriate medication is prescribed, especially antiplatelet, antihypertensive, and lipid-lowering drugs. The nurse liaises with the GPs to up-titrate these medications as required. The nurse also provides education and information to patients and families about their medications to facilitate compliance.

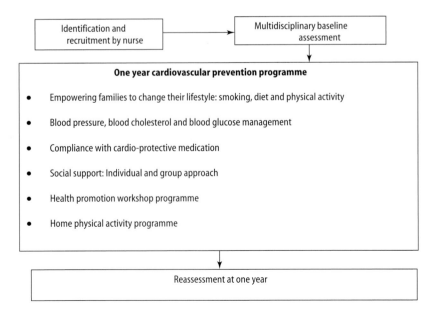

FIGURE 58-2. The process and delivery of care for the primary care cardiovascular prevention program.

TABLE 58-4. Health promotion workshop topics for the primary care cardiovascular prevention program

1. Understanding cardiovascular risk
   a. Adopting healthy lifestyle habits to reduce cardiovascular risk
   b. Smoking and cardiovascular disease
   c. Healthy eating: choosing the right foods
   d. Benefits of physical activity
   e. Other risk factors: Blood pressure, blood cholesterol and blood glucose: how lifestyle change and medication help.
2. Understanding cardioprotective medications
3. Managing stress and learning how to relax: Anxiety and depression – positive thinking

The Health Promotion Workshop Program

The nurse coordinates a rolling program of three workshops which include the topics listed in Table 58-4. The workshops bring high-risk individuals and partners together. They are an important part of the group support provided by the CVP program. The workshops are designed to be interactive, informative, and to provide an open forum for discussion.

Reassessment

One year after identification, the high-risk individuals and their partners are reassessed for lifestyle, risk factor, and therapeutic management.

Outcome Measures

These nurse-led multidisciplinary preventive cardiology programs in hospital and primary care will be evaluated in relation to the following outcome measures:

1. proportions of patients, partners and relatives achieving European and national lifestyle, risk factor, and therapeutic targets for cardiovascular disease prevention
2. psychosocial measures
3. return to work
4. health service use
5. health economics
6. major nonfatal cardiovascular events (myocardial infarction and stroke) and cardiovascular/total mortality.

A summary of these outcome measures and measurement instruments is given in the scientific protocol.[10]

Principles of EUROACTION

Scientific evidence for comprehensive cardiovascular prevention and rehabilitation programs is compelling.[16] They can improve quality of life, reduce cardiovascular morbidity and mortality, and increase life expectancy of coronary patients. A similar strength of evidence exists for lifestyle and risk factor modification in individuals at high risk of developing the disease.[1] However, the professional challenge is translation of that evidence into effective care of patients in every day clinical practice.

The EUROACTION project offers preventive cardiology programs in both hospital and primary care which are based on several important principles.

The first principle is inclusive preventive care. EUROACTION addresses the complete spectrum of preventive cardiology care: from patients with atherosclerotic coronary disease and their families to those among the apparently healthy population who are at high risk of developing CVD. Although cardiac rehabilitation programs have traditionally focused on patients following acute myocardial infarction, or cardiac surgery (principally coronary artery bypass surgery), the EUROACTION project is extending preventive cardiology care to other groups of high-risk patients. Those presenting with angina (unstable or stable) are at high risk of progressing to a myocardial infarction or other major CVD event. Therefore it is logical to offer the same lifestyle, risk factor, and therapeutic interventions to such patients. Similarly, apparently healthy people living in the community who are at high risk of developing CVD (many of whom will have asymptomatic atherosclerotic disease), which includes those with diabetes, also require a similar comprehensive approach to CVD risk factor assessment and management. They all need to have their total CVD risk reduced through lifestyle and appropriate drug therapies. So EUROACTION makes no distinction between those with symptomatic coronary disease (secondary prevention) and those at high risk of developing symptoms (primary prevention). These people are all at high CVD risk and require similar professional support to achieve the same lifestyle and risk factor targets. EuroAction offers total risk management to all these high-risk people in order to reduce their risk of a major cardiovascular event.

The second principle is equity of access. Professional preventive care should be provided for all atherosclerotic disease patients, and also for those who are found to be at high risk of developing CVD. So the EUROACTION project was intentionally set up in busy general hospitals and general practices, not academic or specialist rehabilitation centers. In other words, the EURO-ACTION program is being run in the type of medical facilities that provide cardiovascular care for the vast majority of patients in each country. Doing so gives easy and equitable access to preventive cardiology care for all coronary and high-risk patients seen in everyday clinical practice. Patients need to be able to access local services near where they live in their own community. Traveling to a specialized facility which may be further away can be more difficult and more expensive. This means some patients, and also their families, will not participate in such programs. Integrating the diagnosis and management of both coronary patients and high-risk individuals with continuing preventive care in the same medical facility is more likely to result in higher participation and compliance with the program. So EUROACTION is designed to be appropriate to the everyday clinical setting in which most people who develop coronary disease, or who are found to be at high CVD risk, can be managed. The program is therefore generalizable to all hospitals and general practices which do not have specialized facilities for cardiac rehabilitation.

The third principle is a family-centered program. It actively involves the partners of the patients and other relatives living in the same household. For patients with premature disease the program also reaches out to all first degree relatives, namely siblings and offspring, many of whom are living elsewhere. The principle underlying a family-based intervention is as follows. Married couples show concordance for lifestyle and other risk factors, and there is evidence of concordance for change. Couples can help each other to quit smoking, change their diets and physical activity patterns. For example, in helping a patient to quit smoking it is important to address the partner's smoking habits at the same time. Modification of eating habits depends on the

person who shops and cooks having an understanding of the principles of a healthy diet. Attempting to change the eating habits of a patient in isolation from the rest of the family, and especially if that person neither shops nor cooks, is less likely to be successful. Investing in the family as a whole also includes any offspring living at home. For a patient to become more physically active also depends on the attitude of their partner and the family as a whole. There are many everyday physical activities which can be enjoyed by families together including walking, swimming, and active but non-competitive sports.

The fourth principle is a nurse-led multidisciplinary program. The nurses lead a team involving dietitians and physiotherapists, and they work with cardiologists and general practitioners. The nurses set up and organize the day-to-day running of the programs, actively recruit patients and their families, and undertake the comprehensive lifestyle and risk factor assessment with the other health professionals. They provide weekly one-to-one patient and family reviews, provide smoking cessation support, and organize the weekly educational program. The nurses monitor blood pressure, lipids, and glucose in relation to defined targets and, based on these results, inform the physicians of the need to initiate and up-titrate drugs to protect the heart and circulation. In this central role the nurses in the hospital program are supported by dietitians and physiotherapists who address the other aspects of lifestyle change. Avoidance of all forms of tobacco, achieving a healthy diet, and becoming physically active are all given equal priority. The nurse, dietitian, and physiotherapist are all essential members of the multidisciplinary team who work together to achieve lifestyle change in families. In primary care the nurses also received training to address all aspects of lifestyle. The nurses organize the final assessment of families and write the reports on the patients (and partners) for their specialists and general practitioners.

The fifth principle is that the EUROACTION program does not require specialized hospital or community facilities. All the programs in both hospital and primary care were set up in existing accommodation. Space was provided for the nurses and other health professionals to undertake confidential lifestyle assessments of individual patients and their families. In addition, existing space was used to offer health promotion workshops and to undertake supervised physical activity sessions without specialized equipment. The exercise program was intentionally designed around simple equipment – step blocks, light weights, resistance bands – so it could be easily replicated in the home environment. This was to encourage patients and their families to achieve the frequency of exercise training associated with gains in physical fitness. It is these gains in physical fitness that are associated with improved symptomatology and quality of life and reduced risk of subsequent CVD. So the EuroAction program could be set up in any hospital or general practice with sufficient space but without the need for dedicated specialized facilities.

The sixth principle is addressing total CVD risk. The EUROACTION program assesses total cardiovascular disease risk, not single risk, and manages factors in isolation. The traditional medical silos of "hypertension," "hyperlipidemia," and "diabetes" are replaced by a comprehensive approach targeting those with established coronary disease or who are at high total (multifactorial) risk of developing CVD. The latter are identified in EUROACTION by the Joint European Societies CVD Risk Charts, derived from the SCORE project. This approach requires a comprehensive risk factor assessment, and then integrates age, gender, smoking habit, blood pressure, and lipids (total to HDL cholesterol ratio) into a risk score: the probability of developing fatal CVD over the next 10 years. A SCORE ≥5% for fatal CVD over 10 years is considered to be sufficiently high to justify both pr3ofessional lifestyle intervention and drug therapies to manage risk factors to target. EUROACTION is also targeting patients with medically diagnosed hypertension, dyslipidemia, or diabetes who are already on drug treatment in primary care. It offers them the same comprehensive risk factor assessment and total risk management. The object in all these high-risk patient groups is to reduce total CVD risk in both patients and their partners.

So, in summary, EUROACTION is stepping up to the European-wide professional challenge of translating scientific evidence into effective preventive care for all high-risk patients in everyday clinical practice. The principles of patient inclusiveness, equity of access, nurse-led multidiscipli-

nary family-based lifestyle intervention, and total cardiovascular risk assessment and management are all central to this preventive cardiology program. This innovative model of care is being evaluated in the context of a cluster randomized controlled trial. So it will be possible to quantify what this program is achieving compared to usual care, and at what cost.

References

1. De Backer G, Ambrosioni E, Borch-Johnsen K, et al. European guidelines on cardiovascular disease prevention in clinical practice. Third Joint Task Force of European and other Societies on Cardiovascular Disease Prevention in Clinical Practice (constituted by representatives of eight societies and by invited experts). Eur J Cardiovasc Prev Rehabil 2003;10 (Suppl 1):S1–S78.
2. Needs and priorities in cardiac rehabilitation and secondary prevention in patients with coronary heart disease. WHO Technical Report Series 831. Geneva: World Health Organization; 1993.
3. EUROASPIRE Study Group. EUROASPIRE. A European Society of Cardiology survey of secondary prevention of coronary heart disease: Principal results. Eur Heart J 1997;18:1569–1582.
4. EUROASPIRE Study Group. Lifestyle and risk factor management and use of drug therapies in coronary patients from 15 countries. Principal results from EUROASPIRE II. Euro Heart Survey Programme. Eur Heart J 2001;22:554–572.
5. EUROASPIRE Study Group. Clinical reality of coronary prevention guidelines: a comparison of EUROASPIRE I and II in nine countries. Lancet 2001;357:995–1001.
6. Kotseva K, Wood D, De Bacquer D, et al. on behalf of the EUROASPIRE II Study Group. Cardiac rehabilitation for coronary patients: lifestyle, risk factor and therapeutic management. Results from the EUROASPIRE II survey. Eur Heart J Suppl 2004;6 (Suppl J):J17–J26.
7. De Sutter J, De Bacquer D, Kotseva K, et al. Screening of family members of patients with premature coronary heart disease. Results from the EUROASPIRE II family survey. Eur Heart J 2003;24:249–257.
8. Conroy RM, Pyorala K, Fitzgerald AP, et al. Estimation of ten-year risk of fatal cardiovascular disease in Europe: the SCORE project. Eur Heart J 2003;24:987–1003.
9. Bhatt DL, Steg GP, Ohman EM, et al. International prevalence, recognition, and treatment of cardio-

vascular risk factors in outpatients with atherothrombosis. JAMA 2006;295:180–189.

10. Wood DA, Kotseva K, Jennings C, et al. EUROAC-TION: A European Society of Cardiology demonstration project in preventive cardiology. A cluster randomised controlled trial of a multi-disciplinary preventive cardiology programme for coronary patients, asymptomatic high risk individuals and their families. Summary of design, methodology and outcomes. Eur Heart J Suppl 2004;6(Suppl J):J3–J15.

11. Wood D, De Backer G, Faergeman O, Graham I, Mancia G. Pyörälä K. Prevention of coronary heart disease in clinical practice. Recommendations of the Second Joint Task Force of European and other Societies on coronary prevention. Eur Heart J 1998;19:1434–1503.

12. Wood DA, Roberts TL, Campbell M. Women married to men with myocardial infarction are at increased risk of coronary heart disease. J Cardiovasc Risk 1997;4:7–11.

13. Pyke S, Wood DA, Kinmonth AL, Thompson S on behalf of the British Family Heart Study Group. Concordance of changes in coronary risk and risk factor levels in couples following lifestyle intervention in the British Family Heart Study. Arch Fam Med 1997;6(4):354–360.

14. Prochaska JO, DiClemente CC. Self change processes, self efficacy and decisional balance across five stages of smoking cessation. Prog Clin Biol Res 1984;156:131-140.

15. Miller W, Rollnick S. Motivational interviewing, 2nd edn. London: Guilford; 2002.

16. Taylor RS, Brown A, Ebrahim S, et al. Exercise-based rehabilitation for patients with coronary heart disease: systematic review and meta-analysis of randomized controlled trials. Am J Med 2004;116: 782–792.

59
Outcome Measurement and Audit

Joep Perk

Comprehensive cardiac rehabilitation (CR) is defined as: "The sum of activities required to ensure the best possible physical, mental and social conditions, so that the cardiac patient may resume as normal a place as possible in the life of the community."[1] This implies the use of an individually tailored combination of physiological, clinical, psychological and social methods. Measuring the outcome of a multifaceted intervention is a methodological and logistical challenge. At present quality assurance of CR is relatively uncommon even though guidelines recommend that data are routinely collected and presented.[2] Thus, as CR programs must compete for resources with other healthcare modalities, caregivers will increasingly demand auditing of the service.

When measuring outcome by means of an audit, three different levels are used: clinical outcome of the individual patient, health service outcome of the program, health economic and health management data. Recently a standardized cardiac rehabilitation system for Europe (Euro-CardioRehab) has been proposed under the auspices of the former ESC Working Group on Cardiac Rehabilitation and Exercise Physiology (now: the European Association for Cardiovascular Prevention and Rehabilitation (EACPR)).[3] This system forms the basis of the chapter.

Data Required for the Audit

As not all centers have the means to perform a major audit, we present the following options for quality control: a basic outcome report, the stan-dard EuroCardioRehab audit and an extended version including health economic data. In all three alternatives, data on program content, referral, baseline program entry data, and outcome at the end of the program are needed. For the extended version a cost-analysis is mandatory.

Define Program Content (Table 59-1)

This includes the design of the program, that is, inclusion criteria for participation, description of the different interventions (physical training, psychological support, dietary counseling, smoking cessation, vocational guidance), duration, number of sessions. It should contain a description of the structure of the cardiac rehabilitation staff, facilities (training halls, equipment), and safety precautions. Financial issues should be addressed: costs of the program, costs for the participant, resources available from healthcare providers.

Referral to CR (Table 59-2)

Here an estimate of the annual total patient population eligible for CR from the referral area of the center should be given. For the individual patient, the initiating cardiac event and the demographic data are required as well as information on relevant co-morbidity. Date of referral, referring physician, and reasons for non-referral or not agreeing to attend should be recorded.

TABLE 59-1. Content of the cardiac rehabilitation program

Criteria for participation: initiating event
    All age groups or age limits?
    Contraindications:
        Unstable angina pectoris
        Severe cardiac failure
        Hazardous arrhythmia
        Others

Options (duration, number of sessions)
    Exercise training
        Group exercise
        Individual exercise program
        Home exercise plan
    Lifestyle education
        Written
        Group discussion, video etc.
    Dietary advice
        Group class (practical sessions)
        Individual
    Psychological intervention
        Stress management
        Psychological advice in group
        Individual psychological session
    Vocational assessment
        Occupational therapist: group session
        Occupational therapist: individual session
    Other methods, e.g. Heart Manual, Angina Plan, home visits etc.
    Medication advice

Staff
    Structure: cardiologist, cardiac nurse, physiotherapist, dietitian, occupation therapist, psychologist, others
    Level of competence: targeted education, postgraduate education, research

Facilities, safety
    Training halls, meeting rooms, equipment
    Safety precautions, resuscitation material, emergency medication

Costs
    Total CR program budget
        Staff costs
        Other program costs
        Patient fees
    Main care provider

Pre-Cardiac Rehabilitation Data (Table 59-3)

Upon commencing the program, work status and risk behavior prior to the event, the present risk factor status, relevant biometric data and biochemistry, ongoing medication, physical work capacity, and mental health status should be entered.

TABLE 59-2. Referral to cardiac rehabilitation

Expected annual size of the population eligible for the program: $n = \ldots$

Referral
- Referring physician or clinic
- Date of referral
- If no referral: reason?
- Age
- Gender
- Marital status
- Educational level

Reason for non-inclusion
- Exclusion criteria
- Lack of resources
- Ongoing investigations
- Other

Reasons for non-acceptance
- Not interested
- Too far to travel
- Returned to work
- Mental disorder
- Others

Initiating event
- STEMI/LBBB MI
- NSTEMI
- Unstable angina
- Stable angina
- Percutaneous coronary intervention
- Coronary artery bypass surgery
- Other cardiac surgery
- Chronic heart failure
- Pacemaker
- ICD
- Cardiac transplant
- Congenital heart disease
- Other

Previous cardiac events (as left)

Relevant co-morbidity
- Angina
- Stroke
- Diabetes mellitus
- Hypertension
- Claudication
- Musculoskeletal disorders
- Chronic obstructive pulmonary disease
- Malignancy
- Other

TABLE 59-3. Pre-cardiac rehabilitation data

Work status
- Full-time
- Part-time
- Unemployed
- Permanent sick leave
- Retired
- Housework
- Student

Biometric data and biochemistry
- Height
- Weight
- Waist circumference
- Systolic blood pressure
- Diastolic blood pressure
- Blood lipids
    Total cholesterol
    HDL cholesterol
    LDL cholesterol
    Triglycerides
- Fasting plasma glucose
- Physical work capacity
    Exercise stress test
      METs
    Number of shuttles
    Distance walked

Risk factor status
- Smoking
    Current
    Former
    Never
- Hypertension
- Hyperlipidemia
- Physical inactivity
- Overweight

Mental health status
- History of depression
- Anxiety score on HAD chart
- Depression score on HAD chart

Medication
- Antiplatelet
- Anticoagulant
- Beta-blocker
- ACE inhibitor
- Angiotensin II receptor blocker
- Lipid-lowering drugs
- Antidiabetic drugs
- Others

Post-Cardiac Rehabilitation Data (Table 59-4)

When the patient has completed program work the actual risk factor status (physically active, non-smoker, adequate food habits etc.), relevant biometric data and biochemistry, ongoing medication, physical work capacity, mental health status, and the resumption of work should be recorded. Has the patient complied with the program, discontinued, or was there poor compliance? Any adverse events in the course of the program? Which type of onward referral has been chosen?

Health Economic Data

In the extended version of the audit, the total direct costs of the program and the program costs per patient are required, as are the direct costs for the patient (fees, transport etc.). For a more advanced analysis, other costs must be included, such as the costs of medical care (including drugs and admissions) during the duration of CR and the indirect costs for the patient (absence from work). (See Chapter 60.)

Basic Outcome Report

The basic report consists of an individual patient assessment form and an annual service assessment form. The patient document can act both as direct outcome feedback to the participant and as a base for onward referral after completion of the program. This form should contain a progress report, a summary of the patient's risk factor status, ongoing treatment, and recommendations for a heart-healthy lifestyle.

The basic demands of an annual service assessment form are:

- number of participants entering the CR program as part of the total eligible population
- number of patients completing the program
- percentage of patients reaching the target goals for preventive cardiology[4]
  - total cholesterol <5 mmol/L, LDL cholesterol <3 mmol/L
  - Blood pressure <140/90 mmHg
  - BMI ≤25, waist circumference <102 cm for men, 88 cm for women
  - non-smoking
  - regular physical activity 30 min/day at least 3–5 times weekly
- percentage of patients returning to work
- a summary of adverse events related to the program.

The basic outcome report will give patients, referring physicians, and the recipients of onward referral the key patient data of the program. It may also satisfy the need for annual quality assurance of CR centers in most countries as the main data on production, effects, and side-effects are included.

TABLE 59-4. Post-cardiac rehabilitation data

Program	Compliance
Which options were offered:	Participation rate:
• Exercise training	• 90% of all sessions attended
• Lifestyle education	
• Dietary advice	• 75–90% attended
• Psychological intervention	• 50–75% attended
• Vocational assessment	• <50% attended
• Other methods	
• Medication advice	
	Reasons for drop-out:
Adverse events:	• Poor motivation
• Cardiac events	• Distance
• Orthopedic injuries	• Returned to work
• Psychological complaints	• Intercurrent disease
• Other	• Others
Return to work	Onward referral
• Yes	• General practitioner
• No	• Cardiologist
• Part-time	• Primary care CHD nurse
• Sick leave retirement	• Phase IV maintenance program
	• Other community program
Physical activity	• Patient support group
• Number of times per week	• Smoking clinic
• Duration of the activity	• Other
Food habits	
• Unchanged	
• Partially changed	
• Completely changed	

Standard EuroCardioRehab Audit

This audit provides an in-depth analysis of the program. Detailed data on the population using the service are available: demographic data, the different indications for referral, time lag between initial event and entry in the program, and the reasons for not being or not willing to be enrolled.

There are the necessary data at the start of CR to be compared with the outcome after completing the program: metabolic parameters, blood lipid levels, blood pressure, weight, and exercise capacity. Risk behavior is documented regarding physical activity, smoking and food habits, but even psychological outcomes are all measured.

The EuroCardioRehab model includes an analysis of compliance in which participation in the different CR options can be monitored and related to age, gender, and the initial cardiac event, thus enabling in-program adaptations.

Here, the individual patient assessment form may contain the same elements as in the basic format but the annual service assessment form can be further tailored to the needs of the CR team (e.g. detailed report on adherence and outcome of different interventions). Health authorities will find data regarding access for the eligible population, the size and structure of CR, adherence to guidelines and health policy data.

On an international level, it facilitates a comparison between different national models which may well contribute to improved services. In this respect it should be noted that the dataset in EuroCardioRehab is based upon existing experience from Italy, Ireland, the United Kingdom, and Switzerland. It has been prepared after consultation with 30 European countries.

The format of the annual service assessment form may differ between users and centers: obviously a service manager will need a different type of report than the team dietitian, who will be more interested in the specific nutritional parts of the program. Therefore it is beyond the scope of the textbook to propose detailed audit models. Yet we recommend that the core components of the annual assessment contain:

- demographic data on the participants entering the CR program as part of the total eligible population: age, gender, diagnosis, risk factor levels at entry, work status.

- reasons for non-referral or non-attendance
- numbers of patients attending the options of the program, drop-out rates per option, and reasons for drop-out
- percentage of patients reaching the target goals for preventive cardiology
  - total cholesterol <5 mmol/L, LDL cholesterol <3 mmol/L
  - blood pressure <140/90 mmHg
  - BMI ≤25 kg/m², waist circumference <102 cm for men, 88 cm for women
  - non-smoking
  - regular physical activity of 30 min/day, at least 3–5 times weekly
- basic statistics of the biometric and biochemistry data
- percentage of patients returning to work
- data on quality of life
- an overview of adverse events related to the program
- morbidity data
- actions taken to improve the program during the year
- educational activities for the staff, scientific projects.

Extended Audit Version

Beyond the core components of the audit, extensions can be made for research purposes, for scientific comparison between models, but even for health economic studies. It has been shown that cardiac rehabilitation is an effective use of available means although the competition from other sectors of healthcare is fierce. CR programs vary widely and the differences in health economic results between programs have been insufficiently documented. Only a small proportion of the patients who would benefit are at present invited to participate, which might be explained by a lack of knowledge on the efficiency of the programs. Therefore, the extended annual assessment should include data on the cost of participation per patient and the cost related to the outcomes on risk factors, medication, return to work, and quality of life.

The choice of method of outcome measurement and auditing remains evidently in the hands of the

CR staff, its management and policy makers, but in the light of increasing demands for healthcare, comprehensive cardiac rehabilitation will face difficulties in the near future if no regular quality control, especially an annual service assessment, can be provided.

References

1. WHO. The rehabilitation of patients with cardiovascular diseases. Report on a seminar. EURO 0381. WHO, regional office for Europe, Copenhagen; 1969.

2. Giannuzzi P, Saner H, Bjornstad H, Fioretti P, et al. Secondary prevention through cardiac rehabilitation: position paper of the Working Group on Cardiac Rehabilitation and Exercise Physiology of the European Society of Cardiology. Eur Heart J 2003;24:1273–1278.

3. McGee H, Fioretti P, Saner H, Perk J. EuroCardioRehab: a standardised cardiac rehabilitation information system for Europe. Eur J Cardiovasc Prev Rehabil 2005;12:299.

4. Third Joint Task Force of European and other Societies. European guidelines on cardiovascular disease prevention in clinical practice. Eur J Cardiovasc Prev Rehabil 2003;10(suppl 1):S1–S78.

60
Economic Evaluation of Cardiac Rehabilitation

N.B. Oldridge

Introduction

- Is healthcare service "A" more cost-effective than the alternative service "B" which, most frequently, is usual care?
- What is the cost impact for the healthcare system if service "A" is substituted for service "B"?

The increasing costs of health are driven by factors such as demographic shifts and increased life expectancy, an increased prevalence of chronic disease, increased demands for more and higher quality healthcare, and the greater availability of increasingly costly technological advances. As a result, identifying the most efficient use of the limited and finite resources available for healthcare has become a major challenge. In the European Union the 2003 direct healthcare costs for cardiovascular diseases were €104.7 billion ($108.9 billion), of which €22.9 billion ($23.8 billion) can be accounted for by coronary heart disease.[1] The respective 2005 amounts in the US are estimated to be $241.9 billion and $70.7 billion (€176.6 and €51.6 billion),[2] reinforcing the enormous, and escalating, cost burden of treating chronic diseases and their associated risk factors.

Economic evaluation, defined as "the comparative analysis of alternative courses of action in terms of both costs and consequences,"[3] is one method for evaluating the effectiveness of competing effective health interventions.

The main function of an economic evaluation is to provide a framework for identifying the most efficient use of the limited and finite resources available for alternative healthcare services, in other words, attempting to answer the two key questions posed above. Economic evaluation data are used for both treatment efficiency as well as policy purposes, that is, reimbursement for a particular product or service. However, we know little about the cost-effectiveness of many of our current interventions, making decisions about which alternative to choose from among the many current and emerging healthcare services often problematic and always challenging.[4]

Based on meta-analytic evidence,[5,6] secondary prevention cardiac rehabilitation (CR) is recognized an integral part of the contemporary care of patients with heart disease.[7,8] Although limited, the evidence suggests that supervised CR programs are cost-effective.[9,10] There are, for example, only two randomized controlled trials (RCTs) of CR with estimated quality-adjusted life-years (QALYs) and a cost-utility analysis[11,12] although this is the methodology recommended by the US Public Health Service Panel on Cost-Effectiveness in Health and Medicine[4,13,14] and the National Institute for Health and Clinical Excellence (NICE).[15]

The purpose of this chapter is to provide a brief description of the types of economic evaluations commonly used in healthcare and to summarize the available economic evaluation data for comprehensive CR.

Economic Evaluation, Reference Case Analysis

Economic evaluations provide a balance sheet of the effects, either benefits (i.e., advantages) or harms (i.e., disadvantages), and costs for making choices between alternative healthcare services.[3] Standardization of economic evaluation methodology is important for clinicians, payers, and policy makers such as healthcare administrators and politicians as well as patients in order to make meaningful comparisons of the cost-effectiveness of various treatments. A standard set of economic evaluation methodologies, the "reference case" analysis, has been recommended by the Panel[4,13,14] and by NICE.[15]

The societal perspective is recommended for "reference case" economic evaluations as this represents the public interest rather than that of any specific group when assessing the relative value or merit of alternative healthcare services, and accounting for associated benefits, harms, and costs.[4] The essence of an economic evaluation is the incremental cost-effectiveness ratio (ICER) or the incremental cost-utility ratio (ICUR), a special form of cost-effectiveness[4] where incremental is the difference between the experimental intervention (E) and the alternative healthcare service, usually usual care (UC):

$$ICER = \frac{Cost_E - Cost_{UC}}{LYG_e - LYG_{UC}}$$

$$ICUR = \frac{Cost_E - Cost_{UC}}{QALY_E - QALY_{UC}}$$

The numerator of the ICER or ICUR consists of the costs of a healthcare service, reflecting the resources utilized to provide the healthcare service.

- *Direct costs* are the costs of healthcare services (activities of the institution and health professionals), patients' own costs including non-medical (time, transportation, lodging, food, family care, care-giving) and are usually based on the price of the factors involved.
- *Indirect costs* reflect the impact of the resources lost due to either mortality or morbidity (reflecting premature death and the time lost

from production and/or consumption activities) and may or may not be considered.

- The *health effect or outcome* of the healthcare service is the denominator term in the ICER or ICUR and for the "reference case" is measured in derived units (e.g. QALY) which by convention go into the denominator of either the ICER or the ICUR.

However, the "reference case" will not always address all questions about the cost-effectiveness of alternative interventions and so, depending on the reason for the cost-effectiveness analysis (CEA), it may be more appropriate to use a health outcome other than QALYs such as, for example, years of life gained (LYG) or life-years saved (LYS).[16] The problem with using laboratory outcome measures such as blood pressure, blood lipids, or improvement of angina class or exercise tolerance is that they make comparability between CEA studies of alternative interventions difficult, if not impossible.

When the measure of health effect needs to be comparable across conditions and interventions and capable of capturing the impact of interventions with different effects, the Panel[4] and NICE[15] recommended QALYs as the preferred measure. Preference-based scales are designed to provide preference scores for health states and are used to assess health-related quality of life and estimate QALYs.[4] Preference scores may be measured either indirectly using health-state classification systems such as the Health Utility Index, the Quality of Well-Being (QWB) scale, and the EuroQoL[4] or directly using techniques such as the time trade-off (TTO) and the standard gamble.[13] The "reference case" criteria are recommended to managers of CR programs as the preferred methodology with which to provide cost-effectiveness information to clinicians and patients as well as administrators and policy makers.

Categories of Economic Evaluation

There are two main categories of economic evaluation, partial and full.[3] Partial economic evaluations do not provide a cost/outcome ratio as they

TABLE 60-1. Incremental decision theory modeling cost-effectiveness reported in the original publication, in 2004 US$ and € (adjusted for US medical care inflation and 2004 exchange rates for €) of cardiac rehabilitation for persons with myocardial infarction (MI) or cardiovascular disease (CVD)

Gender	Cost 1995 US$/LYS Mainly male	Cost 1996 US$/LYS	
		Female	Male
Ades[19]			
MI, primarily < 65 years	$4950 (2004 $11,500) (2004 €8400)		
Lowensteyn[20]			
CVD, 35–54 years		$42,367 (2004 $93,700) (2004 €68,400)	$13,719 (2004 $30,300 (2004 €22,100)
CVD, 55–64 years		$12,015 (2004 $26,600) (2004 €19,400)	$8562 (2004 $18,900) (2004 €13,800)
CVD, 65–74 years		$20,307 (2004 $44,900) (2004 €32,800)	$14,464 (2004 $32,000) (2004 €23,400)

report (a) either the costs or outcomes of two or more interventions or (b) both the costs and outcomes but only one alternative.

There are three (or four) forms of full economic evaluation where both costs and outcomes of two or more alternative interventions are evaluated, so providing a cost/outcome ratio with which the efficiency of the healthcare services (effort per effect unit) can be assessed. In *cost minimization analysis* the evidence suggests an equivalent effectiveness of the alternative interventions with the less expensive intervention preferred as it is considered the more efficient. In *cost-benefit analysis* both costs and health effects are given a monetary value but, as there is considerable difficulty in putting a monetary value on the complex outcomes of healthcare, this is seldom performed for healthcare decision-making. The third form, *cost-effectiveness analysis*, comes in two types. The first is where the denominator of the ICER is measured in terms of effect, most commonly expressed as either LYG or LYS. The second is a *cost-utility analysis* (CUA) where the denominator of ICUR is based on the individual's preference (or value) for a specific health state or treatment outcome with an estimation of the QALYs gained. In both cases, incre-

mental costs are determined per unit outcome and the lower the ICER or the ICUR, the greater the cost-effectiveness or cost-utility.

As all costs in the CR economic evaluations were reported in US dollars, it was decided to inflate all costs to 2004 US dollar figures using the US healthcare inflation rate[17] and then these 2004 US dollar figures were converted to euros using the exchange rate on December 31, 2004 for comparison purposes (Tables 60-1, 60-2, and 60-3). While there are no empirical data for defining what ICER or ICUR monetary values are considered highly attractive, relatively attractive, marginally attractive and unattractive, there are guidelines for these categories in US dollars.[18] Care must be taken with the exchange into euros in figures associated with these categories listed below as the impact of healthcare cost inflation has not necessarily been considered and it is not the same in different countries:

Highly attractive: <US$20,000 (€15,000)
Attractive: >US$20,000 (€15,000) up to US$50,000 (€36,000)
Marginally attractive: >US$50,000 (€36,000) up to US$100,000 (€73,000)
Unattractive: >US$100,000 (€73,000)

TABLE 60-2. Incremental cost-effectiveness reported in the original publication, in 2004 US$ and € (adjusted for US medical care inflation and 2004 exchange rates for €) of cardiac rehabilitation for persons with either myocardial infarction (MI), heart failure or angina

	Cost 1991 US$ per LYG	Cost 1999 US$ per LYG	Cost 2002 US$ per CCS class
Oldridge[11] MI < 65 years	$21,800 (2004 $83,300) (2004 €60,800)		
Georgiou[21] Heart failure 55–64 years		$1773 (2004 $3100) (2004 €2300)	
Hambrecht[22] Angina ≤70 years			$2378 (2004 $2600) (2004 €1900)

CCS: Canadian Cardiovascular Society.

Cardiac Rehabilitation

Partial economic evaluations are important but, as they provide no comparison of alternatives, they do not permit an examination of the efficiency of healthcare services which full economic evaluations do. This chapter therefore focuses on the six available full economic evaluation studies of CR[11,12,19–22] as they permit comparison with an alternative.

Chronologically, the first full economic evaluation of CR was published in 1993 by Oldridge and colleagues.[11] The next two full economic evaluations of CR were both modeling studies, the first published in 1997 by Ades and colleagues[19] and the second in 2000 by Lowensteyn and colleagues.[20] The most recent full economic evaluations of CR are each based on RCT data, the first by Georgiou and colleagues[21] in 2001 and the two

TABLE 60-3. Incremental cost-utility reported in the original publication, in 2004 US$ and € (adjusted for US medical care inflation and 2004 exchange rates for €) of cardiac rehabilitation for persons with myocardial infarction using time trade-off (TTO) and quality of well-being (QWB) quality-adjusted life years (QALYs)

	Cost 1991 US$/QALY	Cost 2001 US$/QALY	Cost 2001 US$/QALY
Oldridge[11] TTO QALYs	$9200 (2004 $35,100) (2004 €25,600)		
Oldridge[24] TTO QALYs		$17550 (2004 $24,900) (2004 €18,200)	
QWB QALYs		$63,818 (2004 $90,700) (2004 €66,200)	
Yu[12] TTO QALYs			−$640 (savings) (2004 −$900) (2004 −€700)

published in 2004 by Hambrecht and colleagues[22] and Yu and coworkers.[12] With no universally accepted approach to the delivery of CR services between different countries, let alone within the same country, the generalizability of the data on the cost-effectiveness of comprehensive CR to different healthcare systems is uncertain. Of the full economic evaluation studies, two were carried out in Canada[11,20] and one in each of the US,[19] Italy,[21] Germany,[22] and Hong Kong.[12]

Decision Theory Modeling: Cost-Effectiveness

Ades and colleagues carried out a decision theory modeling exercise of the cost-effectiveness of CR after myocardial infarction (MI) using the perspective of the patient or insurance payer.[19] In this model they used the total of direct medical expenditures (less costs associated with drugs, outpatient care and home care) including cost data derived from 626 operating CR centers minus the direct savings realized from averted medical care. Health outcome data were derived from published results of RCTs on mortality and epidemiological studies of long-term survival. An incremental life expectancy of 0.202 years during a 15-year period following rehabilitation was estimated and, with inflation-adjusted costs in 1995 US$, the ICER for CR was estimated as $4950/LYS (Table 60-1). The authors conclude by stating that "CR is more cost-effective than thrombolytic therapy, coronary bypass surgery, and cholesterol lowering drugs, though less cost-effective than smoking cessation . . . and should stand alongside these therapies as standard of care in the post-MI setting."[19]

Lowensteyn and colleagues[20] carried out a decision theory modeling economic evaluation study in patients with cardiovascular disease. Long-term cardiovascular endpoints were derived from a Canadian life expectancy model with estimated LYS. The model assigns costs to cardiovascular medical events and the CR program with averted medical expenses derived from studies of exercise training CR. The cost-effectiveness per LYS (in 1996 US$) of secondary prevention of cardiovascular disease was estimated for both unsupervised and supervised settings and for men and women by age (35–54, 55–64, and 65–75 years) with the

supervised group-based data also presented in Table 60-1. The ICERs ranged from $8562 to $43,267 by age and gender. The authors conclude that "supervised exercise is highly cost-effective for all men with cardiovascular disease and women with cardiovascular disease between 55 and 64 years of age . . . and relatively cost-effective for older women with cardiovascular disease."[20]

Randomized Controlled Trials: Cost-Effectiveness

Patients with a documented MI, identified as moderately anxious or depressed while in hospital ($n = 201$), were randomized in the late 1980s in Canada to either an 8-week comprehensive CR intervention ($n = 99$) or usual community care (control, $n = 102$).[23] The data collected in this RCT permitted both a CEA and a CUA to be carried out with published meta-analytic mortality data defining the denominator term in the CEA as LYG gained.[11] Using the societal perspective, costs were estimated for the program, the patients, and the provincial healthcare system using Ontario Health Insurance Plan rates. The incremental direct cost in 1991 US$ was $480 (1991)[11] with an incremental 0.022 LYG per rehabilitation patient giving an ICER of $21,800 per LYG (Table 60-2). The investigators in this study concluded that "the data provide evidence that brief CR initiated soon after MI for patients with mild to moderate anxiety or depression, or both, is an efficient use of healthcare resources and can be economically justified."[11]

Patients with class II and III heart failure ($n = 99$) were recruited in Italy and randomized to either a 14-month exercise training program ($n = 50$) or usual community care (control, $n = 49$).[21] Direct costs were estimated per admission and the exercise program with indirect costs as wages lost using US Census Bureau rates. The number of life-years lost was determined directly from the RCT with 10-year mortality estimated from US survey examination data. With incremental costs in 1999 US$ of $3227 and an incremental life expectancy of an additional 1.82 LYS/patient, the ICER for CR was $1773/LYS (Table 60-2). The authors suggest that the cost-utility ratio per QALY would possibly be lower because of the significant improvements in health-related quality of life observed in the RCT and state that "quality adjustment would result in a cost-effectiveness ratio that would more heavily favor exercise training."[21]

As part of a RCT of CR carried out in Germany, 101 patients with Canadian Cardiovascular Society (CCS) class I and II angina pectoris were recruited and randomized to either a 12-month exercise training program or a standard percutaneous coronary intervention with stenting and followed up for 12 months.[22] Direct costs were estimated as the total costs of treatment and the cost of the exercise program while the health effects were estimated as the mean improvement in CCS class. With mean 12-month total costs in 2002 US$ of $3708 per exercise training patient and US$6086 per PCI patient ($P < 0.001$) (Table 60-2), the authors point out that the exercise training CR program "achieved a clinical improvement of 1 CCS class at approximately half the total cost of an interventional strategy."[22]

Randomized Controlled Trials: Cost-Utility

In the Canadian RCT described earlier with 201 patients with MI and moderately anxious or depressed with MI (99 randomized to 8 weeks of CR and 102 to usual community care), directly measured TTO preferences permitted a CUA to be carried out with incremental QALYs gained as the denominator term.[11] The incremental cost in 1991 US$ was $480 per rehabilitation patient together with an incremental 0.052 QALYs gained per rehabilitation patient, resulting in an ICUR of $9200 per QALY gained with CR. The investigators in this study concluded by stating that "the data provide evidence that brief CR initiated soon after MI for patients with mild to moderate anxiety or depression, or both, is an efficient use of healthcare resources and can be economically justified."[11]

The data collected in the RCT, which included both the direct TTO and the indirect, multi-attribute, community-based QWB preference measure, have been re-analyzed recently.[24] Using more up-to-date analytic strategies, patients with CR gained 0.011 more QWB-derived QALYs than the control group while the difference with TTO preference scores was 0.040 more TTO-derived QALYs gained with no significant difference

between the preference scores. With estimated net incremental costs in 2001 US$ of $702 (adjusted for inflation between 1991 and 2001), the mean ICURs were $63,818/QWB-derived QALY and $17,550/TTO-derived QALY. The conclusion of the CUA of CR is that community-based preferences and patient-based preferences give different results. While this cannot be generalized to other studies, it is cause for concern because it suggests that the cost-effectiveness of a particular intervention may well differ depending upon which types of preferences are used.[24]

As part of an RCT of CR carried out in Hong Kong, patients with MI ($n = 193$) or after elective PCI ($n = 76$) were randomized to either an exercise CR program (24 months, supervised and maintenance) or a control group.[12] Direct costs in 2001 US$ were based on local healthcare system costs (hospital, investigations, interventions, and CR program) and the health outcome was the TTO-derived QALYs gained per patient. The direct costs of the 2-year CR in this RCT were US$15,292 compared to US$15,707 for the control group; the incremental mean gain in QALYs was 0.6 QALYs at the end of the 2-year period of time. The ICUR for the 2-year CR program is reported as US$640 saved per QALY gained.[12] The authors state that CR "was highly cost-effective, with a net gain in QALY, whereas direct healthcare expenses were reduced, which was primarily related to the reduction of the subsequent need for PCI. The information provided in this study supports the adoption of CR in addition to the contemporary regimen of managing patients with coronary heart disease."[12]

Discussion

Cost-effectiveness analysis is one of a number of methodological strategies which permit an evaluation of the effectiveness of a given healthcare intervention. In this case, the intervention is CR and the analysis provides a framework for identifying the most efficient use of limited resources and finite healthcare resources. The six full economic evaluations of CR demonstrate incremental CERs and CURs that range from marginally cost-effective[24] to relatively cost-effective[11,20] to highly cost-effective[11,19-22] with cost savings per QALY in one RCT.[12] Although economic evaluation is an important tool in the evaluation of competing health care interventions, little is known about the economic benefits of different CR program delivery models, i.e., supervised, home-based and alternative delivery models of CR. In a recent systematic review, Papadakis and colleagues[25] identified 15 economic evaluations (including the six RCTs discussed in detail in this chapter and nine partial economic evaluations) which provide evidence to support the cost-effectiveness of supervised CR in myocardial infarction and heart failure patients. However, they pointed out that the literature evaluating home-based and alternative delivery models of CR is insufficient to draw conclusions about their relative cost-effectiveness.

For comparison purposes only, the ICER and ICUR reported in each of the six economic evaluations has been converted to 2004 US dollars and euros. Although the actual values of a highly attractive, attractive, marginally attractive, and unattractive ICER or ICUR need to be determined according to national standards, the data on the efficiency of CR services are generally positive. However, this does not negate the need for evidence of the efficiency of CR at the local level and it is incumbent on those responsible for providing the CR services to document the efficiency of their specific program(s) for clinicians, patients, institutional administrators, policy makers, and politicians. Considerations for data to be used in economic evaluations of CR programs include:

- model to be used
- identification of costs and outcomes
- detailed description of methods for obtaining estimates of costs and outcomes
- perspective and the year of the analysis
- description of the alternative interventions.

However straightforward this may seem, it is important to acknowledge the complexities of an economic evaluation and we recommend consulting a health economist before attempting to collect data to demonstrate efficiency of a CR program.

Few countries have considered formal requirements for cost-effectiveness evidence.[26] However, there seems to be some agreement that, at this time, clinical effectiveness may be more important than cost-effectiveness when making decisions about reimbursement for healthcare

services as more evidence is available for clinical effectiveness.[27] This certainly is true of the clinical evidence for CR[5-8] versus the cost-effectiveness evidence for CR.[9,10] However, it is equally clear that cost-effectiveness will be an increasingly important part of decision-making vis-a-vis both reimbursement for a specific healthcare service as well as for treatment efficiency purposes. This means that those responsible for CR services will need to recognize and acknowledge the importance of documenting the efficiency of their CR program for their managers in light of the competing demands from other healthcare services for the limited and finite healthcare resources.

References

1. British Heart Foundation. www.heartstats.org/eucosts. 2005.
2. American Heart Association. Heart and Stroke Statistics – 2005 Update. Dallas: American Heart Association; 2005.
3. Drummond MF, Sculpher MJ, Torrance GW, O'Brien BJ, Stoddart GL. Methods for the Economic Evaluation of Health Care Programs. 3rd ed. Oxford: Oxford University Press; 2005.
4. Russell LB, Gold MR, Siegel JE, Daniels N, Weinstein MC, for the Panel on Cost-Effectiveness in Health and Medicine. The role of cost-effectiveness analysis in health and medicine. JAMA 1996;276:1172–1177.
5. Jolliffe JA, Rees K, Taylor RS, Thompson D, Oldridge N, Ebrahim S. Exercise-based rehabilitation for coronary heart disease. Cochrane Database Syst Rev 2001:CD001800.
6. Taylor RS, Brown A, Ebrahim S, et al. Exercise-based rehabilitation for patients with coronary heart disease: systematic review and meta-analysis of randomized controlled trials. Am J Med 2004;116:682–692.
7. Giannuzzi P, Saner H, Bjornstad H, et al. Secondary prevention through cardiac rehabilitation: position paper of the Working Group on Cardiac Rehabilitation and Exercise Physiology of the European Society of Cardiology. Eur Heart J 2003;24:1273–1278.
8. Leon AS, Franklin BA, Costa F, et al. Cardiac rehabilitation and secondary prevention of coronary heart disease. Circulation 2005;111:369–376.
9. Oldridge NB. Comprehensive cardiac rehabilitation: Is it cost-effective? Eur Heart J 1998;19(Suppl O):O42–O49.

10. Brown A, Taylor R, Noorani H, Stone J, Skidmore B. Exercise-based cardiac rehabilitation programmes for coronary artery disease: A systematic clinical and economic review. Technical overview # 11. Ottawa: Canadian Coordinating Office for Health Technology Assessment; 2003.

11. Oldridge N, Furlong W, Feeny D, et al. Economic evaluation of cardiac rehabilitation soon after acute myocardial infarction. Am J Cardiol 1993;72:154–161.

12. Yu CM, Lau CP, Chau J, et al. A short course of cardiac rehabilitation programme is highly cost effective in improving long-term quality of life in patients with recent myocardial infarction or percutaneous coronary intervention. Arch Phys Med Rehabil 2004;85:1915–1922.

13. Weinstein MC, Siegel JE, Gold MR, et al., for the Panel on Cost-Effectiveness in Health and Medicine. Recommendations of the Panel on Cost-Effectiveness in Health and Medicine. JAMA 1996;276:1253–1258.

14. Siegel JE, Weinstein MC, Russell LB, Gold MR, for the Panel on Cost-Effectiveness in Health and Medicine. Recommendations for reporting cost-effectiveness analyses. JAMA 1996;276:1339–1341.

15. National Institute for Clinical Excellence. Guide to Methods for Technology Appraisal. London; April, 2004:1–54.

16. Lys K, Pernice R. Perceptions of positive attitudes toward people with spinal cord injury. Int J Rehabil Res 1995;18:35–43.

17. Economic Report of the President. Washington, DC: United States Government Printing Office; 2005: Table B-60, p. 279.

18. Mark DB, Hlatky MA. Medical economics and the assessment of value in cardiovascular medicine: Part I. Circulation 2002;106:516–520.

19. Ades PA, Pashkow FJ, Nestor JR. Cost-effectiveness of cardiac rehabilitation after myocardial infarction. J Cardiopulm Rehabil 1997;17:222–231.

20. Lowensteyn I, Coupal L, Zowall H, Grover SA. The cost-effectiveness of exercise training for the primary and secondary prevention of cardiovascular disease. J Cardiopulm Rehabil 2000;20:147–155.

21. Georgiou D, Chen Y, Appadoo S, et al. Cost-effectiveness analysis of long-term moderate exercise training in chronic heart failure. Am J Cardiol 2001;87:984–988.

22. Hambrecht R, Walther C, Mobius-Winkler S, et al. Percutaneous coronary angioplasty compared with exercise training in patients with stable coronary artery disease: a randomized trial. Circulation 2004;109:1371–1378.

23. Oldridge N, Guyatt G, Jones N, et al. Effects on quality of life with comprehensive rehabilitation after acute myocardial infarction. Am J Cardiol 1991;67:1084–1089.

24. Furlong W, Oldridge N, Perkins A, Feeny D, Torrance G. Community or patient preferences for cost-utility analyses: does it matter? Value Health 2003;6:298.

25. Papadakis S, Oldridge N, Coyle D, Mayhew A, Reid R, Angus D. Economic evaluation of cardiac rehabilitation: A systematic review. Eur J Cardiovasc Prev Rehabil 2005;12:513–520.

26. Taylor RS, Drummond MF, Salkeld G, Sullivan SD. Inclusion of cost effectiveness in licensing requirements of new drugs: the fourth hurdle. BMJ 2004;329:972–975.

27. Raftery J. NICE: faster access to modern treatments? Analysis of guidance on health technologies. BMJ 2001;323:1300–1303.

Index

Printed in Singapore